Computational Approaches in Biotechnology and Bioinformatics

Volume 1 of *Computational Approaches in Bioengineering—Computational Approaches in Biotechnology and Bioinformatics*—explores many significant topics of biomedical engineering and bioinformatics in an easily understandable format. It explores recent developments and applications in bioinformatics, biomechanics, artificial intelligence (AI), signal processing, wearable sensors, biomaterials, cell biology, synthetic biology, biostatistics, prosthetics, big data, and algorithms. From applications of biomaterials in advanced drug delivery systems to the role of big data, AI, and machine learning in disease diagnosis and treatment, the book will help readers understand how these technologies are being applied across the areas of biomedical engineering, bioinformatics, and healthcare. The chapters also include case studies on the role of medical robots in surgery and the determination of protein structure using genetic algorithms. The contributors are all leading experts across multiple disciplines and provide chapters that truly represent a complete view of these state-of-the-art technologies.

FEATURES

- Covers a wide range of subjects from biomedical engineering like wearable devices, biomaterials, synthetic biology, phytochemical extraction, and prosthetics
- Explores AI, machine learning, big data analysis, and algorithms in biomedical engineering and bioinformatics in an easily understandable format
- Includes case studies on the role of medical robots in surgery and the determination of protein structure using genetic algorithms
- Discusses genetic diagnosis, classification, and risk prediction in cancer using next-generation sequencing in oncology

This book is ideally designed for biomedical professionals, biomedical engineers, healthcare professionals, data engineers, clinicians, physicians, medical students, hospital directors, clinical researchers, and others who work in the field of artificial intelligence, bioinformatics, and computational biology.

Emerging Trends in Biomedical Technologies and Health Informatics Series

Series Editors

Subhendu Kumar Pani
Orissa Engineering College, Bhubaneswar, Orissa, India

Sujata Dash
North Orissa University, Baripada, India

Sunil Vadera
University of Salford, Salford, UK

Everyday Technologies in Healthcare
Chhabi Rani Panigrahi, Bibudhendu Pati, Mamata Rath, Rajkumar Buyya

Biomedical Signal Processing for Healthcare Applications
Varun Bajaj, G R Sinha, Chinmay Chakraborty

Deep Learning in Biomedical and Health Informatics
M. Jabbar, Ajith Abraham, Onur Dogan, Ana Madureira, Sanju Tiwar

Computational Approaches in Biotechnology and Bioinformatics
Pranav Deepak Pathak, Roshani Raut, Sebastián Jaramillo-Isaza, Pradnya Borkar, and Rutvij H. Jhaveri

Computational Approaches in Biomaterials and Biomedical Engineering Applications
Pranav Deepak Pathak, Roshani Raut, Sebastián Jaramillo-Isaza, Pradnya Borkar, and Rutvij H. Jhaveri

For more information about this series, please visit: www.routledge.com/Emerging-Trends-in-Biomedical-Technologies-and-Health-informatics-series/book-series/ETBTHI

Computational Approaches in Bioengineering

Volume 1: Computational Approaches in Biotechnology and Bioinformatics

Edited by Pranav Deepak Pathak,
Roshani Raut, Sebastián Jaramillo-Isaza,
Pradnya Borkar, and Rutvij H. Jhaveri

CRC Press
Taylor & Francis Group
Boca Raton London New York

CRC Press is an imprint of the
Taylor & Francis Group, an **informa** business

Designed cover image: © iStock. Credit: Kateryna Bereziuk

First edition published 2024
by CRC Press
2385 NW Executive Center Drive, Suite 320, Boca Raton FL 33431

and by CRC Press
4 Park Square, Milton Park, Abingdon, Oxon, OX14 4RN

CRC Press is an imprint of Taylor & Francis Group, LLC

Library of Congress Cataloging-in-Publication Data
Names: Pathak, Pranav Deepak, editor. | Raut, Roshani, 1981– editor. | Jaramillo-Isaza, Sebastián, editor. | Borkar, Pradnya, editor. | Jhaveri, Rutvij, editor.
Title: Computational approaches in biomedical engineering / edited by Pranav Deepak Pathak, Roshani Raut, Sebastian Jaramillo-Isaza, Pradnya Borkar and Rutvij H. Jhaveri.
Description: First edition. | Boca Raton FL : CRC Press, 2024. | Includes bibliographical references and index. | Contents: v. 1. Computational approaches in biotechnology and bioinformatics — v. 2. Computational approaches in biomaterials and biomedical engineering applications.
Identifiers: LCCN 2023048741 (print) | LCCN 2023048742 (ebook) | ISBN 9781032406107 (v. 1 ; hardback) | ISBN 9781032407128 (v. 1 ; paperback) | ISBN 9781032635255 (v. 2 ; hardback) | ISBN 9781032635279 (v. 2 ; paperback) | ISBN 9781003354437 (v. 1 ; ebook) | ISBN 9781032699882 (v. 2 ; ebook)
Subjects: MESH: Biomedical Engineering—methods | Computational Biology—methods | Biotechnology—methods | Biocompatible Materials
Classification: LCC R857.M3 (print) | LCC R857.M3 (ebook) | NLM QT 36 | DDC 610.28/4—dc23/eng/20240301
LC record available at https://lccn.loc.gov/2023048741
LC ebook record available at https://lccn.loc.gov/2023048742

ISBN: 978-1-032-63530-9 (set)
ISBN: 978-1-032-40610-7 (hbk)
ISBN: 978-1-032-40712-8 (pbk)
ISBN: 978-1-003-35443-7 (ebk)

DOI: 10.1201/9781003354437

Typeset in Times
by Apex CoVantage, LLC

Contents

Preface

This book, *Computational Approaches in Biotechnology and Bioinformatics*, is a comprehensive guide to understanding and exploring the cutting-edge applications of computational methods in these interdisciplinary domains. This book is volume 1 of the *Computational Approaches in Bioengineering* set.

This book combines a diverse collection of chapters from leading experts and researchers from academia, industry, and healthcare institutions. It encompasses various topics, including computational modelling of biomaterials, drug discovery, bioinformatics approaches, tissue engineering, cancer treatment, and many more. The chapters in this book provide a holistic perspective on the advancements and applications of computational techniques, covering theoretical concepts and practical implementations. Each chapter highlights the unique contributions of computational methods in addressing specific challenges, presenting case studies, experimental results, and future directions for further exploration.

This book comprises fifteen chapters. The process of structure-based designing for inflammatory and infectious disorders is explained in Chapter 1. This study initially provided examples of computer-aided drug designing (CADD), along with the steps of target identification, homology modelling, active site prediction/identification, ligand preparation, virtual screening, molecular docking, pharmacophore modelling, and molecular dynamics simulation. The author also described the effective candidates for treating inflammatory illnesses that target Janus kinase (JAK), Bruton tyrosine kinase (BTK), sphingosine-1-phosphate (S1P), and spleen tyrosine kinase (SYK), among other therapeutic targets. Dihydrofuran diamine derivatives were synthesised and screened against multi-target (SYK/PDGFR-α/C-kit) for anti-rheumatoid arthritis. Pyrazole-pyrimidine derivatives were found as primary scaffolds exhibiting anti-inflammatory activity. Additionally, case studies of drug targets, including methicillin resistance factor A, protein, and other drug targets, will be used to show essential principles and the significance of drug design.

Chapter 2 explains that bioinformatics approaches provide an excellent opportunity for identifying potential compounds, and its application in cancer research has grown dramatically during the last decade. This study initially provided examples of CADD, along with the steps of target identification, homology modelling, active site prediction/identification, ligand preparation, virtual screening, molecular docking, pharmacophore modelling, and molecular dynamics simulation. It also described the effective candidates for treating inflammatory illnesses that target JAK. The second chapter also merges computer-based methods in 'omics' technologies with the analysis of plant-based anti-neoplastic agents and discusses the sophisticated bioinformatics software and tools adopted in the process. It is strongly believed that the general overview of available databases, current computational methods, and the clinical information of cancer patients will accelerate the drug selection process and help develop cost-effective and accurate cancer therapeutics.

Chapter 3 discusses one of the most prevalent malignant illnesses and essential public health issues today: cancer. Compared to current treatments, better and more potent medications are desperately needed to treat this illness. Given its increased prevalence worldwide, a different approach to treating cancer is necessary. A convenient option for allopathic cancer treatment is herbal therapy. It is well known that several medicinal plants contain phytochemical elements with anticancer effects. These plant-derived chemicals may be lead molecules while developing new medications. Due to the development of high-throughput techniques, bioinformatics methods are increasingly essential for evaluating and combining data to conclusions. These methods are crucial for discovering genes and pathways that may be linked to significant secondary metabolites from medicinal plants with anticancer activities. The development of cancer and phytochemical mechanisms of action, the process of creating phytochemical drugs from plants, the main phytochemical components with anticancer properties, the anticancer activity of medicinal plants, bioinformatics approaches, current developments in indigenous medicinal plant informatics, cancer treatment options, and the regulatory aspects of herbal anticancer drugs are all covered in this chapter.

Chapter 4 talks about a convenient option for allopathic cancer treatment: herbal therapy. The plant-derived chemicals may be used as lead molecules while developing new medications. Due to the growth of high-throughput techniques, bioinformatics methods are becoming increasingly crucial for analysing and combining data to make conclusions. This chapter examines the relationship between the development of cancer and phytochemical mechanisms of action, the process of turning plants into phytochemical drugs, the main phytochemicals with anticancer properties, the anticancer activity of medicinal plants, bioinformatics approaches, current advancements in indigenous medicinal plant informatics, cancer treatment options, and the regulatory aspects of herbal anticancer drugs.

In Chapter 5, the authors attempted to collect information on the phenolic compounds in various plants, extraction methods, and their biological properties, including antiviral and antibacterial properties. The bioinformatics approaches to studying phenolic compounds are reviewed. This chapter proposes to review the drug repurposing strategies and provide an overview of the resources and tools commonly used for repurposing studies. Among them, *in silico* virtual screening is one of the essential tools that has proven to help overcome the problems and challenges of antiviral and antibacterial drug discovery. Compound structure databases, molecular docking tools, and pharmacophore-based screening may also help reduce the number of phytocompounds tested *in vitro* or *in vivo*. The various virtual screening methods used to find new antiviral and antibacterial drugs, with particular emphasis on phenolic compounds reported for multiple biological activities, are described. The chapter also covers the current status and future trends in repurposing phenolic compounds.

The study of tissue engineering is presented in Chapter 6. Tissue engineering is also used in self-healing and regenerative medicine. Screening tools have been modified to detect fundamental component properties for applications requiring an intricate fusion of structural functions. The study describes various advancements in neurological disorders modelling and is mainly centred on animal and human translation for scaffolding technology in multiple neurodegenerative diseases. It analyses the current situation and procedures built around integrating components with computer modelling to reduce trial and error and increase reliance on logical design. This plays a central role in driving future applications in regenerative medicine.

A yeast expression (transcriptome) dataset is used in Chapter 7 to train an artificial neural network (ANN) combined with a genetic algorithm to identify the genes involved in lipase production and categorise yeast cells that produce lipase. The dataset was retrieved from the Gene Expression Omnibus database. A robust ANN model is built using the processed gene expression data to distinguish between lipase-producing yeast (LPY) and non–lipase-producing yeast (NLPY). The overexpressed gene contributes to the robust model since it plays a crucial role in classification. The classification of LPY and NLPY is done by unsupervised learning.

Chapter 8 covers phenolic compounds and their classifications; roles of phenolic compounds in human health; methods for extracting, isolating, and purifying phenolic compounds; plant phenolic compounds with antibacterial activity; synergistic antibacterial activity; phenolic compounds with antiviral and antifungal activities; bioinformatics approaches of molecular mechanisms in antimicrobial resistance; future prospects; and limitations.

The research discussed in Chapter 9 focuses on the substances active in peanut skin and looks at whether they have anticancer qualities. A qualitative investigation of peanut skin using gas chromatography–mass spectrometry (GC-MS) indicated the presence of numerous medicinally valuable chemicals such as azulene, farnasene, and bisabolene. These active peanut compounds were tested for their *in silico* anticancer effects against the non–small lung cancer protein Chromobox protein homolog 3 (CBX3). Every chemical that was looked at showed a high binding potential.

Chapter 10 discusses natural medicinal therapy, such as lichens and their bioactive phytochemicals, as a promising alternative to impede diabetes and its analogous comorbidities. Bioinformatics technologies were used to speed up the screening of medication candidates and lessen the need for experimental animals. To evaluate their potential as anti-diabetic medications, an *in silico* analysis of the three metabolites, calcyin, stictic acid, and physodic acid, as well as the three standard anti-diabetic agents, metformin, repaglinide, and sitagliptin, was conducted against twelve known targets of diabetes. Discovery Studio's visualiser was used to evaluate and annotate ligand-target interactions with Autodockvina 1.1.2 visually. The Molsoft prediction server was used to calculate the molecular characteristics and drug likeness.

In Chapter 11, the effects of lapachol and nickel lapachol on fifty distinct tumour proteins linked to various cancers were examined using data from the Protein Data Bank. Molecular docking against these tumour proteins was done using Autodock 4.2 nickel lapachol had higher binding energies with all receptors than lapachol, but most importantly, it showed the most significant energies and was checked for interactions. Using the Molsoft server and Lipinski's rule of five, nickel lapachol demonstrated drug-likeliness characteristics (0.04). On the AdmetSAR platform, toxicology parameters were evaluated and shown to be neither mutagenic nor carcinogenic. Overall findings indicate that nickel lapachol interacts with tumour proteins in a significant way and may have potential as an anticancer chemical.

The study of the many plant parts used to lessen discomfort, lessen inflammation, and treat scorpion stings is covered in Chapter 12. The functional profile of *Solanum virginianum* was characterised in this study using RNA sequencing technology, with a particular emphasis on the genes involved in the biosynthesis pathway of the vitamin B group. B vitamins and other water-soluble vitamins are required for average cell growth and function. The 196 annotated coding sequences (CDS) that make up this sum translate 121 enzymes involved in synthesising the vitamin B complex, including thiamine, riboflavin, vitamin B_6, pantothenate, biotin, and folate. It was established that most of the CDS discovered matched those of *Solanum tuberosum*. This research sheds light on the transcriptome and functional annotation of *S. virginianum* regarding the vitamin B synthetic pathway as in maize, gut bacteria, *Escherichia coli*, and higher plants.

Chapter 13 is about the identification of compounds present in the ethanolic extract of *Cecropia pachystachya* Trécul leaves by CG-MS and *in silico* studies with the enzymes 5-LOX and α-1-antitrypsin. The objective of this study is to carry out chemical compound identification in the ethyl extract of *C. pachystachya* leaves and to verify the PreADMET properties and the interaction of these compounds with 5-LOX and α-1-antitrypsin enzymes through *in silico* tests. Software such as Chimera, Autodock, and AutoDock Tools 1.5.6 were used to realise the molecular docking calculus. In GC-MS analysis, a total of sixty-two compounds were identified, with the substances ethyl hexadecanoic (32), phytol (37), linoleic acid (42), trident-2-vinyl 2,2-dichloroacetate (43) and ethyl octadecanoate (45) showing the highest relative percentage area. Predictions of Absorption, Distribution, Metabolism, Excretion, and Toxicity (PreADMET) properties were determined for each molecule, and all fit the parameters of the rule of five and can be classified as a drug. Among the molecular docking calculations, the complexes with linoleic acid and phytol showed better interaction energy values for the enzyme 5-LOX and α-1-antitrypsin, respectively.

In Chapter 14, it is discussed how many biotic and abiotic factors have an impact on the grapevine, reducing the composition of the grape and, ultimately, the yield. Numerous transcriptome studies use the transcriptional alterations related to grape development and ripening processes, which exhibit complex gene and protein expression variations, to uncover multiple molecular mechanisms. The metabolic profile of grapes under different environmental circumstances, in multiple environments, and under stress has aided in the understanding and development of crop enhancement initiatives. The integration of genomic, transcriptomic, proteomic, and metabolomics research is required to produce a good crop with increased nutritional quality.

The integration of computation and trials in the study of Vietnamese medicinal plants is discussed in Chapter 15. Simulated calculations have always been preferred and widely used to forecast key characteristics of substances undergoing research. Finding the unique features of chemical structures that enable them to bind to proteins is made easier with the help of molecular docking simulation. It forecasts the structural elements of related compounds that share defined components. Docking simulations can plot the values of different interactions between the investigated compound and the viruses, such as hydrogen bonds, cation-cation interactions, ionic interactions, interaction distances between amino acids and active sites of compounds, and van der Waals interactions, in the search for potential drugs to treat or prevent viral entry.

We want to express our gratitude to all the authors who have contributed their expertise and valuable insights to make this book possible. We extend our appreciation to the reader for their interest in this book.

Editors

About the Editors

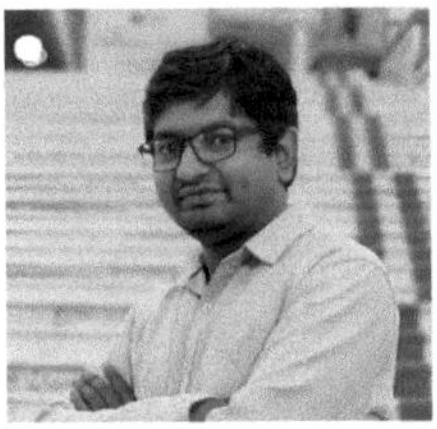

Dr. Pranav Deepek Pathak is an associate professor at the MIT School of Bioengineering Sciences & Research, MIT Art, Design and Technology University, Pune. He has more than 14 years of teaching experience in Fundamentals of Biochemical Engineering, metabolic engineering, Biotransport, Mass transfer, Heat Transfer, and Reaction Engineering. He received his undergraduate and postgraduate degrees in chemical engineering from Sant Gadge Baba Amravati University, India, and a doctoral degree in chemical engineering from Visveswaraya National Institute of Technology, Nagpur, India. His research specializations are bio-refinery, biomass and waste utilization, microbial engineering and fermentation & extraction technology. He has published more than 40 research articles in peer-reviewed international journals/book chapters and has three edited books on his credit. He has also filed several patents to his credit. He participated in various national/international conferences, workshops, and training. His research interests include bioengineering, biorefinery, and wastewater treatment.

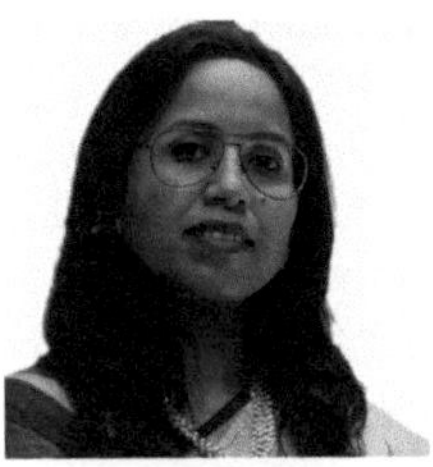

Dr. Roshani Raut obtained her PhD degree in computer science and engineering and ME and BE degrees in computer science and engineering. She has more than 20 years of experience and currently she is working as a professor in the Department of Information Technology and Dean International Relations at Pimpri Chinchwad College of Engineering, Pune, India. She is guiding a PhD research scholar in the University of Technology, Petronas, Malaysia.

She is a member of IEEE and ISTE. She has availed research and workshop grants from BCUD, Pune University. She has presented more than 125 research communications in national and international conferences and journals. She has published 15 patents and has received grants for 10 patents. She worked as a convener for national and international conferences. She has published 10 books, where she worked as an author or editor, of various national and international publications like IGI Global, CRC/Taylor & Francis, and Scrivener Wiley. Her research area includes artificial intelligence, machine learning, data mining, and deep learning, among other areas.

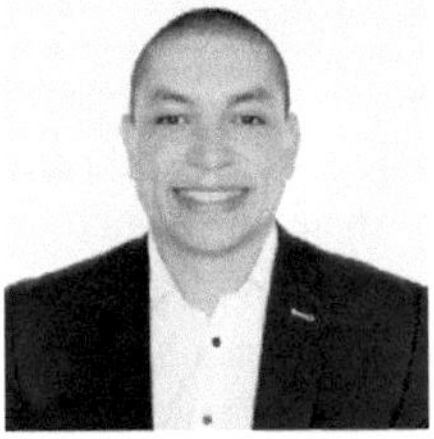

Sebastián Jaramillo-Isaza is a skilled, rigorous, and highly motivated bioengineer. He holds an MSc in mechanics and materials and a doctoral degree in biomechanics, biomaterials, and bioengineering. In addition, he has substantial experience researching and teaching in motion capture and analysis, biomaterials, rehabilitation, bioinstrumentation, and materials characterization. Furthermore, he has participated in and organized national/international conferences and workshops. Currently, he is working as an associate professor in biomedical engineering at Antonio Nariño University in Bogotá, Colombia.

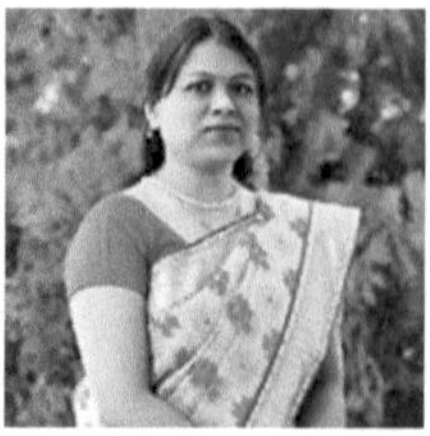

Dr. Pradnya Borkar is an assistant professor at the Department of Computer Science and Engineering, Symbiosis Institute of Technology, Nagpur (Constituent of Symbiosis International University, Pune) She did her BE in computer technology in 2002, M.Tech in computer science and engineering in 2008, and PhD in computer science and engineering in 2018 from Rashtrasant Tukdoji Maharaj Nagpur University (formerly Nagpur University). She has worked with many reputed organizations and has an overall teaching experience of around 19 years. One patent has been granted to her account, and she has filed two more patents. She had handled major responsibilities at the time of accreditation. Her area of interest is high-performance computing, bioinformatics, parallel computing, database management systems, compilers and theory of computation and more. She has presented and published many papers in national/international conferences as well as journals. She has published nine book chapters. She is a reviewer of two international journals and has reviewed book chapters of various publishers of repute. She has chaired sessions at international and national conferences. She is a member of professional societies such as ISTE, CSI, and SDIWC. She worked as a committee member in various capacities at the institute and university level.

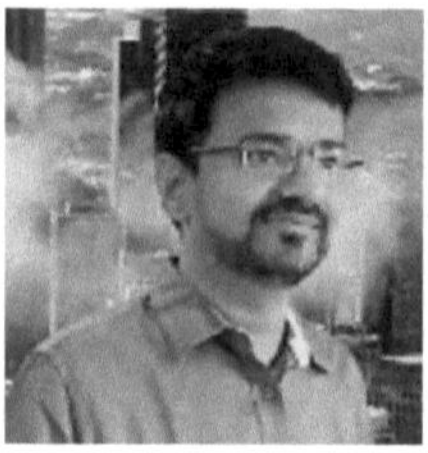

Dr. Rutvij H. Jhaveri (senior member, IEEE) is an experienced educator and researcher working in the Department of Computer Science & Engineering, Pandit Deendayal Energy University, Gandhinagar, India. He conducted his postdoctoral research at Delta-NTU Corporate Lab for Cyber-Physical Systems, Nanyang Technological University, Singapore. He completed his PhD in computer engineering in 2016. In 2017, he was awarded the prestigious Pedagogical Innovation Award by Gujarat Technological University. Currently, he is co-investigating a funded project from GUJCOST. He was ranked among top 2% of scientists around the world in 2021 and 2022. He has 3000+ Google Scholar citations with an h-index of 29. He is an editorial board member in various journals of repute including *IEEE Transactions on Industrial Informatics* and *Scientific Reports*. He also serves as a reviewer in several international journals and as an advisory/TPC member at renowned international conferences. He authored 145+ articles including the IEEE/ACM Transactions and flagship IEEE/ACM conferences. Moreover, he has several national and international patents and copyrights to his name. He also possesses memberships in various technical bodies such as ACM, CSI, ISTE, and others. He is the coordinator of SCAN—Smart Cities Air Quality Network. Moreover, he is a member of the advisory board at the Symbiosis Institute of Digital and Telecom Management and other reputed universities since 2022. He is an editorial board member in several Springer and Hindawi journals. He also served as a committee member in the "Smart Village Project"—government of Gujarat—at the district level during the year 2017. His research interests are cyber security, IoT systems, SDN, and smart healthcare.

Contributors

Achur Rajeshwara
Department of Biochemistry
Jnana Sahyadri Kuvempu University
Shivamogga

Ajiboye Abdulfatai Temitope
Department of Chemistry and Industrial Chemistry
Kwara State University
Malete, Ilorin, Nigeria

Alves Wellington dos S.
State University of Piauí

Ayipo Yusuf Oloruntoyin
Centre for Drug Research
Universiti Sains Malaysia
Pulau Pinang, Malaysia

Badeggi Umar Muhammad
Department of Chemistry
Ibrahim Badamasi Babangida University
Niger State, Nigeria

Bhat Smitha S.
Department of Biotechnology and Bioinformatics
JSS Academy of Higher Education and Research
Mysuru, Karnataka, India

Biswas Sagarika
Department of Genomics and Molecular Medicine
CSIR-Institute of Genomics and Integrative Biology
New Delhi, India

Costa Clara A. C. B
Federal Institute of Alagoas

Dalal Vikram
Department of Genomics and Molecular Medicine
CSIR-Institute of Genomics and Integrative Biology
New Delhi, India

Dieu Nguyen Thi Xuan
Faculty of Pharmacy
University of Medicine and Pharmacy at Ho Chi Minh City
Ho Chi Minh City, Vietnam

D S Gayathri
Department of Zoology
BGS Science Academy
Chikkaballapura, Karnataka, India

Emaikwu Ngozi Georgewill
Department of Biotechnology
Federal University of Technology
Owerri, Nigeria

Freitas Johnnatan D. de
Federal Institute of Alagoas

Gautam Rupesh K.
Department of Pharmacology
Indore Institute of Pharmacy
IIST Campus, Rau, Indore (M.P.), India

Gomes Rafael de O.
State University of Piauí

Hari Somya
Vels Institute of Science, Technology, and Advanced Studies

Hariprasad T P N
Department of Life Science
Bangalore University, Bangalore
Karnataka, India

Hemagirigowda Ravikumar
Department of Life Science
Bangalore University
Bangalore, Karnataka, India

Joshi Chinmayi
Smt. S. S. Patel Nootan Science and Commerce College
Sankalchand Patel University
Visnagar, India

Kamboj Sweta
Guru Gobind Singh College of Pharmacy
Yamunanagar
Haryana, India

Kubera Sumachirayu Chitradurga
Department of Studies and Research in Biochemistry
Tumkur University, Tumakuru

Lima Francisco das C. A.
State University of Piauí

Limbhachiya Viraj
Smt. S. S. Patel Nootan Science and Commerce College
Sankalchand Patel University, Visnagar, India

M A Sundaramahalingam
Chemical and Biochemical Process Engineering Laboratory
Department of Chemical Engineering
National Institute of Technology Tiruchirappalli
Tamilnadu, India

Malhotra Hitesh
Guru Gobind Singh College of Pharmacy
Yamunanagar, Haryana, India

M Likith
Department of Biotechnology
Dayananda Sagar College of Engineering
Bangalore, Karnataka, India

Mordi Mohd Nizam
Centre for Drug Research
Universiti Sains Malaysia
Pulau Pinang, Malaysia

Moura Orlando F. da S.
Federal Institute of Alagoas

Mourão Penina S.
State University of Piauí

Murugan Abirla
University of Pavia

Nhung Nguyen Thi Ai
Department of Chemistry
University of Sciences
Hue University
Vietnam

Ogidi Odangowei Inetiminebi
Department of Biochemistry
Faculty of Basic Medical Sciences
Bayelsa Medical University Yenagoa
Bayelsa State, Nigeria

Sivashanmugam
Chemical and Biochemical Process Engineering Laboratory
Department of Chemical Engineering
National Institute of Technology Tiruchirappalli
Tamilnadu, India

Patel Ritul
Smt. S. S. Patel Nootan Science and Commerce College
Sankalchand Patel University
Visnagar, India

Pathak Deepek Pranav
MIT School of Bioengineering Science and Research
MIT Art, Design and Technology University Pune, India

Prasad Shashanka K.
Department of Biotechnology and Bioinformatics
JSS Academy of Higher Education and Research
Mysuru Karnataka, India

R Sindhu
Department of Microbiology
JSS Academy of Higher Education and Research
Mysuru, Karnataka, India

Ranade Yogita
MIT School of Bioengineering Science and Research
MIT Art, Design and Technology University
Pune

Rao Madhushree M.V.
Defence Institute of Advanced Technology (Deemed to be University)
Girinagar, Pune, India

Ravikumar H
Department of Life Science
Bangalore University
Bangalore, Karnataka, India

Rudraksh
Guru Gobind Singh College of Pharmacy
Yamunanagar, Haryana, India

Sarwara Amrit
Guru Gobind Singh College of Pharmacy
Yamunanagar, Haryana, India

Shivaiah Nagaraju
Department of Studies and Research in Biochemistry
Tumkur University
Tumakuru

Siddaraju Thoyajakshi Ramasamudhra
Department of Studies and Research in Biochemistry
Tumkur University
Tumakuru

Sudharsan Meenambiga Setti
University of Pavia

Tanu Devi
Guru Gobind Singh College of Pharmacy
Yamunanagar, Haryana, India

Teja Relli
Chemical and Biochemical Process Engineering Laboratory
Department of Chemical Engineering
National Institute of Technology Tiruchirappalli
Tamilnadu, India
India Plant Bioactive Compound Laboratory
Faculty of Agriculture
Chiang Mai University
Thailand

Thippeswamy Megha Gowri
Department of Biochemistry
Jnana Sahyadri Kuvempu University
Shivamogga

Triet Nguyen Thanh
Faculty of Traditional Medicine
University of Medicine and Pharmacy at Ho Chi Minh City
Ho Chi Minh City, Vietnam

Uchôa Valdiléia T.
Federal Institute of Alagoas

1 Computational Approaches for the Discovery of New Drugs for Inflammatory and Infectious Diseases

Vikram Dalal and Sagarika Biswas[†]
Department of Genomics and Molecular Medicine, CSIR-Institute of Genomics and Integrative Biology, New Delhi, India
[†]Corresponding Author: sagarika.biswas@igib.res.in

ABBREVIATIONS

ADMET	Absorption, distribution, metabolism, and excretion
AMBER	Assisted model building with energy refinement
***At*SPHK1**	*Arabidopsis thaliana* sphingosine kinase1
BTK	Bruton tyrosine kinase
CADD	Computer-aided drug designing
CAMP	Cationic antimicrobial peptides
CAIs	Carbonate alkylase inhibitors
CHARMM	Chemistry at Harvard Macromolecular Mechanics
CRP	C-reactive protein
DMP	2,6-dimethoxyphenol
DCHP	Dicyclohexyl phthalate
FEL	Free energy landscape
GROMACS	GROningen MAchine for Chemical Simulations
hACMS	Human α-amino-β-carboxymuconate-ε-semialdehyde
HADDOCK	High Ambiguity Driven protein-protein DOCKing
hDHODH	Human dihydroorotate dehydrogenase
hGR	Human glucocorticoid receptor
hTTR	Human transthyretin
HTVS	High-throughput virtual screening
IKK-β	Inhibitor of nuclear factor-kappa B kinase subunit β
JAK	Janus kinases
LLM	Lipophilic membrane protein
MBL	Mannose-binding lectin

DOI: 10.1201/9781003354437-1

MBP	Mono-n-butyl phthalate
MCHP	Mono-cyclohexyl phthalate
MEHP	Mono-2-ethylhexyl phthalate
MEP	Mono-n-ethyl phthalate
MHP	Mono-n-hexyl phthalate
MD	Molecular dynamics
MG	Malachite green
MM-GBSA	Mechanics generalized born surface area
MM-PBSA	Mechanics Poisson-Boltzmann surface area
MV	Methyl violet
Mpro	Main protease
NAMD	Nanoscale molecular dynamics
NEMO	NF-κB essential modulator
NSAIDs	Non-steroidal anti-inflammatory drugs
NTD	N terminal domain
OA	Osteoarthritis
OHPCBs	hydroxylated polychlorinated biphenyls
PA	Phosphatidic acid
PBPs	Penicillin-binding proteins
PCA	Principal component analysis
PDO	Phthalate dioxygenase oxygenase
PDR	Phthalate dioxygenase reductase
PLpro	Papain-like protease
QM/MM	Quantum mechanics/molecular mechanics
PDGFR	Platelet-derived growth factor receptor
PETR-ITC	Pterostilbene-isothiocyanate
RA	Rheumatoid arthritis
RB5	Reactive black 5
RdRp	RNA-dependent RNA polymerase
RF	Rheumatoid factor
Rg	Radius of gyration
RMSD	Root means square deviation
RMSF	Root means square fluctuations
S1P	Sphingosine-1-phosphate
SAR	Structure-activity relationship
SASA	Solvent accessible surface area
SYK	Spleen tyrosine kinase
TTCC	T-type calcium channel
TUM	Tunicamycin
UFF	Universal force field
VA	Veratryl alcohol
WTA	Wall Teichoic Acid

1.1 INTRODUCTION

Drug discovery is a time-consuming, complex, interdisciplinary, and costly process to identify the drugs for life-threatening diseases. In recent years, the process of drug discovery has been increasing rapidly due to the usage of high-throughput virtual screening (HTVS). Drug design is a process that starts with the selection of a target (macromolecule: protein, lipids, DNA, or RNA), preparation of a set of molecules that will be screened with a target, and evaluation of binding affinities of ligands with the receptor, followed by *in vitro* and *in vivo* preclinical analysis to design a drug-like molecule (Figure 1.1). Furthermore, the stability of ligands along with protein complexes will analyze by *in silico* methods like molecular dynamics (MD) simulation, molecular mechanics Poisson-Boltzmann surface area (MM-PBSA), amino acid residues decomposition analysis, mechanics generalized born surface area (MM-GBSA), and quantum mechanics/molecular mechanics (QM/MM). Overall, the aim of drug discovery is to design and develop new drug molecules that can be used for a selective and specific target to combat the pathogenesis of an organism. *In silico* techniques play a vital role in minimizing the cost and time of drug discovery. The study conducted on computers using computational powers to identify drug-like molecules by utilization of bioinformatics approaches is called *in silico* methods. In drug discovery, *in silico* methods consist of several steps which involve a) analysis of the binding (active or allosteric) site of the receptor, b) selection and evaluations of a set of molecules, c) screening and determination of binding affinities of molecules with a receptor, d) ranking of best-scored molecules and cross-verification of the binding affinities, e) Lipinski or absorption, distribution, metabolism, and excretion (ADMET) analysis, f) analysis of the stability of protein-ligand complex, and g) further optimizations. In a nutshell, the most important steps in *in silico* methods are virtual screening, de novo drug designing, Lipinski and ADMET properties, and evaluations of protein-ligand stability (Figure 1.2).

The protein structures of several drug targets of life-threatening diseases like viral diseases, bacterial, tuberculosis, or infectious diseases, etc., are available in the protein databank (www.rcsb.org/) generated via x-ray crystallography, NMR, or cryo-electron microscopy. Experts have claimed that the drug discovery market will grow exponentially in the current decade. Therefore, the development of new algorithms and software is underway to do molecular modeling, docking, and molecular dynamics simulation within a short period of time, which will have a great impact on designing a most promising lead candidate for the desired target.

In the current world, *in silico* approaches for drug designing are extensively utilized to screen and predict the most probable conformation of a ligand at the binding site of the target, along with the determination of binding affinities due to the presence of the non-covalent (hydrogen bonds, hydrophobic interactions, polar interactions, or salt bridge) or covalent interactions between receptor and ligand. There is a long list of available programs like SWISS-MODELLER, Phyre2, Modeller, RaptorX, AutoDock Tools, AutoDock Vina, High Ambiguity Driven protein-protein DOCKing (HADDOCK), Glide, Discovery studio, GROningen MAchine for Chemical Simulations (GROMACS), Assisted Model Building with Energy Refinement (AMBER), DESMOND, SWISS-ADME, Nanoscale Molecular Dynamics (NAMD), pkCSM, etc. for *in silico* work in the field of drug discovery. All these programs may or may not require high computational power (Colovos and Yeates 1993; Schwede et al. 2003; Pettersen et al. 2004; Van Der Spoel et al. 2005; Arnold et al. 2006; Kelley et al. 2015; Van Zundert et al. 2016). But the most important factor for researchers is that they should have fundamental knowledge along with pros and cons of consideration of a specific software or program to get results.

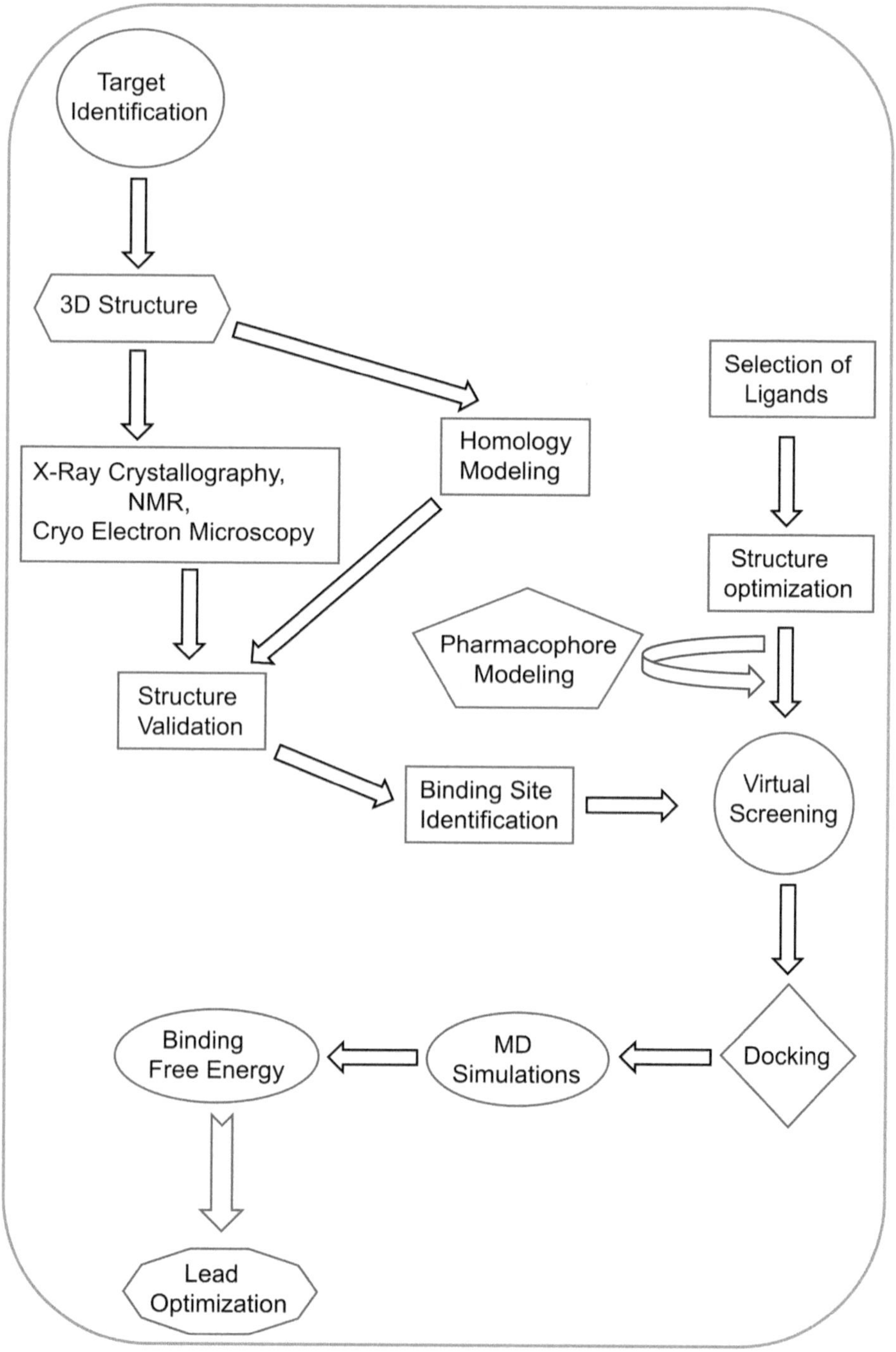

FIGURE 1.1 Summary of general computer-aided drug designing process to identify the lead candidates.

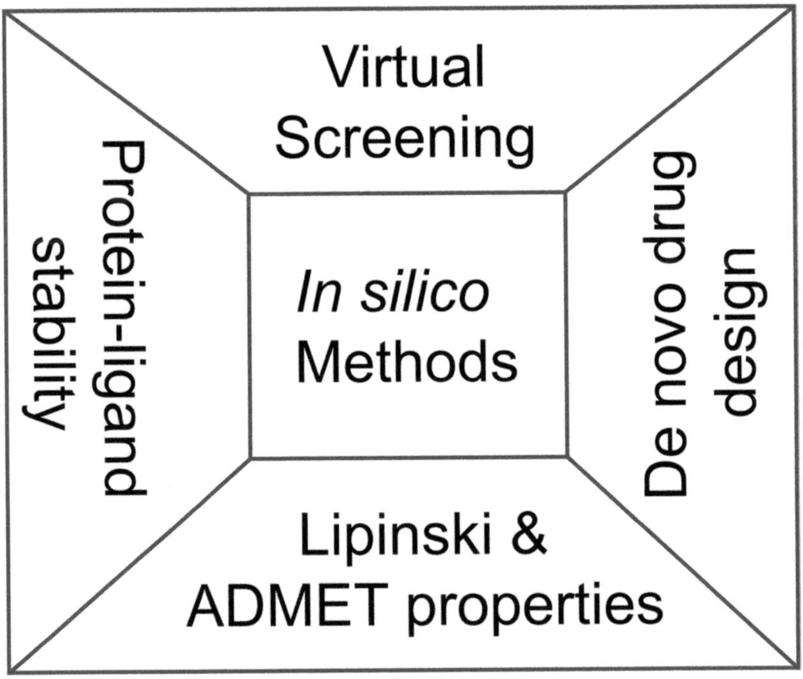

FIGURE 1.2 *In silico* methods of structure-based drug designing.

Additionally, the usage of accurate and up-to-date in silico methods will give precise and reliable results (Weigelt 2010). This chapter sheds light on each step of structure-based drug design, along with case studies in inflammatory and infectious diseases.

1.2 DRUG DISCOVERY METHODS

The ultimate goal of drug discovery is the screening, designing, or identification of promising molecules that have potential to treat diseases along with minimal side effects on living beings. The considered molecules are small organic molecules that have the capability to interact with a specific receptor.

1.2.1 Traditional Drug Discovery

In 1950, the drug discovery method was mainly focused on the synthesis of thousands of small molecules, followed by the screening of synthesized and natural compounds for biological activity against the target (Reddy and Parrill 1999). As soon as a promising lead molecule was screened and considered, hundreds of analogs or similar compounds to potent lead molecules were synthesized and screened again for biological activity. The traditional drug discovery approach was time-consuming and highly expensive. The other risk factors add to the cost and make a total expense of millions for a single novel drug. Other than this, the traditional approach has various other drawbacks, the most challenging of which was why a molecule is active or inactive for the same target in a certain condition. It was unclear how to tackle this situation and improve the lead. This approach has no certainty about which specific molecule is for which specific target, so this was also an obstacle for clinical trials. One lead molecule was identified from a huge synthesized molecular library, and structural optimization was required to enhance the drug's potency and other properties. The most difficult part of this approach was the decision of when to move from the screening to the synthesis stage (Young et al. 1997). Developing new compounds for *in vivo* biological screening methods followed by ADMET profiling was a time-consuming and labor-intensive process (Al Qaraghuli et al. 2017).

1.2.2 Modern Drug Discovery Method

In the current drug discovery approaches, an additional step, i.e., in silico method using computer-aided drug design (CADD), has been incorporated, which has several benefits over the traditional drug discovery method. The usage of *in silico* techniques is valuable in other fields like molecular biology, biochemistry, environmental chemistry, agriculture, nanotechnology, and protein biophysics. *In silico* techniques provide various benefits that reduce the time and cost to improve the drug's affinity, selectivity, specificity, and ADMET properties. Modern techniques are highly interdisciplinary and are used to reduce the challenges in drug discovery. Interestingly, the *in silico* approach can also predict the altered properties (therapeutic effect, affinity, ADMET, or side effects) due to slight modification in the structure of a ligand (Young 2009). Even one can predict which lead may not make it into a clinical trial or will be denied by the FDA for a specific disease. The *in silico* approach is also useful for improving the efficacy or ADMET properties by modifying the basic scaffold. A new drug can also be designed by considering the same pharmacological properties, i.e., chemical imprints and modifications of side groups, followed by assessing the stability of molecules with a receptor (Kalyani et al. 2013).

1.3 COMPUTER-AIDED DRUG DESIGN

In 1989, Plewczynski coined the term *in silico,* which means designing a rational drug by using computational approaches (Plewczynski et al. 2014). The first step is the selection of a protein that is responsible for a specific disease in a pathogenic organism (Young 2009). Furthermore, drug designing steps require a receptor structure either via experimental or 3-D model generation, a set of ligands, binding affinities, molecular docking, experimental assays, and clinical trials (Figure 1.3). Several new techniques/innovations have been made in the field that led to tremendous developments in the drug discovery field (Macalino et al. 2015). Target and hit identification, structure-activity relationship (SAR) modeling, hit-to-lead optimization, and pharmacokinetic and pharmacodynamic property prediction are some of the many useful features of modern computational tools for drug discovery. For this reason, CADD provides significant benefits for researchers by allowing them to avoid the needless screening of countless compounds at random. Experts estimated

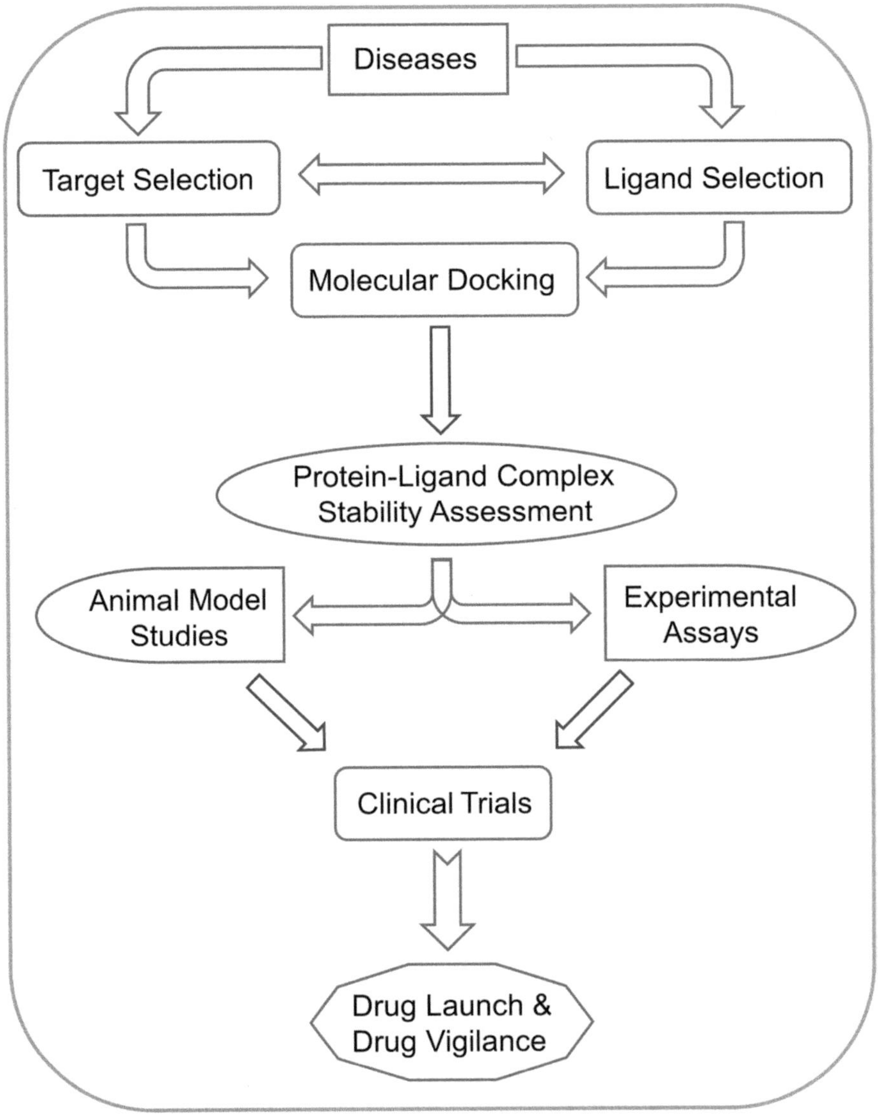

FIGURE 1.3 The schematic representation of drug designing consists of *in silico*, experimental, *in vitro* assays and clinical trials.

that CADD can reduce the drug discovery time and financial investment by 30 percent. The *in silico* methodology has been widely accepted and is a crucial part of the drug development process. As a result, *in silico* approaches were beneficial because they cut down on a) the expense and development time for new pharmaceuticals and b) the number of animals needed for in vivo experiments. New experimental methodologies for analyzing the function and structure of a target and ligand have been made possible by recent advances *in silico*. Structure-based drug designing is the most appropriate approach for identifying novel ligands after structural and functional analysis of a receptor (Gupta et al. 2021; Kumari and Dalal 2021; Kumari et al. 2022b, 2023). Further, MD simulation is an effective and highly utilized technique to assess the dynamics and stability of the protein-ligand complex (Dhankhar et al. 2020a; Bisht et al. 2021; Dalal et al. 2021; Dhankhar et al. 2021a). If the experimental structure of a target is absent, then modeling plays an essential role in generating a 3D model of a receptor (Dhankhar et al. 2020a; Kumari et al. 2020; Saini et al. 2021; Gupta et al. 2022; Rathi et al. 2022; Singh et al. 2022b). In addition, quantum mechanics/molecular mechanics (QM/MM) studies play a vital role in exploring the catalytic mechanism and enzyme kinetics of proteins (Dalal et al. 2022b). QM/MM calculations are also done to explore the stability of the protein along with different ligands (Dalal et al. 2021; Singh et al. 2022b). Overall, all these computational techniques reduce the time and cost significantly in drug discovery.

1.3.1 Target Determination

The identification of a valid drug target that should be essential for cell signaling, metabolic pathways, a cellular process, or directly linked to drug resistance in that specific organism is an initial but crucial step of structure-based drug designing. In SARS-CoV-2, papain-like protease (PLpro) is a protease found to play a major role in the processing of viral polyproteins (Harcourt et al. 2004; Ratia et al. 2008). RNA-dependent RNA polymerase (RdRp) is an essential protein involved in viral replication and transcription (Wang et al. 2020). The N terminal domain (NTD) of nucleocapsid has been reported as a drug target for developing antiviral agents, as it is an essential protein (Chenavas et al. 2013; Lo et al. 2013; Lin et al. 2014b; Monod et al. 2015). Ribosome biogenesis GTP-binding (YsxC) is a GTPase that is essential for translation in *Staphylococcus aureus* (Cooper et al. 2009). Another protein, lipophilic membrane protein (LLM), is involved in peptidoglycan metabolism and affects the bacterial lysis rate also in *S. aureus* (Maki et al. 1994). FmtA is one of the methicillin resistance factors, and its inhibition makes *S. aureus* susceptible to penicillin and methicillin (Sobral et al. 2006; Balibar et al. 2009). The three-dimensional structure of a receptor is required, as either determined by cryo-electron microscopy, x-ray crystallography, or NMR, or by prediction by computer-based modeling (Dalal et al. 2019; Malik et al. 2019; Dhankhar et al. 2020a; Kumari et al. 2021).

1.3.2 Homology Modeling

Homology modeling is most effective in generating the 3D reliable structure of a protein from its primary sequence (Figure 1.4). It is a user-friendly, cost-effective, and safe technique that further helps in the analysis of structural and functional properties of the 3D structure. There are several software programs or online webservers like Modeller, SWISS-MODEL, Phyre2, RaptorX, ITASSER, etc. are available to generate the 3D model of proteins (Schwede et al. 2003; Webb and Sali 2014; Kelley et al. 2015; Wang et al. 2016). Further, model energy minimization can be done by SWISS PDB Viewer, Chimera, GROMACS, or AMBER, etc. (Pettersen et al. 2004;

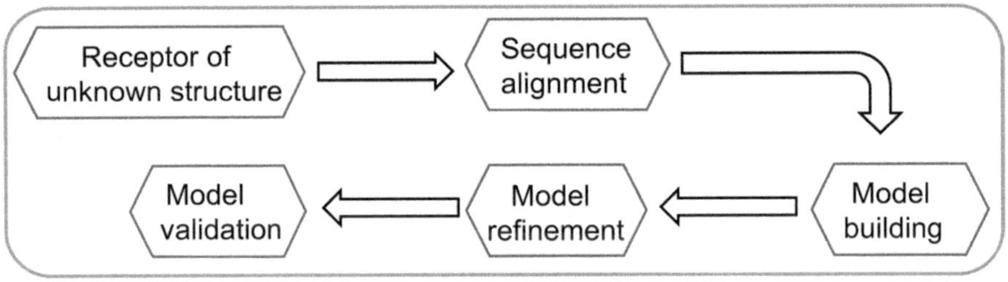

FIGURE 1.4 Different steps of computer-based modelling.

Van Der Spoel et al. 2005; Arnold et al. 2006; Wang et al. 2006). The generated model needs to be validated by Ramachandran plot, ERRAT, VERIFY-3D, ProSA, ProQ, GROMACS, etc. (Colovos and Yeates 1993; Laskowski et al. 1993; Eisenberg et al. 1997; Wallner and Elofsson 2003; Van Der Spoel et al. 2005; Wiederstein and Sippl 2007). For example, three-dimensional models of LLM, YsxC, and GraR from *S. aureus* were generated by RaptorX and SWISS-MODEL, respectively (Kumari et al. 2021; Kumari et al. 2021, 2022b; Kumari et al. 2023). ZnuA1, ESBP, 1 Cys peroxiredoxin, and 2 Cys peroxiredoxin from *Candidatus Liberibacter asiaticus* were predicted by Phyre2 and SWISS-MODEL, respectively (Saini et al. 2019; Gupta et al. 2021; Saini et al. 2021; Gupta et al. 2022). Similarly, the 3D model of the T-type calcium channel (TTCC) from *Homo sapiens* was generated by SWISS-MODEL and validated by Ramachandran plot, ERRAT, ProQ, ProSA, and MD simulation (Kumari et al. 2020).

1.3.3 Active Site Prediction/Identification

The region of the receptor where the substrate or binding partner interacts and performs the biological function is known as an active site. Generally, an active site is a cavity or pocket present at the interface or deep in the receptor (Kahraman and Thornton 2008). This site is lined by amino acid residues, which, directly or indirectly, make interactions with a substrate. The identification of correct information about the active site is crucial and highly desirable, as it is necessary to develop potent candidates to inhibit the interactions and activity of a substrate with a receptor (Szarecka and Dobson 2019). Experimental information on the binding pocket of a receptor is desirable. However, in the absence of any experimental evidence, several tools or webservers like Castp, fpocket, 3DLigandStie, DoGSiteScorer, DeepSite, etc. can predict the cavities with reliability (Le Guilloux et al. 2009; Volkamer et al. 2012; Jiménez et al. 2017; Tian et al. 2018; McGreig et al. 2022). Kumari et al. reported that the structural superposition of the homology model of TTCC with its homologous structures (PDB ID: 5GJV and 6J8G) showed that Glu378, Glu974, Asp975, Asp1504, and Asn1508 are involved in the binding of calcium ions in TTCC (Kumari et al. 2020). Multiple sequence alignment and structural superposition of YsxC with other homologous structures showed a set of amino acid residues are conserved and present at the active site of YsxC in *S. aureus*, as shown in Figure 1.5 (Kumari et al. 2021,

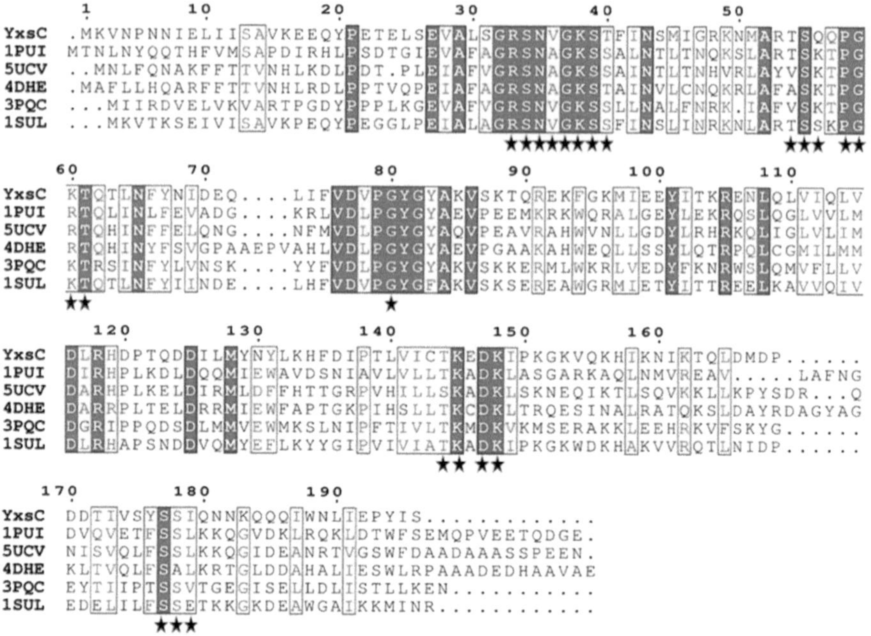

FIGURE 1.5 Multiple sequence alignment (MSA) of YsxC with its homologous structures (PDB ID: 1PUI, 5UCV, 4DHE, 3PQC, and 1SUL). Amino acid residues marked with a star are active site residues in proteins.

2022). Structural superposition of the predicted model of FemC with GlnR (PDB ID: 4R4E) and TnrA (PDB ID: 4R4E) showed that the active site amino acid residues are conserved in FemC and other structures, as shown in Figure 1.6 (Dalal and Kumari 2022).

1.3.4 Ligand Preparation

The virtual screening is an *in silico* approach to identifying potent ligands from a large set of databases. Several databases like ZINC database, selleckchem, asinex, ChemFaces databases, etc. are available free to download fragments, antibacterials, drugs, natural product-like substances, antiviral molecules, etc. to screen against receptors. Saini et al. screened ZnuA1 and ESBP of *Candidatus Liberibacter asiaticus* against the ZINC database (Saini et al. 2019; Saini et al. 2021).

1.3.5 Virtual Screening

Virtual screening is an attractive and effective technique in CADD to screen a large set of small molecule libraries against a receptor. In other words, virtual screening is a process of docking a set of compounds with a receptor for the identification of a potent molecule (Rester 2008). Gupta et al. employed the virtual screening using

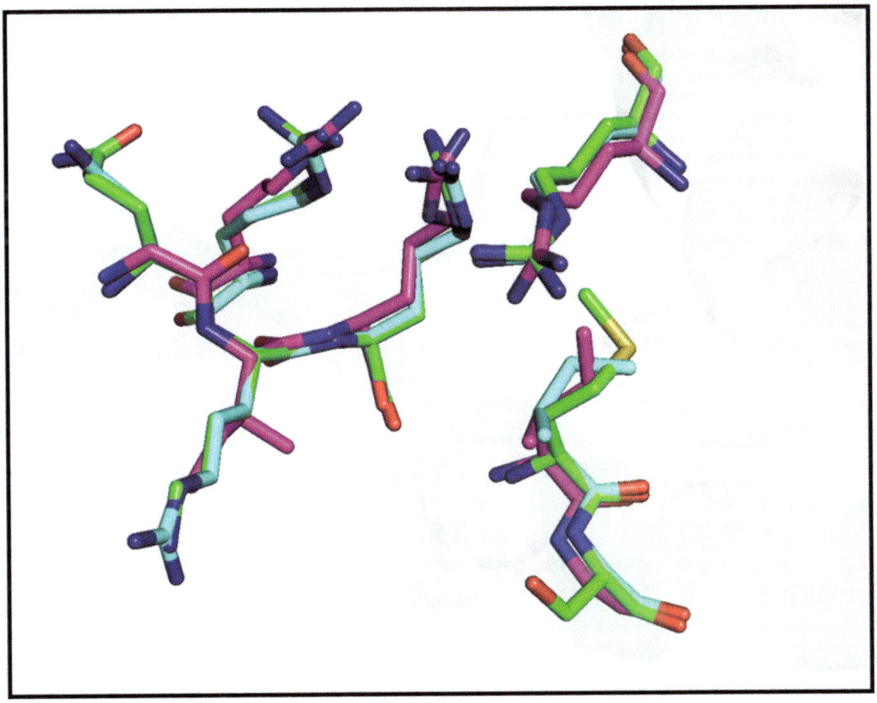

FIGURE 1.6 FemC model (green color) is superposed with its homologous structures (PDB ID: 4R4E-cyan color and 4R22-magenta color).

AutoDock Vina of 1 Cys and 2 Cys peroxiredoxin of *Candidatus Liberibacter asiaticus* against antibacterials and fragment compounds of the asinex and selleckchem database, respectively (Trott and Olson 2010; Gupta et al. 2021; Gupta et al. 2022). The FmtA protein was screened against the e-LEA3D database on the PyRx platform using AutoDock Vina (Dallakyan and Olson 2015; Dalal et al. 2021; Singh et al. 2022a).

1.3.6 Molecular Docking

Molecular docking is a technique in CADD to predict or generate the best promising orientation of a ligand at the specific binding site of a receptor by using an algorithm. Molecular docking is also referred to as the process of predicting ligand conformation along with binding affinity in a protein-ligand complex (Engel et al. 2008). Molecular docking is a most acclaimed approach to evaluate the interactions and binding of a ligand at the binding site of a protein. The usage of molecular docking is increasing day by day due to the atomic resolution structures of receptors solved by x-ray crystallography. Molecular docking is of two types: a) rigid docking (lock and key) and b) flexible docking (induced fit).

1.3.6.1 Rigid Docking

Rigid docking is similar to a lock and key mechanism in which the ligand is flexible (allowed translation and rotation) while the protein is rigid. In rigid docking, amino acid residues of the protein are not allowed to move, while the ligand is free to rotate and translate along with its geometry to predict the best unrestrained conformation of a ligand at the provided binding site or an uncharacterized site of a protein. Singh et al. performed the rigid docking of different phthalates (MEHP, MHP, MBP, and MEP) with MEHP hydrolase by using AutoDock Tools (Singh et al. 2017). AutoDock Tools and Vina were used to dock diphthalates and their corresponding monophthalates with human α-amino-β-carboxymuconate-ε-semialdehyde (hACMS) (Singh et al. 2018). Molecular docking of *Arabidopsis thaliana* Sphingosine kinase1 (*At*SPHK1) with phosphatidic acid (PA) was performed using AutoDock Vina (Pandit et al. 2018). AutoDock Tools was used for molecular docking of dyes and small substrates with dye-decolorizing peroxidases of *Bacillus subtilis* (*Bs*DyP) (Dhankhar et al. 2020b, 2021b). Bisht et al. docked the substrate and product at the active site of alcohol dehydrogenase of *Pichia kudriavzevii* BGY1-γm (*Pk*ADH) by using AutoDock Vina (Bisht et al. 2021). Kumar et al. studied the effect of pterostilbene-isothiocyanate (PETR-ITC) due to interactions with the inhibitor of nuclear factor-kappa B kinase subunit β (IKK-β) and NF-κB essential modulator (NEMO) (Kumar et al. 2021b).

1.3.6.2 Flexible Docking

In flexible docking, the ligand and receptor are both flexible. Few selective amino acid residues or maybe a full protein are also set as flexible in flexible docking. Singh et al. performed the flexible docking of DCHP and MCHP with human glucocorticoid receptor (hGR) using HADDOCK (Singh et al. 2020a). Hydroxylated polychlorinated biphenyls (OHPCBs) were docked at the active site of human transthyretin (hTTR) by using HADDOCK (Kumari et al. 2021). Tri-peptide (Valine Phenylalanine Lysine: VFK) was docked to *Momordica charantia* 7S (*Mc*7S) using HADDOCK (Kesari et al. 2020). The flexible docking approach is not only limited to ligand-to-protein docking; it is also highly used and reliable to evaluate the interactions of a macromolecule (protein, DNA, or RNA) to a receptor. HADDOCK was used to dock phthalate dioxygenase reductase (PDR) with phthalate dioxygenase oxygenase (PDO) (Singh et al. 2019). Single-stranded RNA (ssRNA) was docked with the NTD of nucleocapsid of SARS-CoV-2 using HADDOCK (Dhankhar et al. 2020c). Molecular docking of double-stranded DNA (dsDNA) with pumpkin 2S albumin (rP2SA) was also performed using HADDOCK (Savita et al. 2021).

1.3.7 Pharmacophore Modeling

The steric and electronic properties of a molecule that has abilities to bind with a receptor to inhibit the biological activity of a receptor is known as a pharmacophore. In other words, pharmacophore properties are the chemical imprints of a ligand that are essential to bind with a receptor. Pharmacophore-based virtual screening is a ligand-based virtual screening, i.e., a set of molecules is considered on the basis of chemical imprints of the ligands. Based on the availability of reported ligands, there are two primary ways to generate the library for virtual screening: a) one ligand and b) more than one ligand.

1.3.7.1 One Ligand

In this pharmacophore approach, only one ligand may be either a substrate, product, or inhibitor available for the specific receptor. Here, in this scenario, the interactions of the available ligand with the protein need to be analyzed. The chemical groups that make the essential interactions like catalyzation of reaction, etc., with the protein are considered pharmacophore groups during the pharmacophore modeling. Kumari et al. considered a total of six pharmacophore features of tunicamycin (TUM) for pharmacophore modelling, as these groups exhibit the essential interactions with LLM of *S. aureus* (Figure 1.7) (Kumari et al. 2021). Further, molecules

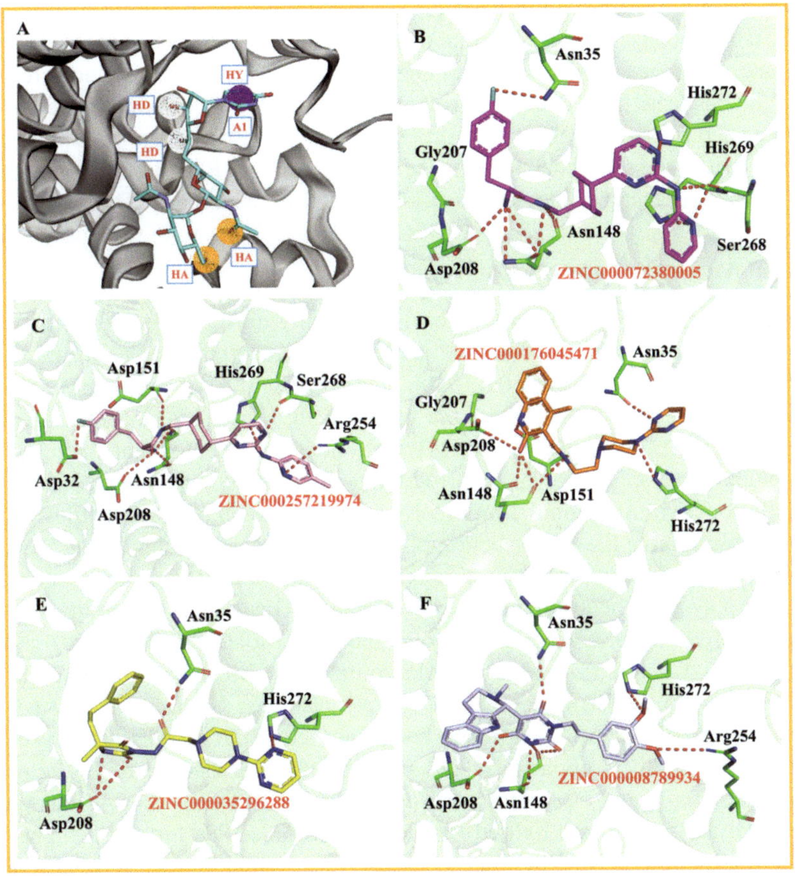

FIGURE 1.7 Identification of five potent molecules (ZINC000072380005, ZINC000257219974, ZINC000176045471, ZINC000035296288, and ZINC000008789934) against the LLM of *S. aureus*. A) Pharmacophore model of tunicamycin (TUM) represented the two hydrogen bond acceptors (HA), two hydrogen bond donors (HD), one hydrophobic (HY), and one aromatic group (A1) shown in orange, white, green, and purple, respectively. Molecular docking results of ZINC000072380005 (B: magenta), ZINC000257219974 (C: pink), ZINC000176045471 (D: orange), ZINC000035296288 (E: yellow), and ZINC000008789934 (F: light blue) with LLM. The protein amino acid residues interacting with ligands are shown in stick format. Hydrogen bonds in protein-ligand complexes are represented in red dashed lines.

were screened out from the ZINC database on the bases of the previously mentioned pharmacophore features of TUM. GTP pharmacophore features showed interactions with YsxC of *S. aureus* that were screened from the ZINC database (Kumari et al. 2021). Furthermore, 13,059 molecules of ZINC databases that exhibited the pharmacophore features of GTP were docked at the active site of YsxC.

1.3.7.2 More Than One Ligand

If more than one ligand (combination of a substrate and a product or two inhibitors) is reported for a receptor, then common groups present among the ligands may be considered pharmacophore features. In other words, it is an approach to selecting similar groups from a set of reported ligands for a specific receptor. Here, similar chemical prints will be considered as pharmacophore features to screen the molecules from a database. Dhankhar et al. considered GMP pharmacophore features and screened the set of ligands from the ZINC database (Dhankhar et al. 2020c). Among the previously mentioned properties, aromatic, hydrophobic, and two hydrogen bond donors were also present in the substrates (GMP, UMP, CMP, and AMP) and inhibitors. All of the pharmacophore features showed essential interactions with the NTD of SARS-CoV-2.

1.3.8 Molecular Dynamics Simulation

Molecular dynamics (MD) simulation is a globally used tool to evaluate the structural, dynamic, and thermodynamic properties of macromolecules in the presence or absence of ligands (Singh et al. 2018; Dhankhar et al. 2020c; Kumar et al. 2020a, 2020b; Kumari et al. 2020; Dhankhar et al. 2021a; Kumari et al. 2021). It is a computer simulation approach that mimics the physical states of atoms of macromolecules to explore the functional and conformational changes in the presence of forces. The overall process of MD simulation involves the conversion of receptor files to an MD software detectable file, construction of periodical boundary conditions (PBCs), the addition of solvents in the PBC, system neutralization, energy minimization, preparation of a system (heating and equilibrations), MD run, and MD analysis. Several programs like GROMACS, AMBER, Nanoscale Molecular Dynamics (NAMD), DESMOND, Chemistry at Harvard Macromolecular Mechanics (CHARMM), etc. are available to perform the MD of macromolecules. Various MD analyses like RMSD, RMSF, Rg, SASA, hydrogen bond numbers, PCA, and FEL analysis can be used to evaluate the compactness and stability of a macromolecule in the presence or absence of a ligand or another macromolecule. RMSD, Rg, SASA, and hydrogen bond analysis results highlighted that identified molecules formed a higher stable RdRP complex than the RdRP-galidesvir complex (Dhankhar et al. 2021a). RMSD, Rg, and SASA results revealed that the antiviral-bound PLpro complex is stable (Kumari et al. 2022a). Protein RMSD, ligand RMSD, Rg, and intermolecular hydrogen bond results were generated to investigate the role of amino acid residues for the catalysis of wall teichoic acid (WTA) by FmtA (Dalal et al. 2022b). The stability of screened molecules with RdRp, main protease (Mpro), and PLpro of SARS-CoV-2 was examined by RMSD, RMSF, Rg, and PCA analysis in MD simulation (Kumar et al. 2021a). RMSD and Rg results suggested that interactions of identified compounds at the active site of LLM formed the higher stable complexes than the LLM-TUM complex, as shown in Figure 1.8 (Rathi et al. 2022). The stability of variants (H106C and D247) of periplasmic metal uptake protein of *Candidatus Liberibacter asiaticus* was studied by RMSD and Rg analysis using AMBER (Kumar et al. 2020b).

1.3.9 Binding Free Energy

MMPBSA and MMGBSA are widely used methods to estimate the binding free energy of small molecules with protein. In both of these approaches, a finite number of trajectories of MD simulation is used to determine the binding energy of a protein-ligand, protein-DNA, protein-RNA, or protein-protein complex. MMPBSA binding affinities of TUM and identified potent antibacterials with LLM were estimated from the trajectories of MD simulation (Kumari et al. 2021; Rathi et al. 2022). The MMPBSA method

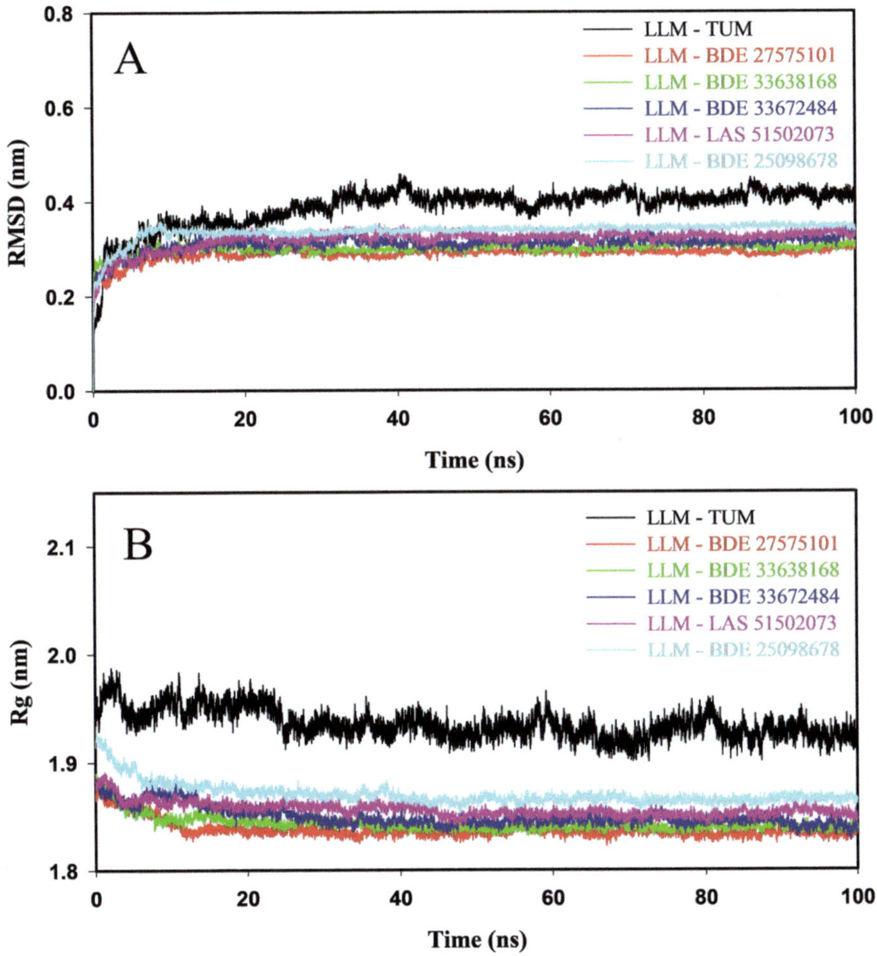

FIGURE 1.8 RMSD (A) and Rg (B) results of LLM-TUM and LLM-inhibitor(s) complexes for the time period of 100 ns.

was also considered to evaluate the binding affinities of RNA along with NTD and its variants (Dhankhar et al. 2020c). MMGBSA was employed to assess the binding affinity of WTA along with wild type and variants FmtA (Dalal et al. 2022b). The MMGBSA approach was also utilized to evaluate the stability of rP2SA-DNA and rP2SA mutants-DNA complex (Savita et al. 2021). In MMPBSA or MMGBSA, per residue decomposition analysis is an important method to examine the importance of critical amino acid residues of a receptor for the stabilization of a ligand, DNA, RNA, or protein with another protein. Gupta et al. performed the amino acid residues decomposition analysis from 2000 frames of MD simulation and confirmed that Pro49, Thr52, Cys55, Lys121, Arg132, and Asp158 of Prx interact with identified compounds to form a stable protein-ligand complex (Gupta et al. 2021). Dhankhar et al. reported the critical and vital amino acid residues to stabilize the NTD-DNA complex (Dhankhar et al. 2020c). Dalal et al. showed that Ser127, Lys130, Tyr211, Asp213, Asn343, and Gly344 are essential amino acid residues for the binding of WTA with FmtA (Dalal et al. 2022b).

1.4 INFLAMMATORY DISEASES

1.4.1 Rheumatoid Arthritis

Rheumatoid arthritis (RA) is an inflammatory disease directly connected to joint and bone destruction. The signs of RA are inflammation like pain, swelling, heat, redness, and loss of function. It can be diagnosed by rheumatoid factor (RF), C-reactive protein (CRP), anti–mannose-binding lectin (MBL), and complete blood count. Various antibodies such as antibodies against heat shock proteins, MBL, heterogenous nuclear RNPs, and elongation factor human cartilage gp39 were reported as biomarkers for RA (Biswas et al. 2013). Proteomic biomarkers, oxidative stress measurements, and nanoparticle mediated approaches can be used to detect and cure RA (Dalal et al. 2017; Dalal and Biswas 2019; Dalal and Biswas 2020; Ramani et al. 2020; Dalal and Biswas 2022; Dalal et al. 2022a, 2022c; Dalal and Biswas 2022). RA treatments include the reduction of joint inflammation and pain that can further lead to inhibition of the destruction of bone. RA treatment involves drug therapy and surgery. Drugs considered for RA treatment are classified into the following categories: a) non-steroidal anti-inflammatory drugs (NSAIDs), b) slow-acting anti-rheumatism drugs, c) glucocorticoids, d) biological agents for therapies, and e) plant drugs. Drugs have been developed like Janus kinase (JAK) inhibitors, Bruton tyrosine kinase (BTK) inhibitors, sphingosine kinase 1 (SphK 1) inhibitors, NSAIDs, spleen tyrosine kinase (SYK) inhibitors, and other types of drugs.

JAK is a cytoplasmic protein tyrosine kinase (JAK 1, JAK 2, and TYK 2) associated with the signaling pathway of cell divisions (De Jonge and Verweij 2006; Bhagwat 2009; Robak and Robak 2012; Hernández-Flórez and Valor 2016). JAK 1 inhibitors can be considered for the treatment of RA, as it is found to be related to interleukin-6 (IL-6) and interferon-γ (IFN-γ) (Giordano and Petrelli 2008). Tofacitinib, a JAK inhibitor, inhibits the activity of JAK 1 and JAK 3, which further block multiple types of inflammation of cytokines (West 2009; Kontzias et al. 2012; Kaur et al. 2017). Chough et *al.* designed, screened, and checked the inhibitory activity of a series of pyrrolidone compounds for JAK. Compound 1 showed the IC_{50} values for 11, 2.4×10^2, and 2.8×10^3 nM against JAK 1, JAK 2, and JAK 3, respectively (Chough et al. 2018). Hamaguchi et al. designed and synthesized pyridine-5-carobxylic amide derivatives and reported that compound 2 had IC_{50} values of 0.49, 1.7, and 0.43 nM against JAK 1, JAK 2, and JAK 3, respectively (Bottini and Firestein 2013; Nugroho and Morita 2014). Compound 3, the designed compound, showed an IC_{50} value of 57 ± 1.21 nM against JAK 3 (He et al. 2017). SYK and JAK 3 inhibitors were designed and synthesized based on the hydroxylindoles (Kaur et al. 2013). Among the designed compounds, compound 4 exhibited a good inhibitory effect on JAK 3 and SYK. BTK is a Tec kinase family, non-receptor cytoplasmic tyrosine kinase that plays a vital role in signal transduction, differentiation, and B-cell proliferation (Harrison 2012; Liu et al. 2013; Young et al. 2015; Young et al. 2016). The series of imidazole quinoxaline compounds showed IC_{50} values in the nanomolar (nM) range (Dixon et al. 2006; Kim et al. 2011). Compound 5 had an IC_{50} value of 1.93 nM against BTK. He et al. developed a series of compounds having 7H-pyrrole pyrimidine-4-amine as a basic skeleton (Bottini and Firestein 2013; Nugroho and Morita 2014; He et al. 2018). Compound 6 revealed inhibition of phosphorylation of BTK Y233 and PLC-γ 2Y1217 with an IC_{50} value of 21.70 ± 0.82 nM against BTK. The structures of JAKs and BTK inhibitors are shown in Figure 1.9.

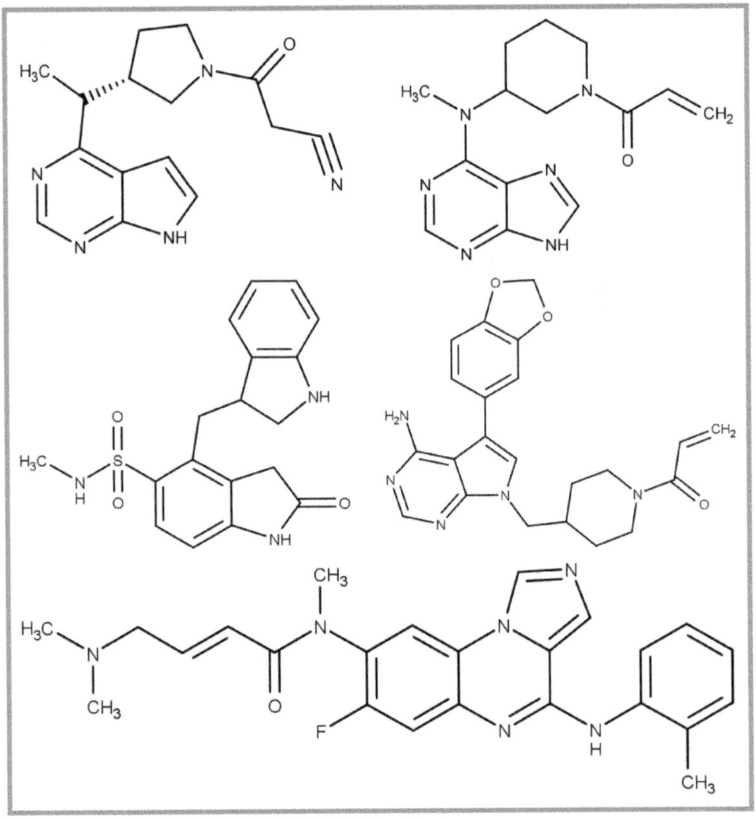

FIGURE 1.9 The structures of JAK and BTK inhibitors.

NSAIDs and carbonate alkylase inhibitors (CAIs) are reported as potential candidates to cure the inflammations and pains of RA (Liu et al. 2012; Witalison et al. 2015; Tanc et al. 2015; Trabocchi et al. 2015; Margheri et al. 2016). NSAID and CAI compounds were developed and tested for anti-rheumatoid activity (Bua et al. 2017). The results showed that synthesized compounds exhibited inhibitory effects for hCA-IV, HCA-XII, and HCA-IX, along with IC_{50} values in the nM range. Akgul et al. synthesized NSAID and CAI compounds and screened for anti-rheumatoid arthritis activity (Akgul et al. 2018). Several NSAID-CAI compounds were reported as potent candidates for the treatment of pain symptoms and RA (Figure 1.10).

Sphingosine kinase 1 and 2 (SphK 1/2) produce sphingosine-1-phosphate (S1P) reportedly associated with bone diseases, RA, and osteoarthritis (OA) (Zhao et al. 2008; Yoshimitsu et al. 2011; Xiao et al. 2018). It has been reported that S1P secretion

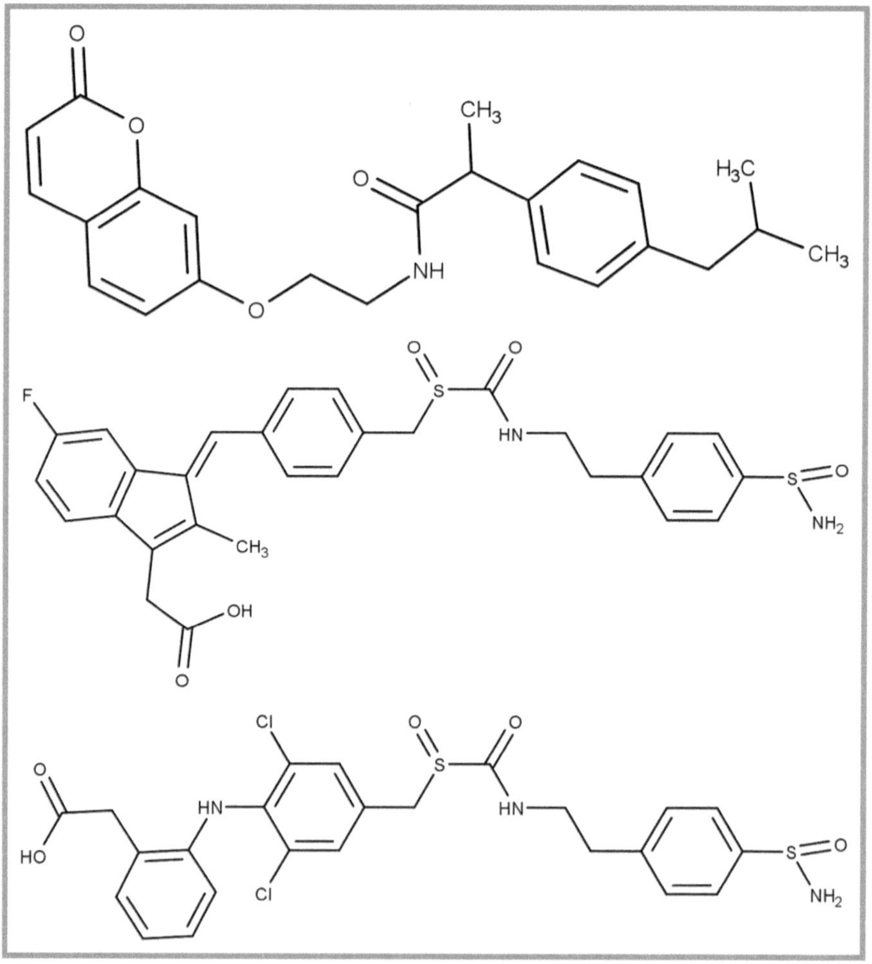

FIGURE 1.10 2D structure of NSAID-CAI compounds.

and SphK 1 expression are enhanced in the synovium of RA patients (Yu et al. 2004; Yoo et al. 2012; Lin et al. 2014a; Pan et al. 2017; Yang et al. 2020). Chiao et al. showed that the hydrochloride of compound 10 exhibits anti-inflammatory activity along with an IC_{50} value of 8.64 ± 0.54 μM (Padilla et al. 2013). SYK is a protein tyrosine kinase, an effective drug target to identify the drug candidates for autoimmune diseases (Singh et al. 2012; Abdel-Magid 2013; He et al. 2017). It has been reported that SYK/platelet-derived growth factor receptor (PDGFR)-α/C-kit inhibitors have anti-inflammatory activity (Wang et al. 2010). Dihydrofuran diamine derivatives were synthesized and screened against multi-target (SYK/PDGFR-α/C-kit) for anti-rheumatoid arthritis (Aggarwal et al. 2012). Compound 11 revealed good inhibitory activity, with IC_{50} values of 2.03 and 3.21 μM against murine bone marrow–derived mast cells and fibroblast-like synovial cells, respectively.

Pyrazole and fused pyrazole membered ring structures were reported as important scaffold characteristics of various different types of NSAIDs (Aggarwal et al. 2015). Pyrazole-pyrimidine was found to be an important skeletal component exhibiting anti-inflammatory activity (Dixon et al. 2006; Kosugi et al. 2012). Novel compounds on the basis of pyrazole-pyrimidine skeletal were synthesized and tested for anti-inflammatory activities (Dixon et al. 2006; Shaaban et al. 2008). Compound 20–25 phosphate compounds showed high anti-inflammatory activity along with ED_{50} values in the range of 0.7 to 10.1 mg/ear (Romero-Estudillo et al. 2019). These compounds had the potency to decrease orbital sinus mononuclear cells and neutrophils in the range of 18.9 to 34.1 percent and 46.7 to 63.0 percent, respectively. Compounds 26 and 27, analogs of double-ring conjugated enones, were designed and synthesized (Zhou et al. 2021a, 2021b). Both of these compounds showed excellent inhibitory activities for the growth of rat synovial cells along with IC_{50} in the range of 2.68 ± 0.16 to 2.71 ± 0.18 μM. Swaminthan et al. performed the pharmacophore screening and reported two compounds (luteolin 7O-glucornide and apigenin 7O-glucornide) against human dihydroorotate dehydrogenase (hDHODH) (Swaminathan and Saleena 2017).

1.5 INFECTIOUS DISEASES

Infectious diseases due to bacteria (*Staphylococcus aureus*, *Acinetobacter baumannii*, *Klebsiella pneumoniae*, *Pseudomonas aeruginosa*, and *Enterococcus faecium*, etc.) or viruses (severe acute respiratory syndrome coronavirus 2, chikungunya, dengue, rotavirus, etc.) are alarming due to their high morbidity and mortality around the globe. *S. aureus* is a pathogenic organism causing infections like skin infections (cellulitis and impetigo), endocarditis (endothelial lining of the heart and valves), and pneumonia (lungs infections) and life-threatening diseases in humans (Lowy 2003) (Rosenbach 1884; Weidenmaier et al. 2005; Stryjewski and Corey 2014; Peacock and Paterson 2015; Tong et al. 2015). The details of various antibiotic resistance in *S. aureus* are mentioned in Table 1.1.

FmtA is one of methicillin resistance factors, which consist of two conserved motifs (SXXK and YXS/N) of penicillin-binding proteins (PBPs) (Komatsuzawa et al. 1999). FmtA is reported to be directly related to cell wall stimulation, and its inactivation makes *S. aureus* susceptible to penicillin and methicillin (Komatsuzawa

TABLE 1.1
Summary of Antibiotic Resistance for *S. aureus*

Gene	Function	Reference
blaR1-balI	It is related to penicillin resistance.	(Ryffel et al. 1992; Abdulgader et al. 2015)
mecR1-mecI	Induction of mecA can cause methicillin resistance.	(Ryffel et al. 1992; Abdulgader et al. 2015)
fmtA	Inactivation of fmtA leads to reduction of methicillin and penicillin resistance.	(Komatsuzawa et al. 1999)
llm	Inactivation of llm can reduce the methicillin resistance.	(Maki et al. 1994)
femC	Inactivation of femC can decrease methicillin resistance.	(Gustafson et al. 1994)
fmtB	Inactivation of fmtB can decrease methicillin resistance.	(De Lencastre et al. 1999; Komatsuzawa et al. 2000)
graR-graS	It regulates the penicillin, methicillin, glycopeptide, and cationic peptide resistance.	(De Lencastre et al. 1999; Meehl et al. 2007; Neoh et al. 2008; Sass and Bierbaum 2009)
lytS-lytR	It regulates the penicillin resistance.	(Bayles 2000)
sigB	It regulates the methicillin and glycopeptide resistance.	(Bischoff and Berger-Bächi 2001; Singh et al. 2003; Bischoff et al. 2004)

et al. 1999; Utaida et al. 2003). FmtA is found to be involved in the removal of D-Ala from WTA (Boles et al. 2010; Rahman et al. 2016). Teichoic acid is directly linked to the attachment to artificial surfaces, biofilm formation, virulence, resistance to cationic antimicrobial peptides, cell division, and metal homeostasis (Neuhaus and Baddiley 2003; Brown et al. 2012). Crystal structure and the mutational study reported that Ser127 and Lys130 may act as a nucleophile and acylation/deacylation, while Tyr211 is necessary to hold the substrate during the catalysis (Dalal et al. 2019). Further, QM/MM studies indicated that Ser127 and Gly344 may play a role as oxyanion hole residues during the catalysis of WTA by FmtA (Dalal et al. 2022b). FmtA was screened against drugs of e-LEA3D: Cheminformatics Tools and database using AutoDock Vina in PyRx0.8 (Singh et al. 2020b; Dalal et al. 2021; Singh et al. 2022b). Molecular docking, MD simulation, MMPBSA/MMGBSA binding free energy, and amino acid residues decomposition analysis showed that drugs (ofloxacin, roflumilast, furazolidone, gemifloxacin, paromomycin, streptomycin, and tobramycin) interact at the active site (Figure 1.11). Activation of GraR causes cationic antimicrobial peptides (CAMP) resistance to *S. aureus* (Fridman et al. 2013). GraR protein was modeled and screened against the ZINC database (Dhankhar et al. 2020a). MD simulation and MMPBSA results suggested that five molecules (ZINC000049170029, ZINC000095509204, ZINC000067688459, ZINC000049169934, and ZINC000095352231) bind efficiently and can be considered as potential lead candidates for GraR.

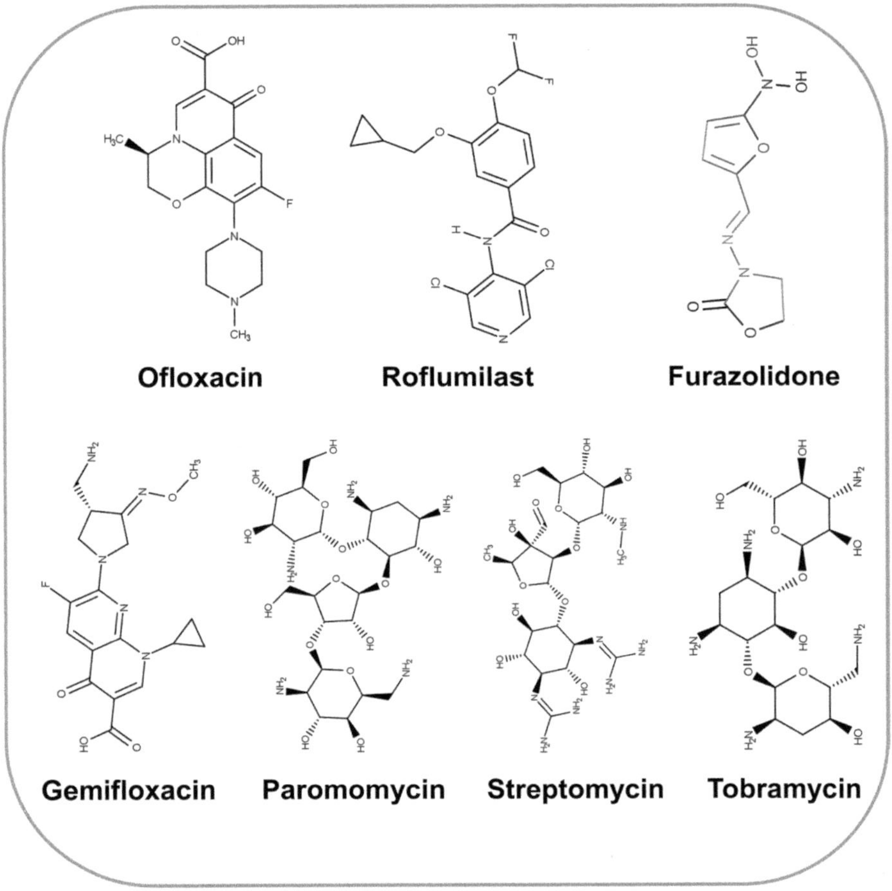

FIGURE 1.11 Seven potent drugs were reported for FmtA of *S. aureus* by structure-based drug designing.

Lipophilic membrane (LLM) protein is associated with the metabolism of peptidoglycan in *S. aureus* (Maki et al. 1994). Pharmacophore modeling and virtual screening were employed, and molecules from the ZINC and asinex database were docked at the active site of the LLM model. Ten molecules were reported as potent molecules which can be used to develop novel antimicrobials for *S. aureus* (Kumari et al. 2021; Rathi et al. 2022). Molecules were screened from the ZINC and asinex database against the YsxC model by using pharmacophore modelling and virtual screening. Molecular docking, dynamics, and MMPBSA results showed that binding of identified molecules with YsxC tend to form a more stable YsxC-ligand(s) complex than the YsxC-GTP complex (Figure 1.12) (Kumari et al. 2023, 2022b). The FemC model was screened against natural product-like compounds (Dalal et al. 2022). Molecular docking, MD simulation, and MMPBSA analysis showed that four compounds resulted in the formation of stable and compact FemC-ligand(s) complexes.

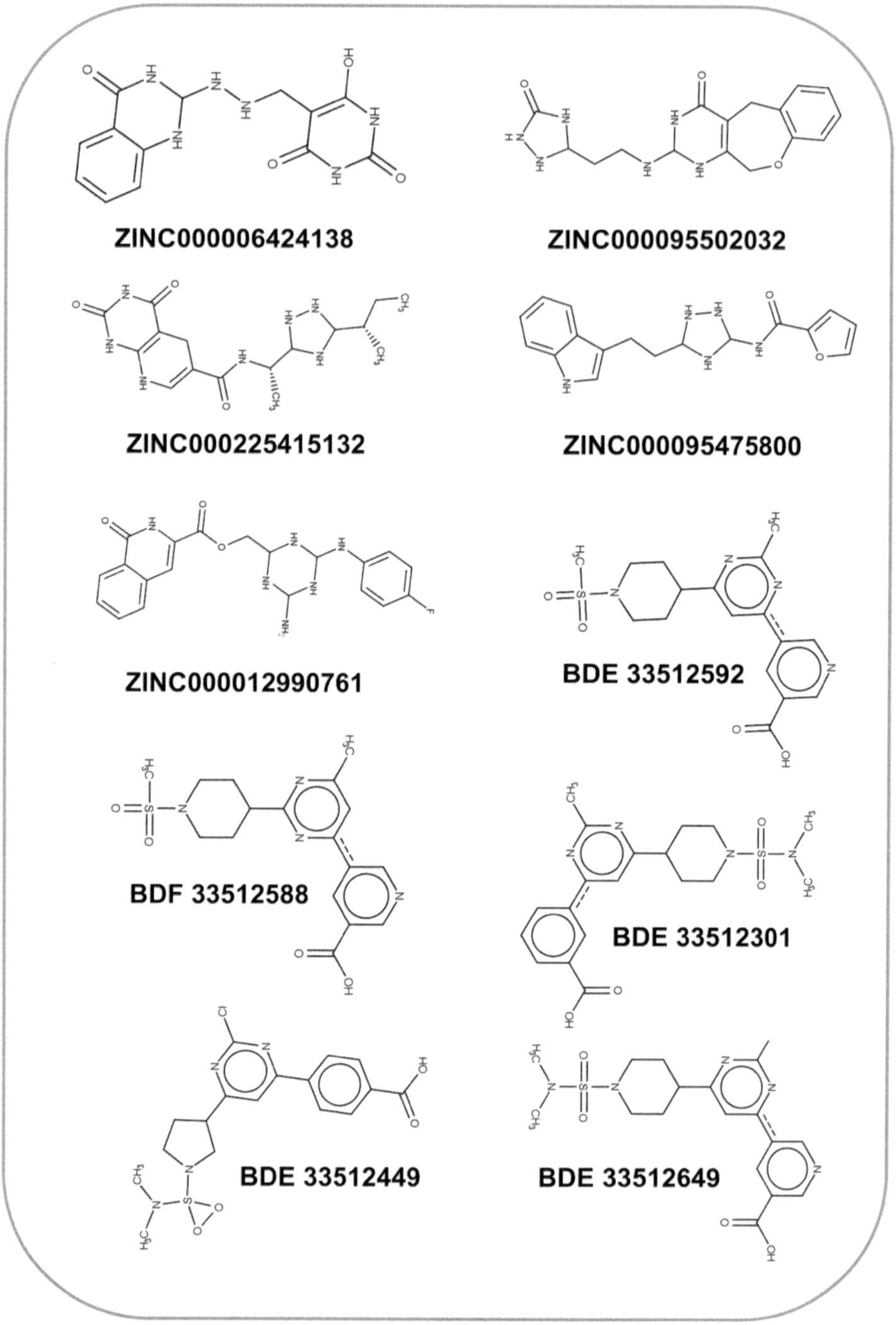

FIGURE 1.12 Potent candidates for YsxC of *S. aureus* identified by pharmacophore modeling and virtual screening.

K. pneumoniae is a gram-negative, rod-shaped organism that can cause various infections like urinary tract infections, meningitis, and pneumonia (Podschun and Ullmann 1998; Navon-Venezia et al. 2017). A hypothetical protein (CP995_08280) model was screened against antibacterial molecules of the asinex database (Singh et al. 2022b). Potent antibacterials were reported for CP995_08280 by using structure-based drug designing.

1.6 FUTURE PROSPECTIVE AND LIMITATIONS

The CADD approach provides tools and software that have accelerated the drug discovery field. It significantly decreases the cost and risk in drug designing and discovery. From a set of biological data, computational methods have been used to predict the molecular and structural properties to derive structure-property relationships. In the current decade, research is underway to develop new tools and software that is less computationally expensive to perform virtual screening, molecular dynamics, and binding free energy analysis. There is still a requirement for new tools to estimate accurate and reliable results so that computational results are comparable to experimental analysis. The usage of machine learning, deep learning, and neural networks may provide a pathway to predict unknown structures with accuracy. Machine learning and artificial intelligence have the potential to collect a large amount of data to screen, design, and develop appropriate and complementary ligands. The overall aim of future drug discovery is to create a set of active ligands followed by the screening and development of effective and non-toxic drugs within a short span of time.

CADD faces several challenges, such as improvement of computational resources; curtailing the time necessary and improving the efficacy of virtual screening, upgrading algorithms to predict reliable orientation, binding energy, and stability of ligand with its target; and most challenging is collaboration with other fields for lead testing, optimization, and identification. In virtual screening, during the generation of libraries, ignorance of the protonation and ionization states of ligands may eventually cause significant hits to be missed or may add false leads as well. In molecular docking, the consideration of a reliable algorithm is still debatable, as the limitation of scoring functions of tools gives an effective assessment of ligand binding affinities; however, it avoids highest confident docking pose and compromises accuracy. Further, there are still other fundamental issues like whether to consider flexible or semi-flexible or rigid targets, consideration of water molecules at the active site, and ions and charges on ligands also make the molecular docking less reliable and widen the gap and decrease the confidence of *in silico* results in relation to accuracy and complementary to experimental studies.

1.7 CONCLUSION

Drug discovery is a time-consuming, complicated, and costly process. The drug discovery process involves target selection, screening of libraries against a target, assessment of binding stability of ligands with protein, cell assays, and *in vitro* and *in vivo* experiments. The modern drug discovery approach uses *in silico* techniques to screen and identify potent molecules from a library of molecules. The usage of *in silico* methods in drug discovery significantly reduces the time and cost of drug discovery. The first step of CADD is identifying the essential target for the pathogenic organism. Then, a 3D structure of the receptor is required, either an experimental structure or prediction of a structure by computer-based modeling. The correct information of the active site or binding site of a receptor is vital in structure-based drug designing. Virtual screening is a process in which the numbers of molecules from libraries are docked at the binding site of a receptor to predict the unrestrained conformation along with binding energy. Molecular docking and dynamics simulation are globally used techniques to evaluate the stability of the protein-ligand, protein-protein, protein-RNA, and protein-DNA complex. Pharmacophore modeling is the generation and screening of similar chemical imprints of ligands with a receptor. The determination of estimation of binding free energies by MMPBSA or MMGBSA is a widely used tool to assess the stability of ligands, proteins, or RNA with a receptor. Amino residue decomposition analysis is an important tool in MMGBSA and MMPBSA to examine a receptor's important amino acid residues in receptor-ligand, receptor-protein, receptor-RNA, and receptor-DNA complexes. New chemical drugs have been synthesized, developed, and identified, such as JAK inhibitors, BTK inhibitors, SphK 1 inhibitors, NSAIDs, SYK inhibitors, and other types of drugs. Several potent candidates such as ofloxacin, roflumilast, furazolidone, gemifloxacin, paromomycin, streptomycin, tobramycin, ZINC000049170029, ZINC000095509204, ZINC000067688459, ZINC000049169934, and ZINC000095352231 have been reported against FmtA, GraR, LLM, YsxC, and FemC of *S. aureus*.

REFERENCES

Abdel-Magid, A. F. (2013). "Spleen tyrosine kinase inhibitors (SYK) as potential treatment for autoimmune and inflammatory disorders: patent highlight." *ACS Publications* 4: 18–19.

Abdulgader, S. M., A. O. Shittu, M. P. Nicol and M. Kaba (2015). "Molecular epidemiology of Methicillin-resistant Staphylococcus aureus in Africa: A systematic review." *Frontiers in Microbiology* 6: 348.

Aggarwal, R., V. Kumar, A. Bansal, D. Sanz and R. M. Claramunt (2012). "Multi-component solvent-free versus stepwise solvent mediated reactions: Regiospecific formation of 6-trifluoromethyl and 4-trifluoromethyl-1H-pyrazolo [3, 4-b] pyridines." *Journal of Fluorine Chemistry* 140: 31–37.

Aggarwal, R., V. Kumar, G. Singh, D. Sanz, R. M. Claramunt, I. Alkorta, G. Sánchez-Sanz and J. Elguero (2015). "An NMR and computational study of azolo [a] pyrimidines with special emphasis on pyrazolo [1, 5-a] pyrimidines." *Journal of Heterocyclic Chemistry* 52(2): 336–345.

Akgul, O., L. Di Cesare Mannelli, D. Vullo, A. Angeli, C. Ghelardini, G. Bartolucci, A. S. Alfawaz Altamimi, A. Scozzafava, C. T. Supuran and F. Carta (2018). "Discovery of novel nonsteroidal anti-inflammatory drugs and carbonic anhydrase inhibitors hybrids (NSAIDs—CAIs) for the management of rheumatoid arthritis." *Journal of Medicinal Chemistry* 61(11): 4961–4977.

Al Qaraghuli, M. M., A. R. Alzahrani, K. Niwasabutra, M. A. Obeid and V. A. Ferro (2017). "Where traditional drug discovery meets modern technology in the quest for new drugs." *Annals of Pharmacology and Pharmaceutics* 2(11): 1–5.

Arnold, K., L. Bordoli, J. Kopp and T. Schwede (2006). "The SWISS-MODEL workspace: A web-based environment for protein structure homology modelling." *Bioinformatics* 22(2): 195–201.

Balibar, C. J., X. Shen and J. Tao (2009). "The mevalonate pathway of Staphylococcus aureus." *Journal of Bacteriology* 191(3): 851–861.

Bayles, K. W. (2000). "The bactericidal action of penicillin: New clues to an unsolved mystery." *Trends in Microbiology* 8(6): 274–278.

Bhagwat, S. S. (2009). "Kinase inhibitors for the treatment of inflammatory and autoimmune disorders." *Purinergic Signalling* 5(1): 107–115.

Bischoff, M. and B. Berger-Bächi (2001). "Teicoplanin stress-selected mutations increasing ςB activity in Staphylococcus aureus." *Antimicrobial Agents and Chemotherapy* 45(6): 1714–1720.

Bischoff, M., P. Dunman, J. Kormanec, D. Macapagal, E. Murphy, W. Mounts, B. Berger-Bächi and S. Projan (2004). "Microarray-based analysis of the Staphylococcus aureus σB regulon." *Journal of bacteriology* 186(13): 4085–4099.

Bisht, N., V. Dalal and L. Tewari (2021). "Molecular modeling and dynamics simulation of alcohol dehydrogenase enzyme from high efficacy cellulosic ethanol-producing yeast mutant strain Pichia kudriavzevii BGY1-γm." *Journal of Biomolecular Structure and Dynamics*: 1–15.

Biswas, S., S. Sharma, A. Saroha, D. Bhakuni, R. Malhotra, M. Zahur, M. Oellerich, H. R. Das and A. R. Asif (2013). "Identification of novel autoantigen in the synovial fluid of rheumatoid arthritis patients using an immunoproteomics approach." *PLoS ONE* 8(2): e56246.

Boles, B. R., M. Thoendel, A. J. Roth and A. R. Horswill (2010). "Identification of genes involved in polysaccharide-independent Staphylococcus aureus biofilm formation." *PLoS ONE* 5(4): e10146.

Bottini, N. and G. S. Firestein (2013). "Duality of fibroblast-like synoviocytes in RA: Passive responders and imprinted aggressors." *Nature Reviews Rheumatology* 9(1): 24–33.

Brown, S., G. Xia, L. G. Luhachack, J. Campbell, T. C. Meredith, C. Chen, V. Winstel, C. Gekeler, J. E. Irazoqui and A. Peschel (2012). "Methicillin resistance in Staphylococcus aureus requires glycosylated wall teichoic acids." *Proceedings of the National Academy of Sciences* 109(46): 18909–18914.

Bua, S., L. Di Cesare Mannelli, D. Vullo, C. Ghelardini, G. Bartolucci, A. Scozzafava, C. T. Supuran and F. Carta (2017). "Design and synthesis of novel nonsteroidal anti-inflammatory drugs and carbonic anhydrase inhibitors hybrids (NSAIDs—CAIs) for the treatment of rheumatoid arthritis." *Journal of Medicinal Chemistry* 60(3): 1159–1170.

Chenavas, S., T. Crépin, B. Delmas, R. W. Ruigrok and A. Slama-Schwok (2013). "Influenza virus nucleoprotein: Structure, RNA binding, oligomerization and antiviral drug target." *Future Microbiology* 8(12): 1537–1545.

Chough, C., M. Joung, S. Lee, J. Lee, J. H. Kim and B. M. Kim (2018). "Development of selective inhibitors for the treatment of rheumatoid arthritis:(R)-3-(3-(Methyl (7H-pyrrolo [2, 3-d] pyrimidin-4-yl) amino) pyrrolidin-1-yl)-3-oxopropanenitrile as a JAK1-selective inhibitor." *Bioorganic & Medicinal Chemistry* 26(8): 1495–1510.

Colovos, C. and T. O. Yeates (1993). "Verification of protein structures: Patterns of non-bonded atomic interactions." *Protein Science* 2(9): 1511–1519.

Cooper, E. L., J. García-Lara and S. J. Foster (2009). "YsxC, an essential protein in Staphylococcus aureus crucial for ribosome assembly/stability." *BMC Microbiology* 9(1): 1–12.

Dalal, V. and S. Biswas (2019). "Nanoparticle-mediated oxidative stress monitoring and role of nanoparticle for treatment of inflammatory diseases." In *Nanotechnology in Modern Animal Biotechnology*. Elsevier: 97–112.

Dalal, V. and S. Biswas (2020). "Nanoscience: Convergence with biomedical and biological applications." In *Functional Bionanomaterials*. Springer: 1–25.

Dalal, V. and S. Biswas (2022). "Erythrocytes model for oxidative stress analysis." In *Nanobioanalytical Approaches to Medical Diagnostics*. Elsevier: 363–390.

Dalal, V., P. Dhankhar and S. Biswas (2022a). "Proteomics as a potential tool for biomarker discovery." In *High Altitude Sickness—Solutions from Genomics, Proteomics and Antioxidant Interventions*. Springer: 119–141.

Dalal, V., P. Dhankhar, V. Singh, G. Rakhaminov, D. Golemi-Kotra and P. Kumar (2021). "Structure-based identification of potential drugs against FmtA of Staphylococcus aureus: Virtual screening, molecular dynamics, MM-GBSA, and QM/MM." *The Protein Journal* 40(2): 148–165.

Dalal, V., D. Golemi-Kotra and P. Kumar (2022b). "Quantum mechanics/molecular mechanics studies on the catalytic mechanism of a novel esterase (FmtA) of Staphylococcus aureus." *Journal of Chemical Information and Modeling* 62(10): 2409–2420.

Dalal, V., P. Kumar, G. Rakhaminov, A. Qamar, X. Fan, H. Hunter, S. Tomar, D. Golemi-Kotra and P. Kumar (2019). "Repurposing an ancient protein core structure: Structural studies on FmtA, a novel esterase of Staphylococcus aureus." *Journal of Molecular Biology* 431(17): 3107–3123.

Dalal, V. and R. Kumari (2022). "Screening and identification of natural product-like compounds as potential antibacterial agents targeting FemC of Staphylococcus aureus: An in-silico approach." *ChemistrySelect* 7(42): e202201728.

Dalal, V., N. K. Sharma and S. Biswas (2017). "Oxidative stress: Diagnostic methods and application in medical science." In *Oxidative Stress: Diagnostic Methods and Applications in Medical Science*. Springer: 23–45.

Dalal, V., V. Singh and S. Biswas (2022c). "High altitude-induced oxidative stress, rheumatoid arthritis, and proteomic alteration." In *High Altitude Sickness—Solutions from Genomics, Proteomics and Antioxidant Interventions*. Springer: 51–69.

Dallakyan, S. and A. J. Olson (2015). "Small-molecule library screening by docking with PyRx." In *Chemical Biology*. Springer: 243–250.

De Jonge, M. and J. Verweij (2006). "Multiple targeted tyrosine kinase inhibition in the clinic: All for one or one for all?" *European Journal of Cancer* 42(10): 1351–1356.

De Lencastre, H., S. Wu, M. Pinho, A. Ludovice, S. Filipe, S. Gardete, R. Sobral, S. Gill, M. Chung and A. Tomasz (1999). "Antibiotic resistance as a stress response: Complete sequencing of a large number of chromosomal loci in Staphylococcus aureus strain COL that impact on the expression of resistance to methicillin." *Microbial Drug Resistance* 5(3): 163–175.

Dhankhar, P., V. Dalal, D. G. Kotra and P. Kumar (2020a). "In-silico approach to identify novel potent inhibitors against GraR of S. aureus." *Frontiers in Bioscience (Landmark Edition)* 25: 1337–1360.

Dhankhar, P., V. Dalal and V. Kumar (2021a). "Screening of severe acute respiratory syndrome coronavirus 2 RNA-dependent RNA polymerase inhibitors using computational approach." *Journal of Computational Biology* 28(12): 1228–1247.

Dhankhar, P., V. Dalal, J. K. Mahto, B. R. Gurjar, S. Tomar, A. K. Sharma and P. Kumar (2020b). "Characterization of dye-decolorizing peroxidase from Bacillus subtilis." *Archives of Biochemistry and Biophysics* 693: 108590.

Dhankhar, P., V. Dalal, V. Singh, A. K. Sharma and P. Kumar (2021b). "Structure of dye-decolorizing peroxidase from Bacillus subtilis in complex with veratryl alcohol." *International Journal of Biological Macromolecules* 193: 601–608.

Dhankhar, P., V. Dalal, V. Singh, S. Tomar and P. Kumar (2020c). "Computational guided identification of novel potent inhibitors of N-terminal domain of nucleocapsid protein of severe acute respiratory syndrome coronavirus 2." *Journal of Biomolecular Structure and Dynamics*: 1–16.

Dixon, S. L., A. M. Smondyrev, E. H. Knoll, S. N. Rao, D. E. Shaw and R. A. Friesner (2006). "PHASE: A new engine for pharmacophore perception, 3D QSAR model development, and 3D database screening: 1. Methodology and preliminary results." *Journal of Computer-Aided Molecular Design* 20(10): 647–671.

Eisenberg, D., R. Lüthy and J. U. Bowie (1997). "[20] VERIFY3D: Assessment of protein models with three-dimensional profiles." *Methods in Enzymology*, Elsevier. 277**:** 396–404.

Engel, S., A. P. Skoumbourdis, J. Childress, S. Neumann, J. R. Deschamps, C. J. Thomas, A.-O. Colson, S. Costanzi and M. C. Gershengorn (2008). "A virtual screen for diverse ligands: Discovery of selective G protein-coupled receptor antagonists." *Journal of the American Chemical Society* 130(15): 5115–5123.

Fridman, M., G. D. Williams, U. Muzamal, H. Hunter, K. M. Siu and D. Golemi-Kotra (2013). "Two unique phosphorylation-driven signaling pathways crosstalk in Staphylococcus aureus to modulate the cell-wall charge: Stk1/Stp1 meets GraSR." *Biochemistry* 52(45): 7975–7986.

Giordano, S. and A. Petrelli (2008). "From single-to multi-target drugs in cancer therapy: When aspecificity becomes an advantage." *Current Medicinal Chemistry* 15(5): 422–432.

Gupta, D. N., V. Dalal, B. K. Savita, M. S. Alam, A. Singh, M. Gubyad, D. K. Ghosh, P. Kumar and A. K. Sharma (2022). "Biochemical characterization and structure-based in silico screening of potent inhibitor molecules against the 1 cys peroxiredoxin of bacterioferritin comigratory protein family from Candidatus Liberibacter asiaticus." *Journal of Biomolecular Structure and Dynamics*: 1–13.

Gupta, D. N., V. Dalal, B. K. Savita, P. Dhankhar, D. K. Ghosh, P. Kumar and A. K. Sharma (2021). "In-silico screening and identification of potential inhibitors against 2Cys peroxiredoxin of Candidatus Liberibacter asiaticus." *Journal of Biomolecular Structure and Dynamics*: 1–15.

Gustafson, J., A. Strässle, H. Hächler, F. H. Kayser and B. Berger-Bächi (1994). "The femC locus of Staphylococcus aureus required for methicillin resistance includes the glutamine synthetase operon." *Journal of Bacteriology* 176(5): 1460–1467.

Harcourt, B. H., D. Jukneliene, A. Kanjanahaluethai, J. Bechill, K. M. Severson, C. M. Smith, P. A. Rota and S. C. Baker (2004). "Identification of severe acute respiratory syndrome coronavirus replicase products and characterization of papain-like protease activity." *Journal of Virology* 78(24): 13600–13612.

Harrison, C. (2012). "BTK inhibitor shows positive results in B cell malignancies." *Nature Reviews Drug Discovery* 11(2): 96.

He, L., H. Pei, T. Lan, M. Tang, C. Zhang and L. Chen (2017). "Design and synthesis of a highly selective JAK3 inhibitor for the treatment of rheumatoid arthritis." *Archiv der Pharmazie* 350(11): 1700194.

He, L., H. Pei, C. Zhang, M. Shao, D. Li, M. Tang, T. Wang, X. Chen, M. Xiang and L. Chen (2018). "Design, synthesis and biological evaluation of 7H-pyrrolo [2, 3-d] pyrimidin-4-amine derivatives as selective Btk inhibitors with improved pharmacokinetic properties for the treatment of rheumatoid arthritis." *European Journal of Medicinal Chemistry* 145: 96–112.

Hernández-Flórez, D. and L. Valor (2016). "Protein-kinase inhibitors: A new treatment pathway for autoimmune and inflammatory diseases?" *Reumatología Clínica (English Edition)* 12(2): 91–99.

Jiménez, J., S. Doerr, G. Martínez-Rosell, A. S. Rose and G. De Fabritiis (2017). "DeepSite: protein-binding site predictor using 3D-convolutional neural networks." *Bioinformatics* 33(19): 3036–3042.

Kahraman, A. and J. M. Thornton (2008). "Methods to characterize the structure of enzyme binding sites." *Computational Structural Biology-Methods and Applications* 1: 189–221.

Kalyani, G., D. Sharma, Y. Vaishnav and V. Deshmukh (2013). "A review on drug designing, methods, its applications and prospects." *International Journal of Pharmaceutical Research and Development* 5(5): 015–010.

Kaur, M., M. Singh and O. Silakari (2013). "Inhibitors of switch kinase 'spleen tyrosine kinase' in inflammation and immune-mediated disorders: A review." *European Journal of Medicinal Chemistry* 67: 434–446.

Kaur, M., M. Singh and O. Silakari (2017). "Oxindole-based SYK and JAK3 dual inhibitors for rheumatoid arthritis: Designing, synthesis and biological evaluation." *Future Medicinal Chemistry* 9(11): 1193–1211.

Kelley, L. A., S. Mezulis, C. M. Yates, M. N. Wass and M. J. Sternberg (2015). "The Phyre2 web portal for protein modeling, prediction and analysis." *Nature Protocols* 10(6): 845–858.

Kesari, P., S. Pratap, P. Dhankhar, V. Dalal, M. Mishra, P. K. Singh, H. Chauhan and P. Kumar (2020). "Structural characterization and in-silico analysis of Momordica charantia 7S globulin for stability and ACE inhibition." *Scientific Reports* 10(1): 1–13.

Kim, K.-H., A. Maderna, M. E. Schnute, M. Hegen, S. Mohan, J. Miyashiro, L. Lin, E. Li, S. Keegan and J. Lussier (2011). "Imidazo [1, 5-a] quinoxalines as irreversible BTK inhibitors for the treatment of rheumatoid arthritis." *Bioorganic & Medicinal Chemistry Letters* 21(21): 6258–6263.

Komatsuzawa, H., K. Ohta, H. Labischinski, M. Sugai and H. Suginaka (1999). "Characterization of fmtA, a gene that modulates the expression of methicillin resistance in Staphylococcus aureus." *Antimicrobial Agents and Chemotherapy* 43(9): 2121–2125.

Komatsuzawa, H., K. Ohta, M. Sugai, T. Fujiwara, P. Glanzmann, B. Berger-Bächi and H. Suginaka (2000). "Tn 551-mediated insertional inactivation of the fmtB gene encoding a cell wall-associated protein abolishes methicillin resistance in Staphylococcus aureus." *Journal of Antimicrobial Chemotherapy* 45(4): 421–431.

Kontzias, A., A. Kotlyar, A. Laurence, P. Changelian and J. J. O'Shea (2012). "Jakinibs: A new class of kinase inhibitors in cancer and autoimmune disease." *Current Opinion in Pharmacology* 12(4): 464–470.

Kosugi, T., D. R. Mitchell, A. Fujino, M. Imai, M. Kambe, S. Kobayashi, H. Makino, Y. Matsueda, Y. Oue and K. Komatsu (2012). "Mitogen-activated protein kinase-activated protein kinase 2 (MAPKAP-K2) as an antiinflammatory target: Discovery and in vivo activity of selective pyrazolo [1, 5-a] pyrimidine inhibitors using a focused library and structure-based optimization approach." *Journal of Medicinal Chemistry* 55(15): 6700–6715.

Kumar, K. A., M. Sharma, V. Dalal, V. Singh, S. Tomar and P. Kumar (2021a). "Multifunctional inhibitors of SARS CoV2 by MM/PBSA, essential dynamics, and molecular dynamic investigations." *Journal of Molecular Graphics and Modelling*: 107969.

Kumar, P., V. Dalal, A. Kokane, S. Singh, S. Lonare, H. Kaur, D. K. Ghosh, P. Kumar and A. K. Sharma (2020a). "Mutation studies and structure-based identification of potential inhibitor molecules against periplasmic amino acid binding protein of Candidatus Liberibacter asiaticus (CLasTcyA)." *International Journal of Biological Macromolecules* 147: 1228–1238.

Kumar, P., V. Dalal, N. Sharma, S. Kokane, D. K. Ghosh, P. Kumar and A. K. Sharma (2020b). "Characterization of the heavy metal binding properties of periplasmic metal uptake protein CLas-ZnuA2." *Metallomics* 12(2): 280–289.

Kumar, V., S. Haldar, N. S. Das, S. Ghosh, P. Dhankhar, D. Sircar and P. Roy (2021b). "Pterostilbene-isothiocyanate inhibits breast cancer metastasis by selectively blocking IKK-β/NEMO interaction in cancer cells." *Biochemical Pharmacology* 192: 114717.

Kumari, N., V. Dalal, P. Kumar and S. N. Rath (2020). "Antagonistic interaction between TTA-A2 and paclitaxel for anti-cancer effects by complex formation with T-type calcium channel." *Journal of Biomolecular Structure and Dynamics*: 1–12.

Kumari, R. and V. Dalal (2021). "Identification of potential inhibitors for LLM of Staphylococcus aureus: Structure-based pharmacophore modeling, molecular dynamics, and binding free energy studies." *Journal of Biomolecular Structure and Dynamics*: 1–15.

Kumari, R., P. Dhankhar and V. Dalal (2021). "Structure-based mimicking of hydroxylated biphenyl congeners (OHPCBs) for human transthyretin, an important enzyme of thyroid hormone system." *Journal of Molecular Graphics and Modelling*: 107870.

Kumari, R., V. Kumar, P. Dhankhar and V. Dalal (2022a). "Promising antivirals for PLpro of SARS-CoV-2 using virtual screening, molecular docking, dynamics, and MMPBSA." *Journal of Biomolecular Structure and Dynamics*: 1–17.

Kumari, R., R. Rathi, S. R. Pathak and V. Dalal (2022b). "Structural-based virtual screening and identification of novel potent antimicrobial compounds against YsxC of Staphylococcus aureus." *Journal of Molecular Structure* 1255: 132476.

Kumari, R., R. Rathi, S. R. Pathak and V. Dalal (2023). "Computational investigation of potent inhibitors against YsxC: Structure-based pharmacophore modeling, molecular docking, molecular dynamics, and binding free energy." *Journal of Biomolecular Structure and Dynamics* 41(3): 930–941.

Laskowski, R. A., M. W. MacArthur, D. S. Moss and J. M. Thornton (1993). "PROCHECK: A program to check the stereochemical quality of protein structures." *Journal of Applied Crystallography* 26(2): 283–291.

Le Guilloux, V., P. Schmidtke and P. Tuffery (2009). "Fpocket: An open source platform for ligand pocket detection." *BMC Bioinformatics* 10(1): 1–11.

Lin, B., Y. Zhao, P. Han, W. Yue, X.-Q. Ma, K. Rahman, C.-J. Zheng, L.-P. Qin and T. Han (2014a). "Anti-arthritic activity of Xanthium strumarium L. extract on complete Freund's adjuvant induced arthritis in rats." *Journal of Ethnopharmacology* 155(1): 248–255.

Lin, S.-Y., C.-L. Liu, Y.-M. Chang, J. Zhao, S. Perlman and M.-H. Hou (2014b). "Structural basis for the identification of the N-terminal domain of coronavirus nucleocapsid protein as an antiviral target." *Journal of Medicinal Chemistry* 57(6): 2247–2257.

Liu, C., Y. Wei, J. Wang, L. Pi, J. Huang and P. Wang (2012). "Carbonic anhydrases III and IV autoantibodies in rheumatoid arthritis, systemic lupus erythematosus, diabetes, hypertensive renal disease, and heart failure." *Clinical and Developmental Immunology* 2012.

Liu, Y., G. Zhou, B. Zhang and Y. Liu (2013). "Bruton's tyrosine kinase: Structure and functions, expression and mutations." *Gene Technology* 2: 106.

Lo, Y.-S., S.-Y. Lin, S.-M. Wang, C.-T. Wang, Y.-L. Chiu, T.-H. Huang and M.-H. Hou (2013). "Oligomerization of the carboxyl terminal domain of the human coronavirus 229E nucleocapsid protein." *FEBS Letters* 587(2): 120–127.

Lowy, F. D. (2003). "Antimicrobial resistance: The example of Staphylococcus aureus." *The Journal of Clinical Investigation* 111(9): 1265–1273.

Macalino, S. J. Y., V. Gosu, S. Hong and S. Choi (2015). "Role of computer-aided drug design in modern drug discovery." *Archives of Pharmacal Research* 38(9): 1686–1701.

Maki, H., T. Yamaguchi and K. Murakami (1994). "Cloning and characterization of a gene affecting the methicillin resistance level and the autolysis rate in Staphylococcus aureus." *Journal of Bacteriology* 176(16): 4993–5000.

Malik, A., V. Dalal, S. Ankri and S. Tomar (2019). "Structural insights into Entamoeba histolytica arginase and structure-based identification of novel non-amino acid based inhibitors as potential antiamoebic molecules." *The FEBS Journal* 286(20): 4135–4155.

Margheri, F., M. Ceruso, F. Carta, A. Laurenzana, L. Maggi, S. Lazzeri, G. Simonini, F. Annunziato, M. Del Rosso and C. T. Supuran (2016). "Overexpression of the transmembrane carbonic anhydrase isoforms IX and XII in the inflamed synovium." *Journal of Enzyme Inhibition and Medicinal Chemistry* 31(sup4): 60–63.

McGreig, J. E., H. Uri, M. Antczak, M. J. Sternberg, M. Michaelis and M. N. Wass (2022). "3DLigandSite: Structure-based prediction of protein-ligand binding sites." *Nucleic Acids Research* 50(W1): W13–W20.

Meehl, M., S. Herbert, F. Götz and A. Cheung (2007). "Interaction of the GraRS two-component system with the VraFG ABC transporter to support vancomycin-intermediate resistance in Staphylococcus aureus." *Antimicrobial Agents and Chemotherapy* 51(8): 2679–2689.

Monod, A., C. Swale, B. Tarus, A. Tissot, B. Delmas, R. W. Ruigrok, T. Crépin and A. Slama-Schwok (2015). "Learning from structure-based drug design and new antivirals targeting the ribonucleoprotein complex for the treatment of influenza." *Expert Opinion on Drug Discovery* 10(4): 345–371.

Navon-Venezia, S., K. Kondratyeva and A. Carattoli (2017). "Klebsiella pneumoniae: A major worldwide source and shuttle for antibiotic resistance." *FEMS Microbiology Reviews* 41(3): 252–275.

Neoh, H.-M., L. Cui, H. Yuzawa, F. Takeuchi, M. Matsuo and K. Hiramatsu (2008). "Mutated response regulator graR is responsible for phenotypic conversion of Staphylococcus aureus from heterogeneous vancomycin-intermediate resistance to vancomycin-intermediate resistance." *Antimicrobial Agents and Chemotherapy* 52(1): 45–53.

Neuhaus, F. C. and J. Baddiley (2003). "A continuum of anionic charge: Structures and functions of D-alanyl-teichoic acids in gram-positive bacteria." *Microbiology and Molecular Biology Reviews* 67(4): 686–723.

Nugroho, A. E. and H. Morita (2014). "Circular dichroism calculation for natural products." *Journal of Natural Medicines* 68(1): 1–10.

Padilla, F., N. Bhagirath, S. Chen, E. Chiao, D. M. Goldstein, J. C. Hermann, J. Hsu, J. J. Kennedy-Smith, A. Kuglstatter and C. Liao (2013). "Pyrrolopyrazines as selective spleen tyrosine kinase inhibitors." *Journal of Medicinal Chemistry* 56(4): 1677–1692.

Pan, T., T.-F. Cheng, Y.-R. Jia, P. Li and F. Li (2017). "Anti-rheumatoid arthritis effects of traditional Chinese herb couple in adjuvant-induced arthritis in rats." *Journal of Ethnopharmacology* 205: 1–7.

Pandit, S., V. Dalal and G. Mishra (2018). "Identification of novel phosphatidic acid binding domain on sphingosine kinase 1 of Arabidopsis thaliana." *Plant Physiology and Biochemistry* 128: 178–184.

Peacock, S. J. and G. K. Paterson (2015). "Mechanisms of methicillin resistance in Staphylococcus aureus." *Annual Review of Biochemistry* 84: 577–601.

Pettersen, E. F., T. D. Goddard, C. C. Huang, G. S. Couch, D. M. Greenblatt, E. C. Meng and T. E. Ferrin (2004). "UCSF Chimera—a visualization system for exploratory research and analysis." *Journal of Computational Chemistry* 25(13): 1605–1612.

Plewczynski, D., A. Philips, M. V. Grotthuss, L. Rychlewski and K. Ginalski (2014). "HarmonyDOCK: The structural analysis of poses in protein-ligand docking." *Journal of Computational Biology* 21(3): 247–256.

Podschun, R. and U. Ullmann (1998). "Klebsiella spp. as nosocomial pathogens: Epidemiology, taxonomy, typing methods, and pathogenicity factors." *Clinical Microbiology Reviews* 11(4): 589–603.

Rahman, M. M., H. N. Hunter, S. Prova, V. Verma, A. Qamar and D. Golemi-Kotra (2016). "The Staphylococcus aureus methicillin resistance factor FmtA is a d-amino esterase that acts on teichoic acids." *MBio* 7(1): e02070–02015.

Ramani, S., A. Pathak, V. Dalal, A. Paul and S. Biswas (2020). "Oxidative stress in autoimmune diseases: An under dealt malice." *Current Protein and Peptide Science* 21(6): 611–621.

Rathi, R., R. Kumari, S. R. Pathak and V. Dalal (2022). "Promising antibacterials for LLM of Staphylococcus aureus using virtual screening, molecular docking, dynamics, and MMPBSA." *Journal of Biomolecular Structure and Dynamics*: 1–13.

Ratia, K., S. Pegan, J. Takayama, K. Sleeman, M. Coughlin, S. Baliji, R. Chaudhuri, W. Fu, B. S. Prabhakar and M. E. Johnson (2008). "A noncovalent class of papain-like protease/deubiquitinase inhibitors blocks SARS virus replication." *Proceedings of the National Academy of Sciences* 105(42): 16119–16124.

Reddy, R. and A. Parrill (1999). "Chapter 1—Overview of rational drug design." In *Rational Drug Design, Novel Methodology and Practical Applications*. ACS Symposium Series. American Chemical Society.

Rester, U. (2008). "From virtuality to reality-Virtual screening in lead discovery and lead optimization: A medicinal chemistry perspective." *Current Opinion in Drug Discovery & Development* 11(4): 559–568.

Robak, T. and E. Robak (2012). "Tyrosine kinase inhibitors as potential drugs for B-cell lymphoid malignancies and autoimmune disorders." *Expert Opinion on Investigational Drugs* 21(7): 921–947.

Romero-Estudillo, I., J. L. Viveros-Ceballos, O. Cazares-Carreño, A. González-Morales, B. F. de Jesús, M. López-Castillo, R. S. Razo-Hernández, G. Castañeda-Corral and M. Ordóñez (2019). "000Synthesis of new α-aminophosphonates: Evaluation as anti-inflammatory agents and QSAR studies." *Bioorganic & Medicinal Chemistry* 27(12): 2376–2386.

Rosenbach, F. (1884). "Microorganisms in the wound infections diseases of man." *Wiesbaden, Germany: JF Bergmann* 18.

Ryffel, C., F. H. Kayser and B. Berger-Bächi (1992). "Correlation between regulation of mecA transcription and expression of methicillin resistance in staphylococci." *Antimicrobial Agents and Chemotherapy* 36(1): 25–31.

Saini, G., V. Dalal, D. N. Gupta, N. Sharma, P. Kumar and A. K. Sharma (2021). "A molecular docking and dynamic approach to screen inhibitors against ZnuA1 of Candidatus Liberibacter asiaticus." *Molecular Simulation*: 1–16.

Saini, G., V. Dalal, B. K. Savita, N. Sharma, P. Kumar and A. K. Sharma (2019). "Molecular docking and dynamic approach to virtual screen inhibitors against Esbp of Candidatus Liberibacter asiaticus." *Journal of Molecular Graphics and Modelling* 92: 329–340.

Sass, P. and G. Bierbaum (2009). "Native graS mutation supports the susceptibility of Staphylococcus aureus strain SG511 to antimicrobial peptides." *International Journal of Medical Microbiology* 299(5): 313–322.

Savita, B. K., V. Dalal, S. Choudhary, D. N. Gupta, N. Das, S. Tomar, P. Kumar, P. Roy and A. K. Sharma (2021). "Characterization of recombinant pumpkin 2S albumin and mutation studies to unravel potential DNA/RNA binding site." *Biochemical and Biophysical Research Communications* 580: 28–34.

Schwede, T., J. Kopp, N. Guex and M. C. Peitsch (2003). "SWISS-MODEL: An automated protein homology-modeling server." *Nucleic Acids Research* 31(13): 3381–3385.

Shaaban, M. R., T. S. Saleh, A. S. Mayhoub, A. Mansour and A. M. Farag (2008). "Synthesis and analgesic/anti-inflammatory evaluation of fused heterocyclic ring systems incorporating phenylsulfonyl moiety." *Bioorganic & Medicinal Chemistry* 16(12): 6344–6352.

Singh, N., V. Dalal and P. Kumar (2018). "Structure based mimicking of Phthalic acid esters (PAEs) and inhibition of hACMSD, an important enzyme of the tryptophan kynurenine metabolism pathway." *International Journal of Biological Macromolecules* 108: 214–224.

Singh, N., V. Dalal and P. Kumar (2020a). "Molecular docking and simulation analysis for elucidation of toxic effects of dicyclohexyl phthalate (DCHP) in glucocorticoid receptor-mediated adipogenesis." *Molecular Simulation* 46(1): 9–21.

Singh, N., V. Dalal, V. Kumar, M. Sharma and P. Kumar (2019). "Characterization of phthalate reductase from Ralstonia eutropha CH34 and in silico study of phthalate dioxygenase and phthalate reductase interaction." *Journal of Molecular Graphics and Modelling* 90: 161–170.

Singh, N., V. Dalal, J. K. Mahto and P. Kumar (2017). "Biodegradation of phthalic acid esters (PAEs) and in silico structural characterization of mono-2-ethylhexyl phthalate (MEHP) hydrolase on the basis of close structural homolog." *Journal of Hazardous Materials* 338: 11–22.

Singh, R., E. S. Masuda and D. G. Payan (2012). "Discovery and development of spleen tyrosine kinase (SYK) inhibitors." *Journal of Medicinal Chemistry* 55(8): 3614–3643.

Singh, V. K., V. Dalal, P. Dhankhar, D. G. Kotra and P. Kumar (2020b). "Molecular docking and simulation study to identify novel potent inhibitors against FmtA in Staphylococcus aureus." *Proceedings of International Conference on Drug Discovery (ICDD).* Available at SSRN: https://ssrn.com/abstract=3529035

Singh, V. K., P. Dhankhar, V. Dalal, S. Tomar, D. Golemi-Kotra and P. Kumar (2022a). "Drug-repurposing approach to combat Staphylococcus aureus: Biomolecular and binding interaction study." *ACS Omega* 7(43): 38448–38458.

Singh, V. K., P. Dhankhar, V. Dalal, S. Tomar and P. Kumar (2022b). "In-silico functional and structural annotation of hypothetical protein from Klebsiella pneumonia: A potential drug target." *Journal of Molecular Graphics and Modelling* 116: 108262.

Singh, V. K., J. L. Schmidt, R. Jayaswal and B. J. Wilkinson (2003). "Impact of sigB mutation on Staphylococcus aureus oxacillin and vancomycin resistance varies with parental background and method of assessment." *International Journal of Antimicrobial Agents* 21(3): 256–261.

Sobral, R., A. Ludovice, H. De Lencastre and A. Tomasz (2006). "Role of murF in cell wall biosynthesis: Isolation and characterization of a murF conditional mutant of Staphylococcus aureus." *Journal of Bacteriology* 188(7): 2543–2553.

Stryjewski, M. E. and G. R. Corey (2014). "Methicillin-resistant Staphylococcus aureus: An evolving pathogen." *Clinical Infectious Diseases* 58(suppl_1): S10–S19.

Swaminathan, P. and L. Saleena (2017). "Evaluation of Cardiospermum halicacabum leaf compounds against human DihydroOrotate Dehydrogenase: A target for rheumatoid arthritis using structure based drug designing." *Journal of Applied Pharmaceutical Science* 7(8): 48–61.

Szarecka, A. and C. Dobson (2019). "Protein structure analysis: Introducing students to rational drug design." *The American Biology Teacher* 81(6): 423–429.

Tanc, M., F. Carta, A. Scozzafava and C. T. Supuran (2015). "α-Carbonic anhydrases possess thioesterase activity." *ACS Medicinal Chemistry Letters* 6(3): 292–295.

Tian, W., C. Chen, X. Lei, J. Zhao and J. Liang (2018). "CASTp 3.0: Computed atlas of surface topography of proteins." *Nucleic Acids Research* 46(W1): W363–W367.

Tong, S. Y., J. S. Davis, E. Eichenberger, T. L. Holland and V. G. Fowler Jr (2015). "Staphylococcus aureus infections: Epidemiology, pathophysiology, clinical manifestations, and management." *Clinical Microbiology Reviews* 28(3): 603–661.

Trabocchi, A., N. Pala, I. Krimmelbein, G. Menchi, A. Guarna, M. Sechi, T. Dreker, A. Scozzafava, C. T. Supuran and F. Carta (2015). "Peptidomimetics as protein arginine deiminase 4 (PAD4) inhibitors." *Journal of Enzyme Inhibition and Medicinal Chemistry* 30(3): 466–471.

Trott, O. and A. J. Olson (2010). "AutoDock Vina: Improving the speed and accuracy of docking with a new scoring function, efficient optimization, and multithreading." *Journal of Computational Chemistry* 31(2): 455–461.

Utaida, S., P. Dunman, D. Macapagal, E. Murphy, S. Projan, V. Singh, R. Jayaswal and B. Wilkinson (2003). "Genome-wide transcriptional profiling of the response of Staphylococcus aureus to cell-wall-active antibiotics reveals a cell-wall-stress stimulon." *Microbiology* 149(10): 2719–2732.

Van Der Spoel, D., E. Lindahl, B. Hess, G. Groenhof, A. E. Mark and H. J. Berendsen (2005). "GROMACS: Fast, flexible, and free." *Journal of Computational Chemistry* 26(16): 1701–1718.

Van Zundert, G., J. Rodrigues, M. Trellet, C. Schmitz, P. Kastritis, E. Karaca, A. Melquiond, M. van Dijk, S. De Vries and A. Bonvin (2016). "The HADDOCK2. 2 web server: User-friendly integrative modeling of biomolecular complexes." *Journal of Molecular Biology* 428(4): 720–725.

Volkamer, A., D. Kuhn, F. Rippmann and M. Rarey (2012). "DoGSiteScorer: A web server for automatic binding site prediction, analysis and druggability assessment." *Bioinformatics* 28(15): 2074–2075.

Wallner, B. and A. Elofsson (2003). "Can correct protein models be identified?" *Protein Science* 12(5): 1073–1086.

Wang, J., W. Wang, P. A. Kollman and D. A. Case (2006). "Automatic atom type and bond type perception in molecular mechanical calculations." *Journal of Molecular Graphics and Modelling* 25(2): 247–260.

Wang, M., R. Cao, L. Zhang, X. Yang, J. Liu, M. Xu, Z. Shi, Z. Hu, W. Zhong and G. Xiao (2020). "Remdesivir and chloroquine effectively inhibit the recently emerged novel coronavirus (2019-nCoV) in vitro." *Cell Research* 30(3): 269–271.

Wang, P., L. Song, H. Yi, M. Zhang, S. Zhu, H. Deng and M. Shao (2010). "Convenient one-pot synthesis of fluorinated DHPs derivatives and their further transformations." *Tetrahedron Letters* 51(30): 3975–3977.

Wang, S., W. Li, S. Liu and J. Xu (2016). "RaptorX-property: A web server for protein structure property prediction." *Nucleic Acids Research* 44(W1): W430–W435.

Webb, B. and A. Sali (2014). Protein structure modeling with MODELLER. *Methods in Molecular Biology* 1137: 1–15.

Weidenmaier, C., A. Peschel, Y.-Q. Xiong, S. A. Kristian, K. Dietz, M. R. Yeaman and A. S. Bayer (2005). "Lack of wall teichoic acids in Staphylococcus aureus leads to reduced interactions with endothelial cells and to attenuated virulence in a rabbit model of endocarditis." *Journal of Infectious Diseases* 191(10): 1771–1777.

Weigelt, J. (2010). "Structural genomics—impact on biomedicine and drug discovery." *Experimental Cell Research* 316(8): 1332–1338.

West, K. (2009). "CP-690550, a JAK3 inhibitor as an immunosuppressant for the treatment of rheumatoid arthritis, transplant rejection, psoriasis and other immune-mediated disorders." *Current Opinion in Investigational Drugs (London, England: 2000)* 10(5): 491–504.

Wiederstein, M. and M. J. Sippl (2007). "ProSA-web: Interactive web service for the recognition of errors in three-dimensional structures of proteins." *Nucleic Acids Research* 35(suppl_2): W407–W410.

Witalison, E., P. R Thompson and L. J. Hofseth (2015). "Protein arginine deiminases and associated citrullination: Physiological functions and diseases associated with dysregulation." *Current Drug Targets* 16(7): 700–710.

Xiao, L., Y. Zhou, L. Zhu, S. Yang, R. Huang, W. Shi, B. Peng and Y. Xiao (2018). "SPHK1-S1PR1-RANKL axis regulates the interactions between macrophages and BMSCs in inflammatory bone loss." *Journal of Bone and Mineral Research* 33(6): 1090–1104.

Yang, H., Y. Li, H. Chai, T. Yakura, B. Liu and Q. Yao (2020). "Synthesis and biological evaluation of 2-epi-jaspine B analogs as selective sphingosine kinase 1 inhibitors." *Bioorganic Chemistry* 98: 103369.

Yoo, H., Y. S. Lee, S. Lee, S. Kim and T. Y. Kim (2012). "Pachastrissamine from Pachastrissa sp. inhibits melanoma cell growth by dual inhibition of Cdk2 and ERK-mediated FOXO3 downregulation." *Phytotherapy Research* 26(12): 1927–1933.

Yoshimitsu, Y., S. Oishi, J. Miyagaki, S. Inuki, H. Ohno and N. Fujii (2011). "Pachastrissamine (jaspine B) and its stereoisomers inhibit sphingosine kinases and atypical protein kinase C." *Bioorganic & Medicinal Chemistry* 19(18): 5402–5408.

Young, D. C. (2009). *Computational Drug Design: A Guide for Computational and Medicinal Chemists*. John Wiley & Sons.

Young, S. S., C. F. Sheffield and M. Farmen (1997). "Optimum utilization of a compound collection or chemical library for drug discovery." *Journal of Chemical Information and Computer Sciences* 37(5): 892–899.

Young, W. B., J. Barbosa, P. Blomgren, M. C. Bremer, J. J. Crawford, D. Dambach, C. Eigenbrot, S. Gallion, A. R. Johnson and J. E. Kropf (2016). "Discovery of highly potent and selective Bruton's tyrosine kinase inhibitors: Pyridazinone analogs with improved metabolic stability." *Bioorganic & Medicinal Chemistry Letters* 26(2): 575–579.

Young, W. B., J. Barbosa, P. Blomgren, M. C. Bremer, J. J. Crawford, D. Dambach, S. Gallion, S. G. Hymowitz, J. E. Kropf and S. H. Lee (2015). "Potent and selective Bruton's tyrosine kinase inhibitors: Discovery of GDC-0834." *Bioorganic & Medicinal Chemistry Letters* 25(6): 1333–1337.

Yu, N., K. D. Lariosa-Willingham, F. F. Lin, M. Webb and T. S. Rao (2004). "Characterization of lysophosphatidic acid and sphingosine-1-phosphate-mediated signal transduction in rat cortical oligodendrocytes." *Glia* 45(1): 17–27.

Zhao, C., M. J. Fernandes, M. Turgeon, S. Tancrède, J. Di Battista, P. E. Poubelle and S. G. Bourgoin (2008). "Specific and overlapping sphingosine-1-phosphate receptor functions in human synoviocytes: Impact of TNF-α." *Journal of Lipid Research* 49(11): 2323–2337.

Zhou, S., G. Huang, G. Chen and J. Liu (2021a). "Synthesis, activity and mechanism for double-ring conjugated enones." *Bioorganic & Medicinal Chemistry Letters* 49: 128315.

Zhou, S., H. Zou, G. Huang, G. Chen, X. Zhou and S. Huang (2021b). "Design, synthesis and anti-rheumatoid arthritis evaluation of double-ring conjugated enones." *Bioorganic Chemistry* 109: 104701.

2 A Bioinformatics Approach Towards Plant-Based Anticancer Drug Discovery

Smitha S. Bhat, Sindhu R**, and Shashanka K. Prasad*,†*

*Department of Biotechnology and Bioinformatics, JSS Academy of Higher Education and Research, Mysuru, Karnataka, India; **Department of Microbiology, JSS Academy of Higher Education and Research, Mysuru, Karnataka, India

†Corresponding Author: shashankaprasad@jssuni.edu.in; shashanka.k@cmu.ac.th

ABBREVIATIONS

ADMET	Absorption, Distribution, Metabolism, Excretion and Toxicity
AI	Artificial Intelligence
CADD	Computer-Aided Drug Design
CMAUP	Collective Molecular Activities of Useful Plants
CVNN DL	Convolutional Neural Networks with Deep Learning
DL	Deep Learning
GPU	Graphics Processing Units
IMPLAD	Indian Medicinal Plants Database
IMPPAT	Indian Medicinal Plants, Phytochemistry and Therapeutics
LS	Ligand SMILES
MD	Molecular Dynamics
ML	Machine Learning
NADI	Natural Product Discovery System
NPACT	Naturally occurring Plant-based Anti-cancer Compound-Activity-Target
QSAR	Qualitative Structure-Activity" Relationship
VS	Virtual Screening

2.1 INTRODUCTION

Cancer, the second leading cause of death worldwide, has increased considerably in recent decades and is defined by unchecked cell growth and proliferation (de Martel et al. 2020). Although there exist many forms of cancer treatments, including chemo-,

DOI: 10.1201/9781003354437-2

immunological, radiation, hormone, and targeted therapies, they all have substantial drawbacks and potential adverse effects. Recently, over 70% of the population in developing countries have switched to using traditional medicines with a hope of minimized associated side effects (Oyebode et al. 2016). A variety of medicinal plants that have significant chemo-protective and anti-carcinogenic properties have recently been advised in cancer patients as an alternative medicine to help prevent and treat cancer and are generally considered safe and possess fewer adverse effects as compared to conventional therapies. Approximately 30% of presently existing medications are derived from natural plant products (Strohl 2000). However, only a handful of natural cancer prevention medications have advanced to the stage of clinical trials, including vinflunine ditartrate, combretastatins, genistein, anhydrovinblastine, tafluposide, and salvicine (Bhat et al. 2022b; Gezici and Şekeroğlu 2019; Khan et al. 2022).

Natural compounds and their derivatives have shown tremendous promising effects in the development of chemotherapeutics due to the virtue of their diverse structural makeup and favorable pharmacological and molecular properties (Greenwell and Rahman 2015). Natural products or their derivatives account for 52% of the chemotherapeutic compounds produced between 1981 and 2014, during which 85 (49%) of the 131 anticancer compounds produced were from natural products and their derivatives (Narsing Rao, Xiao, and Li 2017). Of the 136 novel chemical entities registered, 113 were natural or products based on natural ingredients, accounting for 83% of the total (Newman and Cragg 2007). Some of these medications include paclitaxel and docetaxel, both of which were authorized in the 1990s and used to treat breast cancer. Other examples include the 1960s-era drugs vincristine and vinblastine, both of which are currently utilized to treat a range of malignancies, including testicular, breast, and bladder cancers (X. Wang et al. 2018). Some bioactive anticancer phytochemicals are listed in Table 2.1. From the perspective

TABLE 2.1
Bioactive Anticancer Phytochemicals and Their Targets

Phytochemical Compounds	Type of Cancer	Molecular Target	References
Gefitinib	Non–small-cell lung cancer (NSCLC)	Epidermal growth factor receptor kinase	(Sabbah, Hajjo, and Sweidan 2020; M. Liu et al. 2016)
Erlotinib	Pancreatic cancer, NSCLC	EGFR kinase	(Masago et al. 2010)
Sorafenib	Thyroid cancer, renal cancer, liver cancer	Vascular endothelial growth factor receptor kinase	(Chang et al. 2007; Negrier et al. 2010)
Lapatinib	Breast cancer	Erb-B2 receptor tyrosine kinase 2/EGFR	(Xia et al. 2011; Lu et al. 2012)
Abiraterone	Hormone refractory prostate cancer or metastatic castration-resistant prostate cancer	Inhibitor of androgen synthesis	(Asmane et al. 2011; Jagusch et al. 2008)
Crizotinib	NSCLC	Anaplastic lymphoma kinase	(Rodig and Shapiro 2010)
Genistein	Breast	Tumor necrosis factor-α	(Bhat et al. 2021)

of drug development, finding and creating a new drug can take over a decade and cost an estimated 2.8 billion US dollars. Nevertheless, nine out of ten pharmaceutical substances fail to receive regulatory approval and pass phase II clinical studies (Fleming 2018; Álvarez-Machancoses and Fernández-Martínez 2019). Despite these hindrances, the development of new anticancer phytopharmaceuticals derived from medicinal plants are expected to be beneficial for cancer management and prevention. The creation of new medicines requires an expensive and time-consuming process called 'drug design'. This procedure is rooted in ancient herbal treatments. Although research on plant-based medicines has shown great promise for advancing contemporary medical treatments, it is still lagging behind (Yuan et al. 2016). This might be partly due to the time- and money-consuming nature of traditional plant drug development processes (Yuan et al. 2016). In addition, current pharmaceutical needs cannot be met using traditional, laborious bio-screening techniques for discovering and studying therapeutic plants. Hence, robust technologies that minimize time constraints and provide useful data are needed. Computational biology and systems pharmacology technologies have been used to assess many plant-based anti-cancerous bioactive compounds. Finding new applications for already-approved drugs is significantly less expensive than looking for brand-new cancer treatments. When used as chemotherapeutic treatments, plant-based bioactive chemicals can occasionally have unwanted side effects in addition to improving the effectiveness of chemo medicines (Subramaniam, Selvaduray, and Radhakrishnan 2019). These bioactive substances also modify the immune system and alter cellular pathways, which suppresses cancer (Baraya, Wong, and Yaacob 2017). Bioinformatic techniques offer a great critical set of tools for creating effective and focused pursuits for plant-based medicines. A new age of plant-based medicine discovery may be made possible by merging bioinformatics approaches.

2.2 BIOINFORMATICS APPROACHES IN DRUG DESIGN

In the last decade, the use of computers has extended and so has its prominence in drug discovery. Computer-aided drug design (CADD) is used to define the juncture of computational and pharmaceutical investigations (Lengauer and Rarey 1996; Dallakyan and Olson 2015; Taft, Da Silva, and Da Silva 2008). Over the last decade, the practice of computational techniques for natural product drug discovery has expanded, facilitated by the availability of a wide range of new omics phytochemical structural data, combined with the appearance of new chemo- and bioinformatic approaches, which have paved the way for the investigation of the pharmacological activity of plant bioactive molecules. Many of the strategies use molecular docking, machine learning, pharmacophores, and quantitative or qualitative "structure-activity" connections (QSAR) techniques to facilitate lead discovery for specific targets (Torres et al. 2019; Adelusi et al. 2022). Almost every significant step in the plant-based drug design process involves bioinformatics. In lead compound screening, it is essential to perform extensive biochemical screening of many complex compounds, which is expensive. With the aid of QSAR, it can be determined that substances tend to have pharmacological effects if they have specific chemical structures (Zitnik, Agrawal, and Leskovec 2018; Huang et al. 2005). In target protein discovery, to swiftly determine the potential of new genes to become targets of novel medications, bioinformatics methods could be used to enumerate and analyze identified effective target genes, such as summarizing their properties in nucleotide and amino acid sequences and associating the homology of other succession of human genes with target genes (Ferrari, Losasso, and Costi 2008). To lower the chance of development failure far later in the discovery process, bioinformatics approaches are also utilized to determine whether a target is 'druggable'. In determining the mechanism of drug action, research is aided by bioinformatics technology to compare the mechanisms of action of various medications. Studying the mechanism of action of the medicine in relation to currently available medications has turned out to be a key element of drug development. In the clinical statistical analysis, the outcome of medical application, in which biological information is also crucial, serves as the last evaluation criterion, regardless of whether a molecule has been continually improved and tested to be a successful drug or not. Figure 2.1 is an overview of bioinformatic approaches for the development of phytochemical anticancer drugs.

Bioinformatic approaches for drug development require two types of data. Selecting the best targets from a long list of potential therapeutic targets is one of the biggest obstacles in drug development, which calls for effective, efficient, and methodical research (Patel et al. 2013). Based on resources in databases, researchers can easily find significant cancer-drug interactions by applying gene set enrichment analysis to genes associated with cancer and those sensitive to drugs. In a different way, scientists could create more complex frameworks like machine learning or network analysis to examine the raw information in the databases to investigate any possible relationships between plant-based drugs, their combinations, and cancer, as

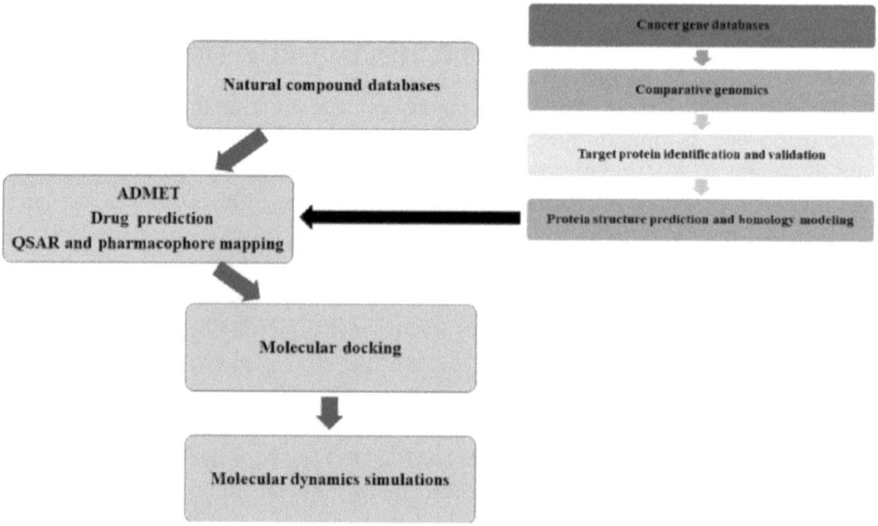

FIGURE 2.1 An overview of bioinformatic approaches and techniques for the development of phytochemical anticancer drugs.

well as to uncover the underlying mechanisms of cancer therapy. To investigate drug repositioning, customized treatment, and medication combinations, various studies have incorporated multi-omics data, for example, transcriptomics, toxico- and functional-genomics, and biological networks (Sachlos et al. 2012; S.-I. Lee et al. 2018; Cheng, Kovács, and Barabási 2019). The drug development pipeline is covered by a wide range of applications for CADD; however, these are heavily clustered in the early stages. CADD's primary goal is to rationalize and expedite the drug design process while also lowering expenses (Taft, Da Silva, and Da Silva 2008). The goal of the initial stage of drug development is to recognize the first-hit ligands. High-throughput screening, which comprises the evaluation of many ligands with an appropriate activity assay, is occasionally used to accomplish this task. By employing computer methods to filter libraries of compounds, virtual screening seeks to prioritize the phytochemicals most likely to be bioactive for a specific target (Bajorath 2002).

Large libraries of small compounds can now be screened using virtual screening (VS), a potent computer method, to find novel hits with desired qualities that can then be evaluated experimentally. The goal of VS, like other computational techniques, is to hasten the process of discovery, to cut down on the number of candidates that need to be evaluated experimentally, and to rationalize the selection of those candidates rather than to replace *in vitro* or *in vivo* experiments. Because it saves time, money, resources, and labor, VS has also become quite popular in pharmaceutical businesses and academic institutions. It is necessary to augment the effectiveness of the hit and lead molecules in the drug discovery pipeline (Hopkins et al. 2014). This can be accomplished using traditional medicinal chemistry methods, in which the strategy can be constructed either on structural data or on observed structure-activity relationships (Thiel 2004). Computational techniques can also be utilized to develop a variety of derivatives founded on various scaffolds and then rated for increased potency (Sun, Tawa, and Wallqvist 2012; Schuffenhauer 2012). In a short span of time, this emphasizes the most optimistic derivatives of phytochemicals (Langdon et al. 2013; Schneider, Schneider, and Renner 2006).

The massive amount of genomic data accumulated in public repositories corresponds to rich reserves for cancer researchers. The literature and resources that are now available in this field are typically dispersed, making it difficult to quickly take advantage of the lack of knowledge on medicinal plants. The diversity of chemicals can be analyzed computationally using a variety of methods. These methods are crucial for CADD (Prachayasittikul et al. 2015). To keep up with the increasing demand for pharmaceuticals, the drug design and discovery of medicinal plants entails the implementation of such methodologies for speedier and more effective advancement. Building databases and tools that report on herbal formulations, medicinal plant bioactive components, and related data is becoming increasingly popular. There are numerous initiatives, including the Collective Molecular Activities of Useful Plants (CMAUP), the Natural Product Discovery System (NADI), Indian Medicinal Plants, Phytochemistry and Therapeutics (IMPPAT), SymMap, Indian Medicinal Plants Database (IMPLAD), and others (Ikram et al. 2015; Zeng et al. 2019; Rajasekharan and Wani 2020; Wu et al. 2019; Mohanraj et al. 2018; Kumar and Arya 2020). Large amounts of data produced by molecular biology-based procedures can be analyzed and interpreted using a variety of vital techniques provided by bioinformatics. Such methods have become increasingly important in data analysis and integration to deduce information as high-throughput techniques have advanced. A detailed examination of the genomic, proteomic, and metabolomic data is necessary to improve the current knowledge of the biological processes related to plants. The identification of genes and specific pathways that could be linked to significant bioactive secondary metabolites from plants with biomedical activity is facilitated by bioinformatic methods (Sharma and Sarkar 2013). Changes in information flow from the genome to the proteome are required to cause manifestations of malignant phenotypes. The cancer phenotype emerges because of molecular changes at several information processing levels. It is necessary to examine neoplastic cells utilizing numerous stages of knowledge flow signified by distinct omics, including genomes, epigenomics, transcriptomics, and proteomics, to recognize the inherent mechanisms that underlie the process of cancer development and therapy (Das et al. 2020; Gamberi et al. 2021). The disadvantage of integrating numerous omics datasets adds another layer of intricacy resulting from the inherently different categories of omics datasets, which render it problematic to incorporate the omics data in a way that is biologically relevant (López de Maturana et al. 2019). If the abundance of cancer-specific online omics data resources can be effectively and methodically incorporated, it may aid in the production of novel biological insights for cancer research. Researchers currently understand more about the cellular processes and pathways connected to cancer thanks to the online omics data repositories. Different datasets can be systematically integrated for quick hypothesis formulation and validation, and the online sources offer researchers the great opportunity to identify changed molecular patterns in either a specific category or across all tumor categories (Cui et al. 2020; Rahman et al. 2022).

The origin and treatment of cancer are the focus of ongoing research. As a result, data on cancer is increasing exponentially and is being stored in appropriate repositories from a variety of sources, including scientific journals, genome-wide association studies, data on gene-gene or protein-protein interactions, immunomics, epigenomics, gene expression experiments, enzymatic assays, and cytogenetics. These data are complicated and assorted, vacillating from raw sequences and polymorphisms, which are unprocessed, unstructured data, to organized data that have been well annotated. As a result, biomedical researchers face a significant problem in effectively storing, mining, retrieving, and analyzing these data. Several databases are available, including the Cancer Genome Atlas, Gene Expression Omnibus, and Cancer-related Pathways and Networks, that include raw high-throughput data which must be examined by bioinformatics methods to recognize genes correlated to cancer (Brennan et al. 2013; Edgar, Domrachev, and Lash 2002). Some open databases provide relevant data sources. Some of these, such as the Online Mendelian Inheritance in Man, Gender and Development database, genome-wide association studies Catalog, and DisGeNET databases, directly provide details on oncogenes or tumor suppressor genes in various types of malignancies (McKusick 2007; Amberger et al. 2015; Piñero et al. 2017; Buniello et al. 2019; Piñero et al. 2015). Other databases offer drug-target gene interactions to FDA-approved or clinically exploratory medications. The DrugBank database offers drug-target interactions (Wishart et al.

2006, 2008; Law et al. 2013; Tran and Pham 2021); the Therapeutic Target Database, the PharmGKB database, and the naturally occurring plant-based anti-cancer compound-activity-target database (NPACT) (Y. H. Li et al. 2018; X. Chen, Ji, and Chen 2002; Whirl-Carrillo et al. 2012; Mangal et al. 2013) are some such examples. Other databases, such as cMAP software, and Cancer Cell Line Encyclopedia, provide extensive gene expression profiles of human malignant cell lines treated with various drugs under various circumstances (Subramanian et al. 2017; Lamb et al. 2006; Barretina et al. 2012; Cancer Cell Line Encyclopedia Consortium 2015; Shoemaker 2006; Abaan et al. 2013).

The strength of the chemicals, however, is not the only factor in the development of anticancer drugs from plant sources. If a chemical is to be clinically beneficial, its pharmacokinetic qualities (absorption, distribution, metabolism, and excretion) as well as toxicity, often known as ADMET, are crucial to know (A. P. Li 2001; Yu and Adedoyin 2003; Ekins et al. 2002). To anticipate the ADMET properties of phytochemical molecules early in the investigative process, virtual approaches have also been developed in addition to a series of *in vitro* and *in vivo* investigations.

2.3 ABSORPTION, DISTRIBUTION, METABOLISM, EXCRETION AND TOXICITY PREDICTION

In addition to ADMET, high potency, affinity, and selectivity against molecular targets are all characteristics of effective and secure medications. A significant barrier to medication R&D is the synchronized honing of these inter-reliant variables (Segall 2014). ADMET prediction via computational methods has a progressively substantial part in drug research and development by offering a useful tool to evaluate various PK features in hit-to-lead and lead optimization campaigns (Kesharwani et al. 2020). The significance of such a technique has magnified with the advancement of chemoinformatics, which entered the big data era after ground-breaking discoveries in the 1960s and notions of drug similarity that were widely used in the 1990s. The boiled egg model is a simple way to predict both blood-brain access and passive gastrointestinal absorption, two essential ADME factors. Although this classification model is conceptually extremely straightforward because it only uses two physicochemical descriptors, it was constructed with great effort to ensure statistical significance and robustness. Figure 2.2 illustrates the egg-shaped categorization plot, which entails the white and yolk (i.e., the physicochemical area for very probable blood-brain barrier permeability; i.e., the physicochemical space for highly probable gastrointestinal absorption). The outside gray zone signifies substances with qualities implying predicted low absorption and restricted brain penetration; however, the two compartments are not mutually exclusive. In a variety of drug discovery circumstances, the boiled egg model has established simple interpretation and effective translation to molecular design (Daina, Michielin, and Zoete 2017; Arulanandam et al. 2022; Kar and Leszczynski 2020).

Cutting-edge machine learning (ML) tactics have shown superiority over conventional chemometrics methods in this progressively difficult situation, given the necessity to handle bigger and more varied datasets. The significance of ML tactics in the field of ADMET modelling is supported by studies, which mainly used

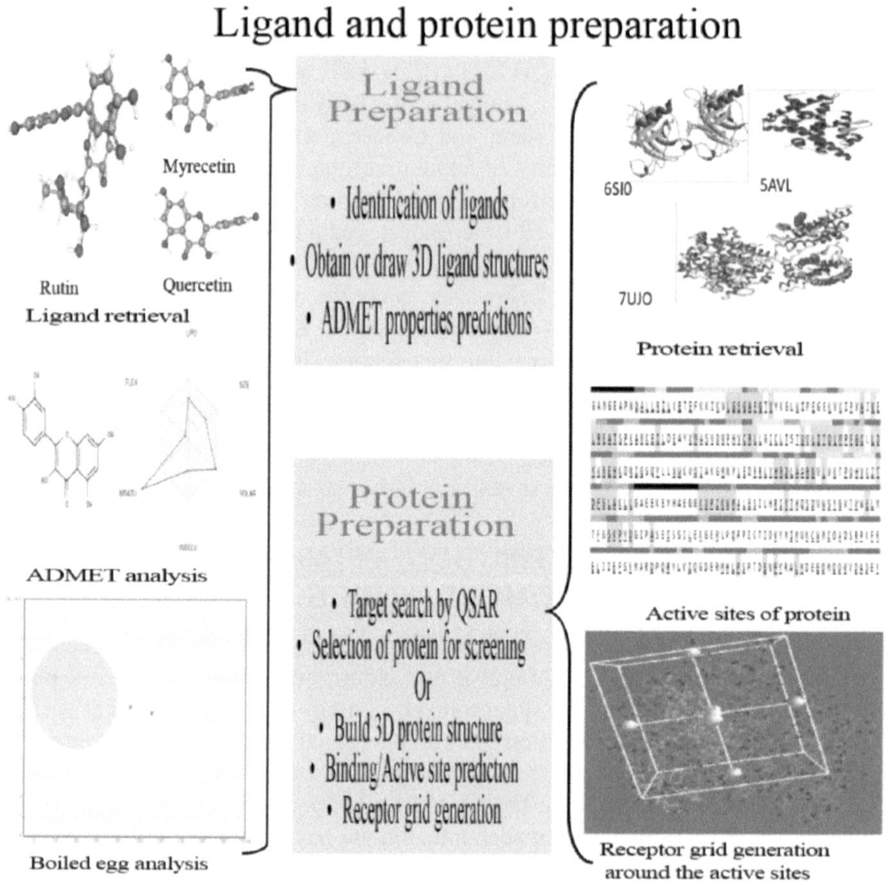

FIGURE 2.2 An overview of ligand and target protein selection processes performed before molecular docking.

random forest, support vector machine, and tree-based techniques. The conversion of generated models into efficient and comprehensible online podiums that can be openly retrieved by the worldwide drug developing community is another crucial consideration. These resources have successfully advanced drug R&D by integrating additional pertinent attributes such as safety endpoints, structural alerts, drug and lead likeness, and physicochemical traits. Understanding how compounds interact with targets is crucial for optimizing lead molecules and producing compounds with high activity and acceptable ADME/T characteristics.

2.4 MOLECULAR DOCKING

Since its introduction in the 1970s, molecular docking is a well-known bioinformatic structure-based technique that is extensively employed in drug development and has emerged as a distinct *in silico* technique to accelerate drug discovery and design.

Docking enables the discovery of new therapeutic phytochemicals, the forecast of ligand-target interactions at the molecular level, and the definition of structure-activity correlations lacking prior knowledge of the chemical composition of other target modulators (Arjmand et al. 2022; S. Singh, Bani Baker, and Singh 2022). Docking was initially established to support the understanding of the molecular mechanisms dictating the acknowledgement between small and large molecules, but in recent years, it has seen a substantial change in its usage and applications in drug development. Through molecular docking, small molecules are inserted into macromolecular structures to measure their complementary values at the binding sites. The most attractive approaches in this burgeoning field of study are structure-based drug design, lead optimization, and biochemical pathways. An efficient docking experiment must have the two elements of correct position and affinity prediction. Since each software package has different rewards and shortcomings in terms of docking precision, ranking precision, and time consumption, generalization is not possible. Additionally, users typically neglect to include test sets with enough diversity, which results in certain systems performing better than others.

Today, docking is frequently used to support an assortment of other drug discovery tasks, such as the identification of new chemicals in large compound libraries to carry out target fishing and profiling for drug repositioning, polypharmacology, adverse effect prediction, and beyond. For instance, to improve prediction performances in de novo virtual screening, target fishing, polypharmacology, and drug repurposing, docking has been utilized in conjunction with ligand-based, molecular dynamics, binding free energy calculations, and artificial intelligence (AI) techniques. Figure 2.2 is an overview of ligand and target protein selection processes performed before molecular docking. However, docking is now frequently utilized to support a range of additional drug discovery tasks outside of the areas for which it was initially designed. Docking, a flexible tool, will undoubtedly be used in more areas of drug discovery. Additionally, automated procedures for screening sizable libraries of chemicals and targets have successfully incorporated docking (H. Li et al. 2006; Y. Z. Chen and Zhi 2001; Xie et al. 2016; J.-C. Wang et al. 2012; Labbé et al. 2015; Irwin et al. 2009). Recent developments in high-performance computing have been crucial in this regard. For instance, it has been made possible to quickly screen millions of chemicals *in silico* (Perez-Sanchez and Wenzel 2011; Dong et al. 2018). Additionally, recent developments in graphics processing units (GPUs) have produced notable gains in both data-driven drug discovery and molecular dynamics simulations (De Vivo et al. 2016; Gawehn et al. 2018). In fact, compared to central processing unit computations, GPU calculations facilitate a thorough examination of the conformational landscape that proteins may be able to access (X.-W. Chen and Lin 2014). GPU computing has opened up big data–driven computation jobs to a wider audience, and it is anticipated to play a significant part in the future of docking and computational drug design (Stone et al. 2010).

Despite being initially created and used as a stand-alone technique, docking methods for assisting various tasks in drug discovery have also evolved and are primarily used in conjunction with other computational techniques inside integrated workflows. The use of approximate scoring methods and non-exhaustive conformational sampling, two of the most important inherent molecular docking constraints, have been made possible as a result. The use of mixed techniques typically leads to higher prediction performance and enables better exploitation of data from various sources. Docking has been used in the application of integrated workflows to help with various drug development activities. One should be aware that each computational approach has its own drawbacks, which may make it difficult for docking to be integrated into combined workflows or even lessen the predictive capacity of the chosen protocol. Ligand-based methods might not be the best option for enhancing the docking forecast if there are not enough ligands for the target(s) being investigated. However, these techniques significantly enhanced docking predictions in terms of both hit rates and enrichment factors when the combination was practical. Figure 2.3 is an overview of the molecular docking procedure for phytochemical screening. Instead, molecular dynamics and binding free energy estimates may be able to help advance docking predictions even for targets that are less well-characterized, for instance, by identifying conformational ensembles that can be used in structure-based analyses and by more precisely determining the ligand-protein

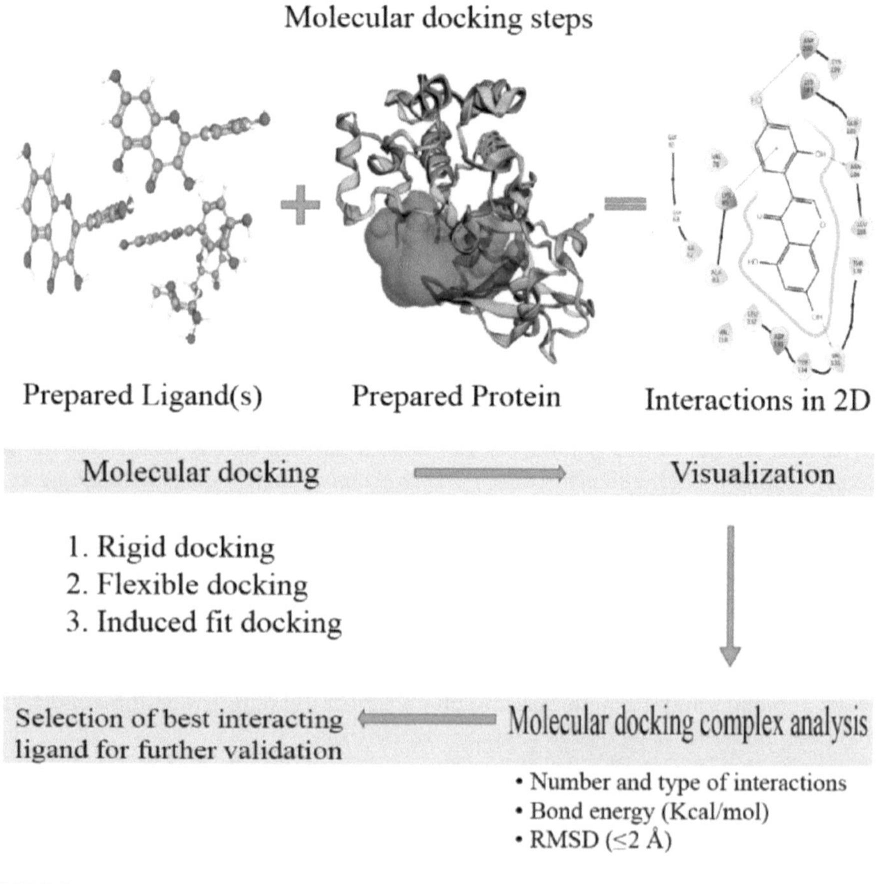

FIGURE 2.3 An overview of the molecular docking procedure for phytochemical screening.

binding affinity (Rastelli and Pinzi 2019; Caporuscio and Rastelli 2016). Even with the abundance of *in silico* tools and methods presently existing in the market, docking still has many potential applications in integrated workflows. Additionally, ongoing advancements in hardware and software engineering will make it easier to integrate them. In addition, the expansion of publicly available structural, chemical, and biological information and its incorporation into databases, web platforms, and automated processes will undoubtedly bring forth unique, useful opportunities for data and technique integration. Further work should go into better integration of various methodologies, with the information reported in these databases being made available to the public. This is anticipated to offer novel and beneficial options for the detection and advancement of new medications in the future, for the creation of difficult and inventive drugs (multi-target ligands), and for ligand profiling and repositioning. Given the high attrition rates that characterize drug discovery, it will be crucial to take advantage of docking's potential in conjunction with the methods described here to speed up the development of clinical candidates with advanced safety profiles and to find new uses for medications that are already on the market (Dowden and Munro 2019).

2.5 MOLECULAR DYNAMICS SIMULATIONS

CADD, particularly VS techniques, has been utilized extensively for the discovery and optimization of new, minimally toxic anticancer drugs, leading to increased productivity (Loukatou et al. 2014; Torres et al. 2019; De Vivo et al. 2016). However, conventional molecular docking techniques do not fully justify the flexibility of the target, which can result in oversight and thereby omission of some bioactive phytochemicals. Molecular dynamics (MD) simulations can offer a plethora of data regarding the interactions between proteins and ligands, along with dynamical structure data on biomacromolecules (Bunker and Róg 2020; Kotzabasaki and Froudakis 2018). Figure 2.4 is an overview of the MD simulations procedure. Such knowledge is crucial for determining the structure-function connection of the target, the fundamentals of protein-ligand interactions, and for directing drug discovery and design processes (X. Liu et al. 2018; Lin 2022; Shukla and Tripathi 2021). Consequently, MD simulations have been efficaciously utilized at every stage of contemporary drug research. The pathogenic mechanisms of ailments induced by protein misfolding, VS, and investigation of drug resistance machineries brought on by target mutations have all benefited greatly from the use of MD simulations (Salo-Ahen et al. 2021; Hidayat et al. 2022).

Comparatively, MD simulations can acquire several target conformations and are often employed in molecular docking to account for the flexibility of the targets. One of the most dynamic expanses of research in the field of VS is the development of effective systems that can accurately score candidates. Because they can augment the prediction precision of binding capability between ligands and the target, MD simulations in conjunction with binding free energy estimates have also proved to be a viable technique to increase the enrichment factor of virtual screening (Alonso, Bliznyuk, and Gready 2006; Rastelli et al. 2010). Numerous studies have used MD simulations and binding free energy designs to examine how phytochemical ligands interact with cancer target proteins (Bhat et al. 2022a; Antony and Vijayan 2016).

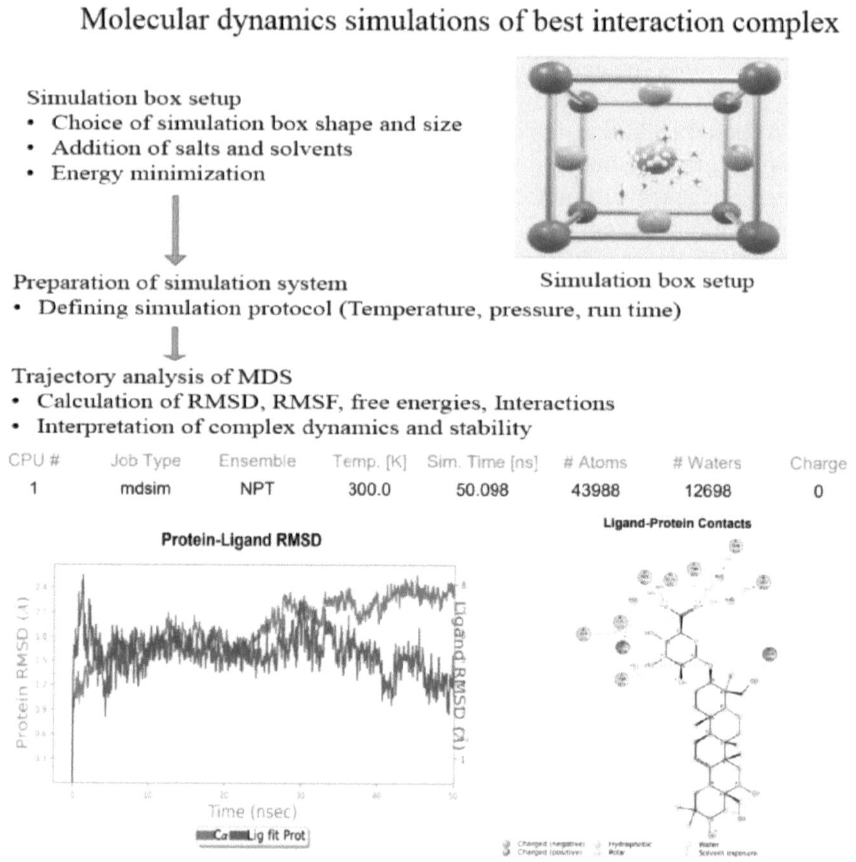

FIGURE 2.4 An overview of molecular dynamics simulations procedure.

2.6 QUANTITATIVE STRUCTURE-ACTIVITY RELATIONSHIP

Due to its high and quick throughput, QSAR analysis is the most effective technique among the VS techniques. QSAR modelling has a nearly 60-year history of rich technique advances and applications. To understand the association of structure and bioactivity in relatively small congeneric chemical series and forecast relatively tiny structural adjustments that would result in higher activity, QSAR modelling was used only as a tool for lead optimization (Neves et al. 2018). Modern QSAR modelling is a very difficult and complex field that calls for in-depth knowledge and much practice to produce reliable models (Ahirwar et al. 2022). The first stage in developing a QSAR model is to gather pertinent chemogenomics data from databases and the literature. Then, using machine learning approaches, chemical descriptors are computed on various representations of the molecular structure, spanning from 1D to nD, and then connected with the biological trait (Crampon et al. 2022). QSAR models are employed to forecast the biotic properties of novel substances after being developed and validated (Mao et al. 2021; Neves et al. 2018). Although it is not a fundamental component of QSAR approach, experimental testing of computational hits is extremely desirable and should be carried out as the last validation of generated models.

The use of QSAR has been expanded in the modern era of drug design and discovery to include molecular design; biological activity prediction; lead compound optimization; VS; classification, diagnosis, and elucidation of drug action mechanisms; toxicity prediction of environmental toxicants; and drug-induced toxicity predictions. QSAR refers to mathematical correlations between chemical structure and pharmacological activity in a quantitative way for a group of chemicals. These approaches associate the molecular structure to a certain bioactive property generated either *in vitro* or *in vivo* (Cherkasov et al. 2014). Structure-activity modelling is important, as it allows researchers to assess and pinpoint the variables that influence the activity that is observed for a given system in order to gain understanding of its functioning and behavior. To do this, a mathematical model is created that links experimental results with a collection of chemical descriptors derived from the molecular structure of a variety of molecules. To forecast the examined biological or physicochemical behavior for novel substances, the generated QSAR model should have the best feasible predictive capabilities. Numerous physicochemical descriptors, including as those that take into consideration hydrophobicity, electrical characteristics, steric effects, structural complexity, and topology, are used to represent the factors controlling the events in biological systems (Johnson et al. 1998). To determine the biochemical basis of drug action prediction for drugs or chemicals, one must have a thorough understanding of the biological system, the innumerable aspects regulating physiological processes and those that contribute to pathological states, a careful inspection of drug molecules and their properties, and the discovery of the aspects that modulate drug biological activity. As a result, QSAR becomes quicker, less expensive, and more dependable while also making financial sense. Such knowledge aids in the scientific development of more efficient and less harmful medications (Perkins et al. 2003).

Regression-based QSAR models, classification-based QSAR models, and machine learning methods can all be considered broad categories of QSAR models. Data preparation and analysis, model validation, and data interpretation are the four processes that make up the QSAR model creation process (Golbraikh et al. 2017). In order to develop better QSAR models that describe and forecast crucial biological reactions, a huge collection of new and conventional descriptors is used. Several chemometric tools, including stepwise multiple linear regression, partial least squares, classification algorithms, genetic function approximation, genetic partial least squares, artificial neural networks, and others are used to create the QSAR models (Deeb and Goodarzi 2012). Since the latter half of the 20th century, the QSAR technique has been successfully used to construct prediction models and design expert systems for a variety of biological activity and toxicity profiles. However, the number of QSAR models developed for natural products is surprisingly small. As previously mentioned, phytochemicals are a known source of medicines, and as QSAR models can aid in better drug design, it is crucial to put special emphasis on the creation of QSAR models using phytochemicals (Kar and Roy 2012). A pharmacophore model for tyrosinase inhibitors was created using the compound (S)-(+)-decursin and its analogues by Lee et al, who found 4'-epi-decursin to be the most active molecule after evaluation of a library of natural products (Kyeong Lee and Jung 2012). Similar investigations were carried out on a series of flavonoids isolated from plants of medicinal importance (*Dalbergia parviflora* and *Belamcanda chinensis*), which identified their anticancer activity both in computational and *in vitro* methods (De-Eknamkul et al. 2011).

Physicochemical properties, such as log P or log D, can be quickly predicted using a computational model based on QSAR. These models, however, are a long way from making accurate predictions about intricate biological characteristics like a compound's effectiveness and unfavorable adverse effects. Small training sets, incorrect investigational data in training sets, and a dearth of experimental validations are further problems QSAR-based models encounter (Daina, Michielin, and Zoete 2017).

2.7 ARTIFICIAL INTELLIGENCE IN DRUG DISCOVERY

Due to a lack of cutting-edge technologies, developing new medications is a laborious and expensive endeavor that can be improved by means of AI. AI can quickly validate therapeutic targets, find hit and lead compounds, and optimize structural design. There is a lot of potential for creating new medicines for diseases that are currently incurable by using AI in medication research (J. W. Lee et al. 2022; Saldívar-González et al. 2022). Additionally, it will cut R&D costs and raise drug discovery success rates. But there is no denying the requirement of continuing innovation in AI platforms. The only way to enhance AI is to either create whole new algorithms or feed existing ones with supplementary data from other sources, the latter of which is highly challenging due to ethical and legal considerations. The failure of AI is also significantly influenced by bad data governance. Although a current method for objective data analysis was published, it will be ineffective due to disorganized data. Even though a chemical database created from traditional medicine would generate more data for the discovery of new pharmaceuticals, sufficient supervision is desired to ensure the superiority of the information produced. Pharmaceutical companies with strong experience in AI systems may therefore have a significant impact on the creation of such databases and their integration with cutting-edge AI-assisted drug discovery platforms. Recent advances in AI, such as deep learning (DL) and pertinent modelling studies, can be employed for safety and efficacy assessments of medicinal ligands based on big data modelling and analysis to overcome the limitations of QSAR-based procedures (Urbina et al. 2022; Roshan Kumar and Purabi Saha 2022). Along with structural and ligand-based tactics, there are many *in silico* techniques for virtual screening of compounds from virtual chemical spaces that offer better profile analysis, quicker non-lead compound elimination, and faster therapeutic molecule selection at a lower cost (Mak and Pichika 2019; Paul et al. 2021) The physical, chemical, and toxicological properties are taken into account by drug design systems like coulomb matrices and molecular fingerprint identification to choose a lead compound (Chan et al. 2019; Walters and Barzilay 2021).

In addition to being utilized for VS based on synthesis feasibility, algorithms like nearest-neighbor classifiers, extreme learning machines, and deep neural networks may also forecast *in vivo* activity and toxicity (Álvarez-Machancoses and Fernández-Martínez 2019; Dana et al. 2018). By taking into account the characteristics or resemblances of the drug and its target, AI-based tactics can estimate a drug's binding affinity (Jiménez-Luna et al. 2021). Feature-based interactions identify the chemical moieties of the medicine and the target to determine the feature vectors. In contrast, similarity-based interactions allow for the study of similarities between the drug and the target and make the assumption that they will interact with the same targets (Öztürk, Özgür, and Ozkirimli 2018). ChemMapper, which employs the molecular 3D similarity ensemble approach is one web-based application that is available to predict drug-target interactions and chemical structure (Lounkine et al. 2012). Because DL approaches use network-based techniques that are independent of the accessibility of the 3D protein structure, they have demonstrated superior performance to ML approaches (Lounkine et al. 2012). Some DL approaches used to assess drug-target binding affinities include DeepDTA, PADME, WideDTA, and DeepAffinity. The amino acid sequence is entered for protein input data and for the one-dimensional illustration of the drug assembly when submitting drug data to DeepDTA in the form of SMILES (Mahmud et al. 2019). WideDTA is a CVNN DL approach that uses input data from protein domains and motifs, amino acid sequences, ligand SMILES (LS), and ligand maximum common substructures to determine the binding affinity (Gao and Huang 2018). Despite its benefits, AI must contend with serious data difficulties such the size, expansion, diversity, and ambiguity of the data (Yang et al. 2019). Millions of molecules may be present in the datasets available to pharmaceutical corporations for the development of new drugs, making them difficult for typical ML systems to handle.

2.8 FUTURE PROSPECTS AND LIMITATIONS

There is no doubt that the production of a vast volume of multi-omics data presents significant opportunities for the economical discovery of precise and effective anti-cancer drugs. Although the effectiveness of the 'prediction approaches' has improved significantly, there exist numerous challenges to overcome in the actual world. To find and create a safe new lead drug that specifically targets cancer cells and enhances therapeutic applications for cancer therapy and prevention, bioinformatics tools indeed may offer a thorough understanding of the cellular processes associated with plant molecules and the target of interest through in-depth analysis of genomic, proteomic, and metabolomic information (Paananen and Fortino 2020). Additionally, to making it easier to analyze high-throughput data, bioinformatics tools provide important information on gathering and collecting the scattered pieces of evidence into meaningful hypotheses and creating prospective candidates for experimental validation. Thus, hybrid technologies that integrate several omics approaches can aid in a better comprehension and interpretation of *in vitro* and *in vivo* results. However, a lot of previous research has taken prior knowledge into account like protein-protein interaction networks and biological pathways which severely restrict the integrality and accurateness of computer predictions. More research may also be needed on context-specific therapy for predicting drug response. Prediction models have mainly been built on pancreatic cancer data studies, which do not consider context specificity, as there are now just a few datasets available for specific tissues or drugs.

Further, both cytotoxic chemotherapy and molecularly targeted cancer therapies have historically relied on compounds produced mostly by plants and will continue to do so in the future. They more frequently require thorough structural optimization to enhance their pharmacokinetic, safety, and accessibility characteristics. Additionally, a thorough comprehension of the interactions between phytochemicals and related signaling pathway targets will help in developing anticancer medications that are more efficient, selective, and less harmful by deciphering their molecular mechanisms of action and pharmacokinetic performances. Most of the current prediction techniques for drug development also rely on the molecular profiles of cancer cell lines known as transcriptomes. It has been shown that cancer cell lines do not faithfully mimic the molecular irregularities observed in patients (Romano and Tatonetti 2019). Bioinformaticians need to be more knowledgeable on the limitations of cell lines to therapeutically experiment on the usefulness of select candidate molecules for further applications. Adopting techniques that depend on sparser data types, such as CMap-based models, where data are only available for a small quantity of cell lines in a narrow range of tissue types, leads to models that are less extensible and usable in clinical applications. The selection of cell lines that do not accurately reflect tumour biology and the unavailability of suitable cell lines for modeling response for some malignancies are the main constraints leading to failure of computational drug development. However, partnerships with clinicians may facilitate the possibility to forecast cancer medications more accurately by incorporating clinical data for therapeutic purposes.

2.9 CONCLUSION

Natural products are gaining popularity due to their low cost and superiority in terms of the side effects of prescription drugs. As bioactive phytochemicals and formulations may be utilized as a basis for the development of safe anticancer drugs, the development of phytopharmaceuticals against cancer is a major emphasis in the field of cancer research. To achieve this goal, many plants and the phytochemicals they contain have been examined, but only a few have reached the clinical stage. It is necessary to produce phytochemical substances in drug forms with sufficient bioavailability. The development of new anticancer medications is facilitated by bioinformatics techniques that include virtual screening, molecular docking, and molecular dynamics simulations in addition to QSAR and ADMET testing methods. Additional study on this subject might result in the creation of novel computational methods that are more suited to the process of discovering phytochemical drugs as well as the evolution of plant-based anticancer drugs.

REFERENCES

Abaan, Ogan D, Eric C Polley, Sean R Davis, Yuelin J Zhu, Sven Bilke, Robert L Walker, Marbin Pineda, et al. 2013. "The Exomes of the NCI-60 Panel: A Genomic Resource for Cancer Biology and Systems Pharmacology." *Cancer Research* 73 (14): 4372–4382. https://doi.org/10.1158/0008-5472.CAN-12-3342.

Adelusi, Temitope Isaac, Abdul-Quddus Kehinde Oyedele, Ibrahim Damilare Boyenle, Abdeen Tunde Ogunlana, Rofiat Oluwabusola Adeyemi, Chiamaka Divine Ukachi, Mukhtar Oluwaseun Idris, et al. 2022. "Molecular Modeling in Drug Discovery." *Informatics in Medicine Unlocked* 29: 100880. https://doi.org/10.1016/j.imu.2022.100880.

Ahirwar, Hemant, Gabbar Kurmi, Rubeena Khan, Basant Khare, Anushree Jain, Prateek Kumar Jain, and Bhupendra Singh Thakur. 2022. "Review on QSAR Using Anticancer Drug." *Asian Journal of Dental and Health Sciences* 2 (4 SE-Review Articles): 59–63. https://doi.org/10.22270/ajdhs.v2i4.27.

Alonso, Hernán, Andrey A Bliznyuk, and Jill E Gready. 2006. "Combining Docking and Molecular Dynamic Simulations in Drug Design." *Medicinal Research Reviews* 26 (5). United States: 531–568. https://doi.org/10.1002/med.20067.

Álvarez-Machancoses, Óscar, and Juan Luis Fernández-Martínez. 2019. "Using Artificial Intelligence Methods to Speed Up Drug Discovery." *Expert Opinion on Drug Discovery* 14 (8). Taylor & Francis: 769–777.

Amberger, Joanna S, Carol A Bocchini, François Schiettecatte, Alan F Scott, and Ada Hamosh. 2015. "OMIM.Org: Online Mendelian Inheritance in Man (OMIM®), an Online Catalog of Human Genes and Genetic Disorders." *Nucleic Acids Research* 43 (Database issue): D789–D798. https://doi.org/10.1093/nar/gku1205.

Antony, Priya, and Ranjit Vijayan. 2016. "Acetogenins from Annona Muricata as Potential Inhibitors of Antiapoptotic Proteins: A Molecular Modeling Study." *Drug Design, Development and Therapy* 10: 1399–1410. https://doi.org/10.2147/DDDT.S103216.

Arjmand, Babak, Shayesteh Kokabi Hamidpour, Sepideh Alavi-Moghadam, Hanieh Yavari, Ainaz Shahbazbadr, Mostafa Rezaei Tavirani, Kambiz Gilany, and Bagher Larijani. 2022. "Molecular Docking as a Therapeutic Approach for Targeting Cancer Stem Cell Metabolic Processes." *Frontiers in Pharmacology*. https://doi.org/10.3389/fphar.2022.768556.

Arulanandam, Charli Deepak, Jiang-Shiou Hwang, Arthur James Rathinam, and Hans-Uwe Dahms. 2022. "Evaluating Different Web Applications to Assess the Toxicity of Plasticizers." *Scientific Reports* 12 (1): 19684. https://doi:10.1038/s41598-022-18327-0.

Asmane, Irène, Jocelyn Ceraline, Brigitte Duclos, Lynn Rob, Valère Litique, Philippe Barthelemy, Jean-Pierre Bergerat, Patrick Dufour, and Jean-Emmanuel Kurtz. 2011. "New Strategies for Medical Management of Castration-Resistant Prostate Cancer." *Oncology* 80 (1–2). Karger Publishers: 1–11.

Bajorath, Jürgen. 2002. "Integration of Virtual and High-Throughput Screening." *Nature Reviews. Drug Discovery* 1 (11). England: 882–894. https://doi.org/10.1038/nrd941.

Baraya, Yusha'u Shu'aibu Baraya, Kah Keng Wong, and Nik Soriani Yaacob. 2017. "The Immunomodulatory Potential of Selected Bioactive Plant-Based Compounds in Breast Cancer: A Review." *Anti-Cancer Agents in Medicinal Chemistry (Formerly Current Medicinal Chemistry-Anti-Cancer Agents)* 17 (6). Bentham Science Publishers: 770–783.

Barretina, Jordi, Giordano Caponigro, Nicolas Stransky, Kavitha Venkatesan, Adam A Margolin, Sungjoon Kim, Christopher J Wilson, et al. 2012. "The Cancer Cell Line Encyclopedia Enables Predictive Modelling of Anticancer Drug Sensitivity." *Nature* 483 (7391): 603–607. https://doi.org/10.1038/nature11003.

Bhat, Smitha S, Shreya D Mahapatra, Sindhu R, Sarana R Sommano, and Shashanka K Prasad. 2022a. "Virtual Screening and Quantitative Structure—Activity Relationship of Moringa Oleifera with Melanoma Antigen A (MAGE-A) Genes Against the Therapeutics of Non-Small Cell Lung Cancers (NSCLCs)." *Cancers*. https://doi.org/10.3390/cancers14205052.

Bhat, Smitha S, Shashanka K Prasad, Chandan Shivamallu, Kollur Shiva Prasad, Asad Syed, Pruthvish Reddy, Charley A Cull, and Raghavendra G Amachawadi. 2021. "Genistein: A Potent Anti-Breast Cancer Agent." *Current Issues in Molecular Biology* 43 (3): 1502–1517. https://doi.org/10.3390/cimb43030106.

Bhat, Smitha S, Shivamallu, Chandan, Kollur, Shiva Prasad, and Prasad, Shashank K. 2022b. "Biomedical Importance of Lablab Purpureus: A Review." *Medicinal Plants* 14 (1): 20–29. https://doi.org/10.5958/0975-6892.2022.00003.X.

Brennan, Cameron W, Roel G W Verhaak, Aaron McKenna, Benito Campos, Houtan Noushmehr, Sofie R Salama, Siyuan Zheng, et al. 2013. "The Somatic Genomic Landscape of Glioblastoma." *Cell* 155 (2): 462–477. https://doi.org/10.1016/j.cell.2013.09.034.

Buniello, Annalisa, Jacqueline A L MacArthur, Maria Cerezo, Laura W Harris, James Hayhurst, Cinzia Malangone, Aoife McMahon, et al. 2019. "The NHGRI-EBI GWAS Catalog of Published Genome-Wide Association Studies, Targeted Arrays and Summary Statistics 2019." *Nucleic Acids Research* 47 (D1): D1005–D1012. https://doi.org/10.1093/nar/gky1120.

Bunker, Alex, and Tomasz Róg. 2020. "Mechanistic Understanding from Molecular Dynamics Simulation in Pharmaceutical Research 1: Drug Delivery." *Frontiers in Molecular Biosciences* 7: 604770. https://doi.org/10.3389/fmolb.2020.604770.

Cancer Cell Line Encyclopedia Consortium. 2015. "Pharmacogenomic Agreement between Two Cancer Cell Line Data Sets." *Nature* 528 (7580): 84–87. https://doi.org/10.1038/nature15736.

Caporuscio, Fabiana, and Giulio Rastelli. 2016. "Exploiting Computationally Derived Out-of-the-Box Protein Conformations for Drug Design." *Future Medicinal Chemistry* 8 (15). Future Science: 1887–1897.

Chan, H C Stephen, Hanbin Shan, Thamani Dahoun, Horst Vogel, and Shuguang Yuan. 2019. "Advancing Drug Discovery via Artificial Intelligence." *Trends in Pharmacological Sciences* 40 (8). Elsevier: 592–604.

Chang, Yong S, Jalila Adnane, Pamela A Trail, Joan Levy, Arris Henderson, Dahai Xue, Elizabeth Bortolon, Marina Ichetovkin, Charles Chen, and Angela McNabola. 2007. "Sorafenib (BAY 43–9006) Inhibits Tumor Growth and Vascularization and Induces Tumor Apoptosis and Hypoxia in RCC Xenograft Models." *Cancer Chemotherapy and Pharmacology* 59 (5). Springer: 561–574.

Chen, X, Z L Ji, and Y Z Chen. 2002. "TTD: Therapeutic Target Database." *Nucleic Acids Research* 30 (1): 412–415. https://doi.org/10.1093/nar/30.1.412.

Chen, Xue-Wen, and Xiaotong Lin. 2014. "Big Data Deep Learning: Challenges and Perspectives." *IEEE Access* 2. IEEE: 514–525.

Chen, Y Z, and D G Zhi. 2001. "Ligand—Protein Inverse Docking and Its Potential Use in the Computer Search of Protein Targets of a Small Molecule." *Proteins: Structure, Function, and Bioinformatics* 43 (2). Wiley Online Library: 217–226.

Cheng, Feixiong, István A Kovács, and Albert-László Barabási. 2019. "Network-Based Prediction of Drug Combinations." *Nature Communications* 10 (1): 1197. https://doi.org/10.1038/s41467-019-09186-x.

Cherkasov, Artem, Eugene N Muratov, Denis Fourches, Alexandre Varnek, Igor I Baskin, Mark Cronin, John Dearden, et al. 2014. "QSAR Modeling: Where Have You Been? Where Are You Going To?" *Journal of Medicinal Chemistry* 57 (12): 4977–5010. https://doi.org/10.1021/jm4004285.

Crampon, Kevin, Alexis Giorkallos, Myrtille Deldossi, Stéphanie Baud, and Luiz Angelo Steffenel. 2022. "Machine-Learning Methods for Ligand—Protein Molecular Docking." *Drug Discovery Today* 27 (1): 151–164. https://doi.org/10.1016/j.drudis.2021.09.007.

Cui, Wenqiang, Adnane Aouidate, Shouguo Wang, Qiuliyang Yu, Yanhua Li, and Shuguang Yuan. 2020. "Discovering Anti-Cancer Drugs via Computational Methods." *Frontiers in Pharmacology*. https://doi.org/10.3389/fphar.2020.00733.

Daina, Antoine, Olivier Michielin, and Vincent Zoete. 2017. "SwissADME: A Free Web Tool to Evaluate Pharmacokinetics, Drug-Likeness and Medicinal Chemistry Friendliness of Small Molecules." *Scientific Reports* 7 (1). Nature Publishing Group: 1–13.

Dallakyan, Sargis, and Arthur J Olson. 2015. "Small-Molecule Library Screening by Docking with PyRx." *Methods in Molecular Biology (Clifton, N.J.)* 1263. United States: 243–250. https://doi.org/10.1007/978-1-4939-2269-7_19.

Dana, Dibyendu, Satishkumar V Gadhiya, Luce G St. Surin, David Li, Farha Naaz, Quaisar Ali, Latha Paka, Michael A Yamin, Mahesh Narayan, and Itzhak D Goldberg. 2018. "Deep Learning in Drug Discovery and Medicine; Scratching the Surface." *Molecules* 23 (9). MDPI: 2384.

Das, Tonmoy, Geoffroy Andrieux, Musaddeque Ahmed, and Sajib Chakraborty. 2020. "Integration of Online Omics-Data Resources for Cancer Research." *Frontiers in Genetics*. https://doi.org/10.3389/fgene.2020.578345.

Deeb, Omar, and Mohammad Goodarzi. 2012. "In Silico Quantitative Structure Toxicity Relationship of Chemical Compounds: Some Case Studies." *Current Drug Safety* 7 (4). United Arab Emirates: 289–297. https://doi.org/10.2174/157488612804096533.

De-Eknamkul, Wanchai, Kaoru Umehara, Orawan Monthakantirat, Radovan Toth, Vladimir Frecer, Lorena Knapic, Paolo Braiuca, Hiroshi Noguchi, and Stanislav Miertus. 2011. "QSAR Study of Natural Estrogen-like Isoflavonoids and Diphenolics from Thai Medicinal Plants." *Journal of Molecular Graphics & Modelling* 29 (6). United States: 784–794. https://doi.org/10.1016/j.jmgm.2011.01.001.

Dong, Dong, Zhijian Xu, Wu Zhong, and Shaoliang Peng. 2018. "Parallelization of Molecular Docking: A Review." *Current Topics in Medicinal Chemistry* 18 (12). Bentham Science Publishers: 1015–1028.

Dowden, Helen, and Jamie Munro. 2019. "Trends in Clinical Success Rates and Therapeutic Focus." *Nature Reviews Drug Discovery* 18 (7): 495–496.

Edgar, Ron, Michael Domrachev, and Alex E Lash. 2002. "Gene Expression Omnibus: NCBI Gene Expression and Hybridization Array Data Repository." *Nucleic Acids Research* 30 (1): 207–210. https://doi.org/10.1093/nar/30.1.207.

Ekins, Sean, Bruno Boulanger, Peter W Swaan, and Maggie A Z Hupcey. 2002. "Towards a New Age of Virtual ADME/TOX and Multidimensional Drug Discovery." *Molecular Diversity* 5 (4). Netherlands: 255–275. https://doi.org/10.1023/a:1021376212320.

Ferrari, Stefania, Valeria Losasso, and Maria Costi. 2008. "Sequence-Based Identification of Specific Drug Target Regions in the Thymidylate Synthase Enzyme Family." *ChemMedChem* 3 (April): 392–401. https://doi.org/10.1002/cmdc.200700215.

Fleming, Nic. 2018. "How Artificial Intelligence Is Changing Drug Discovery." *Nature* 557 (7706). Nature Publishing Group: S55.

Gamberi, Tania, Alessandro Pratesi, Luigi Messori, and Lara Massai. 2021. "Proteomics as a Tool to Disclose the Cellular and Molecular Mechanisms of Selected Anticancer Gold Compounds." *Coordination Chemistry Reviews* 438: 213905. https://doi.org/10.1016/j.ccr.2021.213905.

Gao, H, and H Huang. 2018. "Proceedings of the Twenty-Seventh International Joint Conference on Artificial Intelligence." *International Joint Conferences on Artificial Intelligence*, AAAI Press, Washington, DC, USA.

Gawehn, Erik, Jan A Hiss, John B Brown, and Gisbert Schneider. 2018. "Advancing Drug Discovery via GPU-Based Deep Learning." *Expert Opinion on Drug Discovery* 13 (7). Taylor & Francis: 579–582.

Gezici, Sevgi, and Nazım Şekeroğlu. 2019. "Current Perspectives in the Application of Medicinal Plants Against Cancer: Novel Therapeutic Agents." *Anti-Cancer Agents in Medicinal Chemistry* 19 (1). Netherlands: 101–111. https://doi.org/10.2174/1871520619666181224121004.

Golbraikh, Alexander, Xiang Simon Wang, Hao Zhu, and Alexander Tropsha. 2017. "Predictive QSAR Modeling: Methods and Applications in Drug Discovery and Chemical Risk Assessment." In *Handbook of Computational Chemistry*, edited by Jerzy Leszczynski,

Anna Kaczmarek-Kedziera, Tomasz Puzyn, Manthos G Papadopoulos, Heribert Reis, and Manoj K Shukla, 2303–2340. Cham: Springer International Publishing. https://doi.org/10.1007/978-3-319-27282-5_37.

Greenwell, M, and P K S M Rahman. 2015. "Medicinal Plants: Their Use in Anticancer Treatment." *International Journal of Pharmaceutical Sciences and Research* 6 (10): 4103–4112. https://doi.org/10.13040/IJPSR.0975-8232.6(10).4103-12.

Hidayat, Syahrul, Faisal Maulana Ibrahim, Cecep Suhandi, and Muchtaridi Muchtaridi. 2022. "A Systematic Review: Molecular Docking Simulation of Small Molecules as Anticancer Non-Small Cell Lung Carcinoma Drug Candidates." *Journal of Advanced Pharmaceutical Technology & Research* 13 (3). India: 141–147. https://doi.org/10.4103/japtr.japtr_311_21.

Hopkins, Andrew L, György M Keserü, Paul D Leeson, David C Rees, and Charles H Reynolds. 2014. "The Role of Ligand Efficiency Metrics in Drug Discovery." *Nature Reviews. Drug Discovery*. England. https://doi.org/10.1038/nrd4163.

Huang, Danzhi, Urs Lüthi, Peter Kolb, Karin Edler, Marco Cecchini, Stephan Audetat, Alcide Barberis, and Amedeo Caflisch. 2005. "Discovery of Cell-Permeable Non-Peptide Inhibitors of Beta-Secretase by High-Throughput Docking and Continuum Electrostatics Calculations." *Journal of Medicinal Chemistry* 48 (16). United States: 5108–5111. https://doi.org/10.1021/jm050499d.

Ikram, Nur Kusaira Khairul, Jacob D Durrant, Muchtaridi Muchtaridi, Ayunni Salihah Zalaludin, Neny Purwitasari, Nornisah Mohamed, Aisyah Saad Abdul Rahim, Chan Kit Lam, Yahaya M Normi, and Noorsaadah Abd Rahman. 2015. "A Virtual Screening Approach for Identifying Plants with Anti H5N1 Neuraminidase Activity." *Journal of Chemical Information and Modeling* 55 (2). ACS Publications: 308–316.

Irwin, John J, Brian K Shoichet, Michael M Mysinger, Niu Huang, Francesco Colizzi, Pascal Wassam, and Yiqun Cao. 2009. "Automated Docking Screens: A Feasibility Study." *Journal of Medicinal Chemistry* 52 (18). ACS Publications: 5712–5720.

Jagusch, Carsten, Matthias Negri, Ulrike E Hille, Qingzhong Hu, Marc Bartels, Kerstin Jahn-Hoffmann, Mariano A E Pinto-Bazurco Mendieta, Barbara Rodenwaldt, Ursula Müller-Vieira, and Dirk Schmidt. 2008. "Synthesis, Biological Evaluation and Molecular Modelling Studies of Methyleneimidazole Substituted Biaryls as Inhibitors of Human 17α-Hydroxylase-17, 20-Lyase (CYP17). Part I: Heterocyclic Modifications of the Core Structure." *Bioorganic & Medicinal Chemistry* 16 (4). Elsevier: 1992–2010.

Jiménez-Luna, José, Francesca Grisoni, Nils Weskamp, and Gisbert Schneider. 2021. "Artificial Intelligence in Drug Discovery: Recent Advances and Future Perspectives." *Expert Opinion on Drug Discovery* 16 (9). Taylor & Francis: 949–959. https://doi.org/10.1080/17460441.2021.1909567.

Johnson, T, I A Khan, M A Avery, J Grant, and S R Meshnick. 1998. "Quantitative Structure-Activity Relationship Studies of a Series of Sulfa Drugs as Inhibitors of Pneumocystis Carinii Dihydropteroate Synthetase." *Antimicrobial Agents and Chemotherapy* 42 (6): 1454–1458. https://doi.org/10.1128/AAC.42.6.1454.

Kar, Supratik, and Kunal Roy. 2012. "QSAR of Phytochemicals for the Design of Better Drugs." *Expert Opinion on Drug Discovery* 7 (10). England: 877–902. https://doi.org/10.1517/17460441.2012.716420.

Kar, Supratik, and Jerzy Leszczynski. 2020. "Open Access in Silico Tools to Predict the ADMET Profiling of Drug Candidates." *Expert Opinion on Drug Discovery* 15 (12): 1473–1487. https://doi:10.1080/17460441.2020.1798926.

Kesharwani, Rajesh Kumar, Virendra Kumar Vishwakarma, Raj K Keservani, Prabhakar Singh, Nidhi Katiyar, and Sandeep Tripathi. 2020. "Role of ADMET Tools in Current Scenario: Application and Limitations." In *Computer-Aided Drug Design*, edited by Dev Bukhsh Singh, 71–87. Singapore: Springer Singapore. https://doi.org/10.1007/978-981-15-6815-2_4.

Khan, Haroon, Waqas Alam, Khalaf F Alsharif, Michael Aschner, Samreen Pervez, and Luciano Saso. 2022. “Alkaloids and Colon Cancer: Molecular Mechanisms and Therapeutic Implications for Cell Cycle Arrest.” *Molecules (Basel, Switzerland)* 27 (3). https://doi.org/10.3390/molecules27030920.

Kotzabasaki, Marianna, and George Froudakis. 2018. “Review of Computer Simulations on Anti-Cancer Drug Delivery in MOFs.” *Inorganic Chemistry Frontiers* 5 (March). https://doi.org/10.1039/C7QI00645D.

Kumar, Anil, and Praffulla Kumar Arya. 2020. “Database Resources for Drug Discovery.” In *Computer-Aided Drug Design*, edited by Dev Bukhsh Singh, 89–114. Singapore: Springer Singapore. https://doi.org/10.1007/978-981-15-6815-2_5.

Kumar, Roshan, and Purabi Saha. 2022. “A Review on Artificial Intelligence and Machine Learning to Improve Cancer Management and Drug Discovery.” *International Journal for Research in Applied Sciences and Biotechnology* 9 (3 SE-Articles): 149–156. https://doi.org/10.31033/ijrasb.9.3.26.

Labbé, Céline M, Julien Rey, David Lagorce, Marek Vavruša, Jérome Becot, Olivier Sperandio, Bruno O Villoutreix, Pierre Tufféry, and Maria A Miteva. 2015. “MTiOpenScreen: A Web Server for Structure-Based Virtual Screening.” *Nucleic Acids Research* 43 (W1). Oxford University Press: W448–W454.

Lamb, Justin, Emily D Crawford, David Peck, Joshua W Modell, Irene C Blat, Matthew J Wrobel, Jim Lerner, et al. 2006. “The Connectivity Map: Using Gene-Expression Signatures to Connect Small Molecules, Genes, and Disease.” *Science (New York, N.Y.)* 313 (5795). United States: 1929–1935. https://doi.org/10.1126/science.1132939.

Langdon, Sarah R, Isaac M Westwood, Rob L M van Montfort, Nathan Brown, and Julian Blagg. 2013. “Scaffold-Focused Virtual Screening: Prospective Application to the Discovery of TTK Inhibitors.” *Journal of Chemical Information and Modeling* 53 (5): 1100–1112. https://doi.org/10.1021/ci400100c.

Law, Vivian, Craig Knox, Yannick Djoumbou, Tim Jewison, An Chi Guo, Yifeng Liu, Adam Maciejewski, et al. 2013. “DrugBank 4.0: Shedding New Light on Drug Metabolism.” *Nucleic Acids Research*, November. https://doi.org/10.1093/nar/gkt1068.

Lee, Jai Woo, Miguel A Maria-Solano, Thi Ngoc Lan Vu, Sanghee Yoon, and Sun Choi. 2022. “Big Data and Artificial Intelligence (AI) Methodologies for Computer-Aided Drug Design (CADD).” *Biochemical Society Transactions* 50 (1): 241–252. https://doi.org/10.1042/BST20211240.

Lee, Kyeong, and Sangwon Jung. 2012. “3D-QSAR Study of Melanin Inhibiting (S)-(+)-Decursin and Its Analogues by Pharmacophore Mapping.” *Bulletin of the Korean Chemical Society* 33 (1): 149–152. https://doi.org/10.5012/BKCS.2012.33.1.149.

Lee, Su-In, Safiye Celik, Benjamin Logsdon, Scott Lundberg, Timothy Martins, Vivian Oehler, Elihu Estey, et al. 2018. “A Machine Learning Approach to Integrate Big Data for Precision Medicine in Acute Myeloid Leukemia.” *Nature Communications* 9 (January). https://doi.org/10.1038/s41467-017-02465-5.

Lengauer, T, and M Rarey. 1996. “Computational Methods for Biomolecular Docking.” *Current Opinion in Structural Biology* 6 (3). England: 402–406. https://doi.org/10.1016/s0959-440x(96)80061-3.

Li, A P. 2001. “Screening for Human ADME/Tox Drug Properties in Drug Discovery.” *Drug Discovery Today* 6 (7). England: 357–366. https://doi.org/10.1016/s1359-6446(01)01712-3.

Li, Honglin, Zhenting Gao, Ling Kang, Hailei Zhang, Kun Yang, Kunqian Yu, Xiaomin Luo, Weiliang Zhu, Kaixian Chen, and Jianhua Shen. 2006. “TarFisDock: A Web Server for Identifying Drug Targets with Docking Approach.” *Nucleic Acids Research* 34 (suppl_2). Oxford University Press: W219–W224.

Li, Ying Hong, Chun Yan Yu, Xiao Xu Li, Peng Zhang, Jing Tang, Qingxia Yang, Tingting Fu, et al. 2018. "Therapeutic Target Database Update 2018: Enriched Resource for Facilitating Bench-to-Clinic Research of Targeted Therapeutics." *Nucleic Acids Research* 46 (D1): D1121–D1127. https://doi.org/10.1093/nar/gkx1076.

Lin, Xubo. 2022. "Chapter 27—Applications of Molecular Dynamics Simulations in Drug Discovery." In *Advances in Protein Molecular and Structural Biology Methods*, 455–465. Academic Press. https://doi.org/10.1016/B978-0-323-90264-9.00027-1.

Liu, Minghui, Song Xu, Yuli Wang, Ying Li, Yongwen Li, Hongbing Zhang, Hongyu Liu, and Jun Chen. 2016. "PD 0332991, a Selective Cyclin D Kinase 4/6 Inhibitor, Sensitizes Lung Cancer Cells to Treatment with Epidermal Growth Factor Receptor Tyrosine Kinase Inhibitors." *Oncotarget* 7 (51). Impact Journals, LLC: 84951.

Liu, Xuewei, Danfeng Shi, Shuangyan Zhou, Hongli Liu, Huanxiang Liu, and Xiaojun Yao. 2018. "Molecular Dynamics Simulations and Novel Drug Discovery." *Expert Opinion on Drug Discovery* 13 (1). England: 23–37. https://doi.org/10.1080/17460441.2018.1403419.

López de Maturana, Evangelina, Lola Alonso, Pablo Alarcón, Isabel Adoración Martín-Antoniano, Silvia Pineda, Lucas Piorno, M Luz Calle, and Núria Malats. 2019. "Challenges in the Integration of Omics and Non-Omics Data." *Genes* 10 (3). https://doi.org/10.3390/genes10030238.

Loukatou, Styliani, Louis Papageorgiou, Paraskevas Fakourelis, Arianna Filntisi, Eleftheria Polychronidou, Ioannis Bassis, Vasileios Megalooikonomou, Wojciech Makałowski, Dimitrios Vlachakis, and Sophia Kossida. 2014. "Molecular Dynamics Simulations Through GPU Video Games Technologies." *Journal of Molecular Biochemistry* 3 (2). NIH Public Access: 64.

Lounkine, Eugen, Michael J Keiser, Steven Whitebread, Dmitri Mikhailov, Jacques Hamon, Jeremy L Jenkins, Paul Lavan, Eckhard Weber, Allison K Doak, and Serge Côté. 2012. "Large-Scale Prediction and Testing of Drug Activity on Side-Effect Targets." *Nature* 486 (7403). Nature Publishing Group: 361–367.

Lu, Chafen, Li-Zhi Mi, Thomas Schürpf, Thomas Walz, and Timothy A Springer. 2012. "Mechanisms for Kinase-Mediated Dimerization of the Epidermal Growth Factor Receptor." *Journal of Biological Chemistry* 287 (45). ASBMB: 38244–38253.

Mahmud, S M Hasan, Wenyu Chen, Hosney Jahan, Yongsheng Liu, Nasir Islam Sujan, and Saeed Ahmed. 2019. "IDTi-CSsmoteB: Identification of Drug—Target Interaction Based on Drug Chemical Structure and Protein Sequence Using XGBoost with Over-Sampling Technique SMOTE." *IEEE Access* 7. IEEE: 48699–48714.

Mak, Kit-Kay, and Mallikarjuna Rao Pichika. 2019. "Artificial Intelligence in Drug Development: Present Status and Future Prospects." *Drug Discovery Today* 24 (3). Elsevier: 773–780.

Mangal, Manu, Parul Sagar, Harinder Singh, Gajendra P S Raghava, and Subhash M Agarwal. 2013. "NPACT: Naturally Occurring Plant-Based Anti-Cancer Compound-Activity-Target Database." *Nucleic Acids Research* 41 (Database issue): D1124–D1129. https://doi.org/10.1093/nar/gks1047.

Mao, Jiashun, Javed Akhtar, Xiao Zhang, Liang Sun, Shenghui Guan, Xinyu Li, Guangming Chen, et al. 2021. "Comprehensive Strategies of Machine-Learning-Based Quantitative Structure-Activity Relationship Models." *IScience* 24 (9): 103052. https://doi.org/10.1016/j.isci.2021.103052.

Martel, Catherine de, Damien Georges, Freddie Bray, Jacques Ferlay, and Gary M Clifford. 2020. "Global Burden of Cancer Attributable to Infections in 2018: A Worldwide Incidence Analysis." *The Lancet. Global Health* 8 (2). England: e180–e190. https://doi.org/10.1016/S2214-109X(19)30488-7.

Masago, Katsuhiro, Yosuke Togashi, Masahide Fukudo, Tomohiro Terada, Kaoru Irisa, Yuichi Sakamori, Shiro Fujita, Young Hak Kim, Tadashi Mio, and Ken-ichi Inui. 2010. "Good Clinical Response to Erlotinib in a Non-Small Cell Lung Cancer Patient Harboring Multiple Brain Metastases and a Double Active Somatic Epidermal Growth Factor Gene Mutation." *Case Reports in Oncology* 3 (2). Karger Publishers: 98–105.

McKusick, Victor A. 2007. "Mendelian Inheritance in Man and Its Online Version, OMIM." *American Journal of Human Genetics* 80 (4): 588–604. https://doi.org/10.1086/514346.

Mohanraj, Karthikeyan, Bagavathy Shanmugam Karthikeyan, R P Vivek-Ananth, R P Chand, S R Aparna, Pattulingam Mangalapandi, and Areejit Samal. 2018. "IMPPAT: A Curated Database of Indian Medicinal Plants, Phytochemistry and Therapeutics." *Scientific Reports* 8 (1). Nature Publishing Group: 1–17.

Negrier, S, E Jäger, C Porta, D McDermott, M Moore, J Bellmunt, S Anderson, F Cihon, J Lewis, and B Escudier. 2010. "Efficacy and Safety of Sorafenib in Patients with Advanced Renal Cell Carcinoma with and without Prior Cytokine Therapy, a Subanalysis of TARGET." *Medical Oncology* 27 (3). Springer: 899–906.

Neves, Bruno J, Rodolpho C Braga, Cleber C Melo-Filho, José Teófilo Moreira-Filho, Eugene N Muratov, and Carolina Horta Andrade. 2018. "QSAR-Based Virtual Screening: Advances and Applications in Drug Discovery." *Frontiers in Pharmacology*. https://doi.org/10.3389/fphar.2018.01275.

Newman, David J, and Gordon M Cragg. 2007. "Natural Products as Sources of New Drugs Over the Last 25 Years." *Journal of Natural Products* 70 (3). United States: 461–477. https://doi.org/10.1021/np068054v.

Oyebode, Oyinlola, Ngianga-Bakwin Kandala, Peter J Chilton, and Richard J Lilford. 2016. "Use of Traditional Medicine in Middle-Income Countries: A WHO-SAGE Study." *Health Policy and Planning* 31 (8): 984–991. https://doi.org/10.1093/heapol/czw022.

Öztürk, Hakime, Arzucan Özgür, and Elif Ozkirimli. 2018. "DeepDTA: Deep Drug—Target Binding Affinity Prediction." *Bioinformatics* 34 (17). Oxford University Press: i821–i829.

Paananen, Jussi, and Vittorio Fortino. 2020. "An Omics Perspective on Drug Target Discovery Platforms." *Briefings in Bioinformatics* 21 (6): 1937–1953. https://doi.org/10.1093/bib/bbz122.

Patel, Mishal N, Mark D Halling-Brown, Joseph E Tym, Paul Workman, and Bissan Al-Lazikani. 2013. "Objective Assessment of Cancer Genes for Drug Discovery." *Nature Reviews. Drug Discovery*. England. https://doi.org/10.1038/nrd3913.

Paul, Debleena, Gaurav Sanap, Snehal Shenoy, Dnyaneshwar Kalyane, Kiran Kalia, and Rakesh K Tekade. 2021. "Artificial Intelligence in Drug Discovery and Development." *Drug Discovery Today* 26 (1). England: 80–93. https://doi.org/10.1016/j.drudis.2020.10.010.

Perez-Sanchez, Horacio, and Wolfgang Wenzel. 2011. "Optimization Methods for Virtual Screening on Novel Computational Architectures." *Current Computer-Aided Drug Design* 7 (1). Bentham Science Publishers: 44–52.

Perkins, Roger, Hong Fang, Weida Tong, and William J Welsh. 2003. "Quantitative Structure-Activity Relationship Methods: Perspectives on Drug Discovery and Toxicology." *Environmental Toxicology and Chemistry* 22 (8). United States: 1666–1679. https://doi.org/10.1897/01-171.

Piñero, Janet, Àlex Bravo, Núria Queralt-Rosinach, Alba Gutiérrez-Sacristán, Jordi Deu-Pons, Emilio Centeno, Javier García-García, Ferran Sanz, and Laura I Furlong. 2017. "DisGeNET: A Comprehensive Platform Integrating Information on Human Disease-Associated Genes and Variants." *Nucleic Acids Research* 45 (D1): D833–D839. https://doi.org/10.1093/nar/gkw943.

Piñero, Janet, Núria Queralt-Rosinach, Àlex Bravo, Jordi Deu-Pons, Anna Bauer-Mehren, Martin Baron, Ferran Sanz, and Laura I Furlong. 2015. "DisGeNET: A Discovery Platform for the Dynamical Exploration of Human Diseases and Their Genes." *Database: The Journal of Biological Databases and Curation* 2015: bav028. https://doi.org/10.1093/database/bav028.

Prachayasittikul, Veda, Apilak Worachartcheewan, Watshara Shoombuatong, Napat Songtawee, Saw Simeon, Virapong Prachayasittikul, and Chanin Nantasenamat. 2015. "Computer-Aided Drug Design of Bioactive Natural Products." *Current Topics in Medicinal Chemistry* 15 (18). United Arab Emirates: 1780–1800. https://doi.org/10.2174/1568026615666150506151101.

Rahman, Md Mominur, Md Rezaul Islam, Firoza Rahman, Md Saidur Rahaman, Md Shajib Khan, Sayedul Abrar, Tanmay Kumar Ray, et al. 2022. "Emerging Promise of Computational Techniques in Anti-Cancer Research: At a Glance." *Bioengineering (Basel, Switzerland)* 9 (8). Switzerland. https://doi.org/10.3390/bioengineering9080335.

Rajasekharan, P E, and Shabir Hussain Wani. 2020. "Distribution, Diversity, Conservation and Utilization of Threatened Medicinal Plants." In Rajasekharan, P E, and Shabir Hussain Wani. (eds) *Conservation and Utilization of Threatened Medicinal Plants*. Cham: Springer. https://doi.org/10.1007/978-3-030-39793-7

Rao, Narsing, Manik Prabhu, Min Xiao, and Wen-Jun Li. 2017. "Fungal and Bacterial Pigments: Secondary Metabolites with Wide Applications." *Frontiers in Microbiology*. https://doi.org/10.3389/fmicb.2017.01113.

Rastelli, Giulio, and Luca Pinzi. 2019. "Refinement and Rescoring of Virtual Screening Results." *Frontiers in Chemistry* 7. Frontiers Media SA: 498.

Rastelli, Giulio, Alberto Del Rio, Gianluca Degliesposti, and Miriam Sgobba. 2010. "Fast and Accurate Predictions of Binding Free Energies Using MM-PBSA and MM-GBSA." *Journal of Computational Chemistry* 31 (4). United States: 797–810. https://doi.org/10.1002/jcc.21372.

Rodig, Scott J, and Geoffrey I Shapiro. 2010. "Crizotinib, a Small-Molecule Dual Inhibitor of the c-Met and ALK Receptor Tyrosine Kinases." *Current Opinion in Investigational Drugs (London, England: 2000)* 11 (12): 1477–1490.

Romano, Joseph D, and Nicholas P Tatonetti. 2019. "Informatics and Computational Methods in Natural Product Drug Discovery: A Review and Perspectives." *Frontiers in Genetics*. https://doi.org/10.3389/fgene.2019.00368.

Sabbah, Dima A, Rima Hajjo, and Kamal Sweidan. 2020. "Review on Epidermal Growth Factor Receptor (EGFR) Structure, Signaling Pathways, Interactions, and Recent Updates of EGFR Inhibitors." *Current Topics in Medicinal Chemistry* 20 (10): 815–834. http://dx.doi.org/10.2174/1568026620666200303123102

Sachlos, Eleftherios, Ruth M Risueño, Sarah Laronde, Zoya Shapovalova, Jong-Hee Lee, Jennifer Russell, Monika Malig, et al. 2012. "Identification of Drugs Including a Dopamine Receptor Antagonist That Selectively Target Cancer Stem Cells." *Cell* 149 (6). United States: 1284–1297. https://doi.org/10.1016/j.cell.2012.03.049.

Saldívar-González, F I, V D Aldas-Bulos, J L Medina-Franco, and F Plisson. 2022. "Natural Product Drug Discovery in the Artificial Intelligence Era." *Chemical Science* 13 (6). The Royal Society of Chemistry: 1526–1546. https://doi.org/10.1039/D1SC04471K.

Salo-Ahen, Outi M H, Ida Alanko, Rajendra Bhadane, Alexandre M J J Bonvin, Rodrigo V Honorato, Shakhawath Hossain, André H Juffer, et al. 2021. "Molecular Dynamics Simulations in Drug Discovery and Pharmaceutical Development." *Processes*. https://doi.org/10.3390/pr9010071.

Schneider, Gisbert, Petra Schneider, and Steffen Renner. 2006. "Scaffold-Hopping: How Far Can You Jump?" *QSAR & Combinatorial Science* 25 (12). John Wiley & Sons, Ltd: 1162–1171. https://doi.org/10.1002/qsar.200610091.

Schuffenhauer, Ansgar. 2012. "Computational Methods for Scaffold Hopping." *Wiley Interdisciplinary Reviews: Computational Molecular Science* 2 (November). https://doi.org/10.1002/wcms.1106.

Segall, Matthew. 2014. "Advances in Multiparameter Optimization Methods for de Novo Drug Design." *Expert Opinion on Drug Discovery* 9 (7). Taylor & Francis: 803–817. https://doi.org/10.1517/17460441.2014.913565.

Sharma, Vivekanand, and Indra Neil Sarkar. 2013. "Bioinformatics Opportunities for Identification and Study of Medicinal Plants." *Briefings in Bioinformatics* 14 (2): 238–250. https://doi.org/10.1093/bib/bbs021.

Shoemaker, Robert H. 2006. "The NCI60 Human Tumour Cell Line Anticancer Drug Screen." *Nature Reviews. Cancer.* England. https://doi.org/10.1038/nrc1951.

Shukla, Rohit, and Timir Tripathi. 2021. "Molecular Dynamics Simulation in Drug Discovery: Opportunities and Challenges." In *Innovations and Implementations of Computer Aided Drug Discovery Strategies in Rational Drug Design*, edited by Sanjeev Kumar Singh, 295–316. Singapore: Springer Singapore. https://doi.org/10.1007/978-981-15-8936-2_12.

Singh, Sakshi, Qanita Bani Baker, and Dev Bukhsh Singh. 2022. "Chapter 18—Molecular Docking and Molecular Dynamics Simulation." In *Bioinformatics Pathak*, edited by Dev Bukhsh Singh and Rajesh Kumar, 291–304. Academic Press. https://doi.org/10.1016/B978-0-323-89775-4.00014-6.

Stone, John E, David J Hardy, Ivan S Ufimtsev, and Klaus Schulten. 2010. "GPU-Accelerated Molecular Modeling Coming of Age." *Journal of Molecular Graphics and Modelling* 29 (2). Elsevier: 116–125.

Strohl, W R. 2000. "The Role of Natural Products in a Modern Drug Discovery Program." *Drug Discovery Today* 5 (2). England: 39–41. https://doi.org/10.1016/s1359-6446(99)01443-9.

Subramaniam, Shonia, Kanga Rani Selvaduray, and Ammu Kutty Radhakrishnan. 2019. "Bioactive Compounds: Natural Defense against Cancer?" *Biomolecules* 9 (12). MDPI: 758.

Subramanian, Aravind, Rajiv Narayan, Steven M Corsello, David D Peck, Ted E Natoli, Xiaodong Lu, Joshua Gould, et al. 2017. "A Next Generation Connectivity Map: L1000 Platform and the First 1,000,000 Profiles." *Cell* 171 (6): 1437–1452.e17. https://doi.org/10.1016/j.cell.2017.10.049.

Sun, Hongmao, Gregory Tawa, and Anders Wallqvist. 2012. "Classification of Scaffold-Hopping Approaches." *Drug Discovery Today* 17 (7–8): 310–324. https://doi.org/10.1016/j.drudis.2011.10.024.

Taft, Carlton A, Vinicius Barreto Da Silva, and Carlos Henrique Tomich De Paula Da Silva. 2008. "Current Topics in Computer-Aided Drug Design." *Journal of Pharmaceutical Sciences* 97 (3). United States: 1089–1098. https://doi.org/10.1002/jps.21293.

Thiel, Karl. 2004. "Structure-Aided Drug Design's Next Generation." *Nature Biotechnology* 22 (June): 513–519. https://doi.org/10.1038/nbt0504-513.

Torres, Pedro H M, Ana C R Sodero, Paula Jofily, and Floriano P Silva-Jr. 2019. "Key Topics in Molecular Docking for Drug Design." *International Journal of Molecular Sciences* 20 (18). https://doi.org/10.3390/ijms20184574.

Tran, Tien-Dzung, and Duc-Tinh Pham. 2021. "Identification of Anticancer Drug Target Genes Using an Outside Competitive Dynamics Model on Cancer Signaling Networks." *Scientific Reports* 11 (1): 14095. https://doi.org/10.1038/s41598-021-93336-z.

Urbina, Fabio, Filippa Lentzos, Cédric Invernizzi, and Sean Ekins. 2022. "Dual Use of Artificial-Intelligence-Powered Drug Discovery." *Nature Machine Intelligence* 4 (3): 189–191. https://doi.org/10.1038/s42256-022-00465-9.

Vivo, Marco De, Matteo Masetti, Giovanni Bottegoni, and Andrea Cavalli. 2016. "Role of Molecular Dynamics and Related Methods in Drug Discovery." *Journal of Medicinal Chemistry* 59 (9). ACS Publications: 4035–4061.

Walters, W Patrick, and Regina Barzilay. 2021. "Critical Assessment of AI in Drug Discovery." *Expert Opinion on Drug Discovery* 16 (9). Taylor & Francis: 937–947. https://doi.org/10.1080/17460441.2021.1915982.

Wang, Jui-Chih, Pei-Ying Chu, Chung-Ming Chen, and Jung-Hsin Lin. 2012. "IdTarget: A Web Server for Identifying Protein Targets of Small Chemical Molecules with Robust Scoring Functions and a Divide-and-Conquer Docking Approach." *Nucleic Acids Research* 40 (W1). Oxford University Press: W393–W399.

Wang, Xiaoyu, Linfeng Xu, Yuanzhi Lao, Hongmei Zhang, and Hongxi Xu. 2018. "Natural Products Targeting EGFR Signaling Pathways as Potential Anticancer Drugs." *Current Protein & Peptide Science* 19 (4). United Arab Emirates: 380–388. https://doi.org/10.2174/1389203718666170106104211.

Whirl-Carrillo, M, E M McDonagh, J M Hebert, L Gong, K Sangkuhl, C F Thorn, R B Altman, and T E Klein. 2012. "Pharmacogenomics Knowledge for Personalized Medicine." *Clinical Pharmacology and Therapeutics* 92 (4): 414–417. https://doi.org/10.1038/clpt.2012.96.

Wishart, David S, Craig Knox, An Chi Guo, Dean Cheng, Savita Shrivastava, Dan Tzur, Bijaya Gautam, and Murtaza Hassanali. 2008. "DrugBank: A Knowledgebase for Drugs, Drug Actions and Drug Targets." *Nucleic Acids Research* 36 (Database issue): D901–D906. https://doi.org/10.1093/nar/gkm958.

Wishart, David S, Craig Knox, An Chi Guo, Savita Shrivastava, Murtaza Hassanali, Paul Stothard, Zhan Chang, and Jennifer Woolsey. 2006. "DrugBank: A Comprehensive Resource for in Silico Drug Discovery and Exploration." *Nucleic Acids Research* 34 (Database issue): D668–D672. https://doi.org/10.1093/nar/gkj067.

Wu, Yang, Feilong Zhang, Kuo Yang, Shuangsang Fang, Dechao Bu, Hui Li, Liang Sun, Hairuo Hu, Kuo Gao, and Wei Wang. 2019. "SymMap: An Integrative Database of Traditional Chinese Medicine Enhanced by Symptom Mapping." *Nucleic Acids Research* 47 (D1). Oxford University Press: D1110–D1117.

Xia, Wenle, Zuguo Liu, Rongrong Zong, Leihua Liu, Sumin Zhao, Sarah S Bacus, Yubin Mao, Jia He, Julia D Wulfkuhle, and Emanuel F Petricoin. 2011. "Truncated ErbB2 Expressed in Tumor Cell Nuclei Contributes to Acquired Therapeutic Resistance to ErbB2 Kinase InhibitorsTruncated, Nuclear ErbB2 and Resistance to ErbB2 TKI." *Molecular Cancer Therapeutics* 10 (8). AACR: 1367–1374.

Xie, Tao, Lan Zhang, Shouyue Zhang, Liang Ouyang, Haoyang Cai, and Bo Liu. 2016. "ACTP: A Webserver for Predicting Potential Targets and Relevant Pathways of Autophagy-Modulating Compounds." *Oncotarget* 7 (9). Impact Journals: 10015–10022.

Yang, Xin, Yifei Wang, Ryan Byrne, Gisbert Schneider, and Shengyong Yang. 2019. "Concepts of Artificial Intelligence for Computer-Assisted Drug Discovery." *Chemical Reviews* 119 (18). American Chemical Society: 10520–10594. https://doi.org/10.1021/acs.chemrev.8b00728.

Yu, Hongshi, and Adedayo Adedoyin. 2003. "ADME-Tox in Drug Discovery: Integration of Experimental and Computational Technologies." *Drug Discovery Today* 8 (18). England: 852–861. https://doi.org/10.1016/s1359-6446(03)02828-9.

Yuan, Haidan, Qianqian Ma, Li Ye, and Guangchun Piao. 2016. "The Traditional Medicine and Modern Medicine from Natural Products." *Molecules (Basel, Switzerland)* 21 (5). https://doi.org/10.3390/molecules21050559.

Zeng, Xian, Peng Zhang, Yali Wang, Chu Qin, Shangying Chen, Weidong He, Lin Tao, Ying Tan, Dan Gao, and Bohua Wang. 2019. "CMAUP: A Database of Collective Molecular Activities of Useful Plants." *Nucleic Acids Research* 47 (D1). Oxford University Press: D1118–D1127.

Zitnik, Marinka, Monica Agrawal, and Jure Leskovec. 2018. "Modeling Polypharmacy Side Effects with Graph Convolutional Networks." *Bioinformatics* 34 (13): i457–i466. https://doi.org/10.1101/258814.

3 Recent Advances in Anticancer Activity and Bioinformatics Approach from Potential Plants

Odangowei Inetiminebi Ogidi†
Department of Biochemistry, Faculty of Basic Medical Sciences, Bayelsa Medical University, Yenagoa, Bayelsa State, Nigeria
†Corresponding Author: ogidiodangowei@gmail.com

ABBREVIATIONS

AKBA	Acetyl-11-keto-boswellic acid
Akt/PKB	Protein kinase B
AP-1	Activating protein 1
CMAUP	Collective Molecular Activities of Useful Plants
COX-2	Cyclooxygenase-2
DNA	Deoxyribonucleic acid
EGF	Epidermal growth factor
EMA	European Medicines Agency
FDA	Food and Drug Administration
FTIR	Fourier-transform infrared
HCC	Hepatocellular carcinomas
HNE-2	4-Hydroxy-2-nonenal
HPLC	High-performance liquid chromatography
ID3	Iterative dichotomiser-3
IMPLAD	Indian Medicinal Plants Database
IMPPT	Indian Medicinal Plants, Phytochemistry and Therapeutics
iNOS	Inducible nitric oxide synthase
IO	Intraosseous
LLC	Lewis lung cancer
MCF-7	Michigan Cancer Foundation-7
NF-kB	Nuclear factor kappa B
NMR	Nuclear magnetic resonance
NO	Nitric acid
PC3	Prostate cancer
PD	Pharmacodynamics

DOI: 10.1201/9781003354437-3

PK	Pharmacokinetics
QSAR	Quantitative structure-activity relationship
QSP	Quantitative systems pharmacology
ROS	Reactive oxygen species
SPQSP	Special quantitative systems pharmacology
STAT-3	Signal transducer and activator of transcription 3
TLC	Thin-layer chromatography
TNBC	Triple-negative breast cancer
TPA	Third-party administrator
VEGF	Vascular endothelial growth factor
WHO	World Health Organization

3.1 INTRODUCTION

In 2018, there were 9.6 million cancer-related deaths and 18.1 million new cases (Jemal et al. 2011). Cancer has 36 distinct forms and mostly affects men and women in various ways, including colorectal, liver, lung, stomach, and prostate cancers in men and the breast, cervix, colorectal, lung, and thyroid cancers in women (Bray et al. 2018). The major cause of the rising number of cancer cases is the global population's shifting lifestyle. According to statistics, lung cancer affects men more often than women, accounting for 17% of all cancer cases in men, whereas breast cancer affects roughly 23% of women's cancer cases (Jemal et al. 2011).

Cancer patient survival rates are poor in developing nations due to delayed diagnosis and insufficient treatment options. Therefore, an urgent need is required for more potent treatment and prevention approaches to this pandemic illness. The study of cancer treatment has expanded significantly. Both traditional and very contemporary methods are used to treat cancer. Cancer is treated using a range of methods, including surgery, radiation treatment, and chemotherapy; however, each one has its own disadvantages (Karpuz et al. 2018). The usage of traditional chemicals is hazardous and has adverse effects (Nobili et al. 2009). Therefore, in order to reduce the number of deaths caused by this pandemic illness, innovative cancer preventive and treatment methods are urgently required.

The therapeutic potential of medicinal plants as a source of strong anticancer drugs has recently attracted increased attention from the scientific community. The vast majority of different kinds of bioactive chemicals with a variety of therapeutic characteristics are thought to be stored in medicinal plants. Over a very long time, the medicinal potential of plants has been thoroughly investigated which includes anti-inflammatory, antiviral, anticancer, antimalarial, antibacterial, antifungal, antiplasmodial, antioxidant, and analgesic, to mention just a few of the therapeutic benefits of medicinal plants (Ogidi 2022, 2023; More et al. 2022; Ogidi and Enenebeaku 2023; Vaou et al. 2022; Enenebeaku et al. 2022a, 2022b; Lobiuc et al. 2023; Ogidi et al. 2022).

Herbal medicine has developed into a highly secure, non-toxic, and widely accessible source of chemicals that treat cancer. Due to a variety of properties, herbs are thought to counteract the impact of illnesses on the body (Cheng 1995). For instance, among the various anticancer medicinal plants, *Fagonia indica* (local name: Dhamasa) and *Phaleria macrocarpa* (local name: Mahkota dewa) have historically been employed for the anticancer effects of their active components (Shehab et al. 2011; Faried et al. 2007). The plant material's metabolites are employed to cause cancer cells to undergo apoptosis. Gallic acid, which was isolated as the active ingredient from *P. macrocarpa's* fruit extract, has been shown to have a part in the activation of apoptosis in lung cancer, leukaemia, and colon adenocarcinoma cell lines (Sohi et al. 2003; Inoue et al. 1994). It is a polyhydroxy phenolic chemical that is found in a range of organic foods, including grapes, strawberries, bananas, green tea, and vegetables. It is also a natural antioxidant (Sun et al. 2002). Additionally, it is essential for stopping the growth of cancer and transforming malignancies (Taraphdar 2001).

Similar to this, different substances from other plants, including vinca alkaloids, podophyllotoxin, and camptothecin, are used to treat cancer. The usage of herbs was long forgotten due to the development of the industrial sector and industrial medicine (Pal and Shukla 2003). The development of new procedures has lowered obstacles relating to natural substances, and interest in using such natural constituents in the pharmaceutical business has grown (Koehn and Carter 2005; Saklani and Kutty 2008). The WHO estimates that traditional medical practices are used in 80% of the world's population (Wang et al. 2012). Modern biomolecular research, which identifies certain significant qualities including anticancer, anti-inflammatory, and antiviral, helps us understand the impacts or activities of herbs on numerous targets.

These herbal medicines' actions against various malignancies have also been discovered as our knowledge of their effects grows. For instance, hepatocellular carcinoma (HCC) is the fifth most prevalent cancer in the world, and its frequency is rising (Fattovich et al. 2004; Liovet 2005). It has been shown in several research studies on the treatment and prevention of HCC with herbal medicine that all stages of HCC, including start, development, and progression, may be impacted by herbal components (Rvan et al. 2006).

The literature and resources that are now accessible in this field are often dispersed, which makes it difficult to quickly take advantage of the little knowledge on medicinal plants. The diversity of chemicals may be analysed computationally using a variety of methods. These methods have been crucial to computer-aided drug design (Jorgensen 2004). To keep up with the increasingly demanding pharmaceutical demands, the area of drug design and discovery from medicinal plants necessitates the implementation of methodologies for faster and more effective advancement. Huge amounts of data produced by molecular biology–based procedures may be analysed and interpreted utilising a variety of vital tools provided by bioinformatics. Such methods have become more important in data analysis and integration to infer information from a total systems perspective as high-throughput techniques have advanced.

The identification of genes and pathways that may be linked to significant bioactive secondary metabolites from medicinal plants is facilitated by the use of bioinformatics methods (Saito and Matsuda 2010). The development of cancer and phytochemical mechanisms of action, the process of creating phytochemical drugs from plants, the main phytochemical components with anticancer properties, the anticancer activity of medicinal plants, bioinformatics approaches, current developments in indigenous medicinal plant informatics, cancer treatment options, and the regulatory aspects of herbal anticancer drugs are all covered in this chapter.

3.2 DEVELOPMENT OF CANCER AND PHYTOCHEMICAL PATHWAYS OF ACTION

Over the years, several studies have been done to determine the precise mechanism of carcinogenesis. Carcinogenesis was shown by Sporn and Liby (2020) to be a multi-step process with three primary stages, including start, promotion, and advancement. A carcinogen often undergoes detoxification once it enters the body. It could, however, be triggered by several metabolic pathways. According to Klaunig and Wang (2018), carcinogenic substances cause DNA damage, induce oxidative stress, and start the carcinogenesis process. During the promotion phase, cells begin to proliferate, which results in the buildup of preneoplastic cells. The third and final phase, known as the progression phase, sees the invasion and dissemination of these preneoplastic cells throughout the body (Klaunig 2018).

Due to the involvement of several routes in both the development and progression of cancer, the prevention and treatment of cancer by a single pathway does not seem to be a successful method (Ranjan et al. 2019). A few obstacles affect all treatment plans, such as chemotherapy's adverse effects and medication resistance (Nedeljkovic and Damjanovic 2019). These obstacles have made it challenging for researchers to effectively design diverse cancer therapy options (Chan et al. 2017). Another strategy that is extensively used across the globe is chemoprevention. Some people have even observed that it is effective throughout the promotion and progression stages of carcinogenesis (Koh et al. 2020). The chemopreventive drugs are often divided into two main groups: blocking agents and suppressive agents, both of which are mostly derived from plant phytochemicals (Dewanje et al. 2021). The method by which blocking agents function is different; they stop the metabolic pathway from being activated by carcinogens and prevent them from interacting with the biomolecule. Conversely, suppressive chemicals function in a different manner to stop the growth or spread of malignant cells (Igbai et al. 2019). The majority of the time, chemopreventive drugs control certain enzyme activities and cell cycles or have an antiproliferative and antioxidant impact. Additionally, these substances control signal transduction pathways and stop the development of cancer (Steward and Brown 2013)

3.3 STEPS INVOLVED IN THE DEVELOPMENT OF PHYTOCHEMICAL DRUGS FROM THE MEDICINAL PLANTS

The potency of plants' active phytochemicals dictates how effective they are as medicinal agents. The age of the plants, environment, season, and other crucial variables have an impact on the quality of phytochemicals in plants. On the other hand, certain plant portions contain more bioactive phytochemicals than others. The active phytochemical may be purified using a variety of methods, such as bioassay-guided fractionation, combinatorial chemistry, and isolation tests (Sebastian et al. 2020).

In the case of bioassay-guided fractionation, a variety of analytical methods may be utilised to separate bioactive molecules from a mixture of chemicals. Testing natural extracts from dry or wet plant material is the first step in determining the biological activity (Sebastian et al. 2020). Suitable matrices are employed for the fractionation of active extract, and several analytical methods, including mass spectroscopy, HPLC, TLC, FTIR, and NMR, are used to separate the active chemicals (Sebastian et al. 2020).

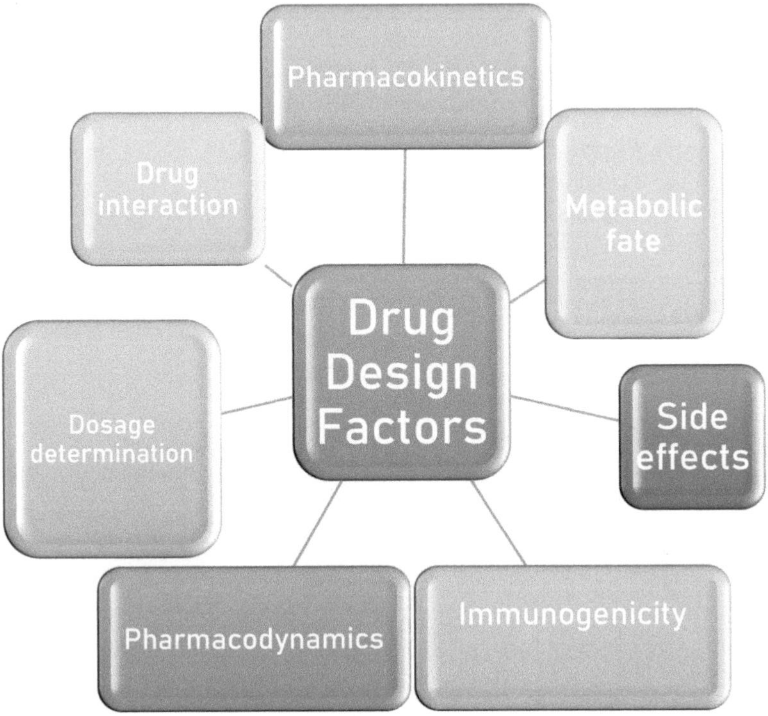

FIGURE 3.1 Factors to be considered in drug design.

The solvents that may be employed for the separation come in a wide range. Silica, superdex, and other suitable matrices may be utilised for the fractionation. The natural bioactive substances present in medicinal plants may be found using a variety of colours. Additionally, when these phytochemicals have been purified, they are examined for *in vivo* or *in vitro* anticancer properties (Sessions et al. 2020). After attaining anticancerous outcomes, future medication design will concentrate on additional factors as shown in Figure 3.1.

3.4 MAJOR PHYTOCHEMICAL CONSTITUENTS WITH ANTICANCER PROPERTIES

Phytochemical compounds with anticancer properties are shown in Figure 3.2.

3.4.1 Flavonoids

Flavonoids are thought to be powerful antioxidants and have antiangiogenic properties (Ogidi et al. 2019b). According to several studies, flavonoids suppress the metabolic activation of carcinogens and halt the formation of aberrant cells that might later turn into malignant cells (Hassan et al. 2014). Some plant families' essential phytochemical components are thought to be flavonoids and their derivatives.

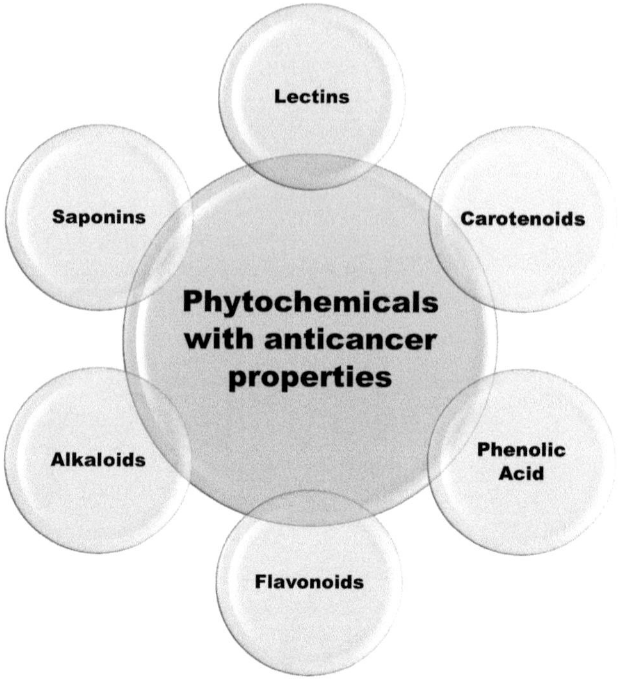

FIGURE 3.2 Phytochemicals with anticancer properties

Chalcone, flavones, flavonol, isoflavones, a flavonol glycoside, prenylated flavonoids, and lavandulyl flavanones are some of the most significant flavonoids that have been identified from the diverse plant groups (Agbo et al. 2015). Prenylated flavonoids from several Fabaceae family members are known to have antioxidant and anticancer effects, according to Krishna et al. (2012). In a study, Kleemann et al. (2011) acknowledged that flavonoids might be utilised as a preventative measure against oxidative stress, cellular inflammation, and certain types of cancer. However, an isoflavones extract from bean sprouts demonstrated inhibitory effects on the breast cancer MCF-7 cell line (Sebastian et al. 2020). Additionally, *Cicer arietinum* L. isoflavone extract was discovered by Wang et al. (2020) to have a suppressive impact on MCF-7 breast cancer cells. Microscopic studies and findings from flow cytometry confirmed the inhibitory impact on MCF-7 cell lines, and *C. arietinum* isoflavones at a concentration of 32 g mL-1 are sufficient to induce MCF-7 to undergo apoptosis.

Clinical investigations have shown that isoflavones have a beneficial impact on human health by avoiding certain malignancies, particularly those that are hormone-dependent. Another significant genus in the Fabaceae family with anticancer properties is *Eriosema chenense* (Cornwell et al. 2004). Lung cancer and oral epidermal carcinoma are two cancers that are inhibited by flavonoids from species including *E. chenense* Vogel, *E. griseum* Baker, and *E. robustum* Baker (Ateba et al. 2021).

According to Aregueta-Robles et al. (2018), *Phaseolus vulgaris* L. extract and its flavonoid components have an inhibitory impact on lymphoma in mice both *in vivo* and *in vitro*. Following treatment with flavonoid fraction, there was an increase in the cellular population in the S phase because flavonoid fraction dose-dependently halted the development of malignant cells. The anticancer activities of *P. vulgaris* flavonoids have also been validated by Ombra et al. (2016). Flavonoids from *P. vulgaris* also inhibit the growth of human MCF-7 cells and human epithelial colorectal adenocarcinoma (Caco-3) cells.

Gatouillat et al. (2015) investigated the anticancer activity from the flavonoids fraction of the *Medicago* genus L. and discovered that the flavonoids millepurpan and medicarpin, isolated from *Medicago sativa* L., inhibit the multiplication of cancer cells. Millepurpan and medicarpin may be used as chemopreventive medicines for breast cancer and cervical cancer, as claimed by Bora and Sharma (2011). In 2007, Stochmal et al. looked at the potential of the Medicago truncatula Gaertn flavone tricin as a chemopreventive drug. Tricin was shown to halt the cell cycle or have an impact that inhibited the development of MDA-MB-468 breast cancer in people. Tricin controls the cyclooxygenase-mediated synthesis of prostaglandins by primarily inhibiting the cyclooxygenase enzyme activity. Tricin may be used as a chemopreventive drug for prostate and intestinal carcinogenesis as a result of this action.

3.4.2 Lectins

Because the majority of the Fabaceae family's plants have anticancer and antitumour properties, communities all over the world utilise them to treat a variety of maladies (Sebastian et al. 2020). Numerous studies have shown that lectins prevent tumour growth in a variety of cell lines, including bone, skin, bile duct, and liver cell lines (Majeed et al. 2021; Bhutia et al. 2019). De Mejia and Prisecaru (2005) claimed that several lectin variants demonstrated anticancer capabilities both *in vivo* and *in vitro* studies. Lectins attached to the membranes of cancer cells or their receptors will causes apoptosis and cytotoxicity and ultimately suppress the proliferation of cancer cells. The anticancer activity of lectin extracted from *Phaseolus vulgaris* L. was evaluated by Fang et al. (2010), who revealed that the lectin had anticancer properties, especially against MCF-7, nasopharyngeal carcinoma cells (HNE-2, CNE-1, CNE-2), and liver cancer cells (Hep G2). Additionally, the *P. vulgaris* lectin controls nitric oxide (NO) production by increasing inducible NO synthase, which is known to cause the introduction of apoptotic bodies and support the anticarcinogenic effect. While researching the anticancer potential of lectin extracted from *P. vulgaris*, Lam and Ng (2010) found similar results.

Ye and Ng (2011), showed that the lectin from *Glycine max* (L.) Merr. had anticancer effects on hepatoma and breast cancer cells. *C. arietinum* has a long history of usage as a medicine in many regions of India due to its abundant lectin content and potent cancer-preventive properties (Gautam et al. 2018). Gondim et al. (2017) also assessed the anticancer efficacy of *Dioclea lasiocarpa* Mart. Ex. DLasiL lectin from seed isolation. The results of the research demonstrated the

DLasiL lectin's efficacy against the PC-3 prostate cancer, A-2780 ovarian cancer, and MCF-7 breast cancer cell lines. According to Lagarda-Diaz et al. (2017), legume lectins exhibited antioxidant and anticancer properties. Lung cancer cell multiplication is inhibited by legume lectins, and eating legume lectins boosts immunity against many cancers. *Griffonia simplicifolia* (DC.) Baill. lectin-1 (GS 1) was successfully employed by Korourian et al. (2008) to inhibit the growth of human breast ductal cancer.

3.4.3 Saponins

Many Fabaceae family members, including the lentil, soybean, and peanut, are high in saponins and are thought to have anticancer qualities. The effectiveness of saponins extracted from Fabaceae family members against colon cancer, melanoma cells, and cervical cancer has been shown by several studies all over the world. Saponins may limit the spread of cancer via a number of methods, including cell cycle arrest, cellular invasion inhibition, antioxidant action, activation of autophagy and apoptosis, and cell invasion inhibition (Elekofehinti et al. 2021). According to Rochfort and Panozzo (2007), eating legume saponins boosts protection against many cancers, such as colon and cervical cancer.

The anticarcinogenic activity of legume saponins was studied by Mudryj et al. (2014), who found that these compounds work through a variety of mechanisms, including immune modulatory effects, acid and neutral sterol metabolism, normalisation of carcinogen-induced cell proliferation, and cytotoxicity of cancerous cells. Saponins interact with cholesterol or free sterols found in cell membranes to affect the permeability of the membrane, which has growth-repressing effects on colon cancer cells (Singh et al. 2017). Gurfinkel and Rao (2003) claimed that bacteria in the colon hydrolyse saponins into sapogenols, which have potent chemopreventive effects against colon cancer and inhibit the spread of the disease.

According to Dai et al. (2002), eating *Glycine max* saponins lowers the chance of developing breast cancer and slows its progression. In the case of premenopausal women in particular, the benefits were more noticeable. Additionally, *Glycine max* saponins suppress prostate cancer; however, additional study is needed to determine the precise mechanism. according to Mujoo et al. (2001), *Acacia victoria* Benth saponins have been found in significant amounts, and they have been shown to significantly reduce the growth of immortalised breast epithelial cells, human foreskin fibroblasts, and mouse fibroblasts at a concentration that also inhibits the proliferation of various tumour cell lines.

3.4.4 Alkaloids

Alkaloids are essential secondary metabolites and are regarded as an excellent source of new medications (Ogidi et al. 2019a). Alkaloids have been shown in several studies to have anticancer and antiproliferative effects (Najjaa et al. 2020). The most effective examples of alkaloids that have previously been successfully as anticancer medications include vindesine, vinorelbine, vinblastine, and vincristine. These are helpful against a variety of cancer types, including melanoma, lung cancer, bladder cancer, brain cancer, and testicular cancer. Most of the over 21,000 known alkaloids are excellent sources of medications, particularly those that have anticancer properties (Mondal et al. 2019).

The phytochemical steroidal alkaloids are the most promising in terms of their ability to fight cancer. With the help of more clinical trials in the future, steroidal alkaloids may be used in the development of safer medications for the treatment of cancer (Dey et al. 2019).

The *Sophora* genus' matrine alkaloid revealed potential anticancer properties against lung cancer and liver cancer (Zhang et al. 2009). One of the few significant quinolizidine alkaloid substances is oxymatrine, which is mostly obtained from the roots of *Sophora flavescens* Aiton. According to reports, oxymatrine may be utilised to boost immunity against a variety of different cancers as well as lung cancer by increasing antitumour defences (Ye et al. 2018). Another alkaloid called cytisine is found naturally in two genera of the Fabaceae family, such as *Cytisus* and *Laburnum* (Zhu et al. 2018). Through the stimulation of mitochondria-mediated apoptosis and cell cycle arrest, cytisine aids in the suppression of lung cancer and implies potential anticancer action (Xu et al. 2020).

3.4.5 Carotenoids

Carotenoids, which predominantly consist of carotenes and also contain lutein, neoxanthin, crocetin, antheraxanthin, violaxanthin, and some others in very little amounts, are an essential component of legume leaves. However, compared to the leaves, legume roots are less abundant in carotenoids (Sri and Erdman 1987). Numerous experimental investigations have pinpointed distinct methods through which carotenoids may regulate the development of various cancer types in people. Retinol, antioxidant effects, communication processes, and cell signalling are a few of these systems. Consequently, carotenoids' assistance for antioxidant defence lowers the likelihood of developing cancer (Fiedor and Burda 2014). According to a thorough research by Nishino et al. (2000), carotene, cryptoxanthin, lycopene, lutein, and zeaxanthin may all be employed as chemopreventative agents. Additionally, beta-cryptoxanthin controls the activity of the *RB* gene, a well-known anti-oncogene. The carotenoids derived from legumes, according to Horvath et al. (2021), have therapeutic, preventive, and even curative actions against several forms of cancer.

Two essential carotenoids that reduce the risk of some malignancies are lutein and zeaxanthin (Krinsky 2005). The protective benefits of both are attributable to their anti-inflammatory and antioxidant capabilities since cancer is connected to inflammatory processes (Bhatt 2008). The proliferation of oesophageal malignant cells is significantly both dose- and time-dependently inhibited by beta-carotene. Another noteworthy finding is that normal oesophageal epithelial Het-1A cells are unaffected by the same dose of beta-carotene, indicating that the substance has substantial anticancer properties (Zhu et al. 2016). Although there are many other mechanisms that carotenoids may employ for their anticancer effect, the activation of apoptosis is thought to be the most frequent one.

Long-term usage of retinol, carotene, lutein, and lycopene lowers the incidence of lung cancer, according to Satia et al. (2009). According to Gong et al. (2018), through processes mediated by reactive oxygen species (ROS), legumes are a substantial source of lutein and greatly suppress the growth of breast cancer cells while enhancing the efficacy of chemopreventive medicines. The impact of lutein on the growth of rat prostate carcinoma cells and human prostate cancer cells (PC3) was studied by Rafi et al. (2015). Lutein's anticancer properties worked against prostate cancer in both rats and people. According to research by Kim et al. (2019), zeaxanthin and lutein reduce the risk of colorectal cancer via the death of malignant cells and antioxidant properties.

3.4.6 Phenolic Acids

Phenolic acids are essential phytochemicals that are abundantly found in various plant family members. Non-flavonoid phenolic chemicals known as phenolic acids come in free, insoluble-bound, and conjugated soluble forms. These phenolic non-flavonoid chemicals are found in a variety of plant species. Ferulic acid, vanillic acid, caffeic acid, benzoic acid, p-hydroxy acid, 3,4-dihydroxybenzoic acid, sinapinic acid, and syringic acid are natural phenolic acids that are found in diverse members of several plant groups (Behbahani et al. 2015).

Secondary chemicals called phenolic acids have lately been studied for their potential to treat different disorders, including cancer. These phenolics target many elements of cancer, including growth, development, and metastasis, and decrease the proliferation of malignant cells while promoting apoptosis (Rashmi and Negi 2020). Due to their anti-inflammatory, antitumour, and antioxidant properties, phenolic acids have recently received substantial research (Aljitan et al. 2018). Anantharaju et al. (2016) showed that phenolic acids have anticarcinogenic activity, which is primarily caused by the following functions: ROS levels are altered; cell cycle arrest is induced; tumour proteins, including p53, are encouraged to be suppressed. oncogenic signalling cascades governing apoptosis, angiogenesis, and proliferation are suppressed; differentiation is enhanced. and eventually the cells change into normal cells.

According to Palko-Labuz et al. (2021), phenolic acids have a variety of positive health effects, including antioxidant, anticancer, and anti-inflammatory properties. Due to their poor bioavailability, phenolic acids often have limited potential medicinal uses. However, conjugating phenolic acids with phospholipids may aid to increase their bioavailability in the biological system. The findings demonstrated the potency of conjugates as apoptosis-inducing, antiproliferative, and cell cycle–affecting agents. Additionally, the majority of metastatic melanoma cell lines responded favourably to the same dose, which, crucially, had no negative effects on healthy fibroblasts. Gallic acid possesses antitumour capabilities because of its antioxidant and anti-inflammatory qualities, according to research by Salem et al. (2011), who extracted bioactive gallic acid from the pod extract of *Acacia nilotica* (L.) Willd. ex Dilile. The summary of selected phytochemicals with various anticancer cell lines are shown in Table 3.1.

TABLE 3.1
Some Phytoconstituents Against Various Cancer Cell Lines

S/N	Phytoconstituents	Cancer Cell Lines	Reference
1	Flavonoids	Breast cancer MCF-7 cell line	Sabastian et al. 2020
2	Lectins	Breast cancer MCF-7 cell line, nasopharyngeal carcinoma cells (HNE-2, CNE-1, CNE-2), liver cancer cell (HepG2), prostate and lung cancer	Lagarda-Diaz et al.2017; Korourian et al. 2008; Lam and Ng 2010; Ye and Ng 2011
3	Saponins	Colon and cervical cancer cell lines	Rochfort and Panozzo 2007
4	Alkaloids	Lung, bladder, brain, testicular cancers	Mondal et al. 2019
5	Carotenoids	Human prostate cancer cell lines, colorectal cancer cell lines	Rafi et al. 2015
6	Phenolic acids	Malignant cell lines	Anantharaju et al. 2016

3.5 SELECTED MEDICINAL PLANTS WITH ANTICANCER ACTIVITIES

Numerous plants and plant-based substances have had their anticancer properties put to the test in research thus far. Some of these plants and the substances they contain show great promise in the fight against one or more cancer types. The following plants in Table 3.2 and discussed later were chosen for their compounds' *in vitro* and *in vivo* anticancer capabilities based on their activities.

3.5.1 *Actaea racemosa*

The Ranunculaceae family, which includes *Actaea racemosa*, has its roots in eastern North America. "Black cohosh" and "black snakeroot" are two of its common names. Cimicifugaside, derivatives of cinnamic acid, and cycloartenol-type triterpenoids are the primary distinctive chemical substances found in this plant. It is generally known that the herb may treat amenorrhea and chronic ovaritis (Mahady et al. 2002). Actein, an active metabolite of this plant, has been shown to have anticancer action by preventing the growth of human breast cancer cells and human liver cancer cells (HepG2). Actein modifies the expression of the p53 pathway, CCND1, ID3, and genes involved in fatty acid and cholesterol synthesis. Reduced amounts of free fatty acids and cholesterol in the liver lead actein to inhibit the development of human HepG2 liver cancer cells (Einbonda et al. 2009).

3.5.2 *Allium sativum*

Garlic, or *Allium sativum*, is a member of the Liliaceae/Alliaceae family. It has 17 amino acids, several enzymes, sulphur compounds, and minerals like selenium. Garlic has a lot of accessible selenium, an antioxidant that may also have

TABLE 3.2
Medicinal Plants and Their Potency Against Various Cancer Cell Lines

S/N	Medicinal Plants	Type of Cancer Cell Lines	Reference
1	*Actaea racemose*	HepG2 liver cancer cell line	Einbonda et al. 2009
2	*Allium sativum*	Breast and prostate cancer cell lines	Sigounas et al. 1997
3	*Artemisia annua*	Lung, colon, renal, and ovarian cancer cell lines	Eferth 2005
4	*Boswellia serrate*	VEGF-induced cell and human prostate tumour	Pang et al. 2009
5	*Catharanthus roseus*	Breast and lung cancer cell line	Nobel 1990
6	*Centella asiatica*	HepG2 cell lines and liver cancer	Lee et al. 2002
7	*Curcuma longa*	NF-B, AP-1 and STAT-3	Plengsuriyakarn et al. 2012
8	*Indigofera tinctoria*	Lewis lung cancer lines	Hoessel et al. 1999
9	*Mangifera indica*	Skin cancer, human epidermoid carcinoma A431 cell lines	Prasad et al. 2009
10	*Morinda citrifolia*	TPA- or EGF-induced cell lines	Liu et al. 2001
11	*Newbouldia laevis*	Pancreatic cancer cell lines	Kuete et al. 2011
12	*Nigella sativa*	NF-BAkt tumour cell lines	Plengsuriyakarn et al. 2012
13	*Solanum incanum*	Lung cancer cell	Liu et al. 2004

chemopreventive properties (Ip and Lisk 1996). Leprosy, severe diarrhoea, fever, stomach aches, deafness, and earaches are among the conditions it is used to treat. One of its main therapeutic benefits is the treatment of cardiovascular disorders via the reduction of cholesterol and blood pressure. Additionally, it functions as a chemopreventive and antibacterial agent. The most significant anticancer component of old garlic extract is S-allylmercaptocysteine. Thioallyl compounds' ability to inhibit cell proliferation has been researched in a variety of cell lines, and the findings have shown that breast and prostate cell lines are particularly susceptible to their effects (Sigounas et al. 1997).

3.5.3 *Artemisia annua*

There are over 400 species in the genus *Artemisia*, which is common in Europe, Asia, North America, and South Africa (Abad et al. 2013). For ages, the genus' plants were used in ancient medicine (Tan et al. 1998). The Asteraceae family includes the annual short-day plant *Artemisia annua*, which has a brownish stiff stem. Old Chinese people employed *A. annua*, often known as sweet wormwood, to make the antimalarial medication artemisinin. It continuously withstands insects and viruses thanks to a special power of environmental adaptability (Lu et al. 2000).

Additionally, *A. annua* produces scopoletin and 1,8-cineole molecules. Similar to this, semisynthetic artemisinin derivatives like arteether, artemether, and artesunate are also produced. According to studies, artesunate is a very potent anticancer substance. Eferth (2005) investigated the effects of artesunate on 55 distinct cancer cell lines, including malignancies of the central nervous system, leukaemia, melanoma, lung cancer, colon cancer, renal cancer, and ovarian cancer. They claimed that leukaemia and colon cancer were the conditions for which artesunate was most helpful. These trials also showed that artesunate was more effective than the medications prescribed for these tumours.

3.5.4 *Boswellia serrate*

The family Burseraceae includes *Boswellia serrata*, which is widely distributed in India, North Africa, and the Middle East. It goes by the names "Indian olibanum tree," "olibanum," "luban," and "gond." It has a variety of chemical components, including terpenoids, carbohydrates, volatile oils, and oils. One of this plant's four pentacyclic triterpene acids, B-boswellic acid, is its main component (Krieglstein et al. 2001). The plant's gummy exudates have astringent, antiarthritic, expectorant, stimulant, and antiseptic actions, among other medicinal benefits. This medicinal plant's key ingredient is acetyl-11-keto-boswellic acid (AKBA), and it has the power to significantly reduce tumour angiogenesis brought on by vascular endothelial growth factor (VEGF) activation. Additionally, it prevents VEGF-induced cell proliferation, migration, invasion, and tube formation at many different stages. According to research, AKBA inhibited tumour development in mice with human prostate tumour xenografts when given daily doses of 10 mg/kg after solid tumours had grown to less than 100 mm^3 ($n = 5$). As a result, the substance AKBA has anticancer properties (Pang et al. 2009).

3.5.5 *Catharanthus roseus*

Catharanthus roseus, sometimes known as Madagascar periwinkle, is a member of the Apocynaceae family. It was first found on the island of Madagascar. Its primary chemical components, alkaloids, are used to treat circulatory disorders, especially to relieve restriction of normal cerebral blood flow. The plant may be used as a cold treatment to relieve lung congestion and inflammation and has medical properties including astringent, diuretic, and antidiabetic effects. The considerable therapeutic benefits of vinblastine and vincristine, which are two pharmacologically active alkaloids that act against human neoplasms, are well documented. In addition to treating acute and chronic leukaemia, vinblastine sulphate (marketed under the name Velban) is used to treat lymphosarcoma, choriocarcinoma, neuroblastoma, and carcinoma of the breasts, lungs, and other organs. As a result of its ability to stop mitosis, vincristine sulphate (marketed under the brand name Oncovin) is used to treat lymphocytic and acute lymphoblastic leukaemia in children. Additionally, Hodgkin disease, Wilkins tumour, neuroblastoma, and reticulum cell sarcoma are treated with vincristine sulphate (Noble 1990).

3.5.6 *Centella asiatica*

Centella asiatica is a member of the Apiaceae family and a tiny perennial herb. Both "gotu kola" and "Asiatic pennywort" are popular names for it. The plant is indigenous to South and Central Africa, Madagascar, Australia, China, India, Indonesia, and the South Pacific. Studies on phytochemistry have shown the existence of the asiatic and madecassic acids, as well as the glycoside asiaticoside. In the Ayurvedic medical system, where it is used as a "brain tonic" for a variety of mental illnesses, its therapeutic value in treating chronic ailments has previously been highlighted. It is used to treat traumatic illnesses, heatstroke, diarrhoea, ulcers, eczema, and heat exhaustion. This plant's medical value as an anticancer agent has been enhanced by the presence of asiatic acid, a pentacyclic triterpene. According to research, asiatic acid has a cytotoxic impact that lowers the viability of HepG2 cells in cases of liver cancer. Increased expression of the tumour-suppressor p53 gene, which is regulated by higher levels of intracellular calcium, is what causes the reduction in cell viability (Lee et al. 2002).

3.5.7 *Curcuma longa*

The Zingiberaceae-related plant *Curcuma longa* is extensively cultivated in Asiatic nations, namely in India and China. It is often referred to as turmeric. Some of the ailments for which the plant has shown therapeutic capabilities include rheumatism, sinusitis, anorexia, coryza, cough, diabetic wounds, hepatic problems, and biliary disorders (Ammon et al. 1992). This plant has a wide range of pharmacological properties, including nematicidal, anti-inflammatory, anti-HIV, antibacterial, and antioxidant actions. Curcumin, its main chemical component, has a variety of biological effects. Additionally, the curcumin component has the capacity to decrease proinflammatory COX-2 and iNOS pathways as well as other events implicated in numerous stages of carcinogenesis, such as transcription factor NF-B, AP-1, and STAT-3 (Plengsuriyakarn et al. 2012).

3.5.8 *Indigofera tinctoria*

The majority of the nations in Africa, Australia, and Asia are home to *Indigofera tinctoria*, which is a member of the Papilionaceae family. It is often referred to as indigo. According to phytochemical screening, the plant's chemical components include flavonoids, terpenoids, alkaloids, and glycosides (Verma and Suresh 2002). The plant has medicinal uses for treating chronic bronchitis, asthma, ulcers, skin conditions, gastropathy, and epilepsy; it also promotes hair growth and has antidepressant properties. The capacity of this plant's metabolite, indirubin, to suppress Lewis lung cancer (LLC) in mice accounts for some of its possible antitumor efficacy. Cyclin-dependent kinases may be effectively inhibited by indurabin as well. A wide variety of cells are prevented from proliferating by indurabin-3'-monoxime, mostly by stopping the cell cycle in the G2/M phase. Antitumor activity is influenced by the inhibition of DNA polymerase I activity and, therefore, DNA synthesis. Indirubin strongly suppresses DNA synthesis according to experimental tests conducted on a variety of cell lines, in cell-free assays, and in rats with Walker 256 sarcoma (Hoessel et al. 1999).

3.5.9 *Mangifera indica*

Mango, scientifically known as *Mangifera indica*, is a member of the Anacardiaceae family. *M. indica*, the most widely farmed Mangifera species, has its roots in both India and Myanmar. It may be used as a treatment for blood diseases, scurvy, vitamin A deficiency, bilious illnesses, and digestive issues (night blindness). Diabetes has also been treated using fresh mango leaves (Shah et al. 2010; Ogidi et al. 2021b). Along with the aforementioned therapeutic value, a recent research found that mango fruit contains lupeol, a triterpene that has been demonstrated to trigger apoptosis in human epidermoid carcinoma A431 cells and has cytotoxic effects against skin cancer. Along with the caspase-dependent mitochondrial cell death pathway, apoptosis is triggered in a dose-dependent manner. It also prevents the phosphorylation of Bad (Ser136), which suppresses the Akt/PKB signalling pathway. As a result, lupeol is an anticancer treatment due to its capacity to inhibit a number of cancer-related molecular targets (Prasad et al. 2009).

3.5.10 *Morinda citrifolia*

The plant *Morinda citrifolia*, sometimes referred to as "noni" in trade, belongs to the Rubiaceae family. It is indigenous to Australia and Southeast Asia (Indonesia). Lignans, oligo- and polysaccharides, iridoids, fatty acids, scopoletin, flavonoids, catechin, sitosterol, damnacanthal, and alkaloids are the main secondary metabolites of this plant (Wang et al. 2002). Its pharmacological advantages include use as a general febrifuge and for analgesic effect, as well as a treatment for malaria, jaundice, hypertension, boils, carbuncles, stomach ulcers, stomach ache, fractures, diabetes, loss of appetite, urinary tract illnesses, abdominal swelling, hernias, and human vitamin A deficiency. In the mouse epidermal JB6 cell line, 6-O-(D-glucopyranosyl)-1-Ooctanoyl-D-glucopyranose and asperulosidic acid, two distinct glycosides, were shown to be very effective in preventing TPA- or EGF-induced cell transformation as well as associated AP-1 activity (Liu et al. 2001).

3.5.11 *Newbouldia laevis*

The African border tree, or *Newbouldia laevis*, is a member of the Bignoniaceae family. Numerous disorders are treated with it. It has the potential to be used as a febrifuge, to cure rheumatism, and to treat epilepsy and convulsions in children. Additionally, its extracts have been shown to have antimalarial and antibacterial activities (Kuete et al. 2007; Eyong et al. 2006). The plant's ability to cause cell death is thought to be due to the chemical 2-acetylfuro-1,4-naphthoquinone, which does so even in the absence of caspase 3/7 activation. It has been recognised that it prevents the development of blood capillaries in pancreatic cancer cell lines (Kuete et al. 2011).

3.5.12 *Nigella sativa*

Nigella sativa, sometimes known as "black caraway," "black cumin," or "black seed," is a member of the Ranunculaceae family. It is widely dispersed across Central Asia. Numerous chemical components, including nigellicine, nigellidine, nigellimine-N-oxide, thymoquinone, dithymoquinone, thymohydroquinone, nigellone, arvacrol, oxy-coumarin, 6-methoxycoumarin, and 7-hydroxycoumarin, hedrin, and steryl glucoside, as well as significant amounts of flavonoids, tannins, are essential. It has medical benefits such as analgesic, anti-inflammatory, antihistaminic, antiallergic, antioxidant, anticancer, immune-stimulating, antiasthmatic, antihypertensive, hypoglycaemic, antibacterial, antifungal, antiviral, and antiparasitic properties (Ali and Bluden 2003). This plant's secondary metabolite, thymoquinone, has lethal properties because it inhibits the signalling pathways for NF-B, Akt activation, and extracellular signal-regulated kinase while inducing apoptosis in tumour cells. It also prevents tumour angiogenesis (Plengsuriyakarn et al. 2012).

3.5.13 *Solanum incanum*

The temperate and tropical parts of the earth are the geographical home of *Solanum incanum*, a plant in the family Solanaceae (nightshade plants). The plant is sometimes referred to as "thorn apple" and "bitter apple." Steroid glycosides, the primary chemical components of the plant, are recognised to have protective properties against infections and plant predators. The steroid alkaloids solanin and solasonine are used to treat cutaneous mycotic infections and other infectious diseases (Al-Fatimi et al. 2007; Ogidi et al. 2021a). Solamargine, a different metabolite, is known to have cytotoxic effects against healthy skin fibroblasts by inducing cell death. In four human lung cancer cell lines, the cytotoxic effects of solamargine have been experimentally investigated. For tumour necrosis factors and Bcl-2–related resistance of human lung cancer cells, this metabolite's molecular actions include the release of cytochrome c, downregulation of antiapoptotic Bcl-2 and Bcl-xL, increased caspase-3 activity (essential for apoptosis), and DNA fragmentation (Liu et al. 2004).

3.6 BIOINFORMATICS APPROACHES

3.6.1 Systems Pharmacology

Systems pharmacology is one of the most popular new methods for researching how medications interact with biological systems (Yue et al. 2017). Network pharmacology, another name for systems pharmacology, may be utilised to identify disease-specific protein-to-protein interaction networks and signalling cascades (Huang et al. 2019a, 2019b). Recent years have seen the identification of several natural compounds and their processes utilising systems pharmacology (Wang et al. 2017). Consequently, network biology also contributes significantly to the discovery of relevant genes linked to a variety of disorders. The systems pharmacology technique was used in recent research to identify wogonoside as a potent angiogenesis inhibitor in TNBC (Huang et al. 2019b). In order to examine the mechanism, a systems pharmacology method was used between the main chemicals of Iranian chrysanthemum cultivars and well-known breast cancer medications with breast cancer–related targets. Rutin, one of these cultivar's principal constituents, has shown anticancer action against the MCF-7 cell line (Hodaei et al. 2021). Aside from the confirmation investigation of the selected target, the systems pharmacology technique provides insight into the target chemical network and the signalling pathways involved in treating complex illnesses like breast cancer (Sakle et al. 2020).

By combining systems biology, pharmacokinetics, and pharmacodynamics (PK/PD), quantitative systems pharmacology (QSP) provides the most comprehensive knowledge of the effectiveness and side effects of a medicine in complex disease systems like breast cancer (Fleisher et al. 2017). Recent studies have shown that it is possible to initialise cell states in special quantitative systems pharmacology (SPQSP) using single-cell data in order to forecast the effectiveness of TNBC treatment (Zhanga et al. 2021). Cancer immunotherapy, commonly referred to as immunological oncology, is a kind of cancer treatment that uses the patient's own immune system to combat the disease. Recent QSP modes will see an increase in usage in IO drug research, while on the other hand, IO will start to perform virtual trials alongside crucial trials. This might provide cancer patients with better medicines more swiftly (Chelliah et al. 2020).

3.6.2 Cheminformatics

Cheminformatics techniques have been developed as a result of the significant increase of epigenetics-related data in recent years. Computational methods might be used to identify hidden allosteric binding sites and protein-protein interaction hotspots for epigenetic targets. Additionally, substantial advances in drug development have been made via cheminformatics and molecular modelling (Sessions et al. 2020). One of the most important techniques for drug discovery is the quantitative structure-activity relationship (QSAR). This makes use of a multi-target strategy that enables the simultaneous prediction of anticancer drugs against several cell lines.

The drug effectiveness and therapeutic index are improved by the cheminformatics-based selection of small molecules as binary weapons that enhance transporter-mediated targeting (Grixti et al. 2017). When repositioning breast cancer medications, cheminformatic techniques and web ontology language may be utilised to explore the pharmacogenomics knowledge base. This improves the performance of potential new indications and contradictory effect predictions for breast cancer medications. Finding new therapeutic applications for already-approved medications is one of the most effective ways to speed up the drug development process (Zhu et al. 2014).

Understanding and identifying the connection between illnesses and medications is a crucial need for repurposing it, and this may be done with the use of cheminformatic techniques. Computational tools that use molecular modelling and cheminformatics techniques may expedite the drug development process for natural products (Medina-Franco and Saldivar-Gonzalez 2020). Cheminformatics has a variety of uses, as shown in Figure 3.3.

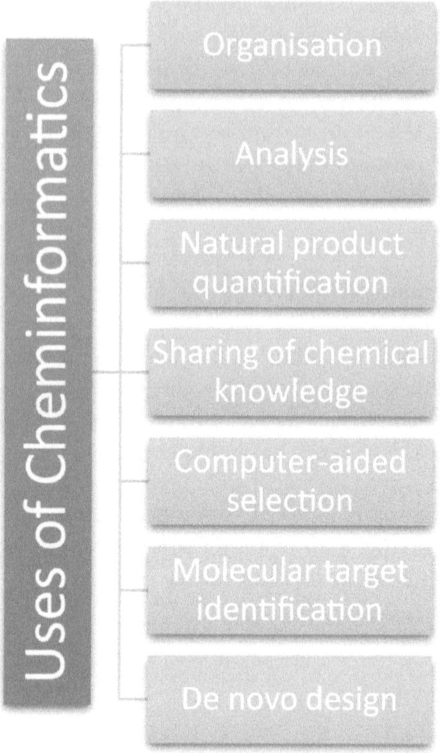

FIGURE 3.3 Cheminformatics uses.

3.7 RECENT TRENDS IN INDIGENOUS MEDICINAL PLANT INFORMATICS AND AVENUES TO COMBAT CANCER

There is a growing tendency to create resources and knowledge bases that provide herbal formulation, bioactive chemicals of medicinal plants, and associated information, thanks to the development of bioinformatics, information technology, and omics. Indian Medicinal Plants, Phytochemistry and Therapeutics (IMPPAT) (Mohanraj et al. 2018), SymMap (Wu et al. 2018), Indian Medicinal Plants Database (IMPLAD) (Venugopalan et al. 2020), and Collective Molecular Activities of Useful Plants (CMAUP) are a few initiatives (Zeng et al. 2018). Additionally, researchers have created cutting-edge methods for simulating the pharmacokinetic features of medicines and bioactive compounds (Jia et al. 2019). These methods are also useful to the virtual screening, plausible and potential mechanisms of action, and drug development of phytochemicals and plant bioactive compounds (Khan et al. 2020). Tools from computational biology and systems pharmacology have been used to analyse several plant-based anticancerous bioactive compounds (Jeyasri et al. 2020).

3.8 REGULATORY ASPECTS OF HERBAL ANTICANCER DRUGS

It is widely accepted that phase III clinical research studies are necessary for the marketing authorisation of all medications, including anticancer substances. For a product to be approved for marketing, the Food and Drug Administration (FDA) and European Medicines Agency (EMA) criteria stipulate that at least one phase III controlled study must have statistically significant findings (Apolone et al. 2005). According to the regulations of international organisations like the FDA and EMA, all pharmaceuticals must go through all rounds of testing, excepting unusual situations. However, it has been noted that pharmaceutical firms stray from the established procedure and begin testing novel substances on humans sooner than the specified time frame. Such actions are taken to hasten the approval of these substances in response to investor demand (Apolone et al. 2005).

This indicates that there are not enough facts about the drug's effectiveness, safety, and quality to support its application for approval. Despite the fact that substances derived from plants have been demonstrated to be less hazardous than traditional synthetic compounds, there is mounting evidence of the negative consequences of using these plants unrestrictedly to treat various disorders. The issue is a lack of information on the effectiveness, safety, and quality of herbal medications. When tested on the MDA-MB-231 cell line, *F. indica*, for instance, had strong anti–breast cancer action (Lam et al. 2012). *F. indica* has long been used to cure a variety of illnesses, and individuals have even begun drinking its herbal tea to prevent breast cancer. The fact that there are only a few studies on the plant's anticancer efficacy raises the issue, nevertheless. Oncology medication research and marketing are controlled on a global scale via the participation of specialists and an advice process facilitated by regulatory bodies (Farrell et al. 2005).

Several regulatory framework models may be used to prescribe these medicines, but there has to be cooperation between the regulatory bodies and advancements in the regulation procedure. For instance, the International Council for Harmonization's questions and answers guidelines on the nonclinical assessment of medications designed to treat cancer have just been accepted by the FDA. In order to harmonise the process of developing anticancer drugs, these recommendations comprise 41 questions and answers that give further information about the topic (Mezher 2018). However, it is recommended that regulatory authorities put more emphasis on merging data from traditional knowledge about that substance and the scientific investigations on it, while maintaining harmony with other organisations working to regulate anticancer herbal chemicals (Calixto 2000).

Furthermore, it is clear that the profile of therapeutic substances in plants of the same species cultivated in various environments varies (Silva et al. 2018). This emphasises the need for concentrating on the cultivation of homogeneous, high-quality plants with a uniform metabolite profile that, after testing, can be definitively classified as safe or dangerous. This might be accomplished with the use of *in vitro* development, biotechnological research, and genetic analysis of these anticancer plants (Khan et al. 2017).

3.9 CONCLUSION

Several phytochemicals and medicinal plants with anticancer properties, as well as the bioinformatics methods used to study them, have been thoroughly discussed in this chapter. These research studies, which mostly use human cell lines, have revealed the suppression of enzymes that inhibit the development of tumours. It has been noted that these plants' various kinds of secondary metabolites serve a significant anticancer function. Due to the phytochemicals' effectiveness in both preventing and treating cancer, eating different species of these plant families reduces the chance of developing cancer. These phytochemicals prevent cancer via a number of pathways, including the inactivation of carcinogens, the stimulation of cell cycle arrest, antioxidant stress, apoptosis, and immune system modulation.

A crucial set of tools for creating effective and focused searches for plant-based treatments is provided by bioinformatics techniques. This chapter also emphasised the many facets of research on medicinal plants where bioinformatics techniques might be used to make substantial advancements. A new phase in the development of plant-based cancer medicines may be made possible by the integration of bioinformatics techniques. The analysis of potential phytochemicals' bioavailability, effectiveness, safety, quality, composition, manufacturing methods, and regulatory and approval procedures must be significantly standardised in order for them to meet the worldwide standard.

REFERENCES

Abad, M.J., L.M. Bedoya, and P. Bermejo. 2013. Essential oils from the asteraceae family active against multidrug-resistant bacteria. In *Fighting Multidrug Resistance with Herbal Extracts, Essential Oils and Their Components*. Eds. Rai, M.K., and K.V. Kon. Academic Press: San Diego, CA, 205–221.

Agbo, M.O., P.F. Uzor, U.N.A. Nneji, C.U.E. Odurukwe, U.B. Ogbatue, and E.C. Mbaoji. 2015. Antioxidant, total phenolic and flavonoid content of selected Nigerian medicinal plants. *Dhaka Univ. J. Pharm. Sci.* 14:35–41.

Al-Fatimi, M., M. Wurster, G. Schroder, and U. Lindequist. 2007. Antioxidant, antimicrobial and cytotoxic activities of selected medicinal plants from Yemen. *J. Ethnopharmacol.* 111: 657–666.

Ali, B.H., and G. Blunden. 2003. Pharmacological and toxicological properties of *Nigella sativa*. *Phytother. Res.* 17: 299–305.

Al Jitan, S., S.A. Alkhoori, and L.F. Yousef. 2018. Phenolic acids from plants: Extraction and application to human health. *Stud. Nat. Prod. Chem.* 58:389–417.

Ammon, H.P.T., M.I. Anazodo, H. Safayhi, B.N. Dhawan, and R.C. Srimal. 1992. Curcumin: A potent inhibitor of leukotriene B4 formation in rat peritoneal polymorphonuclear neutrophils (PMNL). *Planta Med.* 58: 226.

Anantharaju, P.G., P.C. Gowda, M.G. Vimalambike, and S.V. Madhunapantula. 2016. An overview on the role of dietary phenolics for the treatment of cancers. *Nutr. J.* 15: 99.

Apolone, G., R. Joppi, and S. Garattini. 2005. Ten years of marketing approvals of anticancer drugs in Europe: Regulatory policy and guidance documents need to find a balance between different pressures. *Br. J. Cancer.* 93: 504.

Aregueta-Robles, U., O.R. Fajardo-Ramírez, L. Villela, et al. 2018. Cytotoxic activity of a black bean (Phaseolus vulgaris L.) extract and its flavonoid fraction in both in vitro and in vivo models of lymphoma. *Rev. Investig. Clin.* 70: 32–39.

Ateba, S.B., D. Njamen, and L. Krenn. 2021. The genus Eriosema (Fabaceae): From the ethnopharmacology to an evidence-based phytotherapeutic perspective? *Front. Pharmacol.* 12: 641225.

Behbahani, M., J. Abolhasani, M.M. Amini, et al. 2015. Application of mercapto ordered carbohydrate-derived porous carbons for trace detection of cadmium and copper ions in agricultural products. *Food. Chem.* 173: 1207–1212.

Bhatt, D.L. 2008. Anti-inflammatory agents, and antioxidants as a possible "third great wave" in cardiovascular secondary prevention. *Am. J. Cardiol.* 101: S4–S13.

Bhutia, S.K., P.K. Panda, N. Sinha, et al. 2019. Plant lectins in cancer therapeutics: Targeting apoptosis and autophagy-dependent cell death. *Pharmacol. Res.* 144: 8–18.

Bora, K.S., and A. Sharma. 2011. Phytochemical and pharmacological potential of Medicago sativa: A review. *Pharm. Biol.* 49: 211–220.

Bray, F., J. Ferlay, I. Soerjomataram, R.L. Siegel, L.A. Torre, and A. Jemal. 2018. Global cancer statistics 2018: GLOBOCAN estimates of incidence and mortality worldwide for 36 cancers in 185 countries. *CA Cancer J. Clin.* 68: 394–424.

Calixto, J. 2000. Efficacy, safety, quality control, marketing and regulatory guidelines for herbal medicines (phytotherapeutic agents). *Braz. J. Med. Biol. Res.* 33: 179–189.

Chan, C.W., B.M. Law, W.K. So, K.M. Chow, and M.M. Waye. 2017. Novel strategies on personalized medicine for breast cancer treatment: An update. *Int. J. Mol. Sci.* 18: 2423.

Chelliah, V., G. Lazarou, S. Bhatnagar, et al. 2020. Quantitative systems pharmacology approaches for immuno-oncology: Adding virtual patients to the development paradigm. *Clin. Pharmacol. Ther.*: 1–14.

Cheng, H. 1995. *Advanced Textbook on Traditional Chinese Medicine and Pharmacology.* New World Press: Beijing, China.

Cornwell, T., W. Cohick, and I. Raskin. 2004. Dietary phytoestrogens and health. *Phytochemistry.* 65: 995–1016.

Dai, Q., A.A. Franke, F. Jin, et al. 2002. Urinary excretion of phytoestrogens and risk of breast cancer among Chinese women in Shanghai. *Cancer Epidemiol. Biomark. Prev.* 11: 815–821.

De-Mejia, E.G., and V.I. Prisecaru. 2005. Lectins as bioactive plant proteins: A potential in cancer treatment. *Crit. Rev. Food Sci. Nutr.* 45: 425–445.

Dewanjee, S., S. Das, S. Joardar, S. Bhattacharjee, and P. Chakraborty, 2021. Carotenoids as anticancer agents. In *Carotenoids: Structure and Function in the Human Body.* Springer: Berlin/Heidelberg, Germany, 475.

Dey, P., A. Kundu, H.J. Chakraborty, et al. 2019. Therapeutic value of steroidal alkaloids in cancer: Current trends and future perspectives. *Int. J. Cancer.* 145: 1731–1744.

Efferth, T. 2005. Mechanistic perspectives for 1, 2, 4-trioxanes in anti-cancer therapy. *Drug Resist. Updat.* 8: 85–97.

Einbonda, L.S., M. Soffritti, D.D. Esposti, et al. 2009. Actein activates stressand statin-associated responses and is bioavailable in Sprague-Dawley rats. *Fund. Clin. Pharmacol.* 23: 311–321.

Elekofehinti, O.O., O. Iwaloye, F. Olawale, and E.O. Ariyo. 2021. Saponins in cancer treatment: Current progress and future prospects. *Pathophysiology.* 28: 250–272.

Enenebeaku, C.K., C.E. Ogukwe, C.O. Nweke, et al. 2022a. Antiplasmodial and in vitro antioxidant potentials of crude aqueous and methanol extracts of *Chasmanthera dependens* (Hochst). *Bull. Natl. Res. Cent. (Springer Open).* 46(33): 1–12.

Enenebeaku, U.E., C.E. Duru, E.N. Okotcha, et al. 2022b. Phytochemical analysis and antioxidant evaluation of crude extracts from the roots, stem and leaves of dictyandraarborescens (Welw.). *Trop. J. Nat. Prod. Res.* 6(1): 62–70.

Eyong, K.O., G.N. Folefoc, V. Kuete, et al. 2006. Newbouldiaquinone A: A naphthoquinone-anthraquinone ether coupled pigment, as a potential antimicrobial and antimalarial agent from *Newbouldia laevis*. *Phytochemistry* 67: 605–609.

Fang, E.F., P. Lin, J.H. Wong, S.W. Tsao, and T.B. Ng. 2010. A lectin with anti-HIV-1 reverse transcriptase, antitumor, and nitric oxide inducing activities from seeds of Phaseolus vulgaris cv. extralong autumn purple bean. *J. Agric. Food Chem.* 58: 2221–2229.

Faried, A., D. Kurnia, L. Faried, et al. 2007. Anticancer effects of gallic acid isolated from Indonesian herbal medicine, *Phaleria macrocarpa* (Scheff.) Boerl, on human cancer cell lines. *Int. J. Oncol.* 30: 605–613.

Farrell, A., I. Papadouli, A. Hori, et al. 2005. The advisory process for anticancer drug regulation: A global perspective. *Ann. Oncol.* 17: 889–896.

Fattovich, G., T. Stroffolini, I. Zagni, and F. Donato. 2004. Hepatocellular carcinoma in cirrhosis: Incidence and risk factors. *Gastroenterology*. 127: S35–S50.

Fiedor, J., and K. Burda. 2014. Potential role of carotenoids as antioxidants in human health and disease. *Nutrients*. 6: 466–488.

Fleisher, B., K. Andrews, A.A. Brown, and S. Ait-Oudhia. 2017. Application of pharmacometrics and quantitative systems pharmacology to cancer therapy: The example of luminal a breast cancer. *Pharmacol. Res.* 2017: 1–10.

Gatouillat, G., A.A. Magid, E. Bertin, H. Morjani, C. Lavaud, and C. Madoulet. 2015. Medicarpin and millepurpan, two flavonoids isolated from Medicago sativa, induce apoptosis and overcome multidrug resistance in leukemia P388 cells. *Phytomedicine*. 22: 1186–1194.

Gautam, A.K., N. Shrivastava, B. Sharma, and S.S. Bhagyawant. 2018. Current scenario of legume lectins and their practical applications. *J. Crop. Sci. Biotechnol.* 21: 217–227.

Gondim, A.C., I. Romero-Canelon, E.H. Sousa, et al. 2017. The potent anti-cancer activity of Dioclea lasiocarpa lectin. *J. Inorg. Biochem.* 175: 179–189.

Gong, X., J.R. Smith, H.M. Swanson, and L.P. Rubin. 2018. Carotenoid lutein selectively inhibits breast cancer cell growth and potentiates the effect of chemotherapeutic agents through ROS-mediated mechanisms. *Molecules*. 23: 905.

Grixti, J.M., S. Hagan, P.J. Day, and D.B. Kell. 2017. Enhancing drug efficacy and therapeutic index through cheminformatics-based selection of small molecule binaryweapons that improve transporter-mediated targeting: A cytotoxicity system based on gemcitabine. *Front. Pharmacol.* 8: 155.

Gurfinkel, D.M., and A.V. Rao. 2003. Soyasaponins: The relationship between chemical structure and colon anticarcinogenic activity. *Nutr. Cancer.* 47: 24–33.

Hassan, L.E.A., M.B.K. Ahamed, A.S.A. Majid, et al. 2014. Correlation of antiangiogenic, antioxidant, and cytotoxic activities of some Sudanese medicinal plants with phenolic and flavonoid contents. *BMC Complement. Med. Ther.* 14: 406.

Hodaei, M., M. Rahimmalek, and M. Behbahani. 2021. Anticancer drug discovery from Iranian Chrysanthemum cultivars through system pharmacology exploration and experimental validation. *Sci. Rep.* 11: 11767.

Hoessel, R., S. Leclerc, J.A. Endicott, M.E. Nobel, A. Lawrie, P. Tunnah, M. Leost, E. Damiens, D. Marie, D. Marko, et al. (1999). Indirubin, the active constituent of a Chinese antileukaemia medicine, inhibits cyclin dependent kinases. *Nat. Cell Biol.* 1: 60–67.

Horvath, G., E. Csikós, E.V. Andres, et al. 2021. Analyzing the carotenoid composition of melilot (Melilotus officinalis (L.) Pall.) extracts and the effects of isolated (All-E)-lutein-5, 6-epoxide on primary sensory neurons and macrophages. *Molecules*. 26: 503.

Huang, C., R. Li, W. Shi, and Z. Huang. 2019a. Discovery of the anti-tumor mechanism of calycosin against colorectal cancer by using system pharmacology approach. *Med. Sci. Monit.* 25: 5589–5593.

Huang, Y., J. Fang, W. Lu, et al. 2019b. A systems pharmacology approach uncovers wogonoside as an angiogenesis inhibitor of triple-negative breast cancer by targeting Hedgehog signaling. *Cell Chem. Biol.* 26: 1143–1158.

Inoue, M., R. Suzuki, T. Koide, N. Sakaguchi, Y. Ogihara, and Y. Yabu. 1994. Antioxidant, gallic acid, induces apoptosis in HL-60RG cells. *Biochem. Biophys. Res. Commun.* 204: 898–904.

Ip, C., and D.J. Lisk. 1996. The attributes of selenium-enriched garlic in cancer prevention. *Adv. Exp. Med. Biol.* 401: 179–187.

Iqbal, J., B.A. Abbasi, R. Ahmad, et al. 2019. Potential phytochemicals in the fight against skin cancer: Current landscape and future perspectives. *Biomed. Pharmacother.* 109: 1381–1393.

Jemal, A., F. Bray, M.M. Center, J. Ferlay, E. Ward, and D. Forman. 2011. Global cancer statistics. *CA Cancer J. Clin.* 61: 69–90.

Jeyasri, R., P. Muthuramalingam, V. Suba, M. Ramesh, and J.T. Chen. 2020. Bacopa monnieri and their bioactive compounds inferred multi-target treatment strategy for neurological diseases: A cheminformatics and system pharmacology approach. *Biomolecules.* 10: 536.

Jia, C.Y., J.Y. Li, G.F. Hao, and G.F. Yang. 2019. A drug-likeness toolbox facilitates ADMET study in drug discovery. *Drug Discov.* 25: 248–258.

Jorgensen, W.L. 2004. The many roles of computation in drug discovery. *Science.* 303: 1813–1818.

Karpuz, M., M. Silindir-Gunay, and A.Y. Ozer. 2018. Current and future approaches for effective cancer imaging and treatment. *Cancer Biother. Radiopharm.* 33: 39–51.

Khan, T., B.H. Abbasi, M.A. Khan, and M. Azeem. 2017. Production of biomass and useful compounds through elicitation in adventitious root cultures of Fagonia indica. *Ind. Crop. Prod.* 108: 451–457.

Khan, T., M. Ali, A. Khan, et al. 2020. Anticancer plants: A review of the active phytochemicals, applications in animal models, and regulatory aspects. *Biomolecules.* 10: 47.

Kim, J., J. Lee, J.H. Oh, et al. 2019. Dietary lutein plus zeaxanthin intake and DICER1 rs3742330 A > G polymorphism relative to colorectal cancer risk. *Sci. Rep.* 9: 3406.

Klaunig, J.E. 2018. Oxidative stress and cancer. *Curr. Pharm. Des.* 24: 4771–4778.

Klaunig, J.E., and Z. Wang. 2018. Oxidative stress in carcinogenesis. *Curr. Opin. Toxicol.* 7: 116–121.

Kleemann, R., L. Verschuren, M. Morrison, et al. 2011. Anti-inflammatory, antiproliferative, and anti-atherosclerotic effects of quercetin in human in vitro and in vivo models. *Atherosclerosis.* 218: 44–52.

Koehn, F.E., and G.T. Carter. 2005. The evolving role of natural products in drug discovery. *Nat. Rev. Drug Discov.* 4: 206–220.

Koh, Y.C., C.T. Ho, and M.H. Pan. 2020. Recent advances in cancer chemoprevention with phytochemicals. *J. Food Drug Anal.* 28: 14–37.

Korourian, S., E. Siegel, T. Kieber-Emmons, and B. Monzavi-Karbassi. 2008. Expression analysis of carbohydrate antigens in ductal carcinoma in situ of the breast by lectin histochemistry. *BMC Cancer.* 8: 136.

Krieglstein, C.F., C. Anthoni, E.J. Rijcken, et al. 2001. Acetyl-11-keto-beta-boswellic acid, a constituent of a herbal medicine from *Boswellia serrata* resin, attenuates experimental ileitis. *Int. J. Colorectal. Dis.* 16: 88–95.

Krinsky, N.I., and E.J. Johnson. 2005. Carotenoid actions and their relation to health and disease. *Mol. Asp. Med.* 26: 459–516.

Krishna, P.M., R. Knv, and D. Banji. 2012. A review on phytochemical, ethnomedical, and pharmacological studies on genus Sophora, Fabaceae. *Rev. Bras. Farmacogn.* 22: 1145–1154.

Kuete, V., K.O. Eyong, G.N. Folefoc, et al. 2007. Antimicrobial activity of the methanolic extract and of the chemical constituents isolated from *Newbouldia laevis. Pharmazie.* 62: 552–556.

Kuete, V., H.K. Wabo, K.O. Eyong, et al. 2011. Anticancer activities of six selected natural compounds of some Cameroonian medicinal plants. *PLoS ONE.* 6: e21762.

Lagarda-Diaz, I., A.M. Guzman-Partida, and L. Vazquez-Moreno. 2017. Legume lectins: Proteins with diverse applications. *Int. J. Mol. Sci.* 18: 1242.
Lam, M., A.R. Carmichael, and H.R. Griffths. 2012. An aqueous extract of Fagonia cretica induces DNA damage, cell cycle arrest and apoptosis in breast cancer cells via FOXO3a and p53 expression. *PLoS ONE.* 7: e40152.
Lam, S.K., and T.B. Ng. 2010. Isolation and characterization of a French bean hemagglutinin with antitumor, antifungal, and anti-HIV-1 reverse transcriptase activities and an exceptionally high yield. *Phytomedicine.* 17: 457–462.
Lee, Y.S., D.Q. Jin, E.J. Kwon, et al. 2002. Asiatic acid, a triterpene, induces apoptosis through intracellular Ca2+ release and enhanced expression of p53 in HepG2 human hepatoma cells. *Cancer Lett.* 186: 83–91.
Liu, G., A. Bode, W.Y. Ma, S. Sang, C.T. Ho, and Z. Dong. 2001. Two novel glycosides from the fruits of *Morinda citrifolia* (noni) inhibit AP-1 transactivation and cell transformation in the mouse epidermal JB6 cell line. *Cancer Res.* 61: 5749–5756.
Liu, L.F., C.H. Liang, L.H. Shiu, W.L. Lin, C.H. Lin, and K.W. Kuo. 2004. Action of solamargine on human lung cancer cells-enhancement of the susceptibility of cancer cells to TNFs. *FEBS Lett.* 577: 67–74.
Llovet, J.M. 2005. Updated treatment approach to hepatocellular carcinoma. *J. Gastroenterol.* 40: 225–235.
Lobiuc, A., N.E. Pavăl, I.I. Mangalagiu, et al. 2023. Future antimicrobials: Natural and functionalized phenolics. *Molecules.* 28(1114): 1–16.
Lu, H., W.X. Zou, J.C. Meng, J. Hu, and R.X. Tan. 2000. New bioactive metabolites produced by Colletotrichum sp., an endophytic fungus in Artemisia annua. *Plant. Sci.* 151: 67–73.
Mahady, G.B., D. Fabricant, L.R. Chadwick, and B. Dietz. 2002. Black cohosh: An alternative therapy for menopause? *Nut. Clin. Care.* 5: 283–289.
Majeed, M., K.R. Hakeem, and R.U. Rehman. 2021. Mistletoe lectins: From interconnecting proteins to potential tumor inhibiting agents. *Phytomed. Plus.* 1: 100039.
Medina-Franco, J.L., and F.I. Saldívar-González. 2020. Cheminformatics to characterize pharmacologically active natural products. *Biomolecules.* 10: 1566.
Mezher, M. 2018. *FDA Adopts ICH Guideline on Nonclinical Evaluation for Anticancer Drugs.* Regulatory Affairs Professional Society: Rockville, MD.
Mohanraj, K., B.S. Karthikeyan, R.P. Vivek-Ananth, et al. 2018. IMPPAT: A curated database of Indian medicinal plants, phytochemistry and therapeutics. *Sci. Rep.* 8: 4329.
Mondal, A., A. Gandhi, C. Fimognari, A.G. Atanasov, and A. Bishayee. 2019. Alkaloids for cancer prevention and therapy: Current progress and future perspectives. *Eur. J. Pharmacol.* 858: 172472.
More, G.K., J. Vervoort, P.A. Steenkamp, and G. Prinsloo. 2022. Metabolomic profile of medicinal plants with anti-RVFV activity. *Heliyon.* 8: e08936.
Mudryj, A.N., N. Yu, and H.M. Aukema. 2014. Nutritional and health benefits of pulses. *Appl. Physiol. Nutr. Metab.* 39: 1197–1204.
Mujoo, K., V. Haridas, J.J. Hoffmann, et al. 2001. Triterpenoid saponins from Acacia victoriae (Bentham) decrease tumor cell proliferation and induce apoptosis. *Cancer Res.* 61: 5486–5490.
Najjaa, H., B.A. Abdelkarim, E. Doria, et al. 2020. Phenolic composition of some Tunisian medicinal plants associated with an anti-proliferative effect on human breast cancer MCF-7 cells. *Eurobiotech J.* 4: 104–112.
Nedeljkovic, M., and A. Damjanovic. 2019. Mechanisms of chemotherapy resistance in triple-negative breast cancer—How we can rise to the challenge. *Cells.* 8: 957.
Nishino, H., H. Tokuda, M. Murakoshi, et al. 2000. Cancer prevention by natural carotenoids. *Biofactors.* 13: 89–94.
Nobili, S., D. Lippi, E. Witort, M. Donnini, et al. 2009. Natural compounds for cancer treatment and prevention. *Pharmacol. Res.* 59: 365–378.

Noble, R.L. 1990. The discovery of the vinca alkaloids—chemotherapeutic agents against cancer. *Biochem. Cell Biol.* 68: 1344–1351.

Ogidi, O.I. 2022. Phytochemicals of bioactive compounds of brassica juncea (Brown Mustard) seeds. In Ozturk, M. and G.B. Ameenah (eds) *Medicinal and Aromatic Plants of the World.* Encylopedia of Life Support Systems (EOLSS). United Nations Educational, Scientific and Cultural Organization: Abu Dhabi.

Ogidi, O.I. 2023. Sustainable utilization of important medicinal plants in Africa. In Izah, SC and M. C. Ogwu (eds) *Sustainable Utilization and Conservation of Africa's Biological Resources and Environment, Sustainable Development and Biodiversity.* Bugis, Singapore, Springer Nature Singapore Pte Ltd: Germany.

Ogidi, O.I., P. Chukwudi, A.I. Ibe, P.U. Eze, and T.N. Canus. 2021a. Preliminary phytochemical profile and antimicrobial potentials of white-green African garden egg (*solanum macrocarpon*) fruits obtained from Yenagoa. *ASIO J. Pharmace. Herbal Med. Res.* 7(2): 1–5.

Ogidi, O.I. and U.E. Enenebeaku. 2023. Medicinal potentials of Aloe vera (*Aloe barbadensis* Miller): Technologies for the production of therapeutics. In Izah, SC and M. C. Ogwu (eds) *Sustainable Utilization and Conservation of Africa's Biological Resources and Environment, Sustainable Development and Biodiversity.* Bugis, Singapore, Springer Nature Singapore Pte Ltd: Germany.

Ogidi, O.I., N.G. Esie, and O.G. Dike. 2019a. Phytochemical, proximate and mineral compositions of *Bryophyllum Pinnatum* (Never die) medicinal plant. *J. Pharmacogn. Phytochem.* 8(1): 629–635.

Ogidi, O.I., D.G. George, and N.G. Esie. 2019b. Ethnopharmacological properties of *Vernonia amygdalina* (Bitter Leave) Medicinal plant. *J. Medi. Plants Stud.* 7(2): 175–181.

Ogidi, O.I., C.C. Okore, U.M. Akpan, M.N. Ayebabogha, and C.J. Onukwufo. 2021b. Evaluation of antimicrobial activity and bioactive phytochemical properties of mango (*Mangifera Indica*) stem-bark extracts. *Int. J. Pharmacogn.* 8(5): 189–195.

Ogidi, O.I., P.S. Tobia, D.N. Ijere, et al. 2022. Investigation of Bioactive compounds and antimicrobial sensitivity of pawpaw (*carica papaya*) leave extracts against morbific microorganisms. *J. Appl. Pharm. Res.* 10(1): 21–28.

Ombra, M.N., A. d'Acierno, F. Nazzaro, et al. 2016. Phenolic composition and antioxidant and antiproliferative activities of the extracts of twelve common bean (Phaseolus vulgaris L.) endemic ecotypes of Southern Italy before and after cooking. *Oxid. Med. Cell Longev.* 2016: 1398298.

Pal, S.K., and Y. Shukla. 2003. Herbal medicine: Current status and the future. *Asian Pac. J. Cancer Prev.* 4: 281–288.

Palko-Labuz, A., A. Gliszczyńska, M. Skonieczna, et al. 2021. Conjugation with phospholipids as a modification increasing anticancer activity of phenolic acids in metastatic melanoma—In vitro and in silico studies. *Int. J. Mol. Sci.* 22: 8397.

Pang, X., Z. Yi, X. Zhang, et al. 2009. Acetyl-11-keto-b-boswellic acid inhibits prostate tumor growth by suppressing vascular endothelial growth factor receptor 2-mediated angiogenesis. *Cancer Res.* 69: 5893–5900.

Plengsuriyakarn, T., V. Viyanant, V. Eursitthichai, et al. 2012. Anticancer activities against cholangiocarcinoma, toxicity and pharmacological activities of Thai medicinal plants in animal models. *BMC Complement. Altern Med.* 12: 23.

Prasad, S., E. Madan, N. Nigam, P. Roy, J. George, and Y. Shukla. 2009. Induction of apoptosis by lupeol in human epidermoid carcinoma A431 cells through regulation of mitochondrial, Akt/PKB and NFkB signaling pathways. *Cancer Biol. Ther.* 8: 1632–1639.

Rafi, M.M., S. Kanakasabai, S.V. Gokarn, E.G. Krueger, and J.J. Bright. 2015. Dietary lutein modulates growth and survival genes in prostate cancer cells. *J. Med. Food.* 18: 173–181.

Ranjan, A., S. Ramachandran, N. Gupta, et al. 2019. Role of phytochemicals in cancer prevention. *Int. J. Mol. Sci.* 20: 4981.

Rashmi, H.B., and P.S. Negi. 2020. Phenolic acids from vegetables: A review on processing stability and health benefits. *Food Res. Int.* 136: 109298.

Rochfort, S., and J. Panozzo. 2007. Phytochemicals for health, the role of pulses. *J. Agric. Food Chem.* 55: 7981–7994.

Ruan, W.J., M.D. Lai, and J.G. Zhou. 2006. Anticancer effects of Chinese herbal medicine, science or myth? *J. Zhejiang Univ. Sci. B.* 7: 1006–1014.

Saito, K., and F. Matsuda. 2010. Metabolomics for functional genomics, systems biology, and biotechnology. *Annu. Rev. Plant Biol.* 61: 463–489.

Saklani, A., and S.K. Kutty. 2008. Plant-derived compounds in clinical trials. *Drug Discov. Today.* 13: 161–171.

Sakle, N.S., S.A. More, and S.N. Mokale. 2020. A network pharmacology-based approach to explore potential targets of Caesalpinia pulcherima: An updated prototype in drug discovery. *Sci. Rep.* 10: 17217.

Salem, M.M., F.H. Davidorf, and M.H. Abdel-Rahman. 2011. In vitro anti-uveal melanoma activity of phenolic compounds from the Egyptian medicinal plant Acacia nilotica. *Fitoterapia.* 82: 1279–1284.

Satia, J.A., A. Littman, C.G. Slatore, J.A. Galanko, and E. White. 2009. Long-term use of _-carotene, retinol, lycopene, and lutein supplements and lung cancer risk: Results from the Vitamins and Lifestyle (VITAL) study. *Am. J. Epidemiol.* 169: 815–828.

Sebastian, R., B. Jaykar, and V. Gomathi, 2020. Current status of anticancer research in Fabaceae family. *Pathways.* 6: 7.

Sessions, Z., N. Sanchez-Cruz, F.D. Prieto-Martinez, et al. 2020. Recent progress on chemin-formatics approaches to epigenetic drug discovery. *Drug Discov.* 25: 2268–2276.

Shah, K.A., M.B. Patel, R.J. Patel, and P.K. Parmar. 2010. *Mangifera indica* (mango). *Pharmacogn. Rev.* 4: 42–48.

Shehab, N.G., A. Mahdy, S.A. Khan, and S.M. Noureddin. 2011. Chemical constituents and biological activities of *Fagonia indica* Burm F. *Res. J. Med. Plant.* 5: 531–546.

Sigounas, G., J. Hooker, A. Anagnostou, and M. Steiner. 1997. S-Allylmercaptocysteine inhibits cell proliferation and reduces the viability of erythroleukemia, breast, and prostate cancer cell lines. *Nut. Cancer.* 27: 186–191.

Silva, T.C.D., J.M.D. Silva, and M.A. Ramos. 2018. What factors guide the selection of medicinal plants in a local pharmacopoeia? A case study in a rural community from a historically transformed atlantic forest landscape. *Evid.-Based Complement. Altern. Med.* 2018: 2519212.

Singh, B., J.P. Singh, N. Singh, and A. Kaur. 2017. Saponins in pulses and their health-promoting activities: A review. *Food Chem.* 233: 540–549.

Sohi, K.K., N. Mittal, M.K. Hundal, and K.L. Khanduja, 2003. Gallic acid, an antioxidant, exhibits antiapoptotic potential in normal human lymphocytes: A Bcl-2 independent mechanism. *J. Nutr. Sci. Vitaminol. (Tokyo)* 49: 221–227.

Sporn, M.B., and K.T. Liby. 2020. Chemoprevention of cancer: Past, present, and future. In *Natural Products for Cancer Chemoprevention.* Springer: Berlin/Heidelberg, Germany, 1–18.

Sri, K.S., and J.W. Erdman. 1987. Legume carotenoids. *Crit. Rev. Food Sci. Nut.* 26: 137.

Steward, W.P., and K. Brown. 2013. Cancer chemoprevention: A rapidly evolving field. *Br. J. Cancer.* 109: 1–7.

Stochmal, A., I. Kowalska, and W. Oleszek. 2007. Medicago sativa and Medicago truncatula as plant sources of the chemopreventive flavone tricin. *Planta Med.* 73: 304.

Sun, J., Y.F. Chu, X. Wu, and R.H. Liu. 2002. Antioxidant and antiproliferative activities of common fruits. *J. Agric. Food Chem.* 50: 7449–7454.

Tan, R.X., W. Zheng, and H. Tang. 1998. Biologically active substances from the genus Artemisia. *Planta Med.* 64: 295–302.

Taraphdar, A.K., M. Roy, and R. Bhattacharya. 2001. Natural products as inducers of apoptosis: Implication for cancer therapy and prevention. *Curr. Sci.* 1387–1396.

Vaou, N., E. Stavropoulou, C. Voidarou, et al. 2022. Interactions between medical plant-derived bioactive compounds: Focus on antimicrobial combination effects. *Antibiotics.* 11(1014): 1–23.

Venugopalan Nair, S.N., D.K. Ved, K. Ravikumar, et al. 2020. Indian medicinal plants database (IMPLAD) and threatened medicinal plants of India. In *Conservation and Utilization of Threatened Medicinal Plants.* Eds. Rajasekharan, P., and S. Wani. Springer: Cham, Switzerland.

Verma, S.M., and K.B. Suresh. 2002. Phytochemical investigation of *Indigofera tinctoria* Linn leaves. *Anc. Sci. Life.* 21: 235–239.

Wang, C.Z., T. Calway, and C.S. Yuan. 2012. Herbal medicines as adjuvants for cancer therapeutics. *Am. J. Chin. Med.* 40: 657–669.

Wang, J., H. Yu, A. Yili, et al. 2020. Identification of hub genes and potential molecular mechanisms of chickpea isoflavones on MCF-7 breast cancer cells by integrated bioinformatics analysis. *Ann. Transl. Med.* 8: 86.

Wang, J.H., Y. Li, Y.F. Yang, J. Du, M.Q Zhao, and F. Lin. 2017. Systems pharmacology dissection of multi-scale mechanisms of action for herbal medicines in treating rheumatoid arthritis. *Mol. Pharmacol.* 14: 7b00505.

Wang, M.Y., B.J. West, C.J. Jensen, et al. 2002. *Morinda citrifolia* (noni): A literature review and recent advances in noni research. *Acta Pharmacol. Sin.* 23: 1127–1141.

Wu, Y., F. Zhang, K. Yang, et al. 2018. SymMap: An integrative database of traditional Chinese medicine enhanced by symptom mapping. *Nucleic. Acids Res.* 47: D1110–D1117.

Xu, W.T., T.Z. Li, S.M. Li, et al. 2020. Cytisine exerts anti-tumor effects on lung cancer cells by modulating reactive oxygen species-mediated signaling pathways. *Artif. Cells Nanomed. Biotechnol.* 48: 84–95.

Ye, J., M.M. Zou, P. Li, et al. 2018. Oxymatrine and cisplatin synergistically enhance the anti-tumor immunity of CD8+ T cells in non-small cell lung cancer. *Front. Oncol.* 8: 631.

Ye, X.J., and T.B. Ng. 2011. Antitumor and HIV-1 reverse transcriptase inhibitory activities of hemagglutinin and a protease inhibitor from mini-black soybean. *Evid.-Based Complement. Altern. Med.* 2011: 12.

Yue, S.J., J. Liu, W.W. Feng, et al. 2017. System Pharmacology based dissection of the synergistic mechanism of Huangqi and Huanglian for diabetes mellitus. *Front. Pharmacol.* 8: 694.

Zeng, X., P. Zhang, Y. Wang, et al. 2018. CMAUP: A database of collective molecular activities of useful plants. *Nucleic. Acids Res.* 47: D1118–D1127.

Zhang, Y., H. Zhang, P. Yu, et al. 2009. Effects of matrine against the growth of human lung cancer and hepatoma cells as well as lung cancer cell migration. *Cytotechnology.* 59: 191–200.

Zhanga, S., C. Gonga, A. Ruiz-Martinez, et al. 2021. Integrating single cell sequencing with a spatial quantitative systems pharmacology model spQSP for personalized prediction of triple-negative breast cancer immunotherapy response. *Immunoinformatics.* 1–2: 100002.

Zhu, Q., C. Tao, F. Shen, and C.G. Chute. 2014. Exploring the pharmacogenomics knowledge base (pharm GKB) for repositioning breast cancer drugs by leveraging web ontology language (OWL) and cheminformatics approaches. *Pac. Symp. Biocomput.* 172–182.

Zhu, X., Y. Zhang, Q. Li, et al. 2016. β-carotene induces apoptosis in human esophageal squamous cell carcinoma cell lines via the Cav-1/AKT/NF-_B signaling pathway. *J. Biochem. Mol. Toxicol.* 30: 148–157.

Zhu, X.M., L.D. Du, and G.H. Du. 2018. Cytisine. In *Natural Small Molecule Drugs from Plants.* Springer: Berlin/Heidelberg, Germany, 685–689.

4 Extraction of Phenolic Compounds from Some Ayurvedic Botanicals (*Nigella sativa, Andrographis paniculata, and Phyllanthus amarus*) and Evaluation of Their Antibacterial and Antiviral Properties Using Bioinformatics Approaches

*Yusuf Oloruntoyin Ayipo**,†,
*Umar Muhammad Badeggi***,
*Abdulfatai Temitope Ajiboye****,
*and Mohd Nizam Mordi*****
*Centre for Drug Research, Universiti Sains Malaysia, Pulau Pinang, Malaysia; **Department of Chemistry, Ibrahim Badamasi Babangida University, Niger State, Nigeria; ***Department of Chemistry and Industrial Chemistry, Kwara State University Malete, Ilorin, Nigeria; ****Centre for Drug Research, Universiti Sains Malaysia, Pulau Pinang, Malaysia
†Corresponding Author: yusuf.ayipo@kwasu.edu.ng

ABBREVIATIONS

CADD	computer-aided drug design
PDB	protein data bank
RCSB	Research Collaboratory for Structural Bioinformatics

 DOI: 10.1201/9781003354437-4

SMILES	simplified molecular-input line-entry system
MD	molecular dynamics
DFT	density functional theory
HM	homology model
ADMET	absorption, distribution, metabolism, excretion and toxicity
RMSD	root means square deviation
MMGB/SA	molecular mechanics-generalized Born surface area
MMPB/SA	molecular mechanics Poisson-Boltzmann surface area
2D	2-dimensional
3D	3-dimensional
OPLS	Optimized Potentials for Liquid Simulations
RNA	ribonucleic acid
RNAp	RNA polymerase
SARS-CoV2	severe acute respiratory syndrome coronavirus 2
COVID-19	coronavirus 2019
S	spike
E	envelope
M	membrane
N	nucleocapsid
ORF	open reading frame
Nsp	non-structural protein
Mpro	main protease
CLpro	chymotrypsin-like protease
PLpro	Papain-like protease
TMPRSS2	transmembrane protease serine 2
ACE2	angiotensin-converting enzyme
RBD	RNA-binding domain
RdRp	RNA-dependent RNA polymerase
SCP	steroy carrier protein
CHIKV	Chikungunya virus
DENV	dengue virus
HIV	immunodeficiency virus
AP	*Andrographis paniculata*
NS	*Nigella sativa*
PA	*Phyllanthus amarus*
BASA	biaryl succinic acid
HCQ	hydroxychloroquine
CF	cystic fibrosis
TB	tuberculosis
RP-HPLC	reversed-phase high-performance liquid chromatography
UV	ultra violet
LC-ESI-QTOF/MS	liquid chromatography coupled with electrospray ionization-quadrupole-time of flight-mass spectrometry
UHPLC	ultra-high-performance liquid chromatography
UPLC	ultra-performance liquid chromatography
GC-MS	gas chromatography-mass spectrometry

AR	antibiotic resistance
NDM	New Delhi metallo-β-lactamase
IMP	Imipenemase
VIM	Verona integron-encoded metallo-β-lactamase

4.1 INTRODUCTION

Introducing a new drug to the market generally requires a lengthy time of at least 13 years with capitalized cost, exorbitant resource and expertise demands, and high investment risks. The process is oftentimes complicated by adherence to certain regulations and policies, making it a complex operation (Wooller et al. 2017; Reddy 2017). The science of computer-aided drug design (CADD) enhances the discovery of promising drug candidates from large resources in a faster, more economical, and environmentally friendly process. It extensively incorporates the applications of bioinformatics, cheminformatics, molecular modelling and simulations, and quantum techniques for scanning chemical libraries via de novo fragment- or structure-based designs. It represents an essential core of drug discovery (the discovery phase) in modern days, involving the study of the mechanistic biological events regarding the plausible molecular targets and interactivity with drug molecules. The potentials discovered in this phase including the targets, identified hits, and lead-like candidates are optimized for the next stage, i.e., the development phase. In this phase, they are validated through pre-clinical and clinical I-III *in vitro* and *in vivo* experimental models. The third stage is the registry where the distribution, marketing, and clinical usage of the newly discovered drug are established. These earmark the cumbersomeness of the entire traditional drug discovery process. Interestingly, the applications of the CADD significantly ameliorate most of the limitations including lengthy time, high cost, and resource implications (including animal and human subjects) (Prieto-Martínez et al. 2019; Sliwoski et al. 2014; Schaduangrat et al. 2020; Brogi et al. 2020; Wooller et al. 2017).

Bacteria and viruses are mostly implicated in the emergence and spread of infectious diseases and are responsible for most of the global pandemics including cholera, flu, and the ravaging coronaviruses (Piret and Boivin 2021). Bacterial and viral pathogens constitute the mainsprings of human disease-–elated death globally (Lewis et al. 2022). Therefore, the search for effective antibacterial and antiviral agents to mitigate their effects and maintain human wellness remains a global scientific exploration. Moreover, since the inception of humanity, plants have been recognized as the main sources of traditional medicine. In their various forms, they are naturally enriched with bioactive phytochemicals of different classes, amenable for controlling viral and microbial pathogens and their devastating effects in man (Joshi 2023; Stuper-Szablewska et al. 2023). Notably, Ayurveda is a historical traditional system of medicine predominantly traceable to India thousands of years ago. In the system, medicinal plants in various parts and constituents have been formulated in different forms, including extracts, into medicines for preventing and treating human diseases including those induced by pathogenic bacteria and viruses (Kuralkar and Kuralkar 2021). In particular, *Andrographis paniculata* (AP), *Nigella sativa* (NS), and *Phyllanthus amarus* (PA) are among the renowned botanical constituents in extract formulations of Ayurveda for treating various diseases and ailments. The phytochemicals from these plants have been reported with interesting activities against several pathogenic infections (Gyawali et al. 2021; Kumar, Dobos, and Rampp 2017; Chattopadhyay et al. 2022).

Therefore, in this chapter, the phenolic phytochemicals of the aforementioned Ayurvedic botanicals have been showcased for antibacterial and antiviral potential using bioinformatics approaches. The chapter significantly provides first-hand information on the medicinal potency of some notable phenolic compounds extractable from the highlighted plants based on several biomodelling studies from the bioinformatics perspective. In addition to the impacts of bioinformatics in drug and vaccine development, the traditional medicinal system of Ayurveda, extraction methods for the phenolic constituents of three selected plants, and interesting antibacterial and antiviral potential of some notable phenolic phytochemicals of the plants are further explored.

4.1.1 Bioinformatics in Drug Discovery

Bioinformatics typically involves the application of computational methods and software tools to analyse a large variety of biological data for research reproducibility, distinctively supporting biomedical research. Creation of large databases and high-throughput biodata processing and analysis via relevant scientific applications such as omics (citromics, genomics, proteomics, transcriptomics), epigenetics, genomic architecture, and ribosome profiling have been extensively applied for mechanism-based drug discovery. Other relevant aspects such as homology protein/receptor modelling, structural analysis of protein and ribonucleic acids (RNAs), and identification of distinct drug targets/biomarkers have aided modern drug discovery through robust protein-ligand docking, virtual screening, and molecular simulations. (Schaduangrat et al. 2020; Xia 2017; Wooller et al. 2017). Recently, artificial intelligence, machine learning, and other modern bioinformatics applications have been successfully employed for the modelling of biomedical datasets and network-based prediction of drug-target and/or drug-drug interactions (Abbas et al. 2021). In addition to the accelerated identification and validation of drug targets, drug screening, and drug optimization, bioinformatics also aids the characterization of side effects and prediction of drug resistance (Xia 2017; Reddy 2017). As such, bioinformatics has become essentially indispensable in translational drug discovery within research institutions and pharmaceutical industries (Wooller et al. 2017), although applications and pipelines of bioinformatics essentially require capital investments in sophisticated computing and data processing resources and expertise and skill for protocol configuration (Schaduangrat et al. 2020; Wooller et al. 2017). Moreover, its successful application in therapeutic designs depends largely on the nature of the disease and aetiologies. As such, an extensive understanding of the diseases' biochemistry is crucial for selecting appropriate bioinformatics tools for minimizing failure in the processes (Wooller et al. 2017).

4.1.2 Bioinformatics in Vaccine Development for Bacterial and Viral Diseases

The sudden emergence of new and/or re-emergence of mutated strains of pathogenic bacterial and viral organisms usually constitute a pandemic. Thus, due to the almost unbearable time and resources required for the discovery of effective therapeutics to meet the urgent global demands by healthcare systems during the episodes, the development of vaccines remains essential. For instance, the unexpected outbreak of coronavirus 2019 (COVID-19) has overwhelmingly affected human wellness and the global economic systems in an unpredictable fashion, causing morbidity and mortality now and then. Up-to-date, effective therapeutics for its treatment remain arduous despite the ceaseless concerted scientific efforts expanded in this direction globally. However, the timely development of various vaccines has drastically reduced the infection rates and subsequently improved the COVID-19–related health challenges worldwide (Yusuf Oloruntoyin Ayipo, Ahmad et al. 2022; Yusuf Oloruntoyin Ayipo, Bakare et al. 2022). In particular, the enormous applications of bioinformatics in the development of these vaccines and others for pre-existing bacterial and viral diseases cannot be overlooked. Similar to other pathogenic diseases, the viral genomic data of the severe acute respiratory syndrome coronavirus 2 (SARS-CoV-2), antigenic epitopes, antibody structural and protein-protein docking analyses, and simulation of the antigen-antibody reactions have been employed as bioinformatics approaches towards vaccine development for COVID-19 (Chukwudozie et al. 2021).

4.2 AYURVEDIC MEDICINE

Ayurveda, translated in English as "knowledge of life", is a traditional system of medicine of Hindu extraction. It represents one of the oldest medicinal systems, dating back to the Vedic era (around 3000 years ago) in India. The science of Ayurveda is believed to be centred around three main texts: "Ashtanga Hridaya", "Charaka Samhita", and "Sushruta Samhita" and other minor texts detailing the natures of various diseases, diagnostic interventions, and therapeutic recommendations. It covers contextual disease management with medicinal applications of over 700 herbs in about 6000 formulations (single and combination) including decoctions, extracts, juices, powders, and tablets (Gyawali et al. 2021). Interestingly, AP, NS, and PA are among the common plant constituents of Ayurveda formulations for medicinal purposes (Gyawali et al. 2021; Kumar, Dobos, and Rampp 2017; Chattopadhyay et al. 2022).

4.3 ANTIBACTERIAL AND ANTIVIRAL POTENCIES OF EXTRACTS OF SELECTED AYURVEDIC BOTANICALS

4.3.1 *Andrographis paniculata*

AP is also known as "create" or "king of bitter" in the English language because of its extremely bitter taste. It is widely used in traditional medicines including Ayurveda. Phytoconstituent evaluations of AP showed active compounds including flavonoids and andrographolides with multi-faceted therapeutic properties such as anticancer, antibacterial, and antiviral activities (Atu et al. 2022; Mohmmed Arifullah et al. 2013). The aqueous extract of the herb was evaluated against *Staphylococcus aureus, Porphyromonas gingivalis, Actinomyces viscosus, Streptococcus mutans,* and *Streptococcus sobrinus*. Moderate inhibition was recorded with the concentration of 1.0 g/mL across the pathogens, while the dilution of 1:2 and 1:4 gave significantly higher inhibition on all the pathogenic organisms tested (Mohamad et al. 2021). Some constituents of AP were also examined for antibacterial activity on *E. coli, Pseudomonas aeruginosa, S. aureus, Klebsiella pneumonia,* and

Streptococcus thermophilus. They mostly demonstrated significant inhibition against all the tested bacterial strains (Mohmmed Arifullah et al. 2013). Methanol and chloroform extracts of AP have been studied for inhibitory effects on quorum sensing for fighting *P. aeruginosa*. Both extracts showed good inhibition, especially the chloroform fraction, suggesting that most of the effective phytoconstituents must have been partitioned into the chloroform portion (Banerjee et al. 2017). The biochemical studies conducted on the extract of AP showed that the extract is rich in terpenes. Further screening suggested that the terpenoids are non-toxic, and it was therefore applied in the antibacterial evaluation on TEM-1 β-lactamase. The result shows significant inhibition of the enzyme, confirming its efficacy in fighting bacteria (Hajong and Sarma 2021). Leaf extracts of AP were tested at different concentrations (5 μL, 10 μL, 20 μL) for antibacterial activities against some gram-positive and gram-negative bacteria strains. They showed significant and similar inhibition in the tested organisms except for *S. aureus*, having a very low inhibition at low to moderate concentrations (Nayak, Pavithera, and Nanda 2015). The bactericidal effects of aqueous, ethanol, and acetone fractions of AP extracts also showed potent inhibitory activity on *K. pneumonia, P. aeruginosa,* and *Bacillus subtilis*, though the acetone fraction showed better activity than the aqueous and ethanol extracts, possibly due to the type of phytoconstituents of the extract (Rajeshkumar 2015).

4.3.2 Phyllanthus amarus

PA is an Indian medicinal herb belonging to the Euphorbiaceae family. It is widespread across the tropical countries of the world. This plant is commonly used in Ayurvedic medicine to treat diseases such as intestinal infections, kidney disorders, hepatitis, and stomach and liver problems. Some phytoconstituents of this plant are alkaloids, lignans, flavonoids, triterpenes, and tannins. These have conferred pharmacological properties on PA extracts such as anticancer, anti-inflammatory, analgesic, hepatoprotective, antibacterial, and antiviral agents (Sundaram et al. 2016; Sousa et al. 2017). Using the disc diffusion method, the aqueous extract of the leaf and root of PA were screened for antibacterial activities and were found to be bactericidal at concentrations of 10 and 20 μg/mL. Appreciable effects were recorded against gram-positive bacterial strains such as *B. subtilis, S. aureus, Streptococcus faecalis,* and *Staphylococcus albus* and gram-negative strains including *Proteus vulgaris, E. coli, K. pneumonia,* and *P. aeruginosa*. The preliminary phytochemical examinations showed the presence of saponins, tannins, polysterols, amino acids, alkaloids, lignins, and most importantly, the phenolic compounds which may be responsible for the interesting antibacterial activities of these extracts (Dhandapania, Balakrishnanb, and Anandhakumar 2007). Another extract of PA was tested for antibacterial activities against *S. aureus* and *P. aeruginosa*. The results indicated that the extract moderately inhibited *S. aureus* but showed no activity against *P. aeruginosa* (Corciovă et al. 2018). The PA extract as well as phyllanthin, a phytoconstituent isolated from PA, were both employed in the evaluation of their antibacterial potentials against bacterial strains. The extract demonstrated significant antibacterial activity against all gram-negative bacterial strains but was inactive against the gram-positives (Maria et al. 2019).

4.3.3 Nigella sativa

NS, commonly called black seed in English, is of the *Nigella* genus belonging to the family Ranunculaceae. This genus is widespread in Asia, Europe, and North Africa. The black seed is an important plant that has been utilized over the years in traditional medicine to treat several ailments. Notably, its usefulness includes as a diuretic, stomach problems, liver tonic, and diaphoretic diseases in cultures such as those of the Chinese and the Arabs. Reports have also shown that extracts of NS possess anticarcinogenic, anti-inflammatory, antioxidant, memory enhancement, and antibacterial activities, facilitated by the bioactive phytoconstituents (Alshwyeh et al. 2022) available in all parts of the plant, including the root (Maity et al. 2013). The plant houses many phytoconstituents including non-volatile compounds and phenolic compounds. Apigenin, chlorogenic acid, rutin, gallic acid, catechin, and vanillic acid are phenolic compounds isolated from NS (Dalli et al. 2022). In evaluating the antibacterial efficacy of *NS,* researchers have often partitioned the extract into fractions. Thus, Dalli and colleagues reportedly evaluated the antibacterial potentials of extracts of NS against some bacteria strains. The essential oil from the plant was also investigated alongside the extracts. The results showed generally moderate to high inhibitory activities against the gram-positive and gram-negative bacteria strains tested (Dalli et al. 2022). Several other studies have also demonstrated the interesting antibacterial activities of various extracts and essential oils of NS against many bacterial strains including multi-drug-resistant isolates (Muhammad Torequl Islam, Khan, and Kumar 2019; Benlafya et al. 2014; Shafodino, Lusilao, and Id 2022).

These pieces of experimental evidence have validated the claim of antibacterial phytochemicals in Ayurvedic botanicals. Polyphenols are renowned potent antimicrobial agents, as shown by a recent review of the literature (Manso, Lores, and de Miguel 2022). As such, the study of extraction and antibacterial and antiviral properties of phenolic compounds in Ayurvedic botanicals for identifying promising future drugs remains essential. In this regard, the application of bioinformatics tools at the preliminary stages of such worthy investigation could enhance the efficiency of the processes by saving time, being more cost-effective, and being less hazardous.

4.4 EXTRACTION OF PHENOLIC COMPOUNDS FROM SELECTED AYURVEDIC BOTANICALS

Various methods have been employed to extract phenolic phytoconstituents from several parts of the selected Ayurvedic botanicals AP, PA, and NS. These include the conventional methods such as decoction, digestion, and infusion (Matou et al. 2021); maceration (Hameed et al. 2019; Bourgou et al. 2008); maceration-homogenization (Feng, Dunshea, and Suleria 2020); maceration-rotary shaker (Muthusamy et al. 2018); percolation, serial exhaustive, and temperature-modified Soxhlet extraction (Guha et al. 2010); and the non-conventional modern ultrasound method (Gueffai et al. 2022) and sonication (Rafi et al. 2020). These and other commonly employed methods are summarized in Table 4.1. The chemical structures of the extracted phenolic compounds are presented in Figures 4.1 to 4.3.

TABLE 4.1
Summary of Extraction Methods for Phenolic Phytoconstituents in Selected Ayurvedic Botanicals

Part of the Plant	Extraction Methods	Methods for Identifying the Phenolic Contents	Phenolic Compounds	References
Nigella sativa				
Shoots	Maceration	RP-HPLC-UV-vis	Gallic acid (NS1), (—)-*p*-hydroxybenzoic acid (NS2), chlorogenic acid (NS3), vanillic acid (NS4), *trans* 2-hydroxycinnamic acid (NS5), epicatechin/(+)-catechin (NS6), quercetin (AP8/NS7), apigenin (NS8), amentoflavone (NS9)	(Bourgou et al. 2008)
Roots	Maceration	RP-HPLC-UV-vis	NS1, NS2, NS3, NS4, NS5, NS6, NS7, NS8, *p*-coumaric (NS10), ferulic acid (NS11)	(Bourgou et al. 2008)
Seeds	Maceration-homogenize	LC-ESI-QTOF/MS	Kaempferol-3-glucoside (NS12), diosmin (NS13), NS7, kaempferol (AP12/NS14), protocatechuic acid (NS15), NS2–3	(Feng, Dunshea, and Suleria 2020)
Seeds	Maceration	HPLC-UV	NS3, NS14, caffeic acid (NS16)	(Hameed et al. 2019)
Seeds	Conventional method	HPLC-UV	NS6, NS16, rutin (NS17)	(Gueffai et al. 2022)
Seeds	Optimized ultrasound-assisted	HPLC-UV	NS6, AP8/NS7, NS16, NS17	(Gueffai et al. 2022)
Andrographis paniculata				
Leaves and stem	Sonication	LC-MS/MS UHPLC-Orbitrap-MS/MS	NS16	(Rafi et al. 2020)
Leaves	Conventional	UPLC	NS1, NS3, NS15, salicylic acid (AP18), veratric acid (AP19)	(Praveen, Poornananda, and Nayeem 2014)

(Continued)

TABLE 4.1 (*Continued*)
Summary of Extraction Methods for Phenolic Phytoconstituents in Selected Ayurvedic Botanicals

Nigella sativa

Part of the Plant	Extraction Methods	Methods for Identifying the Phenolic Contents	Phenolic Compounds	References
Phyllanthus amarus				
Aerial	Ultrasonication	HPLC-UV-MS	NS3, NS10, NS11, NS16, quercitrin (PA2), gentisic acids (PA12), isoquercitrin (PA13) and rutoside (PA14)	(Corciovă et al. 2018)
Whole plant	Hot Soxhlet extraction	HPLC-analysis	NS3, NS10, NS16, NS17, PA13	(Guha et al. 2010)
Aerial	Conventional (infusion and decoction)	UHPLC-HRMS	NS1, corilagin (PA6), geranilin (PA15), brevifolin carboxylic acid (PA16), phyllanthusiin C (PA17), amariinic acid (PA19)	(Matou et al. 2021)
Whole plant	Maceration-rotary shaker	HPLC/LCMS	Ellagic acid (PA8)	(Muthusamy et al. 2018)
roots	maceration	HPLC/LCMS	NS1, NS6, PA12, galloyl methoxycinnamic acid hexoside (PA18), quercetin 3-malonylglucoside (PA20), naringin (PA21), epicatechin gallate (PA22)	(Maity et al. 2013)
Aerial	Ultrasound-assisted and pressurized liquid extraction	UPLC-ESI-QTOF-MS/MS	NS1, PA6, PA8, PA16, PA17, PA19	(Sousa et al. 2016)

4.5 EVALUATION OF ANTIBACTERIAL ACTIVITIES OF AYURVEDIC BOTANICALS USING BIOINFORMATICS APPROACHES

4.5.1 *Andrographis paniculata*

Cystic fibrosis (CF) is a biofilm-mediated chronic infection of the lung usually caused by *P. aeruginosa*. A methanolic extract of AP experimentally demonstrated effective inhibition of the biofilm and growth of clinical isolates of *P. aeruginosa*. The major (32) phytochemicals in the extract identified by gas chromatography–mass spectrometry (GC-MS) were evaluated for quorum sensing on the organism using molecular docking. Notably, three phenolic phytochemicals, 6H-dibenzo(b,d) pyran-1-ol (AP1), 2-methoxy-4-(1-phenylpropan-2-ylamino)methylphenol (AP2), and 2-methyl-5-(6-methylhept-en-2-yl)phenol (AP3) (Figure 4.1) were among the compounds with the strongest binding affinities for possibly inducing antibiofilm- and quorum quenching–like effects. These were indicated by the high docking scores and interactive poses with relevant biological structures of *P. aeruginosa* including the RhIG (PDB entry 2B4Q), pseudaminidase (PDB entry 2W38), and LasR (PDB entry 3JPU). The selected compounds displayed interesting drug-like properties, promoting them as promising future antibiotics for CF upon further study (Murugan et al. 2013).

4.5.2 *Phyllanthus amarus*

Leptospirosis is a bacterial disease caused by acute or chronic infections of the pathogenic *Leptospira* species. Its ability to evade immune systems and colonize within renal tubules constitutes challenges to treatment. An investigation of phytochemicals isolated from PA including flavonoids and phenolic 4-(3-(3,4dimethoxybenzyl)-4-methoxy-2-(methoxymethyl)butyl)-3,6-dimethoxybenzene-1,2-diol (PA23) (Figure 4.2)

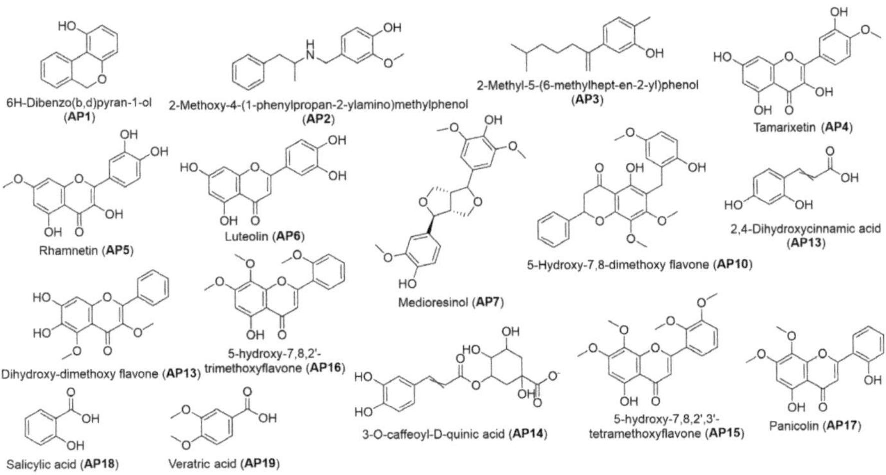

FIGURE 4.1 Chemical structures of some phenolic compounds in *Andrographis paniculate*.

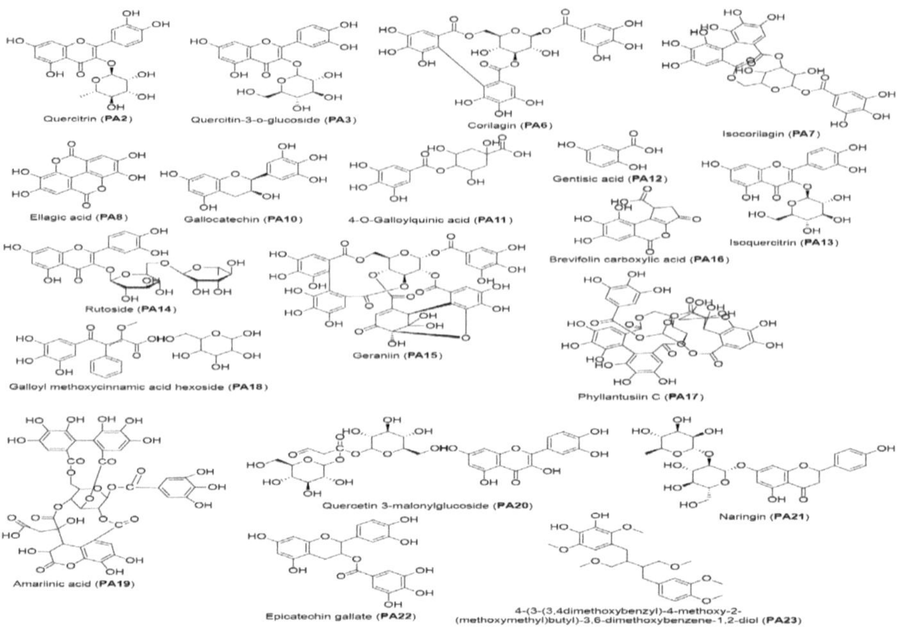

FIGURE 4.2 Chemical structures of some phenolic compounds in *Phyllanthus amarus*.

showed interesting anti-leptospiral performance of the compounds. Specifically, bioinformatic *in silico* studies involving homology modelling of the *Leptospira* protein (*L. interrogans* serovar Lai str. 56601) from the relevant FASTA sequence were obtained from NCBI using RaptorX software. Molecular docking of PA23 onto the active binding pocket of the structure displayed potent binding to amino acid residues essential for inhibition, including Lys 30, Thr 40, Val 47, Lys 48, Leu 50, Arg 83, Asp 168, and Thr 169. Further validation through *in vitro* and *in vivo* analyses confirmed the excellent anti-leptospiral activities of the phenolic compound, making it worthy of therapeutic consideration (Chandan et al. 2022).

4.5.3 Nigella sativa

Tuberculosis (TB) remains notorious among bacterial infections. It is caused by *Mycobacterium tuberculosis* with its RNA polymerase (RNAp) essentially aiding replications, as such recognized as a plausible therapeutic target. In exploration for potential inhibitors of the target, some major phytoconstituents of NS were screened for prospective candidates using the bioinformatics method of molecular docking against the RNAp of *M. tuberculosis* (PDB entry 5UHB). In particular, carvacrol (NS18), nigellidine (NS19), thymol (NS20), and thymohydroquinone (NS21) (Figure 4.3) were recorded with docking scores of −5.0, −6.4, −4.6, and −4.6 kcal/mol, respectively, although the binding affinities were significantly lower than those of α-hederin, a non-phenolic content, and rifampicin, a positive control which

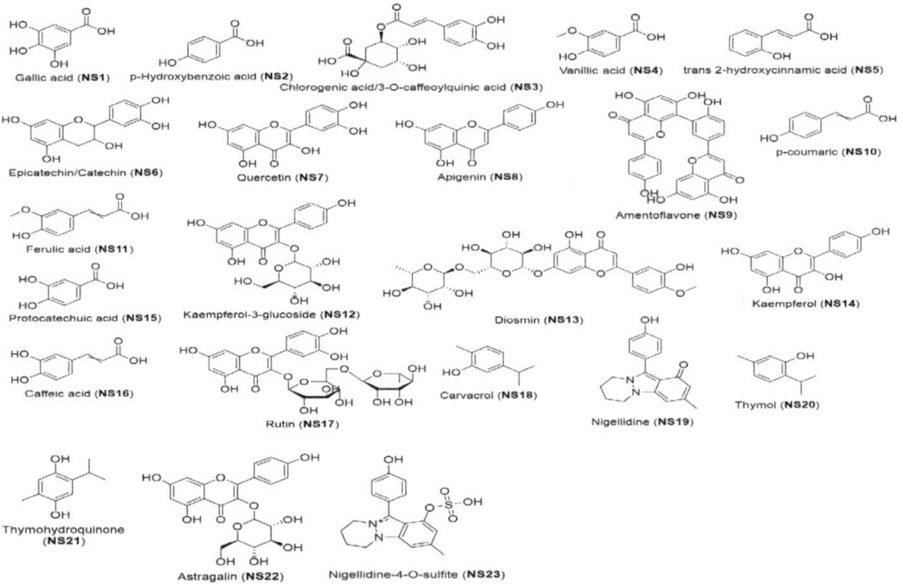

FIGURE 4.3 Chemical structures of some major phenolic compounds in *Nigella sativa*.

was recorded with −8.9 and −10.5 kcal/mol, respectively (Ahmad Mir et al. 2022). However, the synergistic effects of the compounds could cover therapeutic effects on the NS extract amenable for effective prevention and treatment of TB upon further evaluation. The summary of antibacterial activities of some phenolic compounds from the selected Ayurvedic botanicals evaluated using bioinformatics approaches is represented by Table 4.2.

4.6 ANTIBIOTIC RESISTANCE BY METALLO-Β-LACTAMASES AND INHIBITORY INTERACTIONS OF SOME PHENOLIC COMPOUNDS FROM THE SELECTED BOTANICALS USING BIOINFORMATICS APPROACHES

Antibiotic resistance (AR) remains a major public health challenge of the 21st century and is currently among the leading causes of death worldwide. The burden of its rapid spread globally has become critical and could trigger the emergence of much more deadly pathogenic organisms than the existing ones if left unchecked (CDC 2019; Murray et al. 2022). Metallo-β-lactamases are notorious chromosomal AR-inclined enzymes produced by carbapenem-resistant gram-negative bacteria (Tan et al. 2021; Kar et al. 2021). They are predominantly implicated in nosocomial infections mediated by deadly bacterial superbugs: the *Enterobacterales* including *E. coli, K. pneumonia, P. aeruginosa, Acinetobacter baumannii,* and *S. aureus*, making the organisms among the leading causes of AR-attributed deaths (Murray et al. 2022). The New Delhi metallo-β-lactamase (NDM-1), imipenemase (IMP-1), and Verona

TABLE 4.2
Summary of Antibacterial Investigation of Polyphenols and Some Other Metabolites from Selected Ayurvedic Botanicals Using a Bioinformatics Approach

Ayurvedic Botanical	Phenolic Phytochemicals	Target Organism	Mechanisms of Antimicrobial Action	Bioinformatics Tool	Interactive Structure	PDB Entry	Reference
AP	6H-dibenzo(b,d)pyran-1-ol, 2-methoxy-4-[(1-phenylpropan-2-ylamino)methylphenol and 2-methyl-5-(6-methylhept-en-2-yl)phenol	*P. aeruginosa*	Induction of antibiofilm and quorum quenching effects	Molecular docking	RhIG LasR Pseudaminidase	2B4Q 3JPU 2W38	(Murugan et al. 2013)
NS	Carvacrol, nigellidine, thymol and thymohydroquinone	*M. tuberculosis*	Inhibition of bacterial polymerase activities for replication	Molecular docking; MD	RNAp	5UHB	(Ahmad Mir et al. 2022)
PA	4-(3-(3,4dimethoxybenzyl)-4-methoxy-2-(methoxymethyl) butyl)-3,6-dimethoxybenzene-1,2-diol	*Leptospira* sp.	Inhibition of *Leptospira* protein	Molecular docking	HM of *Leptospira* protein		(Chandan et al. 2022)

Hint: AP = *Andrographis paniculata;* PA = *Phyllanthus amarus;* NS = *Nigella sativa;* MD = molecular dynamics; HM = homology model integron-encoded metallo-β-lactamase (VIM-1) represent the most relevant MBLs. They were first discovered in 1988, 1997, and 2008, respectively, and currently have over 1000 variants overwhelming the global healthcare systems through incessant bacterial epidemic diseases. More worrisomely, they evade almost all labelled β-lactam antibiotics even in combinations despite their therapeutic strength, limiting successful inhibitors for clinical applications up to the present day (Boyd et al. 2020; J. Chen, Wang, and Zhu 2017; Kar et al. 2021; Tan et al. 2021). Some recent scientific opinions detailed the insufficiency in the explorations for identifying potent inhibitors of MBLs, making the expansion of the scientific quest for therapeutic interventions to overturn the menace a critical need (CDC 2019; Mojica et al. 2022).

Mechanisms of MBL-mediated AR include the covalent binding of the enzymes to β-lactam antibiotics at the Zn(II) coordination site, thereby inducing the catalytic hydrolysis and eventual cleavage of the β-lactam ring, an active pharmacophore in their structures (Yusuf Oloruntoyin Ayipo, Osunniran et al. 2022; Lima et al. 2020). Thus, effective inhibition of MBLs by covalent inhibitors, especially with structural affinities to the Zn cofactor for coordination-inclined sequestration, could weaken the catalytic functions of the enzymes and promote the therapeutic integrity of antibiotics. Recently, some putative inhibitors of the MBLs, including NDM-1, were identified from natural product phytochemicals using a bioinformatics approach (Kar et al. 2021; Salari-jazi et al. 2021). However, little is known about the propensity of phenolic compounds from Ayurvedic botanicals for inhibiting the notorious enzymes.

In this chapter, inhibitory potentials of the identified phenolic constituents of NS were investigated against the renowned MBLs, NDM-1, IMP-1, and VIM-1 using molecular docking as a bioinformatic tool. The representative compounds (Figure 4.3) were drawn as 2D molecular structures and converted to the simplified molecular-input line-entry system (SMILES) using the cheminformatics tool ChemDraw 20.1.1 version. Then ligands were prepared using Maestro 12.2 (LigPrep, Schrodinger, LCC, New York, NY, 2019) embedded with Optimized Potentials for Liquid Simulations-3e (OPLS-3e) force fields (Harder et al. 2016). The crystal structures for NDM-1, IMP-1, and VIM-1 were retrieved from the open-access Research Collaboratory for Structural Bioinformatics (RCSB) Protein Data Bank (PDB) with respective annotations, PDB entry 5YPL, PDB entry 1JT, and PDB entry 5N5H (Burley et al. 2021). The structures were then prepared in the workspace of Maestro 12.2 using Protein Preparation Wizard (Protein Preparation, Schrodinger, LCC, New York, NY, 2019). These were followed by molecular ligand-receptor Glide docking available in Maestro 12.2 (Ligand Docking, Schrodinger, LCC, New York, NY, 2019). The interactive potentials of the phenolic compounds were assessed in terms of scoring algorithms and binding poses for bonding and non-bonding interactions in comparison with imipenem and meropenem, standard reference inhibitors. Being theoretical procedures, the docking protocols were validated by redocking a co-crystallized inhibitor of IMP-1, biaryl succinic acid (BASA), onto the active pocket of the crystal structure (PDB entry 1JJT). Both the co-crystallized and redocked structures were then superimposed and the root means square deviation (RMSD) between them was estimated. The structures showed a good alignment at the active pocket of IMP-1 with an RMSD value of 0.6013 Å (Figure 4.4), a value much less than 2.0 Å, validating the docking procedures as precise and reliable (Castro-Alvarez,

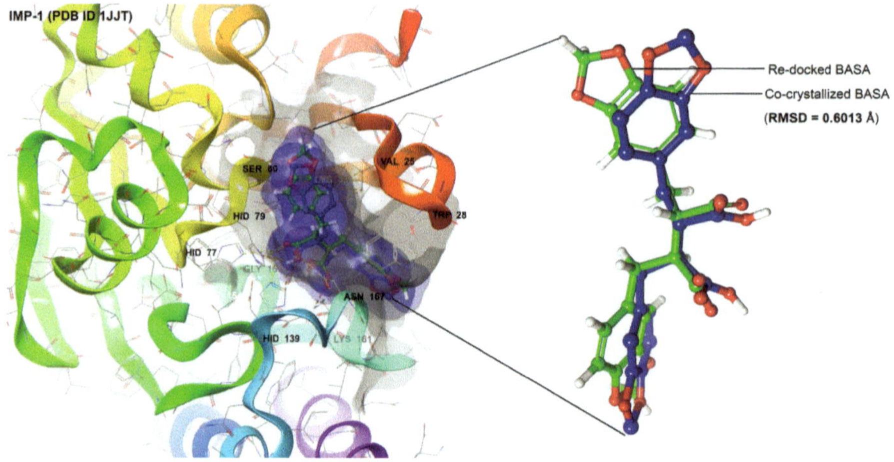

FIGURE 4.4 Validation of docking procedures. Both co-crystallized and redocked biaryl succinic acid superimposed at the active pocket of IMP-1 produced an aligned structure with an RMSD value of 0.6013 Å.

Costa, and Vilarrasa 2017; Ramírez and Caballero 2018; Yusuf Oloruntoyin Ayipo, Alananzeh et al. 2022).

The binding affinities of the phytochemicals to the probed enzymes are represented by the docking scores, arranged in descending order of negative values. The more negative the number, the higher the affinity. From the results against the enzymes (Tables 4.3–4.5), imipenem and meropenem are the clinical inhibitors of the enzymes, even though they are susceptible to their hydrolytic deactivation. Among the three enzymes, imipenem showed the highest affinity, indicated by the consistent top-ranked docking scores. Among the phenolic compounds of NS, compounds 3, 12, 17, and 22 displayed consistently high docking scores across the probed enzymes competitively with imipenem and higher than meropenem in all cases. The scores are functions of their binding interactions with amino acid residues and Zn co-factor at the active pockets of the enzymes. The highlighted phenolic compounds bonded to various active site residues via H-bonding, π-cation, and the salt bridge as hydrophilic interactions. They showed more hydrophobic π-π and non-bonding van der Waals interactions with other amino acid residues, as well as coordinate covalent bonds to Zn(II) ions. These synergistically confer high binding affinities on them and promote them as potential inhibitors for further study. In addition, their coordinate covalent bond formations to the cationic Zn(II) ions indicate propensities for Zn-chelation effects mostly favoured by electron-rich ligands such as carbonate, sulphate, and acetate, along with hydroxide and succinate groups. In particular, this Zn-sequestration has been recognised as one of the most potent strategies for deactivating the enzymes to conserve the antibiotic actions of drugs and defeat AR (Legru et al. 2021; Yusuf Oloruntoyin Ayipo, Osunniran et al. 2022).

The 2D and 3D diagrams of bonding and non-bonding interactions of the selected compounds 3, 12, 17, and 22 at the active pockets of the enzymes under probe are

TABLE 4.3
Docking Results of Representative Phenolic Compounds with VIM-1 (PDB Entry 5N5H)

Compound	Docking Score (kcal/mol)	H-bond Interactions	Other Bonding Interactions
Imipenem	−12.960	Asp 118, Glu 146, Asp 213(2)	Zn 301, Asp 213, Glu 146
NS17	−12.163	Asp 117, Asp 118	His 201
NS22	−11.323	Asp 118, Glu 146, Asn 210, Asp 213	Phe 62, His 116
NS12	−11.301	Asp 118, Glu 146, Asn 210, Asp 213	Phe 62, His 116
NS3	−10.796	Glu 201, Asn 210, His 240	Zn 301, His 201, His 240
Meropenem	−10.699	Asp 117, Asn 148	Zn 301, Phe 62
NS13	−10.337	Ser 61, Asp 81, Tyr 87, Asp 118	Phe 62(2)
NS6	−8.291	Asp 17	Tyr 67, His 116, His 240
NS14	−7.836	Asp 117	Zn 302
NS7	−7.543	Asp 117, Glu 146	His 116
NS1	−6.704	Asp 118, Asn 210	His 240
NS16	−6.702	Asp 118, Asn 210	
NS8	−6.301	Glu 146	Phe 62, His 116(2)
NS9	−6.238	Glu 146	Phe 62(2), His 116
NS10	−6.236	–	Zn 301, Zn 302, Phe 62, His 116
NS11	−6.117	Asp 118, Asn 210	–
NS15	−6.054	Asp 118, Asn 210	His 240
NS4	−5.879	Asn 210	Zn 301
NS21	−5.544	Asp 118, Asn 210	His 240
NS23	−5.363	Asn 210	His 240
NS19	−5.316	Asp 117	Zn 302
NS2	−5.149	–	Zn 301
NS20	−4.981	Asp 118	His 240
NS18	−4.715	Asp 118	His 240
NS5	−3.574	Trp 87, Asp 117, Asp 118	His 240

TABLE 4.4
Docking Results of Representative Phenolic Compounds with IMP-1 (PDB Entry 1JJT)

Compound	Docking Score (kcal/mol)	H-bond Interactions	Other Bonding Interactions
Imipenem	−10.169	Lys 161, Asn 167	Zn 251
NS17	−11.082	Asp 81, Asp 109, Asn 167, Asp 170	–
NS22	−10.774	Ile 160, Lys 161, Gly 164, His 197	His 197
NS12	−8.170	Gly 164, Asn 167	Zn 252, His 197

(Continued)

TABLE 4.4 (*Continued*)
Docking Results of Representative Phenolic Compounds with IMP-1 (PDB Entry 1JJT)

Compound	Docking Score (kcal/mol)	H-bond Interactions	Other Bonding Interactions
NS3	−12.082	Asn 167	Zn 251, Trp 28
Meropenem	−11.193	Ser 80. Asn 167	Zn 251, His 79
NS13	−9.287	Tyr 163, Gly 166	–
NS6	−7.898	Gly 164(2)	–
NS14	−7.318	Asp 81	Trp 28(2)
NS7	−7.820	Trp 28, Lys 161	Trp 28
NS1	−9.268	Asn 167	Zn 251, His 197
NS16	−9.529	Asn 167	Zn 251
NS8	−6.718	Lys 161	Trp 28
NS9	−10.033	Val 30, Asp 81	Trp 28(2), His 197
NS10	−8.522	Asn 167	Zn 251
NS11	−9.183	Asn 167	Zn 251
NS15	−8.930	Asn 167	Zn 251, His 197
NS4	−8.610	Asn 167	Zn 251
NS21	−4.769	–	–
NS23	−6.722	Asn 167, Asp 170	Zn 251(2)
NS19	−5.154	–	–
NS2	−7.900	Asn 167	Zn 251
NS20	−4.872	–	–
NS18	−4.863	–	–
NS5	−9.062	Asn 167	Zn 251

TABLE 4.5
Docking Results of Selected Phenolic Compounds with NDM-1 (PDB Entry 5YPL)

Compound	Docking Score (kcal/mol)	H-bond Interactions	Others Bonding Interactions
Imipenem	−12.165	Glu 152, Asn 220, Asp 223	Zn 301, Asp 223
NS17	−9.650	Asp 124, Glu 152, Asp 223	His 250
NS22	−8.653	Gln 123(2), Lys 211	–
NS12	−8.527	Gln 123(2), Asp 124, Lys 211	His 250
NS3	−10.157	Asp 212(2), Asn 220	Zn 301
Meropenem	−11.523	Gln 123, Asn 220, Lys 211	Zn 301
NS13	−10.177	Glu 152(2), Ser 217(2)	–
NS6	−7.848	Gln 123, Asp 124, Glu 152	–

TABLE 4.5 (*Continued*)
Docking Results of Selected Phenolic Compounds with NDM-1 (PDB Entry 5YPL)

Compound	Docking Score (kcal/mol)	H-bond Interactions	Others Bonding Interactions
NS14	−8.248	Gln 123, Lys 211	–
NS7	−7.927	Gln 123, Asp 124	–
NS1	−7.498	Lys 211, Asn 220	Zn 301
NS16	−8.674	Lys 211, Asn 220	Zn 301, His 250
NS8	−6.202	Gln 123, Lys 211	–
NS9	−7.278	Phe 70, Asp 124, Asp 212	Lys 211
NS10	−8.320	Gln 123	Zn 301, His 122, Lys 211
NS11	−8.526	Gln 123	Zn 301(2), His 122
NS15	−7.035	Lys 211, Asn 220	Zn 301
NS4	−6.709	Lys 211, Asn 220	Zn 301
NS21	−4.884	Asp 124	–
NS23	−5.412	Gln 123, Asn 220	Zn 301(2)
NS19	−5.563	Gln 123	Zn 301
NS2	−6.570	Asn 220	Zn 301
NS20	−4.792	Asp 124	–
NS18	−4.649	Asp 124	–
NS5	−7.189	Asn 220	Zn 301

presented in Figures 4.5–4.7. Accordingly, Zn1 and Zn2 are renowned metal co-factors in the active substrate-binding pockets of binuclear MBLs in addition to relevant amino acid residues such as Tyr 67, Trp 87, His 201, Glu 202, His 116, Asp 117, Asp 118, Ala 208, Asn 210, and His 240 (Tooke et al. 2019; Kar et al. 2021). These are consistent with the catalytic active site of VIM-1 (PDB entry 5N5H) herein defined (Figure 4.5).

The selected phenolic compounds displayed bonding and non-bonding interactions with the active site residues comparably to the reference inhibitors, indicating similar functional binding affinities. The hydrophobic pocket of IMP-1 (PDB entry 1JJT) inclusively contains Glu 23, Val 25, and Phe 51 in the proximity of the Zn(II) ion, while Trp 28 on the flexible loop 1 enhances the stabilization of the hydrophobic binding of ligands (Yamaguchi et al. 2021). The key amino acid residues for substrate sensitivity of the enzymes include Trp 28, Lys 161, Asn 167, and Zn ions for catalytic coordination (Toney et al. 2001; Arjomandi, Kavoosi, and Adibi 2019; Yamaguchi et al. 2021). As shown in Table 4.4 and Figure 4.6, the selected phenolic compounds 3, 12, 17, and 22 interacted with a good number of the enlisted residues via the hydrophilic H-bonding, π-cation, salt-bridge formation, and coordinate covalent bonds to the metal site. In addition, they displayed hydrophobic properties to some of the enlisted amino acid residues through π-π stacking and non-bonding van der Waals forces. These confer strong binding affinities on them, as shown in docking scores and support their inhibitory potentials against the enzymes.

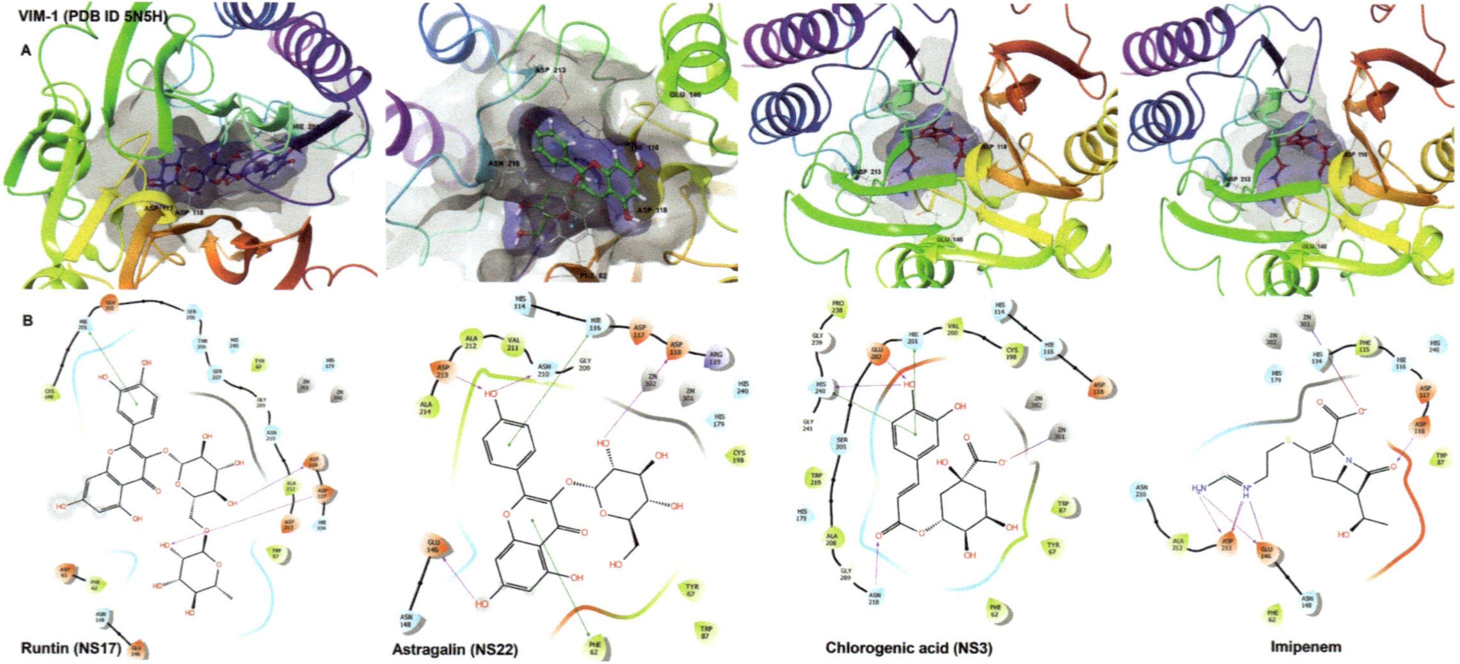

FIGURE 4.5 2D and 3D binding pose showing bonding and non-bonding interactions of rutin, astragalin, and chlorogenic acid with active site residues of VIM-1 (PDB entry 5N5H). Amino acid colours: Red—charged negative; deep blue—charged positive; pale blue—polar; yellow-green—hydrophobic. Bonds: Purple arrow—H-bond; blue-red line—salt bridge; Red line—π-cation; green line—π-π stacking.

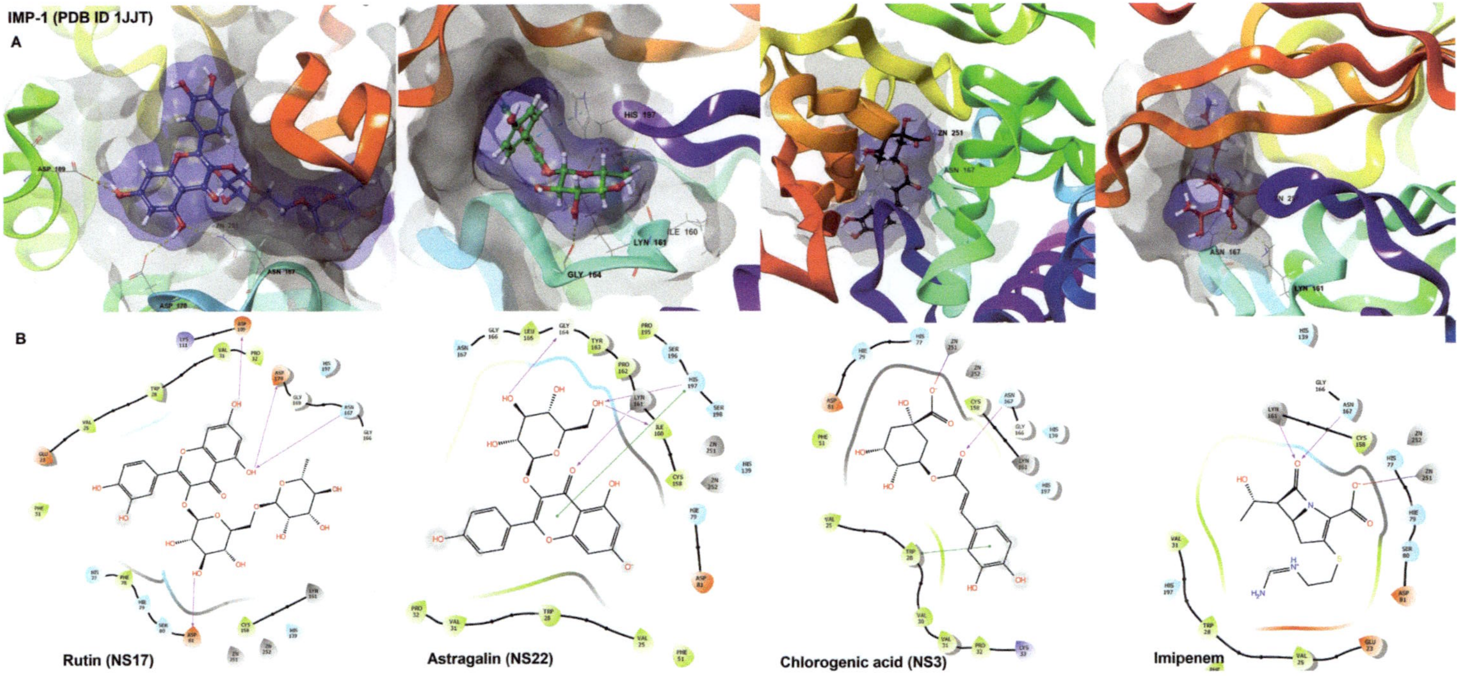

FIGURE 4.6 2D and 3D binding pose showing bonding and non-bonding interactions of rutin, astragalin, and chlorogenic acid with active site residues of IMP-1 (PDB entry 1JJT). Amino acid colours: Red—charged negative; deep blue—charged positive; pale blue—polar; yellow-green—hydrophobic. Bonds: Purple arrow—H-bond; blue-red line—salt bridge; red line—π-cation; green line—π-π stacking.

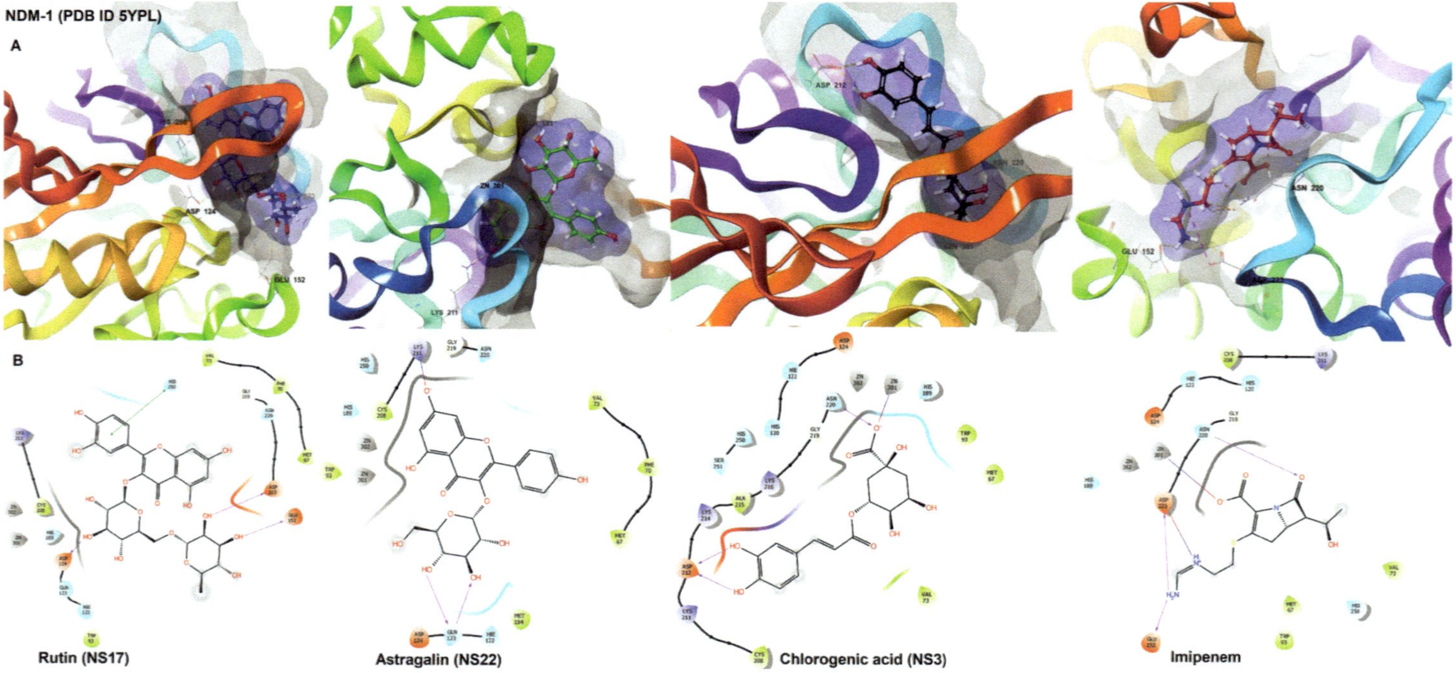

FIGURE 4.7 2D and 3D binding pose showing bonding and non-bonding interactions of rutin, astragalin, and chlorogenic acid with active site residues of NDM-1 (PDB entry 5YPL). Amino acid colours: Red—charged negative; deep blue—charged positive; pale blue—polar; yellow-green—hydrophobic. Bonds: Purple arrow—H-bond; blue-red line—salt bridge; red line—π-cation; green line—π-π stacking.

The catalytic activities of NDM-1 and MBLs generally are influenced by the coordination of Zn ions to some active site residues such as His 120, 122, 189, and 250. Other amino acid residues including Gln 123, Asp 124, Glu 152, Cys 208, Lys 211, Asn 220, and 223 inclusively constitute the binding pocket of NDM-1 and mediate the Zn-dependent catalytic functions (Salari-jazi et al. 2021; Kar et al. 2021; Wang et al. 2020). Hypothetically, the binding of inhibitors to these critical residues could limit their flexibility for antibiotic inactivation and distort the catalytic integrity of the enzymes to promote antibiotic effects (Moreira et al. 2021). From Table 4.5 and Figure 4.7, the selected phenolic compounds bind to many of the relevant residues, including Zn(II) ions, in similar patterns to the reference inhibitor imipenem. This indicates plausibility for covalent bonding and Zn-targeting inhibitory interactions in some cases, whereas shreds of experimental pieces of evidence have shown that Zn-sensitive ligands could be ideal selective inhibitors of MBLs (Bush 2018; A. Y. Chen 2020). Overall, the application of a bioinformatic tool, molecular docking, has revealed the inhibitory potentials of phenolic compounds in NS on MBLs. The results promote them as promising candidates amenable to combating the global AR challenges upon experimental validation and other translational studies.

4.7 ANTIVIRAL ACTIVITIES USING BIOINFORMATICS APPROACHES

4.7.1 ANDROGRAPHIS PANICULATA

About 650 flavonoids from some medicinal plants of Pakistan and India were evaluated for inhibitory potentials against the non-structural protein (nsp) 1–4 of chikungunya virus (CHIKV) using bioinformatics techniques. The crystal structures for nsp 2 and nsp 3, PDB entry 3TRK, and PDB entry 3GPG were retrieved from the RCSB PDB (Burley et al. 2021), while the homology protein structures for nsp 1 and nsp 4 were modelled using I-TASSER (Zhang 2008) and validated by Ramachandran plots using the RAMPAGE server (Lovell et al. 2003). In particular, some phenolic compounds from AP, 3',4',5,7-tetrahydroxyflavone 4',5,7-trihydroxyflavone, tamarixetine (AP4), rhamnetin (AP5), luteolin (AP6), and medioresinol (AP7) showed excellent binding affinities to nsp 1 and nsp 3, especially the first two compounds. For instance, the first interacted with some key amino acid residues at the conserved binding pocket of nsp 1 including Ala 19, Ala 21, Arg 22, Asp 27, Arg 28, and Lys 29 with an overall binding energy of –9.4 kcal/mol. Both highlighted compounds bonded strongly to nsp 3 with the respective binding energy of –9.0 and –8.9 kcal/mol, engaging Ala 22, Val 33, Leu 108, Thr 111, Gly 112, and Tyr 114 via various bonding interactions. Further analyses through the density functional theory (DFT) calculations and *in silico* predictions of properties for absorption, distribution, metabolism, excretion, and toxicity (ADMET) support the two compounds as potent inhibitors of CHIKV replication acting through interactions with the nsps for experimental validation (Hussain, Amir, and Rasool 2020).

Similarly, 5-hydroxy-7,6,2',3'-tetramethoxy flavone (AP8), 5-hydroxy-7,8,2',5'-tetramethoxy flavone (AP9), and 5-hydroxy-7,8-dimethoxy flavone (AP10) from AP also displayed strong binding energies ranging from –7.20 to –9.0 kcal/mol, while remdesivir, a nucleotide inhibitor of SARS-CoV-2, in clinical application scored between 7.60 and 9.50 kcal/mol against the targets. The predicted ADMET profiles of the phenolic compounds also support their use as drugs, suggesting them worthy of further evaluation as promising candidates for the ravaging SARS-CoV-2 (Hiremath et al. 2021). Similarly, AutoDock Vina and Chimera bioinformatics software tools were also employed to investigate the inhibitory potentials of phytochemicals from AP against the 3CLpro of SARS-CoV-2 (PDB entry 6LU7). Among the phytochemicals, two flavonoids, 5,4'-dihydroxy-7-O-β-D-pyran-glycuronate butyl ester (AP11) and 7,8-dimethoxy-2'-hydroxy-5-O-β-d-glucopyranosyloxyflavone (AP12), displayed strong binding affinities to the protease. This was indicated by the docking scores of −8.37 and −8.20 kcal/mol, respectively, whereas the positive control inhibitor, remdesivir and indinavir each were recorded with −8.23 kcal/mol. The predicted toxicological profiles favour the two compounds relative to others and, as such, portray them as putative candidates for further study as inhibitors of SARS-CoV-2 Mpro (Sukardiman et al. 2020). In another study, Glide molecular docking, in silico ADMET predictions, and binding free energy calculation by molecular mechanics-generalized Born surface area (MMGB/SA) support dihydroxy-dimethoxy flavone from AP as a more potent inhibitor of SARS-CoV-2 Mpro (PDB entry 5R82) than hydroxychloroquine and nelfinavir, and comparably to remdesivir (Kalirajan et al., 2020).

To further express the multi-target therapeutic potentials of phytoconstituents of AP, some phenolic contents, 2,4-dihydroxycinnamic acid (AP13), 3-O-caffeoyl-D-quinic acid (AP14), 5-hydroxy-7,8,2',3'-tetramethoxyflavone (AP15), and 5-hydroxy-7,8,2'-trimethoxyflavone (AP16) were reported with inhibitory interactions for mitigating several activities in terms of SARS-CoV-2 infection, the life cycle, and virulent factors. The activities targeted for suppression include viral entry, replication/synthesis, transcription, RNA binding, promotion of cytokines, formation of ion channels for viral particle release, and blocking of the host's RNA translation and dominant immunogens. The interactive implications for such effects were expressed *in silico* using molecular docking, targeting some relevant viral accessory, structural, and non-structural proteins, including the envelope (E) protein (PDB entry 5X29), membrane (M) protein (PDB entry 3I6G), S protein (PDB entry 6CRV), Mpro (PDB entry 6LU7), nsp 3 (PDB entry 6VXS), nsp 9 (PDB entry 6WXD), nsp 15 (PDB entry 6VWW), Open Reading Frame (ORF) 1a (PDB entry 2G9T) and ORF3a polyprotein (PDB entry 6XDC), and RNA binding domain (RBD) (PDB entry 6M0J). The complexes of the compounds with the proteins' structures were established for stability upon molecular dynamics (MD) simulations, while the predicted ADMET profiles support their candidacy as promising multi-target–directed inhibitors of SARS-CoV-2 amenable for further translational assessments (Swaminathan et al. 2021).

Eighty-two phytochemicals detected in extracts of AP and *Tinospora cordifolia* were investigated for larvicidal activities via *in silico* and experimental models. The compounds were observed for interactions with the sterol-carrying protein-2 (SCP-2) of *Aedes aegypti*, a mosquito vector of the dengue virus (DENV). Among the phytochemicals, panicolin (AP17), a phenolic compound in AP, displayed a strong binding affinity for SCP-2 (PDB entry 1PZ4) with an energy score of −9.86 kcal/mol and interacted with essential amino acid residues for disrupting the viral life cycle upon molecular docking analysis. The *in silico* results further support the experimental outcomes, suggesting the compound as a potential larvicidal agent for controlling the spread of DENV through *A. aegypti* (Paul et al. 2021).

Again, phenolic phytoconstituents of some medicinal plants were investigated for inhibitory potentials against some relevant crucial structures for replication and transcription of DENV using molecular docking. The selected targets include the DENV NS3 protease-helicase (PDB entry 2VBC), DENV 1 NS2/NS3 protease (PDB entry 3L6P), DENV NS2B/NS3 protease (PDB entry 2FOM), DENV 3 protease (PDB entry 3U1J), the second conformation of DENV NS3 protease-helicase (PDB entry 2WHX), DENV 1 E protein (PDB entry 3UZQ), DENV 2 E protein (PDB entry 1TG8), DENV 3 E protein (PDB entry 1UZG), DENV 4 E protein (PDB entry 3UYP), and DENV NS5 RdRp (PDB entry 2J7W). In particular, AP8/NS7 and caffeic acid (AP18/NS16) from AP were among the mostly strongly bound ligands to the targets indicated by high binding energies. The two compounds also interacted with key amino acid residues essential for anti-dengue pharmacology, comparable to the standard inhibitors, thus representing promising multi-target–directed candidates for preventing and treating DENV infections upon further study (Pawar and Patravale 2020).

4.7.2 Phyllanthus amarus

Thirty-five phytochemicals from PA and AP were investigated for inhibitory potentials against some key life cycle– and virulence- determining proteins of SARS-CoV-2, spike glycoprotein opened (PDB entry 6VYB) and closed form (PDB entry 6VXX), 3-main protease (Mpro)/3-chymotrypsin-like protease (3CLpro; PDB entry 6LU7), papain-like protease (PDB entry 4OVZ), and RNA-dependent RNA polymerase (RdRp; PDB entry 6NUS) using the AutoDock Vina molecular docking tool. Notably, five phenolic compounds, quercetin (PA1/NS7), quercitrin (PA2), quercetin-3-*O*-glucoside (PA3), astragalin (PA4/NS22), and kaempferol (PA5/NS14) from PA, interestingly bound potently to the active pockets of the crystal structures quantitatively with binding affinities between −7.50 and −10.30 kcal/mol. Some phenolic phytochemicals from PA of Nigerian extraction were investigated for inhibitory interactions against the nsp 16 of SARS-CoV-2 (PDB entry 6YZ1) using the AutoDock Vina bioinformatic approach, followed by *in silico* ADMET prediction. The relevant phytochemicals include corilagin (PA6), isocorilagin (PA7), ellagic acid (PA8), gallic acid (PA9/NS1), gallocatechin (PA10), and 4-O-galloylquinic acid (PA11). Although the compounds showed weaker binding energy than the six hits selected by the authors, including andrographolide from AP, whose docking score was recorded as −7.9 kcal/mol. The latter displayed strong H-bond interactions with relevant active pocket residues such as Asn 43, Asp 99, and Asp 130 and was predicted with ideal ADMET properties for drug likeness (Saliu et al. 2021).

4.7.3 Nigella sativa

Historically, NS is renowned for its anti-inflammatory, antibacterial, and immunomodulatory effects among its vast medicinal properties (Shawky, Nada, and Ibrahim 2020; Pandey et al. 2021). Employing bioinformatics techniques, including molecular docking, with relevant targets CTN and GO enrichment analyses, a recent study revealed the influence of interesting network pharmacological pathways and other potential therapeutic approaches for combating SARS-CoV-2, aided by NS phytochemicals (Shawky, Nada, and Ibrahim 2020). The infusion of SARS-CoV-2 into host cells understandably occurs through the interactions between the viral S protein and the human angiotensin-converting enzyme 2 (ACE2). The process is primarily mediated by the activation of the enzyme ACE2 by the transmembrane protease serine 2 (TMPRSS2). As such, the protease is recognized as a therapeutic target for preventing viral entry and replication, and its renowned inhibitor, camostat, has been reported as active against SARS-CoV-2 (Y.O. Ayipo et al. 2021). The extract of NS reportedly enhanced the helper T-cell as well as suppressor T-cell ratio. Hence, it has increased natural killer cell activity in humans. The extract has also inhibited murine cytomegalovirus and the human immunodeficiency virus (HIV) (Muhammad Torequl Islam, Khan, and Kumar 2019). In a related study, the extract of NS decreased the replication of the virus when the Hela-epithelial carcinoembryonic antigen-related cell adhesion molecule cell was infected with the mouse hepatitis virus (Muhammad T. Islam et al. 2020). In the treatment of SARS-COV-2, the extract of NS was listed among the famous natural immune boosters (Boozari and Hosseinzadeh 2020).

From bioinformatic perspectives, in an *in silico* evaluation of some spice-derived phytochemicals as prospects for COVID-19, NS18 was shown to interact more potently with the active pocket of the homology model of TMPRSS2, with a docking score of –3.90 kcal/mol, than camostat, which scored –3.19. The compound reportedly bound tightly to the oxyanion hole and catalytic triad of the enzyme, engaging the catalytic domain residues His 296, Asp 345, and Ser 441 in bonding interactions. The MD simulation and ADMET prediction also support the drug potential of the phenolic compound as a promising candidate for prophylaxis and treatment of SARS-CoV-2, deserving further scientific attention (Yadav, Jaiswal, and Singh 2021). Similarly, in an exploration of NS for identifying potent chemotherapeutics for COVID-19 using bioinformatics approaches of molecular docking, MD, and ADMET predictions, NS18, NS20, and NS21 displayed strong inhibitory interactions with the SARS-CoV-2 RBD-ACE2 interface (PDB entry 6VW1). Their affinities were quantified by the docking scores of –7.0, –6.0, and –6.1 kcal/mol, respectively, consistently supported by post-MD molecular mechanics Poisson-Boltzmann surface area (MMPB/SA) scores. In particular, NS18 scored closely to chloroquine, a reference control which was recorded at –7.2 kcal/mol. The MD simulations favour their stability with the protein structures, and the predicted ADMET properties support their drug likeness and safety, making them worthy of further consideration (Ahmad et al. 2021). Although NS7, NS20, and NS22 were not among the selected 10 candidates when 25 phytochemicals of NS were investigated against the nucleocapsid (N) protein (PDB entry 6M3M), Mpro (PDB entry 6M03), and PLpro (PDB 6W9C) for SARS-CoV-2 replication using bioinformatic techniques. However, the compounds also displayed fair binding interactions indicated by respective docking scores of −7.15, −4.04, and −7.22 kcal/mol with Mpro and −5.16, −4.95, and −5.31 kcal/mol with PLpro and ideal ADMET profiles (Siddiqui et al. 2022). Similarly, remdesivir and α-hederin, non-phenolic phytoconstituents of NS, showed higher binding affinities to the RdRp of SARS-CoV-2 (PDB entry 6M71) with docking scores of −7.6 and −8.6 kcal/mol, respectively, compared to the phenolic NS18, NS19, NS20, and NS21, which scored −4.5, −6.0, −4.3, and −4.6 kcal/mol, respectively, upon molecular docking analysis (Mir et al. 2022). However, their interactions with RdRp deserve further scientific attention through experimental validation in the quest for RdRp inhibitors for treating COVID-19. Interestingly, the four compounds again expressed higher binding affinities than remdesivir and hydroxychloroquine (HCQ) when investigated against some key targets for suppressing viral infusion, replication, and transcription. These include the 3CLpro (PDB entry 6LU7), RBD-ACE2 interface (PDB entry 6VW1), prefusion S protein (PDB entry 6VSB), and S protein (PDB entry 6VXX). The four phenolic phytochemicals were recorded with docking scores ranging from −6.01 to −4.30 kcal/mol against the receptors, whereas remdesivir and HCQ showed binding energies in the range of −4.09 to 16.82 kcal/mol and −4.83 to −3.61 kcal/mol against the same target. Further, NS18, NS20, and NS21 were selected phenolic phytochemicals among the 13 major phytoconstituents of NS screened for inhibitory potentials against the 3CLpro and nsp 15 of SARS-CoV-2 using bioinformatics approaches involving molecular docking, MD simulation, and ADMET prediction. The compounds were recorded with docking scores of −5.20, −5.19 and −5.35, respectively, against the 3CLpro (PDB entry 6LU7), although the values were lower than −7.95 kcal/mol for lopinavir, a control inhibitor of the target. However, the compounds with the respective binding affinities of −5.50, −5.27, and −5.90 kcal/mol, also bound potently to nsp 15 (PDB entry 6VWW) comparably to the selected control, benzopurpurin B, which scored −5.87 kcal/mol. The predicted physicochemical and ADMET properties, as well as stability with the proteins upon MD simulation, suggest the compounds worthy of further study as prospective candidates for mitigating SARS-CoV-2 replication and transcription (Rizvi et al. 2021). Moreover, an investigation of 58 phytochemicals reportedly extractable from NS using bioinformatics approaches including molecular docking and ADMET predictions favoured NS17, NS19, and NS22 as promising multi-target–directed inhibitors of SARS-CoV-2 among other phenolic contents. The compounds were recorded with respective binding affinities in the ranges of −6.9 to −9.8 kcal/mol, −6.3 to −8.8 kcal/mol, and −6.2 to −8.7 kcal/mol, respectively, when virtually screened against some relevant viral proteins for replication and transcription. These include the crystal structures for Mpro free enzyme (PDB entry 6Y2E), PLpro (nsp 3; PDB entry 6W9C), RdRp (nsp 12; PDB entry 6M71), RBD (PDB entry 6M17), endoribonuclease (nsp 15; PDB entry 6VWW), RNA-binding protein (nsp 9; PDB entry 6W4B), RBD of N protein (PDB entry 6VYO), and nsp 13 helicase (PDB entry 6ZSL). Meanwhile, chloroquine, a reference drug, scored significantly lower with binding affinities ranging from −4.7 to −6.3 kcal/mol against the enlisted targets. Interestingly, the selected compounds were predicted with ideal profiles for drug potential and safety, making them promising therapeutic prospects for COVID-19 with network pharmacological effects amenable for further investigation (Baig and Srinivasan 2022).

Another study was conducted using a bioinformatics approach to promote therapeutic effects of the "miraculous herb" NS for all diseases including emerging ones such as COVID-19 according to prophetic and biblical assertions. In the study, the results from the molecular docking, MD simulations, and predictions of physicochemical properties projected NS19 and NS23 as promising inhibitors of SARS-CoV-2 Mro (PDB entry 6LU7). For instance, the compounds showed respective higher docking scores of −7.8 kcal/mol and −8.2 kcal/mol than a renowned Mpro ligand, leupeptin, with −7.6 kcal/mol, although N3, another Mpro ligand, scored the highest with −9.1 kcal/mol (Hardianto et al. 2021). The voluminous interesting reports from the *in silico* and bioinformatics evaluation of NS further support the worthiness of the medicinal plant as a promising candidate for COVID-19.

To further express the inhibitory potential of NS, its major phytochemicals were screened for interaction with ACE2 using molecular docking analysis. Two phenolic compounds, NS18 and NS21, displayed strong binding affinities to the active pocket of ACE2 (PDB entry 1R4L), especially the latter, whose docking score (−5.466 kcal/mol) was very close to that of the top-ranked non-phenolic ligand, α-hederin (−6.263 kcal/mol). Meanwhile, bioinformatic tools for network interaction analysis have been explored to further validate the molecular correlations between the ACE2 and some relevant biomolecules for hypoxia- and inflammatory-related mechanisms associated with COVID-19. The interaction of the ligands with ACE2 further suggests the propensity of NS phytochemicals for therapeutic designs against the virulent checkpoint in the COVID-19 episode (Jakhmola Mani et al. 2022). The summary of antiviral activities of some phenolic phytochemicals from the three selected Ayurvedic botanicals as investigated using bioinformatics is presented in Table 4.6.

4.8 CONCLUSION AND FUTURE PROSPECTS

Bacterial and viral diseases continuously pose serious threats to human wellness, and they have been responsible for most of the pandemics the world has witnessed. Incessant resistance development by the relevant pathogens, low efficacy, accessibility, and unbearable effects of the currently available medications inclusively constitute therapeutic challenges. This makes continuous scientific efforts towards the discovery of improved alternatives essential. Although the entire process of introducing a new drug for clinical applications is cumbersome, demanding exorbitant costs and other resources, lengthy time frames, and environmental risks, the incorporation of CADD, specifically the bioinformatics approach, ameliorates the challenges and facilitates the process. In this chapter, investigations of antibacterial and antiviral performances of major phenolic phytoconstituents of three Ayurvedic botanicals, *A. paniculata, P. amarus,* and *N. sativa,* were showcased through bioinformatics techniques. Several active phenolic compounds, notably, rutin, astragalin, kaempferol-3-glucoside, and chlorogenic acid, have demonstrated interesting broad-spectrum inhibitory interactions against relevant therapeutic targets of major pathogenic organisms including the multi-drug-resistant metallo-β-lactamase–producing Enterobacteriaceae and the ravaging SARS-CoV-2. The extracts bearing the

TABLE 4.6
Summary of Antiviral Investigations of Representative Polyphenols and Some Other Metabolites from Selected Ayurvedic Botanicals Using a Bioinformatics Approach

Ayurvedic Botanica	Phenolic Phytochemicals	Target Organism	Mechanisms of Antiviral Action	Bioinformatics Tool	Interactive Structure	PDB Entry	Reference
AP	5,7,3',4'-Tertahydroxyflavone, 5,7,4'-trihydroxyflavone, tamarixetin, rhamnetin, luteolin and medioresinol	CHIKV	Inhibition of viral replication	Homology protein structure modelling; Molecular docking; ADMET prediction	nsp 1 nsp 2 nsp 3 nsp 4	HM 3TRK 3GPG HM	(Hussain, Amir, and Rasool 2020)
AP	Panicolin	DENV	Larvicidal effect of *A. aegypti*	Molecular docking	SCP-2	1PZ4	(Paul et al. 2021)
AP	Quercetin and caffeic acid	DENV	Inhibition of viral replication and transcription	Molecular docking	NS3 protease-helicase NS2/NS3 protease NS2B/NS3 protease DENV 3 protease 2nd conformation NS3 protease-helicase DENV 1 E protein DENV 2 E protein DENV 3 E protein DENV 4 E protein NS5 RdRp	2VBC 3L6P 2FOM 3U1J 2WHX 3UZQ 1TG8 1UZG 3UYP 2J7W	(Pawar and Patravale 2020)

(Continued)

TABLE 4.6 (*Continued*)
Summary of Antiviral Investigations of Representative Polyphenols and Some Other Metabolites from Selected Ayurvedic Botanicals Using a Bioinformatics Approach

Ayurvedic Botanica	Phenolic Phytochemicals	Target Organism	Mechanisms of Antiviral Action	Bioinformatics Tool	Interactive Structure	PDB Entry	Reference
AP	2,4-dihydroxycinnamic acid, 3-O-caffeoyl-D-quinic acid, 3,7,8-trimethoxy-2-(2-methoxyphenyl)-4 H, 5-hydroxy-7,8,2',3'-tetramethoxyflavone and 5-hydroxy-7,8,2'-trimethoxyflavone	SARS-CoV-2	Suppression of viral entry, replication/synthesis, transcription, RNA-binding, promotion of cytokines, formation of ion channels for viral particles release, blocking of host's RNA translation and dominant immunogens	Molecular docking; Molecular dynamics; ADMET prediction	Mpro nsp 3 nsp 9 nsp 15 E protein M protein S protein ORF1a ORF3a RBD	6LU7 6VXS 6WXD 6VWW 5X29 3I6G 6CRV 2G9T 6XDC 6M0J	(Swaminathan et al. 2021)
AP	5,4'-Dihydroxy-7-O-β-D-pyran-glycuronate butyl ester and 7,8-dimethoxy-2'hydroxy-5-O-β-d-glucopyranosyloxyflavone	SARS-CoV-2	Inhibition of viral replication and transcription.	Molecular docking; Toxicity prediction	3CLpro	6LU7	(Sukardiman et al. 2020)
AP	Dihydroxy-dimethoxy flavone	SARS-CoV-2	Inhibition of viral replication and transcription.	Molecular docking; ADMET prediction; MMGB/SA	Mpro	5R82	(Kalirajan and Varakumar 2020)
AP	5-Hydroxy-7,6,2',3'-tetramethoxy flavone, 5-hydroxy-7,8,2',5'-tetramethoxy flavone and 5-hydroxy-7,8-dimethoxy flavone	SARS-CoV-2	Inhibition of viral replication and transcription.	Molecular docking; ADMET prediction	S-protein (opened) S-protein (closed) 3CLpro PLpro RdRp	6VYB 6VXX 6LU7 4OVZ 6NUS	(Hiremath et al. 2021)

NS	Carvacrol	SARS-CoV-2	Inhibition of viral entry	Molecular docking; ADMET prediction	TMPRSS2	HM	(Yadav, Jaiswal, and Singh 2021)
NS	Carvacrol, nigellidine, thymol, thymohydroquinone	SARS-CoV-2	Disruption of viral-host entry interface; inhibition of viral replication	Molecular docking; ADMET prediction	RBD-ACE2 3CLpro Prefusion S protein S protein (opened)	6VW1 6LU7 6VSB 6VXX	(Ahmad et al. 2021; Pandey et al. 2021)
NS	Carvacrol and thymohydroquinone	SARS-CoV2	Inhibitory interactions with hypoxia- and inflammatory-related checkpoint for COVID-19 virulence	Network interaction analysis; Molecular docking	ACE2	1R4L	(Jakhmola Mani et al. 2022)
NS	Astragalin, quercetin, and thymol	SARS-CoV-2	Inhibition of viral replication and transcription	Molecular docking; MD; ADMET prediction	N protein Mpro PLpro	6M3M 6M03 6W9C	(Siddiqui et al. 2022)
NS	Rutin, nigellidine, and astragalin	SARS-CoV-2	Inhibition of viral entry, replication/synthesis, transcription, RNA binding, and RNA translation	Molecular docking; ADMET prediction	Mpro PLpro RdRp RBD nsp 15 nsp 9 RBD of N protein nsp 13 helicase	6Y2E 6W9C 6M71 6M17 6VWW 6W4B 6VYO 6ZSL	(Baig and Srinivasan 2022)
NS	Carvacrol, nigellidine, thymol, and thymohydroquinone	SARS-CoV-2	Inhibition of viral replication and synthesis	Molecular docking	RdRp	6M71	(Mir et al. 2022)
NS	Carvacrol, nigellidine, nigellidine-4-O-sulfite, thymol, and thymohydroquinone	SARS-CoV-2	Inhibition of viral replication and transcription	Molecular docking; MD; ADMET prediction	3CLpro nsp 15	6LU7 6VWW	(Rizvi et al. 2021; Hardianto et al. 2021)

Abbreviations: AP = *Andrographis paniculata;* HM = homology model.

representative phytochemicals have also been reported with attractive activities implicating the synergistic effects of the phytoconstituents. The activities of the extracts further validate the results from bioinformatics investigation of individual phenolic compounds, posing them as promising future antibiotic and antiviral alternatives. As such, they represent promising candidates for future antibiotic and antiviral designs.

Considering the unwavering pool of applications in the literature, the bioinformatics approach has become almost inevitable in modern drug discovery. Consistently in this context, it has promoted the therapeutic potentials of phenolic phytochemicals in selected Ayurvedic botanicals for further study as worthy candidates for antibacterial and antiviral drug alternatives. This chapter represents a model for knowledge-based therapeutic science for combating bacterial and viral diseases through the incorporation of bioinformatics techniques.

Despite its enormous advantages, the application of bioinformatics essentially requires capital investments, especially in sophisticated computing and data processing resources, and expertise and skills for protocol configuration. Moreover, an extensive understanding of the diseases' biochemistry is crucial for selecting appropriate bioinformatics tools to minimize failure. In addition, being theoretical, its reliability for accuracy and precision necessarily require experimental validation. Therefore, the enlisted phenolic phytochemicals from the selected Ayurvedic botanicals are hereby presented for experimental scientists for further validation as bona fide antibacterial and antiviral prospects through more robust *in vitro* and *in vivo* investigations.

4.9 ACKNOWLEDGEMENT

This project was financially supported by the Tertiary Education Fund Nigeria, Fundamental Research Grant Scheme, Ministry of Higher Education of Malaysia (grant no. 203.CDADAH.6711955). YOA is thankful to the Universiti Sains Malaysia for GA Scheme (grant no. 308.AIPS.415401).

REFERENCES

Abbas, Khushnood, Alireza Abbasi, Shi Dong, Ling Niu, Laihang Yu, Bolun Chen, Shi Min Cai, and Qambar Hasan. 2021. "Application of Network Link Prediction in Drug Discovery." *BMC Bioinformatics* 22 (1): 1–21. https://doi.org/10.1186/s12859-021-04082-y.

Ahmad, Sajjad, Hyder Wajid Abbasi, Sara Shahid, Sana Gul, and Sumra Wajid Abbasi. 2021. "Molecular Docking, Simulation and MM-PBSA Studies of Nigella Sativa Compounds: A Computational Quest to Identify Potential Natural Antiviral for COVID-19 Treatment." *Journal of Biomolecular Structure and Dynamics* 39 (12): 4225–4233. https://doi.org/10.1080/07391102.2020.1775129.

Ahmad Mir, Shabir, Mohammed Alaidarous, Bader Alshehri, Bilal Ahmad Mir, Abdul Aziz Bin D, Saeed Banawas, Ahmad Firoz, et al. 2022. "Identification of Mycobacterial RNA Polymerase Inhibitors from the Main Phytochemicals of Nigella Sativa: An in Silico Study." *International Journal of Pharmacology* 18 (5): 1015–1025. https://doi.org/10.3923/ijp.2022.1015.1025.

Alshwyeh, Hussah Abdullah, Sahar Khamees Aldosary, Muna Abdulsalam Ilowefah, Raheem Shahzad, Adeeb Shehzad, Saqib Bilal, In-jung Lee, et al. 2022. "Biological

Potentials and Phytochemical Constituents of Raw and Roasted Nigella Arvensis and Nigella Sativa." *Molecules* 27 (550): 1–10. https://doi.org/10.3390/molecules27020550.

Arifullah, Mohmmed, Nima Dandu Namsa, Manabendra Mandal, Paritala Vikrama, Kishore Kumar Chiruvella, and Ghanta Rama Gopal. 2013. "Evaluation of Anti-Bacterial and Anti-Oxidant Potential of Andrographolide and Echiodinin Isolated from Callus Culture of A Ndrographis Paniculata Nees." *Asian Pacific Journal of Tropical Biomedicine* 3 (8): 604–610. https://doi.org/10.1016/S2221-1691(13)60123-9.

Arjomandi, Khalili Omid, Mahboubeh Kavoosi, and Hadi Adibi. 2019. "Synthesis and Enzyme-Based Evaluation of Analogues L-Tyrosine Thiol Carboxylic Acid Inhibitor of Metallo-β-Lactamase IMP-1." *Journal of Enzyme Inhibition and Medicinal Chemistry* 34 (1): 1414–1425. https://doi.org/10.1080/14756366.2019.1651314.

Atu, Sri, Kartika R Pertiw, Mahclisatul Qolbia, and Salsabila Saf. 2022. "Phytochemical Analysis Both of Water and Ethanol Extract from Some Herbs Combinations, Nanoemulsion Formulation, and Antioxidant Effects." *Open Access Macedonian Journal of Medical Sciences* 10: 95–100.

Ayipo, Yusuf Oloruntoyin, Iqrar Ahmad, Yahaya Sani Najib, Sikirat Kehinde Sheu, Harun Patel, and Mohd Nizam Mordi. 2022. "Molecular Modelling and Structure-Activity Relationship of a Natural Derivative of o-Hydroxybenzoate as a Potent Inhibitor of Dual NSP3 and NSP12 of SARS-CoV-2: In Silico Study." *Journal of Biomolecular Structure and Dynamics*: 1–19. https://doi.org/10.1080/07391102.2022.2026818.

Ayipo, Yusuf Oloruntoyin, Waleed A Alananzeh, Iqrar Ahmad, Harun Patel, and Mohd Nizam Mordi. 2022. "Structural Modelling and in Silico Pharmacology of β-Carboline Alkaloids as Potent 5-HT1A Receptor Antagonists and Reuptake Inhibitors." *Journal of Biomolecular Structure and Dynamics*: 1–17. https://doi.org/10.1080/07391102.2022.2104376.

Ayipo, Yusuf Oloruntoyin, Ajibola Abdulahi Bakare, Umar Muhammad Badeggi, Akeem Adebayo Jimoh, Amudat Lawal, and Mohd Nizam Mordi. 2022. "Recent Advances on Therapeutic Potentials of Gold and Silver Nanobiomaterials for Human Viral Diseases." *Current Research in Chemical Biology* 2: 100021. https://doi.org/10.1016/j.crchbi.2022.100021.

Ayipo, Yusuf Oloruntoyin, Wahab Adesina Osunniran, Halimah Funmilayo Babamale, Monsurat Olabisi Ayinde, and Mohd Nizam Mordi. 2022. "Metalloenzyme Mimicry and Modulation Strategies to Conquer Antimicrobial Resistance: Metal-Ligand Coordination Perspectives." *Coordination Chemistry Reviews* 453: 214317. https://doi.org/10.1016/j.ccr.2021.214317.

Ayipo, Yusuf Oloruntoyin, SN Yahaya, WA Alananzeh, HF Babamale, and MN Mordi. 2021. "Pathomechanisms, Therapeutic Targets and Potent Inhibitors of Some Beta-Coronaviruses from Bench-to-Bedside." *Infection, Genetics and Evolution* 93. https://doi.org/10.1016/j.meegid.2021.104944.

Baig, Asma, and Hemalatha Srinivasan. 2022. *SARS-CoV-2 Inhibitors from Nigella Sativa. Applied Biochemistry and Biotechnology.* Vol. 194. Springer US. https://doi.org/10.1007/s12010-021-03790-8.

Banerjee, Malabika, Soumitra Moulick, Kunal Kumar Bhattacharya, Debaprasad Parai, Subrata Chattopadhyay, and Samir Kumar Mukherjee. 2017. "AC SC." *Microbial Pathogenesis.* https://doi.org/10.1016/j.micpath.2017.10.023.

Benlafya, Kamal, Khalid Karrouchi, Yassine Charkaoui, Miloud El Karbane, and Youssef Ramli. 2014. "Extracts and Essential Oil of Nigella Sativa Seeds Antimicrobial Activity of Aqueous, Ethanolic, Methanolic, Cyclohexanic Extracts and Essential Oil of Nigella Sativa Seeds." *Journal of Chemical and Pharmaceutical Research* 6 (8): 4–7.

Boozari, Motahareh, and Hossein Hosseinzadeh. 2020. "Natural Products for COVID-19 Prevention and Treatment Regarding to Previous Coronavirus Infections and Novel Studies." *Phytotherapy Research* 35 (2): 864–876. https://doi.org/10.1002/ptr.6873.

Bourgou, Soumaya, Riadh Ksouri, Amor Bellila, Ines Skandrani, Hanen Falleh, and Brahim Marzouk. 2008. "Phenolic Composition and Biological Activities of Tunisian Nigella Sativa L. Shoots and Roots." *Comptes Rendus—Biologies* 331 (1): 48–55. https://doi.org/10.1016/j.crvi.2007.11.001.

Boyd, Sara E, David M Livermore, David C Hooper, and William W Hope. 2020. "Metallo-β-Lactamases: Structure, Function, Epidemiology, Treatment Options, and the Development Pipeline." *Antimicrobial Agents and Chemotherapy* 64 (10): 1–20. https://doi.org/10.1128/AAC.00397-20.

Brogi, Simone, Teodorico Castro Ramalho, Kamil Kuca, José L Medina-Franco, and Marian Valko. 2020. "Editorial: In Silico Methods for Drug Design and Discovery." *Frontiers in Chemistry* 8: 1–10. https://doi.org/10.3389/fchem.2020.00612.

Burley, Stephen K, Charmi Bhikadiya, Chunxiao Bi, Sebastian Bittrich, Li Chen, et al. 2021. "RCSB Protein Data Bank: Powerful New Tools for Exploring 3D Structures of Biological Macromolecules for Basic and Applied Research and Education in Fundamental Biology, Biomedicine, Biotechnology, Bioengineering and Energy Sciences." *Nucleic Acids Research* 49: D437–D451. https://doi.org/http://doi.org/10.1093/nar/gkaa1038.

Bush, Karen. 2018. "Past and Present Perspectives on β-Lactamases." *Antimicrobial Agents and Chemotherapy* 62 (10): 1–20. https://doi.org/10.1128/AAC.01076-18.

Castro-Alvarez, Alejandro, Anna M Costa, and Jaume Vilarrasa. 2017. "The Performance of Several Docking Programs at Reproducing Protein-Macrolide-like Crystal Structures." *Molecules* 22 (1). https://doi.org/10.3390/molecules22010136.

CDC. 2019. "Antibiotic Resistance Threats in the United States, 2019." *U.S. Department of Health and Human Services*, CDC. https://doi.org/10.15620/cdc:82532.

Chandan, S, S Umesha, Prasad K Shiva, V Balamurugan, S Chandrashekar, Kumar SR Santosh, Ramu Ramith, S Shirahatti Prithvi, Syed Asad, and Abdallah M Elgorban. 2022. "Potential Antileptospiral Constituents from Phyllanthus Amarus." *Pharmacognosy Magazine* 16: S371–S378. https://doi.org/10.4103/pm.pm.

Chattopadhyay, Kaushik, Haiquan Wang, Jaspreet Kaur, Gamze Nalbant, Abdullah Almaqhawi, Burak Kundakci, Jeemon Panniyammakal, et al. 2022. "Effectiveness and Safety of Ayurvedic Medicines in Type 2 Diabetes Mellitus Management: A Systematic Review and Meta-Analysis." *Frontiers in Pharmacology* 13 (June): 1–31. https://doi.org/10.3389/fphar.2022.821810.

Chen, Allie Yingyao. 2020. "Conversion of Metal Chelators to Selective and Potent Inhibitors of New Delhi Metallo-Beta-Lactamase." *UC San Diego*. https://escholarship.org/uc/item/8xk949p6.

Chen, Jianzhong, Jinan Wang, and Weiliang Zhu. 2017. "Zinc Ion-Induced Conformational Changes in New Delphi Metallo-β-Lactamase 1 Probed by Molecular Dynamics Simulations and Umbrella Sampling." *Physical Chemistry Chemical Physics* 19 (4): 3067–3075. https://doi.org/10.1039/c6cp08105c.

Chukwudozie, Onyeka S, Vincent C Duru, Charlotte C Ndiribe, Abdullahi T Aborode, Victor O Oyebanji, and Benjamin O Emikpe. 2021. "The Relevance of Bioinformatics Applications in the Discovery of Vaccine Candidates and Potential Drugs for COVID-19 Treatment." *Bioinformatics and Biology Insights* 15. https://doi.org/10.1177/11779322211002168.

Corciovă, Andreia, Cornelia Mircea, Cristina Tuchiluş, Oana Cioancă, Ana Flavia Burlec, Bianca Ivănescu, Laurian Vlase, et al. 2018. "Phenolic and Sterolic Profile of a Phyllanthus Amarus Extract and Characterization of Newly Synthesized Silver Nanoparticles." *Farmacia* 66 (5): 831–838. https://doi.org/10.31925/farmacia.2018.5.13.

Dalli, Mohammed, Oussama Bekkouch, Salah Eddine Azizi, Ali Azghar, Nadia Gseyra, and Bonglee Kim. 2022. "Nigella Sativa L. Phytochemistry and Pharmacological Activities: A Review (2019–2021)." *Biomolecules* 12 (1). https://doi.org/10.3390/biom12010020.

Dhandapania, R, D Lakshmia, S Jayakumarc, V Balakrishnanb, and Anandha Kumar. 2007. "Preliminary Phytochemical Investigation and Antibacterial Activity of *Phyllanthus Amarus Schum & Thorn*." *Ancient Science of Life* 27 (1): 1–5.

Feng, Yuying, Frank R Dunshea, and Hafiz AR Suleria. 2020. "LC-ESI-QTOF/MS Characterization of Bioactive Compounds from Black Spices and Their Potential Antioxidant Activities." *Journal of Food Science and Technology* 57 (12): 4671–4687. https://doi.org/10.1007/s13197-020-04504-4.

Gueffai, Abdelkrim, Diego J Gonzalez-Serrano, Marios C Christodoulou, Jose C Orellana-Palacios, Maria Lopez S Ortega, Aoumria Ouldmoumna, Fatima Zohra Kiari, et al. 2022. "Phenolics from Defatted Black Cumin Seeds (Nigella Sativa L.): Ultrasound-Assisted Extraction Optimization, Comparison, and Antioxidant Activity." *Biomolecules* 12 (9). https://doi.org/10.3390/biom12091311.

Guha, Gunjan, V Rajkumar, R Ashok Kumar, and Lazar Mathew. 2010. "Aqueous Extract of Phyllanthus Amarus Inhibits Chromium(VI)-Induced Toxicity in MDA-MB-435S Cells." *Food and Chemical Toxicology* 48 (1): 396–401. https://doi.org/10.1016/j.fct.2009.10.028.

Gyawali, Dinesh, Rini Vohra, David Orme-Johnson, Sridharan Ramaratnam, and Robert H Schneider. 2021. "A Systematic Review and Meta-Analysis of Ayurvedic Herbal Preparations for Hypercholesterolemia." *Medicina (Lithuania)* 57 (6): 1–24. https://doi.org/10.3390/medicina57060546.

Hajong, Siddharth, and Sangeeta Sarma. 2021. "Study of Antibacterial Efficacy of Andrographis Paniculata against TEM-1 Beta-Lactamase Producing Escherichia Coli." *Journal of Pharmaceutical Sciences and Research* 13 (9): 590–596.

Hameed, Saleha, Ali Imran, Mehr un Nisa, Muhammad Sajid Arshad, Farhan Saeed, Muhammad Umair Arshad, and Muhammad Asif Khan. 2019. "Characterization of Extracted Phenolics from Black Cumin (Nigella Sativa Linn), Coriander Seed (Coriandrum Sativum L.), and Fenugreek Seed (Trigonella Foenum-Graecum)." *International Journal of Food Properties* 22 (1): 714–726. https://doi.org/10.1080/10942912.2019.1599390.

Harder, Edward, Wolfgang Damm, Jon Maple, Chuanjie Wu, Mark Reboul, Jin Yu Xiang, Lingle Wang, et al. 2016. "OPLS3: A Force Field Providing Broad Coverage of Drug-like Small Molecules and Proteins." *Journal of Chemical Theory and Computation* 12 (1): 281–296. https://doi.org/10.1021/acs.jctc.5b00864.

Hardianto, Ari, Muhammad Yusuf, Ika Wiani Hidayat, Safri Ishmayana, and Ukun Mochammad Syukur Soedjanaatmadja. 2021. "Exploring the Potency of Nigella Sativa Seed in Inhibiting Sars-Cov-2 Main Protease Using Molecular Docking and Molecular Dynamics Simulations." *Indonesian Journal of Chemistry* 21 (5): 1252–1262. https://doi.org/10.22146/IJC.65951.

Hiremath, Shridhar, HD Vinay Kumar, M Nandan, M Mantesh, KS Shankarappa, V Venkataravanappa, CR Jahir Basha, and CN Lakshminarayana Reddy. 2021. "In Silico Docking Analysis Revealed the Potential of Phytochemicals Present in Phyllanthus Amarus and Andrographis Paniculata, Used in Ayurveda Medicine in Inhibiting SARS-CoV-2." *3 Biotech* 11 (2): 1–18. https://doi.org/10.1007/s13205-020-02578-7.

Hussain, Waqar, Anam Amir, and Nouman Rasool. 2020. "Computer-Aided Study of Selective Flavonoids Against Chikungunya Virus Replication Using Molecular Docking and DFT-Based Approach." *Structural Chemistry* 31 (4): 1363–1374. https://doi.org/10.1007/s11224-020-01507-x.

Islam, Muhammad Torequl, Roich Khan, and Siddhartha Kumar. 2019. "An Updated Literature – Based Review: Phytochemistry, Pharmacology and Therapeutic Promises of Nigella Sativa L." *Oriental Pharmacy and Experimental Medicine*, no. 0123456789. https://doi.org/10.1007/s13596-019-00363-3.

Islam, Muhammad Torequl, Chandan Sarkar, Dina M El-Kersh, Sarmin Jamaddar, Shaikh J Uddin, Jamil A Shilpi, and Mohammad S Mubarak. 2020. "Natural Products and Their Derivatives Against Coronavirus: A Review of the Non-Clinical and Pre-Clinical Data." *Phytotherapy Research* 34 (10): 2471–2492. https://doi.org/10.1002/ptr.6700.

Jakhmola Mani, Ruchi, Nikita Sehgal, Nitu Dogra, Shikha Saxena, and Deepshikha Pande Katare. 2022. "Deciphering Underlying Mechanism of Sars-CoV-2 Infection in Humans and Revealing the Therapeutic Potential of Bioactive Constituents from Nigella Sativa to Combat COVID19: In-Silico Study." *Journal of Biomolecular Structure and Dynamics* 40 (6): 2417–2429. https://doi.org/10.1080/07391102.2020.1839560.

Joshi, Rajesh K. 2023. "Bioactive Usual and Unusual Triterpenoids Derived from Natural Sources Used in Traditional Medicine." *Chemistry and Biodiversity* 20 (2). https://doi.org/10.1002/cbdv.202200853.

Kalirajan, Rajagopal, Varakumar Potlapati, Baliwada Aparma, and Byran Gowramma. 2020. "Activity of Phytochemical Constituents of Curcuma longa (Turmeric) Against SARS-CoV-2 Main Protease (Covid19): An in-Silico Approach." *International Journal of Pharmacy* 6 (104): 1–10. https://doi.org/10.1186/s43094-020-00126-x.

Kar, Bipasa, Chanakya Nath Kundu, Sanghamitra Pati, and Debdutta Bhattacharya. 2021. "Discovery of Phyto-Compounds as Novel Inhibitors against NDM-1 and VIM-1 Protein Through Virtual Screening and Molecular Modelling." *Journal of Biomolecular Structure and Dynamics*: 1–14. https://doi.org/10.1080/07391102.2021.2019125.

Kumar, Syal, Gustav J Dobos, and Thomas Rampp. 2017. "The Significance of Ayurvedic Medicinal Plants." *Journal of Evidence-Based Complementary and Alternative Medicine* 22 (3): 494–501. https://doi.org/10.1177/2156587216671392.

Kuralkar, Prajakta, and SV Kuralkar. 2021. "Role of Herbal Products in Animal Production—An Updated Review." *Journal of Ethnopharmacology* 278 (5): 114246. https://doi.org/10.1016/j.jep.2021.114246.

Legru, Alice, Federica Verdirosa, Jean François Hernandez, Giusy Tassone, Filomena Sannio, Manuela Benvenuti, Pierre Alexis Conde, et al. 2021. "1,2,4-Triazole-3-Thione Compounds with a 4-Ethyl Alkyl/Aryl Sulfide Substituent Are Broad-Spectrum Metallo-β-Lactamase Inhibitors with Re-Sensitization Activity." *European Journal of Medicinal Chemistry* 226: 113873. https://doi.org/10.1016/j.ejmech.2021.113873.

Lewis, AL, CM Szymanski, RL Schnaar, et al. 2022. "Bacterial and Viral Infections." In *Essentials of Glycobiology [Internet]*, edited by A Varki, RD Cummings, JD Esko, et al., 4th ed. New York: Cold Spring Harbor Laboratory Press. https://doi.org/10.1101/glycobiology.4e.42.

Lima, Lidia Moreira, Bianca Nascimento Monteiro da Silva, Gisele Barbosa, and Eliezer J Barreiro. 2020. "β-Lactam Antibiotics: An Overview from a Medicinal Chemistry Perspective." *European Journal of Medicinal Chemistry* 208: 112829. https://doi.org/10.1016/j.ejmech.2020.112829.

Lovell, SC, IW Davis, WB Adrendall, PIW de Bakker, JM Word, MG Prisant, JS Richardson, and DC Richardson. 2003. "Structure Validation by C Alpha GeomF. Altschul, S., Gish, W., Miller, W., W. Myers, E., & J. Lipman, D. (1990). Basic Local Alignment Search Tool. Journal of Molecular Biology.Etry: Phi,Psi and C Beta Deviation." *Proteins-Structure Function and Genetics* 50 (August 2002): 437–450. http://onlinelibrary.wiley.com/store/10.1002/prot.10286/asset/10286_ftp.pdf?v=1&t=gwhx9jy0&s=b3b0f129a5acf7f4513aea04d22aad7ee4f4a89d.

Maity, Soumya, Suchandra Chatterjee, Prasad Shekhar Variyar, Arun Sharma, Soumyakanti Adhikari, and Santasree Mazumder. 2013. "Evaluation of Antioxidant Activity and Characterization of Phenolic Constituents of Phyllanthus Amarus Root." *Journal of Agricultural and Food Chemistry* 61 (14): 3443–3450. https://doi.org/10.1021/jf3046686.

Manso, Tamara, Marta Lores, and Trinidad de Miguel. 2022. "Antimicrobial Activity of Polyphenols and Natural Polyphenolic Extracts on Clinical Isolates." *Antibiotics* 11 (1): 1–18. https://doi.org/10.3390/antibiotics11010046.

Maria, Alessandra, Braga Ribeiro, Jonas Nascimento, De Sousa, Luciana Muratori, Felipe Araújo, De Alcântara Oliveira, et al. 2019. "Microbial Pathogenesis Antimicrobial Activity of Phyllanthus Amarus Schumach & Thonn and Inhibition of the NorA e Ffl Ux Pump of Staphylococcus Aureus by Phyllanthin." *Microbial Pthogenesis* 130 (January): 242–246. https://doi.org/10.1016/j.micpath.2019.03.012.

Matou, Mélissa, Sylvie Bercion, Thérèse Marianne-Pepin, Pierre Haddad, and Patrick Merciris. 2021. "Phenolic Profiles and Biological Properties of Traditional Phyllanthus Amarus Aqueous Extracts Used for Diabetes." *Journal of Functional Foods* 83 (June). https://doi.org/10.1016/j.jff.2021.104571.

Mir, Shabir Ahmad, Ahmad Firoz, Mohammed Alaidarous, Bader Alshehri, Abdul Aziz Bin Dukhyil, Saeed Banawas, Suliman A Alsagaby, et al. 2022. "Identification of SARS-CoV-2 RNA-Dependent RNA Polymerase Inhibitors from the Major Phytochemicals of Nigella Sativa: An in Silico Approach." *Saudi Journal of Biological Sciences* 29 (1): 394–401. https://doi.org/10.1016/j.sjbs.2021.09.002.

Mohamad, Suharni, Tuan Nadrah, Naim Tuan, Ismail Tuan, Mohamad Ezany Yusoff, Rosmaniza Abdullah, Siti Asma Hassan, Zeti Norfidiyati Salmuna, and Nusaadatun Nisak Ahmad. 2021. "Antibacterial Activity of Andrographis Paniculata Aqueous Extract Against Oral Pathogens." *MAB Malaysian Applied Biology* 50: 163–167.

Mojica, Maria F, Maria Agustina Rossi, Alejandro J Vila, and Robert A Bonomo. 2022. "The Urgent Need for Metallo-β-Lactamase Inhibitors: An Unattended Global Threat." *The Lancet Infectious Diseases* 22 (1): e28–e34. https://doi.org/10.1016/S1473-3099(20)30868-9.

Moreira, Jonatham Souza, Danilo Santana Galvão, Carolina Ferreira Cavalcanti Xavier, Silvio Cunha, Samuel Silva da Rocha Pita, Joice Neves Reis, and Humberto Fonseca de Freitas. 2021. "Phenotypic and in Silico Studies for a Series of Synthetic Thiosemicarbazones as New Delhi Metallo-Beta-Lactamase Carbapenemase Inhibitors." *Journal of Biomolecular Structure and Dynamics*: 1–13. https://doi.org/10.1080/07391102.2021.2001379.

Murray, Christopher JL, Kevin Shunji Ikuta, Fablina Sharara, Lucien Swetschinski, Gisela Robles Aguilar, Authia Gray, Chieh Han, et al. 2022. "Global Burden of Bacterial Antimicrobial Resistance in 2019: A Systematic Analysis." *The Lancet* 399 (10325): 629–655. https://doi.org/10.1016/s0140-6736(21)02724-0.

Murugan, K, S Sangeetha, VB Kalyanasundaram, and Saleh Al-sohaibani. 2013. "In Vitro and in Silico Screening for Andrographis Paniculata Quorum Sensing Mimics: New Therapeutic Leads for Cystic Fibrosis Pseudomonas Aeruginosa Biofilms." *Plant OMICS* 6 (5): 340–346.

Muthusamy, A, ER Sanjay, HN Nagendra Prasad, M Radhakrishna Rao, B Manjunath Joshi, S Padmalatha Rai, and K Satyamoorthy. 2018. "Quantitative Analysis of Phyllanthus Species for Bioactive Molecules Using High-Pressure Liquid Chromatography and Liquid Chromatography—Mass Spectrometry." *Proceedings of the National Academy of Sciences India Section B—Biological Sciences* 88 (3): 1043–1054. https://doi.org/10.1007/s40011-017-0839-y.

Nayak, BK, S Pavithera, and Anima Nanda. 2015. "Soxhlet Extraction of Leaf Extracts of Andrographis Paniculata and Its Antibacterial Efficacy against Few Pathogenic Bacterial Strains." *Der Pharmacia Lettre* 7 (4): 250–253.

Pandey, Pratibha, Fahad Khan, Avijit Mazumder, Ansh Kumar Rana, and Yashvi Srivastava. 2021. "Inhibitory Potential of Dietary Phytocompounds of Nigella Sativa against Key Targets of Novel Coronavirus (Covid-19)." *Indian Journal of Pharmaceutical Education and Research* 55 (1): 190–197. https://doi.org/10.5530/ijper.55.1.21.

Paul, Anubrata, V Samuel Raj, Arpana Vibhuti, and Ramendra Pati Pandey. 2021. "Larvicidal Efficacy of Andrographis Paniculata and Tinospora Cordifolia against Aedes Aegypti: A Dengue Vector." *Pharmacognosy Research*: 352–360. https://doi.org/10.4103/pr.pr.

Pawar, Rohit, and Vandana Patravale. 2020. "A Step towards Treating Dengue Viral Infection: An in Silico Approach to Identify Potential Antidengue Phytoconstituents." *ChemistrySelect* 5 (44): 13837–13854. https://doi.org/10.1002/slct.202004137.

Piret, Jocelyne, and Guy Boivin. 2021. "Pandemics Throughout History." *Frontiers in Microbiology* 11 (January). https://doi.org/10.3389/fmicb.2020.631736.

Praveen, N, M Naik Poornananda, and Abdul Nayeem. 2014. "Polyphenol Composition and Antioxidant Activity of Andrographis Paniculata L. Nees." *Mapana—Journal of Sciences* 13 (4): 33–46. https://doi.org/10.12723/mjs.31.4.

Prieto-Martínez, Fernando D, Edgar López-López, K Eurídice Juárez-Mercado, and José L Medina-Franco. 2019. "Computational Drug Design Methods—Current and Future Perspectives." *In Silico Drug Design* 3: 19–44. https://doi.org/10.1016/b978-0-12-816125-8.00002-x.

Rafi, Mohamad, Alfi Hudatul Karomah, Rudi Heryanto, Dewi Anggraini Septaningsih, Wisnu Ananta Kusuma, Muhammad Bachri Amran, Abdul Rohman, and Bambang Prajogo. 2020. "Metabolite Profiling of Andrographis Paniculata Leaves and Stem Extract Using UHPLC-Orbitrap-MS/MS." *Natural Product Research*: 1–5. https://doi.org/10.1080/14786419.2020.1789637.

Rajeshkumar, S 2015. "Antimicrobial Effect of King of Bitter Andrographis Paniculata and Traditional Herb Aegle Marmelos against Clinical Pathogens." *International Journal of PharmTech Research* 7 (2): 325–329.

Ramírez, David, and Julio Caballero. 2018. "Is It Reliable to Take the Molecular Docking Top Scoring Position as the Best Solution without Considering Available Structural Data?" *Molecules* 23 (5): 1–17. https://doi.org/10.3390/molecules23051038.

Reddy, MA. 2017. "Bioinformatics-Key to Drug Discovery and Development." *Open Access Journal of Pharmaceutical Research* 1 (5). https://doi.org/10.23880/oajpr-16000126.

Rizvi, SMD, Talib Hussain, Afrasim Moin, Sheshagiri R Dixit, Subhankar P Mandal, and Rahamat Unissa. 2021. "Identifying the Most Potent Dual-Targeting Compound(s) against 3CLprotease and NSP15exonuclease of SARS-CoV-2 from Nigella Sativa: Virtual Screening via Physicochemical Properties, Docking and Dynamic Simulation Analysis." *Processes* 9: 1814.

Salari-Jazi, Azhar, Karim Mahnam, Parisa Sadeghi, and Mohamad Sadegh Damavandi. 2021. "Discovery of Potential Inhibitors against New Delhi from Natural Compounds: In Silico – Based Methods." *Scientific Reports* 0123456789: 1–20. https://doi.org/10.1038/s41598-021-82009-6.

Saliu, Tolulope Peter, Haruna I Umar, Olawale Johnson Ogunsile, Micheal O Okpara, Noriyuki Yanaka, and Olusola Olalekan Elekofehinti. 2021. "Molecular Docking and Pharmacokinetic Studies of Phytocompounds from Nigerian Medicinal Plants as Promising Inhibitory Agents against SARS-CoV-2 Methyltransferase (Nsp16)." *Journal of Genetic Engineering and Biotechnology* 19 (1). https://doi.org/10.1186/s43141-021-00273-5.

Schaduangrat, Nalini, Samuel Lampa, Saw Simeon, Matthew Paul Gleeson, Ola Spjuth, and Chanin Nantasenamat. 2020. "Towards Reproducible Computational Drug Discovery." *Journal of Cheminformatics* 12 (1): 1–30. https://doi.org/10.1186/s13321-020-0408-x.

Shafodino, Festus S, Julien M Lusilao, and Lamech M Mwapagha Id. 2022. "Phytochemical Characterization and Antimicrobial Activity of Nigella Sativa Seeds." *PLoS ONE*: 1–20. https://doi.org/10.1371/journal.pone.0272457.

Shawky, Eman, Ahmed A Nada, and Reham S Ibrahim. 2020. "Potential Role of Medicinal Plants and Their Constituents in the Mitigation of SARS-CoV-2: Identifying Related Therapeutic Targets Using Network Pharmacology and Molecular Docking Analyses." *RSC Advances* 10 (47): 27961–27983. https://doi.org/10.1039/d0ra05126h.

Siddiqui, Sahabjada, Shivbrat Upadhyay, Rumana Ahmad, Anamika Gupta, Aditi Srivastava, Anchal Trivedi, Ishrat Husain, Bilal Ahmad, Maqusood Ahamed, and Mohsin Ali Khan. 2022. "Virtual Screening of Phytoconstituents from Miracle Herb Nigella Sativa Targeting Nucleocapsid Protein and Papain-like Protease of SARS-CoV-2 for COVID-19 Treatment." *Journal of Biomolecular Structure and Dynamics* 40 (9): 3928–3948. https://doi.org/10.1080/07391102.2020.1852117.

Sliwoski, Gregory, Sandeepkumar Kothiwale, Jens Meiler, and Edward W Lowe. 2014. "Computational Methods in Drug Discovery." *Pharmacological Reviews* 66 (1): 334–395. https://doi.org/10.1124/pr.112.007336.

Sousa, Adriana Dutra, Ana Isabel Vitorino Maia, Tigressa Helena Soares Rodrigues, Kirley Marques Canuto, Paulo Riceli Vasconcelos Ribeiro, Rita de Cassia Alves Pereira, Roberto Fontes Vieira, and Edy Sousa de Brito. 2016. "Ultrasound-Assisted and Pressurized Liquid Extraction of Phenolic Compounds from Phyllanthus Amarus and Its Composition Evaluation by UPLC-QTOF." *Industrial Crops and Products* 79: 91–103. https://doi.org/10.1016/j.indcrop.2015.10.045.

Sousa, Adriana Dutra, Paulo Riceli Vasconcelos Ribeiro, Kirley Marques Canuto, Guilherme Julião Zocolo, Rita de Cassia Alves Pereira, and Fabiano André Narciso Fernandes. 2017. "Drying Kinetics and Effect of Air-Drying Temperature on Chemical Composition of Phyllanthus Amarus and Phyllanthus Niruri Drying Kinetics and Effect of Air-Drying Temperature on Chemical Composition of Phyllanthus Amarus and Phyllanthus Niruri." *Drying Technology* 36 (5): 609–616. https://doi.org/10.1080/07373937.2017.1351454.

Stuper-Szablewska, Kinga, Tomasz Szablewski, Anna Przybylska-Balcerek, Lidia Szwajkowska-Michałek, Michał Krzyżaniak, Dariusz Świerk, Renata Cegielska-Radziejewska, and Zbigniew Krejpcio. 2023. "Antimicrobial Activities Evaluation and Phytochemical Screening of Some Selected Plant Materials Used in Traditional Medicine." *Molecules* 28 (1): 1–20. https://doi.org/10.3390/molecules28010244.

Sukardiman, Martha Ervina, Mohammad Rizki Fadhil Pratama, Hadi Poerwono, and Siswandono Siswodihardjo. 2020. "The Coronavirus Disease 2019 Main Protease Inhibitor from Andrographis Paniculata (Burm.f) Ness." *Journal of Advanced Pharmaceutical Technology and Research* 11 (4): 157–162. https://doi.org/10.4103/japtr.JAPTR_84_20.

Sundaram, Dinesh, Karthikeyan Kesavan, Hemalatha Kumaravel, Roohi Fatima Mohammed, Mekata Tohru, Itami Toshiaki, and Sudhakaran Raja. 2016. "Protective Efficacy of Active Compounds from Phyllanthus Amarus against White Spot Syndrome Virus in Freshwater Crab (Paratelphusa Hydrodomous)." *Aquaculture Research* 47 (7): 2061–2067. https://doi.org/10.1111/are.12660.

Swaminathan, Karthikeyan, Kavinkumar Nirmala Karunakaran, Jeevitha Priya Manoharan, and Subramanian Vidyalakshmi. 2021. "SARS-CoV2 Multiple Target Inhibitors from *Andrographis Paniculata*: An in-Silico Report." *European Journal of Molecular & Clinical Medicine* 8 (3): 1653–1685. https://ejmcm.com/article_10126.html.

Tan, Xing, Hwan Seung Kim, Kimberly Baugh, Yanqin Huang, Neeraja Kadiyala, Marisol Wences, Nidhi Singh, Eric Wenzler, and Zackery P Bulman. 2021. "Therapeutic Options for Metallo-β-Lactamaseproducing Enterobacterales." *Infection and Drug Resistance* 14: 125–142. https://doi.org/10.2147/IDR.S246174.

Toney, Jeffrey H, Gail G Hammond, Paula MD Fitzgerald, Nandini Sharma, James M Balkovec, Gregory P Rouen, Steven H Olson, Milton L Hammond, Mark L Greenlee, and Ying Duo Gao. 2001. "Succinic Acids as Potent Inhibitors of Plasmid-Borne IMP-1 Metallo-β-Lactamase." *Journal of Biological Chemistry* 276 (34): 31913–31918. https://doi.org/10.1074/jbc.M104742200.

Tooke, Catherine L, Philip Hinchliffe, Eilis C Bragginton, Charlotte K Colenso, Viivi HA Hirvonen, Yuiko Takebayashi, and James Spencer. 2019. "β-Lactamases and β-Lactamase Inhibitors in the 21st Century." *Journal of Molecular Biology* 431 (18): 3472–3500. https://doi.org/10.1016/j.jmb.2019.04.002.

Wang, Xiyan, Yanan Yang, Yawen Gao, and Xiaodi Niu. 2020. "Discovery of the Novel Inhibitor against New Delhi Metallo-β-Lactamase Based on Virtual Screening and Molecular Modelling." *International Journal of Molecular Sciences* 21 (10). https://doi.org/10.3390/ijms21103567.

Wooller, Sarah K, Graeme Benstead-Hume, Xiangrong Chen, Yusuf Ali, and Frances MG Pearl. 2017. "Bioinformatics in Translational Drug Discovery." *Bioscience Reports* 37 (4): 1–13. https://doi.org/10.1042/BSR20160180.

Xia, Xuhua. 2017. "Bioinformatics and Drug Discovery." *Current Topics in Medicinal Chemistry* 17 (15): 1709–1726. https://doi.org/10.2174/1568026617666161116143440.

Yadav, Pradeep Kumar, Amit Jaiswal, and Rajiv Kumar Singh. 2021. "In Silico Study on Spice-Derived Antiviral Phytochemicals against SARS-CoV-2 TMPRSS2 Target." *Journal of Biomolecular Structure and Dynamics*: 1–11. https://doi.org/10.1080/07391102.2021.1965658.

Yamaguchi, Yoshihiro, Koichi Kato, Yoshimi Ichimaru, Wanchun Jin, Misa Sakai, Miki Abe, Jun Ichi Wachino, et al. 2021. "Crystal Structures of Metallo-β-Lactamase (IMP-1) and Its D120E Mutant in Complexes with Citrate and the Inhibitory Effect of the Benzyl Group in Citrate Monobenzyl Ester." *Journal of Medicinal Chemistry* 64 (14): 10019–10026. https://doi.org/10.1021/acs.jmedchem.1c00308.

Zhang, Yang. 2008. "I-TASSER Server for Protein 3D Structure Prediction." *BMC Bioinformatics* 9: 1–8. https://doi.org/10.1186/1471-2105-9-40.

5 Phenolic Compounds

A Systematic Review of Extraction Methods and a Bioinformatics Approach for Their Antibacterial and Antiviral Properties

Chinmayi Joshi[†], *Ritul Patel, and Viraj Limbhachiya*
Smt. S. S. Patel Nootan Science and Commerce College,
Sankalchand Patel University, Visnagar, India
[†]Corresponding Author: joshichinmayi@gmail.com

ABBREVIATIONS

ADMET	Absorption, distribution, metabolism, elimination, and toxicity
EA	Evolutionary algorithms
EI	Electron ionization (EI)
FDA	Food and Drug Administration
GAE	Gallic acid equivalent
GBS	Genotyping-by-sequencing (GBS)
GC	Gas Chromatography
HHPE	High hydrostatic pressure extraction
HPLC	High-performance liquid chromatography
LLE	Liquid-liquid extraction
MAE	Microwave-assisted extraction
MC	Monte Carlo simulations
MD	Molecular dynamics
PDBML	Protein Data Bank Markup Language
RMSD	Root mean square deviation
SBDD	Structure-based drug design
SBVS	Structure-based virtual screening
SCWE	Subcritical water extraction
SFE	Supercritical fluid extraction
SNPs	Single nucleotide polymorphisms
TB	Tuberculosis
TPC	Total phenolic content
UAE	Ultrasound-assisted extraction
WHO	World Health Organization

DOI: 10.1201/9781003354437-5

5.1 PHENOLICS: THE MOST ABUNDANT SECONDARY METABOLITES

Infectious diseases were an important global cause of various disease conditions and deaths before the beginning of 20th century. There were numerous contagious illnesses present, including the plague, smallpox, cholera, diphtheria, pneumonia, typhoid, TB, syphilis, etc. (Nelsons and Williams, 2013). Prior to the discovery of antibiotics, *Streptococcus pyogenes* was a significant contributor to burn-related mortality and was responsible for half of all postnatal deaths; 80% of wound infections caused by *Staphylococcus aureus* resulted in death (www.abc.net.au/science/slab/antibiotics/history.htm). Sir Alexander Fleming's discovery of penicillin in 1928 signaled the start of the antibiotic revolution. Following this discovery, the antibiotic era saw the development of numerous more antibiotics, and antibiotics were widely employed for the treatment of infectious diseases all around the world. Antibiotics experienced their "golden age" between the 1950s and the 1970s; since then, no noteworthy new antibiotic classes have been created. In the present scenario, modern medicine and molecular biotechnology have helped a lot in the elimination of infections, but because of the rising prevalence of potentially fatal microbial infections, as well as the potential for these human diseases to acquire resistance to existing treatment methods (El-Saadony et al., 2021). In the face of difficulties and obstacles such as treatment failure and drug ineffectiveness, there is a clear need to find alternative tactics that can target resistant microorganisms. Early on in the development of modern medicine, active ingredients from natural products were used (Katiyar et al., 2012; Dias et al., 2012), but natural products were undervalued as a result of high-throughput screening and combinatorial chemistry over-optimization, which accepted only a single active component that could target a single cellular function of a pathogen rather than a multi-target drug. The need for alternative therapies is currently great, so contemporary medicine from natural products is being trusted as an antimicrobial drug (Yuan et al., 2016). Furthermore, according to the WHO, complementary medicine serves as the major source of treatment for 80% of the community in developed countries. The medicinal plants contain a large number of bioactive compounds with low toxicity, specific activity, and high bioavailability. Many studies have reported the effectiveness of numerous plants in combating respiratory viruses when used as their raw extracts or active ingredients. Plants contain a diversity of compounds, including triterpenoids, alkaloids, phenols, and flavonoids, with antimicrobial, antiviral, and various biological activities (Stan et al., 2021; El-Saadony et al., 2021; Khan et al., 2021).

Among the bioactive compounds present in plants, phenolics are the most abundant group of plant metabolites with antibacterial and antiviral activities. Plant phenols are commonly known as phenolics and are made up by bonding between hydroxyl groups and an aromatic hydrocarbon group. Cereals, coffee beans, fruits, olives, vegetables, tea leaves, and other foods contain phenolic chemicals. Fruits, berries, and vegetables are significant sources of natural phenols in human nutrition. Plant polyphenols have drawn increasing interest because of their effective antioxidant abilities and significant contributions as a prophylaxis for many oxidative stress-related disorders, such as cancer (Dai et al., 2010). Many studies have reported the biological activities of plants containing phenols as their constituents; a few of them are summarized in Table 5.1.

TABLE 5.1
Biological Activities of Plants Possessing Phenolic Compounds as Constituents

Plant	Biological Effect	Major Present Phenolic Compounds	Reference
Batatas: *Bauhinia variegata L.*	Iron binding, radical neutralization, and reducing power capabilities as antioxidant	Anthraquinones, terpenoids, phenolics, flavonoids, saponins, tannins, alkaloids	Mishra et al., 2013
Rhizome extracts of *Polygonatum verticillatum (L.)*	Antioxidant activity which was correlated with the quantity of phenolic composition	Petroleum ether, dichloromethane, chloroform, ethanol	Singh et al., 2018
The fern, *Asplenium Nidus nidus L.*	Antibacterial activity against, e.g., *Proteus mirabilis* Hauser, *P. vulgaris* Hauser, and *Pseudomonas aeruginosa* (Schroeter) Migula	Flavonoids	Jarial et al., 2018
Zingiber officinale Roscoe and *Curcuma longa L.*	Anticancer	Ethanol, polyphenol	Danciu et al., 2015
Trianthema decandra L.	Antibacterial activity against *Propionibacterium* acnes, a skin pathogen	Flavonoid	Geethalakhsmi et al., 2018
Cassia fistula	Antimicrobial against bacterial and fungal pathogens	Ethanol	Bhalodia and Shukla, 2011
Cassia italica	Bacteriostatic for *Bacillus anthracis*, *Corynebacterium pseudodiphthericum*, and *P. aeruginosa* and bactericidal for *P. pseudomalliae*	Anthraquinone	Kazmi et al., 1994
Vitis vinifera	Fight against SARS-COV-2 and herpes simplex virus (HSV-1)	Apigenin, isorhamnetin, myricetin, chrysoeriol, biochanin, catechin, isookain, quercetin, luteolin, kaempferol, scutellarein	Zannella et al., 2021
Kei apple (*Dovyalis caffra*)	Anticancer, antioxidant, antiviral, and antimicrobial activities	7-nonynoic acid and methanol, levoglucosenone, isochiapin B, dotriacontane, and tert-hexadecanethiol	Qanash et al., 2022

Plant phenolics comprise several bioactivities, i.e., antioxidant, cytotoxic, antimicrobial, etc., and are reported to be biosynthesized from the shikimate pathway. In addition to plants, phenolic secondary metabolites are also being synthesized by endophytic fungi. Lunardelli et al. (2016) reviewed 124 phenolic secondary metabolites produced by endophytic fungi. However, due to the structural diversity of plant phenolics and the traditional use of plant products since ancient times, phenolics serve as one of the most productive sources of pharmaceuticals. Therefore, research on phenolics can aid in bridging the gap between conventional wisdom and contemporary medicine. The search results for the keyword "plant phenolics" demonstrate the international scientific community's keen interest in phenolics research. In PubMed, for instance, such a search returns more than 65,000 hits, whereas in Google Scholar, such a search returns more than 1.8 million hits. A year-by-year search in PubMed using the same keyword reveals an increase in count from 3296 in 2017 to >4800 in 2022, which clearly states the potential of phenolic compounds as medicine. Kumar et al. (2021) summarized the presence of the major phenolic compounds with reference to the plant part. Among them, caffeic acid, coumaric acid, ellagic acid, ferulic acid, gallic acid, quercetin, etc., are a few common phenolic compounds that are being explored for their therapeutic efficacy. For example, amla, the Indian gross berry plant, is an essential component of popular Ayurvedic formulations, including chyawanprash and triphala. Phenolic compounds such as flavonoids, tannins, ellagic acid, and lupeol are present in various plant parts. These Ayurvedic formulations are being used for the treatment of various disease conditions and to boost immunity (Kumar et al., 2021).

On the basis of the biological activity of phenolic compounds and their numerous implementations in the food, agriculture, chemical, and pharmaceutical industries, studying various methods of extracting these substances from plants has garnered more interest. This chapter will cover information about the extraction techniques that have been employed to date to isolate phenolic compounds from various plants, MAE, UAE, LLE, and SFE. Quantification methods and bioinformatics methods are also discussed, which are being used to study phenolic chemicals. Since it takes a long time to repurpose phytocompounds using traditional methods, bioinformatics approaches are gaining popularity since they are less expensive and time-consuming. The repurposing or validation of phenolics for varied biological possibilities in the context of investigating them for their antibacterial and antiviral activity requires biological, biomedical, and electronic health-related data, which computational algorithms may exploit. Both drug-based tactics and disease-based strategies, in which drug development is based on knowledge associated with either medications or disorders, can be employed with bioinformatics approaches to validate the phenolics.

We reviewed tools and resources frequently employed in repurposing research. One of the crucial strategies that has been shown to be useful in overcoming the issues and difficulties of finding new antiviral and antibacterial drugs is *in silico* virtual screening. Molecular docking methods, chemical structure databases, and pharmacophore-based screening may also be helpful in limiting the number of phytocompounds that need to be investigated *in vitro* or *in vivo*. With a focus on phenolic compounds reported for various biological actions, we propose to describe how various virtual screening techniques might be used to find new antiviral and antibacterial drugs.

5.2 PREPARATION OF EXTRACTS TO EXTRACT THE PHENOLIC COMPOUNDS

The extraction of phenolic compounds from plants is a crucial step in phenolic research. The most popular methods for the extraction of phenolics use organic or inorganic solvents. In plants with different levels of stability, phenolics are not always distributed evenly. This has made the extraction processes more difficult, demonstrating that using a single step or an inefficient extraction technique may have an impact on the yield of phenolic components from plant samples. In order to recover the desired phenolic chemicals, it is crucial to choose the right extraction technique. This will enable significant yields to be recovered from the sample matrix. Duration of extraction, temperature, solvent to sample ratio, and type of solvent can affect the yield of phenolics. Moreover, good recovery and extraction efficiency are determined by the type of plant and active constituents present in the plant. Therefore, selection of extraction solvent, time, temperature, and sample are the important parameters for extracting the phenolic compounds.

Many studies demonstrated various methods for the extraction of phenolic compounds and also studied the factors that affect the phenolic extraction. According to Naczk et al. (2005), 2 minutes (2*1 minute) at room temperature is the ideal extraction time and temperature for extracting phenolics from canola meal, which possesses a significantly higher phenolic content than other oil seeds. Defatted canola meal is a by-product of oil waste that is thrown in thousands of metric tons each year and is also a significant source of phenolic and antioxidant compounds. Therefore, in their study, the recovery of phenolics was influenced by the solvent-to-sample ratio and the number of repeat extractions carried out for each sample. Phenolic extraction from plant samples was encouraged by increasing the solvent-to-sample ratio, but finding the ideal ratio is advised to reduce solvent intake and solvent saturation effects on the phenolics. According to Al-Farsi et al. (2008), the majority of phenolics may be extracted from plant tissues using a two-stage process with a solvent to sample ratio of 60:1. In the study of Pinelo et al. (2008), phenolic extraction from plant materials was significantly influenced by sample matrix and particle size due to the binding of phenolics to additional sample components such as proteins and carbohydrates. Pinelo et al. (2008) added the enzymes to dissolve the linkages and promote the release of bound phenolics. Haghi and Hatami (2010) and Vichapong et al. (2010) employed acidic and alkaline hydrolysis for the isolation of phenolics from plants. In the study, flavonoid aglycones were identified by acidic hydrolysis. In another study by Davidov-Pardo et al. (2011), catechins and their isomers were shown to be more stable in more alkaline or acidic environments at a pH of 4–5. Here, we have collected information about some common phenolic extraction methods.

5.2.1 Conventional Extraction Methods for Phenolics

It has been common practice to extract phenolic chemicals using traditional extraction techniques such as Soxhlet, maceration, infusion, and digesting for many years (Alara et al., 2021; Abubakar and Haque, 2020). The most widely used techniques are Soxhlet extraction and maceration (Caldas et al., 2018; Osorio-Tobón, 2020). For thorough extraction of all phytochemicals from a matrix, Soxhlet extraction and maceration often use high solvent/feed (S/F) ratios (over 20) and lengthy extraction durations. As a result, these techniques are frequently used as models to compare the efficacy of different techniques. Phenolic compounds have been extracted using Soxhlet extraction and maceration for periods of up to 360 and 720 min, respectively.

A dried sample is placed in a thimble for Soxhlet extraction, followed by placing the solvent into the thimble and heated in a distillation flask to get it to evaporate. Reflux and condensate flow back to the thimble holder until they overflow and may be sucked by a syphon. The bulk liquid is where the chemicals are extracted. The solvent continuously refluxes as the flask is heated, keeping the compounds inside while doing so. Before extraction is finished, the reflux procedure is repeated multiple times (Azmir et al., 2013; Alara et al., 2021). In the procedure of maceration, the raw material is extracted over time using a particular solvent. Agitation may or may not be used during maceration. Maceration is carried out at lower temperatures than Soxhlet extraction. For instance, under ideal conditions at room temperature, phenolic compounds are extracted from oil mixes by maceration (Ji et al., 2018).

If we look at this in more detail, one of the main benefits of Soxhlet extraction is that, in contrast to maceration, the matrix could continually come into contact with new solvent because the sample is packaged inside a thimble, eliminating the need for extract filtration. But as phenolic compounds are extracted using longer extraction durations and higher temperatures, the chemicals are degraded, which reduces the bioactivity of the extracts. The main benefits of maceration include the low temperatures used throughout the procedure and the low cost of the operation due to the simple equipment needed. However, maceration uses longer extraction times and produces poorer yields (Alara et al., 2021).

A modified maceration approach, which uses mild heating to ensure that the active phytochemicals in the plant sample are not affected by the temperature, is another conventional method, i.e., digestion technique. This method is typically used for plant materials containing polyphenolic chemicals or poorly soluble components. To extract a wider range of phytochemicals, serial exhaustive extraction requires fractionating crude extracts with higher polarity solvents, such as butanol (a polar solvent) from hexane (a non-polar solvent). Because of the prolonged heating, this method cannot be used to extract thermolabile compounds (Alara and Abdurahman, 2019).

In addition to Soxhlet extraction, maceration, and digestion, the decoction technique has also been used as a conventional extraction method. The decoction approach involves either rapidly boiling the plant samples or pouring boiling water over them and letting the mixture sit for a set amount of time. The majority of heat-stable and water-soluble phytochemicals derived from crude medicines are acceptable for this approach. In a closed system with a ground-up sample, the percolation method drops the solvent gradually from the top to the bottom. This is comparable to the maceration method (Kaufmann and Christen, 2002; Sticher, 2008). Filtration is not compulsory in this case because the percolator devices contain filters that allow only the solvent that actually comprises the extract to go through. The drawbacks of a percolation method include sample size, extraction time, and solubility of the polyphenols, in addition to the time-consuming, large solvent volume drawbacks of the maceration method. Additionally, infusion is utilized to extract volatile plant samples whose phytochemicals easily dissolve in an organic solvent. To achieve this, just briefly macerate the plant sample in hot or cold water and then allow it to soak in the solvent for a while (Alara et al., 2021).

Prior to the main procedure, it is vital to test and adapt the optimum solvent due to the impact of numerous parameters on the extraction of polyphenols, including the degree of conjugation and the presence of numerous hydroxyl groups. Therefore, even though it appears to be concluded that solvent systems that allow the maximization of the polyphenol yield without significantly changing the targets' chemical nature must be considered good, choosing a suitable solvent for the development of a consistent procedure for all types of polyphenols might be a challenging task. In this condition, choosing a solvent for extraction must take into consideration the following factors: safety considerations, legal compliance for food usage, potential reusability, solvent power, solvent polarity, boiling temperature, solvent reactivity, solvent viscosity, and solvent stability (Khoddami et al., 2013; Osorio-Tobón, 2020; Alara et al., 2021).

5.2.2 Alternative Extraction Methods

Contrary to standard procedures, alternative approaches can yield extracts high in phenolic compounds in a shorter amount of time at moderate temperatures with solvents that are generally regarded as safe. UAE, MAE, SFE, SCWE, and HHPE are the popular modern extraction methods for phenolics. All extraction procedures share some key elements, despite the fact that the varieties, cultivars, and stages of maturity of the raw materials all have a substantial impact on the extraction of phenolic chemicals. The choice of solvent, temperature, and extraction time may behave similarly in all extraction methods. Higher temperatures and longer extraction times speed up the diffusion of chemicals, and mass transfer rates provide a more direct and efficient interaction between solvent and matrix. Phenolic chemicals are more soluble in polar solvents like water and ethanol or their combinations (Khoddami et al., 2013; Osorio-Tobón, 2020; Alara et al., 2021).

UAE is a simple, affordable technique that may be used in both small- and large-scale settings, among modern extraction methods (Shirzad et al., 2017). For the extraction of bioactive compounds, conventional power ultrasound is employed, which produces pressure fluctuations as well as the development and dissolution of bubbles in the liquid medium through successions of compressions and rarefactions (Tiwari, 2015). The properties of the solvent and sample, as well as the sonication time, temperature, and ultrasonic wave frequency, all have an impact on the UAE process. For instance, it has been claimed that UAE is more effective than traditional extraction methods at obtaining rosmarinic and carnosic acids. According to a recent study, the UAE approach produced a maximum yield of 13.20 mg/g dry weight (DW) of polyphenols from spruce wood bark. Further, Mojerlou and Elhamirad (2018) optimized UAE conditions for olive cake extract and measured the antioxidant activity. They found 68.9% antioxidant activity. By using UAE, the authors were able to characterize protocatechuic acid and cinnamic acid. Using 48 °C as well as 56.71 W for 40 min as the optimum extracting conditions, Nipornram et al. (2018) established a UAE method for extracting the phenolic compounds (flavonoid, hesperidin) from mandarin (*Citrus reticulata* Blanco cv. ainampueng) peel, with a maximum production of 26.52%, total phenolic (15,263.32 mg eq. gallic/100 g DW) and hesperidin (6435.53 mg/100 g DW). Various studies have reported the use of UAE for phenolic extraction (Espada-Bellido et al., 2017; Pandey et al., 2018; Martinez-Patino et al., 2019). In conclusion, UAE is a quick, effective, and inexpensive way to extract phenolic compounds (Zhang et al., 2022).

MAE is one of the most effective ways to extract phenolic chemicals, much like UAE. MAE is the process of separating analytes from the sample matrix into the solvent by heating solvents in contact with the sample. The key benefit of MAE is its ability to rapidly heat the sample-solvent mixture. Numerous studies have reported the use of MAE for phenolic extraction. For instance, Routray and Orsat (2014) extracted phenolic compounds from blueberry leaves using MAE, which produced a higher yield in less time. Likewise, Radojković et al. (2018) optimized the MAE method for the extraction of phenolic compounds from mulberry leaves. Di Meo et al. (2021) demonstrated the MAE of olive leaf from five Italian cultivars and obtained a higher yield. Based on the unique research in the field of MAE, it is possible to claim that MAE is a quick and effective technique with superior results to other conventional techniques. The microwave is one of the most popular assisted extraction tools due to the volume of material recovered, the decrease in solvent, and the amount of time required. Additionally, typical Soxhlet extraction's heat deterioration of phytoconstituents is minimized by MAE's short extraction time.

SFE and SCWE are also considered important extraction methods. SFE, which uses a supercritical solvent to produce a selective extraction of phenolic chemicals, is regarded as an environmentally benign extraction method. As crucial supercritical fluids, supercritical CO_2, ethane, pentane, butane, nitrous oxide, trifluoromethane, ammonia, and water are frequently employed. The phenolic components in *Hibiscus sabdariffa* can be extracted by supercritical CO_2 extraction, which was developed by Pimentel-Moral et al. (2019). SFE can increase the recovery of hibiscus acid and its derivatives as compared to other traditional and green extraction techniques. Using response surface methodology (RSM), Yang et al. (2019) enhanced the SFE of phenolic compounds from peach blossom (*Amygdalus persica*), confirming that 64 °C, 30 MPa, 143 min, and 35 mL of 100% ethanol as a modifier exhibit the maximum total phenolic contents (54.10 mg GAE/g DW), which is higher than the yield attained by ultrasonic-assisted extraction (44.04 mg GAE/g DW). Additionally, an efficient approach for extracting *Medicago sativa* has been devised employing enzyme-assisted SFE and RSM based on the Box-Behnken design. SFE may use less hazardous organic reagents, require shorter extraction durations than other traditional and novel procedures, improve safety and selectivity, and prevent sample oxidation in the presence of air (Zhang et al., 2022).

Another extraction method is SCWE, which is a relatively new and effective method that works at temperatures between 100 and 374 °C and pressures high enough to keep liquids in that state. Three distinctive characteristics of the extraction method are its high dielectric constant, strong polarity, and, excessively for its mass, a high boiling temperature. As the temperature rises, the diffusion rate increases, the viscosity and surface tension decrease, the permittivity continuously and considerably lowers, and the permittivity also reduces. Due to the need for a less polar medium produced by an increase in temperature, more polar compounds of interest are retrieved successfully at lower temperatures than moderately polar and non-polar compounds. Under normal conditions, more polar compounds have a high solubility in water (Munir et al., 2018; Ko et al., 2020). Additionally, investigations on the extraction of phenolic compounds from various plant sections utilizing a range of extraction procedures have been conducted (Zabidi et al., 2019; Zakaria et al., 2020; Ko et al., 2020).

Among the modern extraction methods, HHPE is a unique method that can be used to extract phenolics from plants. This technique relies on the principles of mass transport phenomena and uses non-thermal super-high hydraulic pressure (1000–8000 bar). According to mass transfer and phase behavior theories, the pressure applied enhances plant cell permeability, resulting in cell component diffusivity (Khoddami et al., 2013). With HHPE, a significant pressure differential is created between the interior and outside of the cell membrane, allowing solvent to enter the cell and cause cell component leakage. Additionally, HHPE can deform cells and denature proteins, which can lessen cell selectivity and boost extraction yield. Depending on the bioactive molecules to be extracted, HHPE is typically carried out at room temperature using various solvents ranging from polar to non-polar. Some researchers have made a strong case for the viability of using HHPE to extract phenolic chemicals from plant material. Comparing HHPE to traditional extraction techniques, higher yields of flavonoids from propolis, anthocyanins from grape by-products, and phenolic compounds from *Maclura pomifera* fruits have all been attained. It has also been claimed that HHPE is effective at removing polyphenols from green tea leaves (Khoddami et al., 2013).

However, these techniques are sensitive and require expensive equipment, such as a pressure vessel and system controller, an extract collection device, and a solvent conveying pump, which is a major drawback of techniques like HHPE, SCWE, and SFE. In addition to these techniques, it is also very important to determine which compound needs to be extracted. Specific protocols need to be standardized to extract the compounds. The extraction of phenolic compounds depends heavily on the use of organic solvents and the length of the treatment process. For example, in plants, phenolic acids are often found free, esterified, or glycosylated. In this case, free and esterified phenolic acids can be extracted using diethyl ether, whereas for the extraction of glycosylated phenolic acids, plant samples can be treated with HCL and N_2, followed by the extraction with diethyl ether. In addition, ethanol, water, and combinations of methanol, acetone, and chloroform can be used to extract phenolic acid from plants (Alara et al., 2021). Among the phenolic compounds, flavonoids are also abundant in edible and non-edible plants. They are typically extracted with organic solvents or mixtures of the solvents using heated reflux extraction procedures. During extraction with HCl under N_2, the flavonoid glycosides frequently break down into their aglycone forms. In order to extract flavonoids from various herbal plant materials, Haghi and Hatami (2010) used 50% methanol that had been acidified with 1.2 M HCl. For the purpose of preventing oxidation, ascorbic acid was added. The flavonoid glycosides were hydrolyzed for 2 hours at 80 °C. In addition to flavonoids and phenolic acids, anthocyanins and proanthocyanidins are also included in the group of polyphenols, which can be extracted using aqueous solvent combinations such as water, acetone, ethanol, or methanol as acidified solvents. The natural anthocyanin structure could be destroyed by the harsh chemical process, though. Anthocyanins are released from cell membranes when the acid in the solvents breaks them. The substitution of mineral acids, such as 0.1% HCl, with organic acids (such as formic or acetic acid) to acidify solvents is crucial (Castaneda-Ovando et al., 2009). According to Bridgers et al. (2010), acidified methanol and ethanol were more successful than non-acidified solvents at extracting anthocyanin from purple-fleshed sweet potatoes. Awika et al. (2004) found that acidified methanol greatly increased anthocyanin extraction from black sorghum over aqueous acetone, whereas organic solvents, such as ethanol, methanol, and acetone, are frequently employed to extract proanthocyanidins.

In total, care should be taken at the time of selecting the method as well as the solvent for phenolic extraction because the structural variations of polyphenols have an impact on their solubility and separation capabilities. Due to the effect of their structural changes on their solubility, high-molecular-weight phenolics are frequently not soluble. Due to the non-uniform distribution of phenolic compounds in plants, there are differences in their stability as well. For example, while certain phenolic compounds are stable, others are either volatile, thermolabile, or prone to oxidation. The recovery of polyphenols from their source is a time-consuming process due to high degree of enzyme activity in the majority of foods and plants. There is currently no widely accepted method for recovering all phenolics or those of a specific category from plant materials. As a result, in order to create the best technique for recovering phenolic compounds from plant materials, the following considerations must be made: An analysis's findings are influenced by the following variables: the sample type, the targeted compounds, the analysis's use of quantification or structural elucidation, the technique, and the targeted compounds, such as total phenolics, a particular class of phenolics, or a specific phenolic. Because most samples are complicated, the way they are prepared typically has a significant impact on the outcomes of the entire extraction process (Robards, 2003; Selvamuthukumaran and Shi, 2017; Alara et al., 2021). Another important point is to remove the unwanted phenolics and interfering substances via appropriate cleaning methods like DCCC and CC. However, in addition to the extraction of phenolics, it is still challenging to quantify different phenolic structural groups.

5.3 QUANTIFICATION AND CHARACTERIZATION OF PHENOLICS

On the basis of phenolic group type, numerous measuring techniques are available for the quantification and characterization of phenolics. The most frequently used methods for quantifying phenolic compounds are HPLC and GC or their combinations with mass spectrometry (Proestos et al., 2013; López-Cobo et al., 2017). Spectrophotometry is another pertinent method for the quantification and characterization of phenolics.

Among the listed methods, a quick and easy method for determining the number of phenolic compounds in plant materials is spectrophotometry, which primarily relies on several measurement techniques for the phenolic compounds' many structural variations. The Folin-Ciocalteu assay has been extensively used for many years to determine phenolic compounds in plants. This test is based on a chemical reduction that makes use of reagents that contain tungsten and molybdenum. The Folin-Ciocalteu method is a Folin-Denis assay version that alters the reagent's composition just a little. The phenolic constituents of the sample are extracted, followed by the addition of the Folin-Ciocalteu reagent, sodium carbonate (7–35%

or 0.1 N), and distilled water. This solution is made, and it is then given 15 to 120 min to react. Generally, spectrophotometry is used to determine the flavonoid concentration. It can also be used to measure the condensed tannin concentration as well as the total phenolic quantity. Owing to its low cost and easy use, spectroscopy is a widely used method for quantifying many types of phenolic chemicals (Zhang et al., 2022). Moreover, proanthocyanidin (condensed tannin), hydrolysable tannin, total flavonoid concentration, and total phenolic quantitation can all be determined using colorimetric techniques. $AlCl_3$ allows for the measurement of total flavonoids in the 410–423 nm range when used with methanolic or ethanolic plant phenolic extracts. Proanthocyanidin determination is also done using butanol-HCl and bovine serum albumin (BSA) techniques. In addition, hydrolysable tannins can be evaluated using the sodium nitrite, rhodanine, and potassium iodate methods. Potassium iodate is the method that is most frequently used for screening samples. The interaction between methyl gallate and potassium iodate produces the red color with a maximum absorption of 500–550 nm. The rhodanine and sodium nitrite procedures can also be used to determine hydrolyzable tannins based on the presence of gallic and ellagic acids in the sample, respectively. The interaction of flavonones and dihydroflavonols with acidic 2,4-dinitrophenylhydrazine is the basis of yet another spectrophotometric technique used to measure them. The standard used in this experiment is pinocembrin, and the absorbance is calculated at 486 nm (Khodammi et al., 2013; Mythili et al., 2014). In total, spectrophotometry is used for the quantification of various groups of phenolic compounds, where GC and HPLC are the most exploited analytical techniques for separation, identification, and quantification of phenolic compounds.

Although HPLC separates the chemicals based on their soluble nature and/or the interactions among a less polar stationary phase and a more polar mobile phase, GC separates the sample between an inert gas under pressure and a thin layer of non-volatile liquid coated with an inert substrate inside the heated column. However, because of its great selectivity and sensitivity in quantification, GC combined with an MS detector has recently become popular in assessing complex substances. For instance, GC-MS has been used to characterize the low-molar-mass fraction of hydrophilic extracts, which are primarily lignans, in Norway spruce knotwood. The columns that are most frequently used in the GC method to study phenolic compounds are capillary columns that are 30 m long and have an inner diameter of 0.25 m and an outer diameter of 0.25 to 0.30 mm. The carrier gas of choice is often helium, whereas in case of HPLC, column types, applied detectors, mobile phase, and the properties of the tested compounds are the major factors that affect HPLC analysis (Zhang et al., 2022).

Since these sophisticated techniques are capable of running a batch of studies and rapidly distinguishing metabolite peaks, the development of a rapid data analysis tool is crucial. Peak identification and annotation are performed using manual techniques, which create major issues with peak detection and annotation accuracy depending on the knowledge and experience of individual researchers. Peak annotation is particularly challenging since it necessitates in-depth familiarity with electron ionization (EI) fragmentation patterns (Tsugawa et al., 2011). At this point, bioinformatics can help identify and annotate metabolites quickly and reliably.

5.4 BIOINFORMATICS: AN EFFECTIVE APPROACH FOR THE BIOPROSPECTING OF PHENOLICS

Bioinformatics is an important discipline that collects, stores, and analyzes biological data using computers. In the current scenario, bioinformatics has become a global approach as it has multiple applications in the biological field. In particular, "omics" tools can help in various ways. For example, if we use omics tools to study the genome, proteome, and transcriptome, the field is respectively called genomics, proteomics, and transcriptomics (Abdurakhmonov et al., 2016). Likewise, bioinformatics tools can also be used to study the plant metabolites, i.e., phenolics. The understanding of the total phenolics and biological activities of wild fruits can be expanded through bioinformatics analysis. The genetic diversity of plants containing phenolics as their secondary metabolites, molecular regulation of phenolic chemical content, and genetic variation analysis of plant species can be done using the genotyping-by-sequencing (GBS) method. Single nucleotide polymorphisms among the plant species and their association with phenolic compounds and their biological activities can also be determined using omics tools. In this chapter, we have summarized the use of bioinformatics approaches for antibacterial and antiviral drug discovery by repurposing phenolic compounds (Nalbantoglu, 2019).

5.4.1 A Bioinformatics Approach for Antibacterial and Antiviral Drug Discovery

The diagnosis of diseases with clearly defined symptoms that reduce the quality of life is the first stage in the process of identifying a medicine. A chemical (which could be a simple molecule or a sophisticated protein) or chemical combination that decreases symptoms without having a significant negative impact on the patient is often regarded as a desirable treatment. An attractive drug should also be affordable and profitable for pharmaceutical corporations and have minimal negative environmental impact, such as no reactivation of bacterial or viral species after human use and a low likelihood of drug resistance (Xia, 2017). Currently, this desirable drug discovery is difficult because it requires a lot of money, effort, and thorough scientific research. Moreover, antimicrobial resistance is a developing issue, and the current pipeline of antimicrobials is still insufficient to address it. A strong pipeline of fresh drugs with novel mechanisms of action is required to combat antimicrobial-resistant "superbugs." In general, bacteria can resist the effects of antibiotics by altering or reducing the number of entryways, employing efflux pumps in their cell envelopes to remove antibiotics that enter the cell, neutralizing antibiotics with enzymes, or switching the antibiotics' targets. The common mechanisms used by existing antimicrobials to target microorganisms include preventing the formation of cell walls, rupturing cell membranes, preventing the synthesis of proteins, and preventing the synthesis of nucleic acids in pathogens. These infections can be managed by utilizing a wider range of modes of action of antimicrobials, but in the current scenario, that is not the case. Due to the common mechanisms of existing drugs, novel compounds as well as novel targets should be identified to tackle drug resistance (Joshi and Kothari, 2022).

Bioinformatics can play a major role at this stage, where the identification of new compounds and new targets is required. This decade has seen enormous biological data produced due to the advent of contemporary sequencing technology, which has provided a new window for clinical diagnostics and therapies for complicated diseases. In order to find and identify new therapeutic targets, bioinformatics may extract, evaluate, and transmit hidden information from sequences and structures, as well as functional knowledge of nucleic acids and proteins. The development of therapeutic drugs that may either activate or inhibit the biological activities of biomolecules may be aided by this, as may the development of a number of prediction models to facilitate virtual bioactive screening (Sliwoski et al., 2014). As a result, safer and more effective therapeutic drugs that can either stimulate or prevent the biological functions of biomolecules will be easier to develop and find (Gashaw et al., 2011; Woller et al., 2017; Xia, 2017). The bioinformatics approach can be exploited in two ways for the investigation of the antibacterial and antiviral potential of phenolics: structure-based drug design and target-based drug design.

5.4.1.1 Structure-Based Drug Design for Antimicrobial Discovery from Phenolics

SBDD is utmost promising *in silico* techniques for drug discovery and uses scoring algorithms to assess the potency of the non-covalent interactions between a ligand and a molecular target. Consequently, the scoring capabilities of SBDD software are the main determinant of success or failure. Due to the large number of software programs used for SBDD and the fact that each one uses a different algorithm, it is likely to obtain various results from the same input while using different software. The most often used computational techniques in SBDD include molecular docking, molecular dynamics simulations, and structure-based virtual screening (SBVS). Numerous analyses of binding energetics, ligand-protein interactions, and assessments of the conformational changes that take place throughout the docking process can all benefit from these techniques (Kalyaanamoorthy and Chen, 2011; Xia, 2017; Maia et al., 2020).

5.4.1.2 *In Silico* Virtual Screening in Antibacterial and Antiviral Discovery Using Phenolics

High-throughput synthesis and combinatorial chemistry-based drug discovery have recently been shown to be less successful overall, and it is commonly acknowledged that while spending much more on R&D now than it did 20 years ago, the pharmaceutical industry is producing fewer novel compounds. It was predicted that from medication development to marketing, *in silico* technologies would take the lead as a tool to handle this issue. Recent developments in computational methodologies and hardware have made it possible for *in silico* methods to accelerate lead optimization and identification. These methods have so far helped create roughly 50 drugs that have gone through clinical trials, some of which have received FDA approval (Zoete et al., 2009; Xu et al., 2022). *In silico* drug design can instantly suggest a small number of drugs with good pharmacokinetic and pharmacodynamic properties and high affinity and selectivity for the target macromolecule, starting from only the

3D structure of the target. Molecular docking is a method that anticipates a ligand's natural position, orientation, and conformation. In order to estimate affinity prior to synthesis and to develop ligand optimization tactics, docking offers a fundamental understanding of the interactions between the ligands and protein receptors. In the process of molecular docking, the ligand-binding modes are sampled using a variety of techniques, and in some cases, the flexibility of the protein is also addressed. Systematic searching, stochastic methods, and simulation techniques can be used to classify these sample algorithms into three main groups (Zoete et al., 2009).

Depending on the molecule size, incremental reconstruction of the ligand is a strategy used by systematic search algorithms. There are essentially two ways to perform incremental reconstruction. The molecule in the first is split into a single stiff fragment and multiple flexible extension shells. The stiff fragment gets docked first because it can interact with the receptor with the greatest frequency. Following that, the flexible moieties are gradually rejoined. The scoring algorithm is exploited to choose the best solutions that are used for the subsequent extension stage after one flexible component has been introduced. New interactions are then sought after in accordance with the torsional database. The molecule is divided into different fragments in the second iteration of incremental reconstruction, which are then individually docked and then joined together into the active site using a hinge-bending method. Along with these reconstruction procedures, other programs simulate a thorough, systematic search of the ligand binding pose space by condensing it using a number of filters. In stochastic approaches, the ligand is taken into account as a whole, and a starting position or a population of poses is subjected to gradual alterations. These methods then assess the novel postures at each stage in an effort to enhance protein interactions and, ideally, reach the native binding mode. These include MC simulations and evolutionary algorithms (EAs) (Friesner et al., 2004; Zoete et al., 2009). The EA replicates the Darwinian evolution process. The starting population, also known as the seeds, is a set of poses that correspond to feasible ligand-receptor complexes. After assigning a score to each binding mode, new poses are generated via computational methods called operators, which are applied to the poses chosen from the population's fittest members in the hopes of producing even fitter solutions, whereas MC-based techniques begin with a single randomly generated pose and proceed to perform random motions such as rotating one dihedral angle and translating or rotating the entire ligand globally. The algorithm either continues from the prior posture after each modification, as determined by the Metropolis criteria, or it preserves the new posture as a starting point for the following modification. The new pose is scored after each change. The algorithm comes to a similar conclusion to EA-based methods.

After the systematic searching, the scoring functions, i.e., knowledge-based, empirical, and force-field-based are implemented in ligand-protein docking. Force-field-based scoring functions evaluate the binding of free energy by physically sound energy functions as well as intramolecular interactions. Knowledge-based scoring functions use inter-atomic interaction potentials using Boltzmann analysis, while empirical scoring functions calculate free energies as a weighted sum of uncorrelated terms (Eldridge et al., 1997; Bohm, 1998; Muegge and Martin, 1999; Huey et al., 2007). Molecular docking is a very useful technique to find the root mean square deviation (RMSD) between the protein and ligand, and it is generally used when ligand and proteins are known, but when the structure of the target is not known, ligand-based virtual high-throughput screening is useful, as it creates a pharmacophore model using measured activities for several well-known substances. Important characteristics like hydrophobic groups and hydrogen bonds are summarized in relation to potential ligands. The most promising options from the library can be chosen using a model (Klebe, 2006). Another approach is structure-based virtual high-throughput screening, which can be used to determine the interaction of protein targets for a whole database of compounds (Li and Shah, 2017).

Another crucial method is called "molecular dynamics," which uses a computer simulation methodology to generate atomic trajectories for a system using numerical integration of Newton's equation of motion for a certain interatomic potential specified by a starting condition and boundary condition. This method allows for the prediction of the time evolution of a particular system that interacts with its environment. This approach offers a framework to predict future behaviour and state changes inside the system through analysing the dynamics of the system and taking into consideration the impact of outside variables including forces, energy exchanges, or other interacting elements. Its ability to forecast the future makes it a useful tool in many different disciplines, improving planning, optimisation, and comprehension of complex systems (Roy et al., 2015). The activity of proteins and other biomolecules is captured in complete atomic detail and at extremely fine temporal resolution by MD simulations. The appeal of biomolecular modeling to experimentalists has expanded thanks to significant advancements in simulation speed, accuracy, and accessibility, as well as the abundance of experimental structural data—a development that is especially apparent in, but not limited to, neurology. Simulations have been useful in understanding the workings of proteins and other biomolecules, identifying the structural underpinnings of disease, and designing and optimizing small molecules, peptides, and proteins. Here, we give a concrete explanation of the kinds of data that MD simulations might produce as well as how they often inspire additional experimental research (Hollingsworth and Dror, 2018).

5.4.2 Workflow for Investigation of the Antibacterial and Antiviral Potential of Phenolic Compounds

Antimicrobial resistance is a persistent danger to our ability to treat common diseases due to the creation and spread of drug-resistant bacteria that have developed new resistance mechanisms. The increasing global development of multi-resistant and extremely drug-resistant bacteria, commonly referred to as "superbugs," which cause diseases that cannot be treated with current antimicrobial medications like antibiotics or antivirals, is particularly concerning. Therefore, it is crucial to discover a new alternative to replace the current ones. Natural substances have been used for a long time, and in particular, plants have a large variety of phytochemicals that are classified as phenolics and are covered in the section earlier. Here, we provide a summary of the actions necessary to improve the workflow for research on the development of antibacterial or antiviral drugs.

5.4.2.1 Target Identification and Protein Preparation

Target identification is the first step in *in silico* virtual screening. This step involves the determination of the function of a particular protein in disease, which is followed by the characterization of the molecular mechanisms addressed by the target. Data mining, genetic association, expression profiling, *in vitro* cell-based mechanistic studies, knockout studies, etc., can be used for target identification (Schenone et al., 2013). For example, in *Pseudomonas aeruginosa,* the LasR protein is a major transcriptional activator, and it is associated with two proteases, i.e., LasB elastase and LasA protease, which have a significant role in virulence. Kiratisin et al. (2002) demonstrated the role of LasR in *P. aeruginosa.* They proved that only when 3O-C_{12}-HSL is present does LasR form multimers using a LexA-based protein interaction assay. This study clearly stated that the LasR functions as a multimer *in vivo.* LasR can be used as a protein target for antimicrobial drug discovery. Likewise, in the case of antiviral lead optimization, various proteins of viruses involved in initiation, penetration, biosynthesis, maturation, and release of viral particles in host cells can be selected as targets for virtual screening (Joshi et al., 2021).

After protein target identification, protein preparation is the next step. For *in silico* studies, proteins should be prepared according to the requirements of the docking software. But before that, structural data on the target protein should be required. To promote protein-related information management, data-driven hypothesis creation, and biological knowledge discovery, numerous publicly accessible data repositories and services have been created. Among them, RCSB PDB (www.wwpdb.org) is a 3D structure database of proteins, which was established in 2003 to keep a single archive of macro-molecular structural data that is accessible to the public, the Protein Data Bank Archive (PDB Archive). The Protein Data Bank Markup Language (PDBML) format, the PDBx/mmCIF (http://deposit.pdb.org/mmcif/), and the classic PDB format are all included as flat files in the "PDB Archive." Each member site offers a unique perspective on the primary data as well as a range of tools and services, acting as a deposition, data processing, and distribution site for the PDB Archive. The 3D structure of a protein can be downloaded from PDB.

5.4.2.2 Lead Identification and Optimization

In the context of phenolics-based drug discovery, phenolics from natural sources can serve as lead compounds. The ideal starting point or source for obtaining promising leads with increased biological activity, selectivity, etc., could be natural compounds. To increase selectivity, boost activity, and lessen adverse effects, lead optimization aims to maximize bonded and non-bonded interactions with the active sites of chosen pharmacological targets. In lead optimization and identification, structural bioinformatics is essential. The lead compounds are then grouped according to predetermined standards, like acceptable pharmacological characteristics gathered using data mining from the lead identification step. Additional screens are applied to particular lead compounds. Structure-activity relationships (SARs) start to form early. A chemistry program is launched to manufacture analogues to improve their molecular characteristics. The fundamental objective of this phase of discovery is to choose the best drug candidate by optimizing the lead series' structure in terms of potency, selectivity, absorption, distribution, metabolism, elimination, and toxicity (ADMET) (deMontigny et al., 2015). Here, to investigate the antibacterial or antiviral potential of phenolics, the structure of the phenolic compound should be known, or the 3D structure of the compound can be downloaded from the various databases, i.e., PubChem (https://pubchem.ncbi.nlm.nih.gov), ChemIDplus (www.nlm.nih.gov/pubs/techbull/ma00/ma00_chemid.html), ChemSpider (www.chemspider.com/), etc. These databases are useful to retrieve the 3D structure of the compounds in the required format. For docking studies, it is essential to convert or prepare the ligand structure according to the software's requirements. In addition to this, bioinformatics tools such as LS-MIDA, Isotopo, and Lipid-Pro can also help in analyzing mass spectrometric, GC, or HPLC data.

5.4.2.3 Molecular Docking and Molecular Dynamics

After retrieving 3D structures of proteins and ligands, structures should be prepared before docking and dynamics. In general, hydrogen atoms are added, hydrogen bonds are optimized, atomic conflicts are eliminated, and structure refinement processes are carried out on protein crystal structures prior to docking. Prior to virtual screening, ligands must also be ready to establish accessible tautomer and ionization states, assign correct bond ordering, and create 3D geometries (Madhavi et al., 2013). For protein-ligand docking and molecular dynamics, various tools are available, i.e., AutoDock Vina, FlexX, Glide, NAMD, Gromacs, etc. Additionally, for visualization of protein-ligand interactions, various tools such as Pymol, Discovery Studio Visualizer, VMD, etc., can be used. Further, molecular dynamics simulates the dynamic behavior of molecular systems as a function of time while treating all the objects in the simulation box (ligands, proteins, and fluids, if explicit) as flexible (Salmaso and Moro, 2018). In pandemic situations, lots of reviews and research studies have been reported by various authors for the repurposing of herbal formulations against SARS-CoV2. (Singh et al., 2021; Jukic et al., 2021; Joshi et al., 2021; Omer et al., 2022). Likewise, numerous studies have reported the activities of phenolics using molecular docking and molecular dynamics (Gurung et al., 2021; Saqallah et al., 2022; Chigurupati et al., 2022).

5.5 APPLICATIONS OF THIS STUDY

The previously mentioned flow of work can be used to study the efficacy of phenolic compounds against various pathogens. Using bioactivity of phenolic compounds, we can also create databases of phenolic compounds and provide the information about the source plant and link the literature reported such compounds as active ingredients. Additionally, we can also use this pipeline for antimicrobial/antiviral drug discoveries. Various targets involved in disease as well as leads having biological activities can be explored for their antimicrobial potential against the proteins of pathogens using molecular docking and dynamics studies.

5.6 FUTURE PROSPECTS AND LIMITATIONS

By facilitating the discovery of potential targets for drug development and the design of novel therapeutics, bioinformatics has revolutionized the study of infectious diseases. With the emergence of drug-resistant bacterial and viral pathogens, the development of effective antibacterial and antiviral drugs is of utmost importance. In this context, the bioinformatics approach has great potential in identifying and developing new drugs with antimicrobial properties. The discovery of new therapeutic targets is a promising field of bioinformatics research for drug development. By analyzing the genomic and protein sequences of bacteria and viruses, bioinformatic techniques can identify prospective therapeutic targets. This method can be used to find proteins, receptors, or enzymes that are crucial for bacterial or viral growth and survival. Researchers can use computer simulations and other techniques to generate small molecules that attach to possible targets and hinder their function after potential targets have been identified. Additionally, bioinformatics can also be helpful in drug designing. In order to develop molecules that specifically target specific regions of the protein, researchers must first analyze the structure of proteins and how they interact with tiny molecules. This strategy may lead to more effective medications with fewer negative effects than conventional broad-spectrum antibiotics or antivirals using bioinformatics.

Although using bioinformatics for drug development has numerous benefits, it also has limitations. The limited availability of high-quality data is one problem. Although there are huge databases containing genetic and protein sequences, many of these sequences are not well annotated, which can reduce the precision of bioinformatics analysis. Additionally, due to the quick development of bacteria and viruses, bioinformatics tools need to be updated frequently to take into account brand-new strains and mutations. The difficulty in forecasting the safety and efficacy of drugs in people is another drawback of bioinformatics. Computer simulations can be a useful tool for understanding how proteins and small molecules interact, but they can never fully capture the complexity of biological systems. In total, bioinformatics serves as a promising approach for antibacterial and antiviral drug discovery, but there are also significant challenges to overcome, such as the limited availability of high-quality data and the difficulty in predicting the efficacy and safety of drugs in humans. Addressing these challenges will require ongoing innovation and collaboration among researchers in the field.

5.7 CONCLUSION

The study of bioactive phenolic compounds is a highly active field worldwide. The concern of antibiotic resistance among harmful bacteria is drawing increasing attention to phenols with antimicrobial and/or anti-infective potential. As medication resistance becomes more difficult to manage, phenolics in particular are being looked at with great optimism, particularly those having antibacterial and antiviral potential. Plant phenolics may strengthen the effects of antibiotic therapy by increasing the susceptibility of the target pathogen population and enhancing the host immunity by lowering the effect of virulence. The development of these active phenolics as useful therapeutic agents will be the true challenge, notwithstanding the abundance of data on the antibacterial and antiviral potential of phenolics. There are many reasons to think that phenolics will eventually make up a sizable portion of the list of approved pharmaceuticals, despite the fact that phenolics research is a complicated field with its own set of challenges. High-throughput virtual screening has the potential to be a key component in bridging the gap between conventional and modern medical practices.

REFERENCES

Abdurakhmonov, Ibrokhim Y. *Bioinformatics: Basics, Development, and Future.* Rijeka: InTech, 2016.

Abubakar, Abdullahi R., and Mainul Haque. "Preparation of medicinal plants: Basic extraction and fractionation procedures for experimental purposes." *Journal of Pharmacy & Bioallied Sciences* 12, no. 1 (2020): 1.

Alara, Oluwaseun Ruth, and Nour Hamid Abdurahman. "Microwave-assisted extraction of phenolics from Hibiscus sabdariffa calyces: Kinetic modelling and process intensification." *Industrial Crops and Products* 137 (2019): 528–535.

Alara, Oluwaseun Ruth, Nour Hamid Abdurahman, and Chinonso Ishamel Ukaegbu. "Extraction of phenolic compounds: A review." *Current Research in Food Science* 4 (2021): 200–214.

Al-Farsi, Mohamed Ali, and Chang Yong Lee. "Optimization of phenolics and dietary fibre extraction from date seeds." *Food Chemistry* 108, no. 3 (2008): 977–985.

Awika, J. M., L. W. Rooney, and R. D. Waniska. "Anthocyanins from black sorghum and their antioxidant properties." *Food Chem* 90 (2005): 293–301. https://doi.org/10.1016/j.foodchem.2004.03.058.

Azmir, Jannatul, Islam Sarker Mohamed Zaidul, Mohd M. Rahman, K. M. Sharif, A. Mohamed, F. Sahena, M. H. A. Jahurul, K. Ghafoor, N. A. N. Norulaini, and A. K. M. Omar. "Techniques for extraction of bioactive compounds from plant materials: A review." *Journal of Food Engineering* 117, no. 4 (2013): 426–436.

Bhalodia, Nayan R., and V. J. Shukla. "Antibacterial and antifungal activities from leaf extracts of Cassia fistula l.: An ethnomedicinal plant." *Journal of Advanced Pharmaceutical Technology & Research* 2, no. 2 (2011): 104.

Böhm, Hans-Joachim. "Prediction of binding constants of protein ligands: A fast method for the prioritization of hits obtained from de novo design or 3D database search programs." *Journal of Computer-Aided Molecular Design* 12, no. 4 (1998): 309.

Bridgers, E. N., M. S. Chinn, and V.-D. Truong. "Extraction of anthocyanins from industrial purple-fleshed sweet potatoes and enzymatic hydrolysis of residues for fermentable sugars." *Industrial Crops and Products* 32 (2010): 613–620. https://doi.org/10.1016/j.indcrop.2010.07.020.

Caldas, Thais W., Karen E. L. Mazza, Aline S. C. Teles, Gabriela N. Mattos, Ana Iraidy S. Brígida, Carlos A. Conte-Junior, Renata G. Borguini, Ronoel L. O. Godoy, Lourdes M. C. Cabral, and Renata V. Tonon. "Phenolic compounds recover from grape skin using conventional and non-conventional extraction methods." *Industrial Crops and Products* 111 (2018): 86–91.

Castaneda-Ovando, A., M. de Lourdes Pacheco-Hernandez, Ma E. Paez-Hernandez, J. A. Rodriguez, and C. A. Galan-Vidal. "Chemical studies of anthocyanins: A review." *Food Chemistry* 113 (2009): 859–871. https://doi.org/10.1016/j.foodchem.2008.09.001.

Chigurupati, Sridevi, Atheer Al-Murphy, Suliman A. Almahmoud, Yosif Almoshari, Amira Saber Ahmed, Shantini Vijayabalan, Shatha Ghazi Felemban, and Vasanth Raj Palanimuthu. "Molecular docking of phenolic compounds and screening of antioxidant and antidiabetic potential of Moringa oleifera ethanolic leaves extract from Qassim region, Saudi Arabia." *Saudi Journal of Biological Sciences* 29, no. 2 (2022): 854–859.

Dai, Jin, and Russell J. Mumper. "Plant phenolics: Extraction, analysis and their antioxidant and anticancer properties." *Molecules* 15, no. 10 (2010): 7313–7352.

Danciu, Corina, Lavinia Vlaia, Florinela Fetea, Monica Hancianu, Dorina E. Coricovac, Sorina A. Ciurlea, Codruţa M. Şoica, et al. "Evaluation of phenolic profile, antioxidant and anticancer potential of two main representants of Zingiberaceae family against B164A5 murine melanoma cells." *Biological Research* 48, no. 1 (2015): 1–9.

Davidov-Pardo, Gabriel, Iñigo Arozarena, and María R. Marín-Arroyo. "Stability of polyphenolic extracts from grape seeds after thermal treatments." *European Food Research and Technology* 232, no. 2 (2011): 211–220.

deMontigny, Pierre, David Harris, Chris Ho, Franz Weiberth, Bruno Galli, and Bernard Faller. "Discover a drug substance, formulate, and develop it to a product." In Camille Georges Wermuth, David Aldous, Pierre Raboisson, Didier Rognan (eds) *The Practice of Medicinal Chemistry*, pp. 793–803. Academic Press, Elsevier, Cambridge, Massachusetts. USA, (2015). Pages 793-803, ISBN 9780124172050, https://doi.org/10.1016/B978-0-12-417205-0.00033-X.

Dias, Daniel A., Sylvia Urban, and Ute Roessner. "A historical overview of natural products in drug discovery." *Metabolites* 2, no. 2 (2012): 303–336.

Di Meo, Maria Chiara, Giuseppa Anna De Cristofaro, Roberta Imperatore, Mariapina Rocco, Daniela Giaquinto, Antonio Palladino, Tiziana Zotti, Pasquale Vito, Marina Paolucci, and Ettore Varricchio. "Microwave-assisted extraction of olive leaf from five Italian cultivars: Effects of harvest-time and extraction conditions on phenolic compounds and in vitro antioxidant properties." *ACS Food Science & Technology* 2, no. 1 (2021): 31–40.

Eldridge, Matthew D., Christopher W. Murray, Timothy R. Auton, Gaia V. Paolini, and Roger P. Mee. "Empirical scoring functions: I. The development of a fast empirical scoring function to estimate the binding affinity of ligands in receptor complexes." *Journal of Computer-Aided Molecular Design* 11, no. 5 (1997): 425–445.

El-Saadany, Mohamed T., Nidal M. Zabermawi, Nehal M. Zabermawi, Maryam A. Burollus, Manal E. Shafi, Mahmoud Alagawany, Nahed Yehia, et al. "Nutritional aspects and health benefits of bioactive plant compounds against infectious diseases: A review." *Food Reviews International* (2021): 1–23.

Espada-Bellido, Estrella, Marta Ferreiro-González, Ceferino Carrera, Miguel Palma, Carmelo G. Barroso, and Gerardo F. Barbero. "Optimization of the ultrasound-assisted extraction of anthocyanins and total phenolic compounds in mulberry (Morus nigra) pulp." *Food Chemistry* 219 (2017): 23–32.

Friesner, Richard A., Jay L. Banks, Robert B. Murphy, Thomas A. Halgren, Jasna J. Klicic, Daniel T. Mainz, Matthew P. Repasky, et al. "Glide: A new approach for rapid, accurate docking and scoring. 1. Method and assessment of docking accuracy." *Journal of Medicinal Chemistry* 47, no. 7 (2004): 1739–1749.

Gashaw, I., P. Ellinghaus, A. Sommer, and K. Asadullah. "What makes a good drug target?" *Drug Discovery Today* 16 (2011): 1037–1043.

Geethalakshmi, Rajarathinam, Jagadish Chandrabose Sundaramurthi, and Dronamraju V. L. Sarada. "Antibacterial activity of flavonoid isolated from Trianthema decandra against Pseudomonas aeruginosa and molecular docking study of FabZ." *Microbial Pathogenesis* 121 (2018): 87–92.

Gurung, Arun Bahadur, Mohammad Ajmal Ali, Joongku Lee, Mohammad Abul Farah, and Khalid Mashay Al-Anazi. "Molecular docking and dynamics simulation study of bioactive compounds from Ficus carica L. with important anticancer drug targets." *PLoS ONE* 16, no. 7 (2021): e0254035.

Haghi, Ghasem, and Alireza Hatami. "Simultaneous quantification of flavonoids and phenolic acids in plant materials by a newly developed isocratic high-performance liquid chromatography approach." *Journal of Agricultural and Food Chemistry* 58, no. 20 (2010): 10812–10816.

Hollingsworth, Scott A., and Ron O. Dror. "Molecular dynamics simulation for all." *Neuron* 99, no. 6 (2018): 1129–1143.

Huey, Ruth, Garrett M. Morris, Arthur J. Olson, and David S. Goodsell. "A semiempirical free energy force field with charge-based desolvation." *Journal of Computational Chemistry* 28, no. 6 (2007): 1145–1152.

Jarial, Rini, Sveta Thakur, Mimi Sakinah, A. W. Zularisam, Amit Sharad, S. S. Kanwar, and Lakhveer Singh. "Potent anticancer, antioxidant and antibacterial activities of isolated flavonoids from Asplenium nidus." *Journal of King Saud University-Science* 30, no. 2 (2018): 185–192.

Ji, Youan, Yucui Hou, Shuhang Ren, Congfei Yao, and Weize Wu. "Highly efficient extraction of phenolic compounds from oil mixtures by trimethylamine-based dicationic ionic liquids via forming deep eutectic solvents." *Fuel Processing Technology* 171 (2018): 183–191.

Joshi, Chinmayi, Armi Chaudhari, Chaitanya Joshi, Madhvi Joshi, and Snehal Bagatharia. "Repurposing of the herbal formulations: Molecular docking and molecular dynamics simulation studies to validate the efficacy of phytocompounds against SARS-CoV-2 proteins." *Journal of Biomolecular Structure and Dynamics* (2021): 1–15.

Joshi, Chinmayi, and Vijay Kothari. "Bacterial stress-response machinery as a target for next-generation antimicrobials." *Infectious Disorders Drug Targets* 22, no. 6 (2022): 1–9.

Jukič, Marko, Katarina Kores, Dušanka Janežič, and Urban Bren. "Repurposing of drugs for SARS-CoV-2 using inverse docking fingerprints." *Frontiers in Chemistry* 9 (2021).

Kaliyamoorthy, Subha, and Yi-Ping Phoebe Chen. "Structure-based drug design to augment hit discovery." *Drug Discovery Today* 16, no. 17–18 (2011): 831–839.

Katiyar, Chandrakant, et al. "Drug discovery from plant sources: An integrated approach." *Ayu* 33, no. 1 (2012): 10.

Kaufmann, Béatrice, and Philippe Christen. "Recent extraction techniques for natural products: Microwave-assisted extraction and pressurised solvent extraction." *Phytochemical Analysis: An International Journal of Plant Chemical and Biochemical Techniques* 13, no. 2 (2002): 105–113.

Kazmi, Mehdi H., Abdul Malik, Saira Hameed, Nargis Akhtar, and Samina Noor Ali. "An anthraquinone derivative from Cassia Italica." *Phytochemistry* 36, no. 3 (1994): 761–763.

Khan, Tariq, Mubarak Ali Khan, Nazif Ullah, and Akhtar Nadhman. "Therapeutic potential of medicinal plants against COVID-19: The role of antiviral medicinal metabolites." *Biocatalysis and Agricultural Biotechnology* 31 (2021): 101890.

Khoddami, Ali, Meredith A. Wilkes, and Thomas H. Roberts. "Techniques for analysis of plant phenolic compounds." *Molecules* 18, no. 2 (2013): 2328–2375.

Kiratisin, Pattarachai, Kenneth D. Tucker, and Luciano Passador. "LasR, a transcriptional activator of Pseudomonas aeruginosa virulence genes, functions as a multimer." *Journal of Bacteriology* 184, no. 17 (2002): 4912–4919.

Klebe, Gerhard. "Virtual ligand screening: Strategies, perspectives and limitations." *Drug Discovery Today* 11, no. 13–14 (2006): 580–594.

Ko, Min-Jung, Hwa-Hyun Nam, and Myong-Soo Chung. "Subcritical water extraction of bioactive compounds from Orostachys japonicus A. Berger (Crassulaceae)." *Scientific Reports* 10, no. 1 (2020): 1–10.

Kumar, Bhanu, Ankita Misra, and Sharad Srivastava. "Bioactive phenolic compounds from Indian medicinal plants for pharmaceutical and medical aspects." In *Phenolic Compounds-Chemistry, Synthesis, Diversity, Non-Conventional Industrial, Pharmaceutical and Therapeutic Applications*. London: IntechOpen, 2021.

Li, Qingliang, and Salim Shah. "Structure-based virtual screening." In *Protein Bioinformatics*, pp. 111–124. New York: Humana Press, 2017.

López-Cobo, Ana, Vito Verardo, Elixabet Diaz-de-Cerio, Antonio Segura-Carretero, Alberto Fernández-Gutiérrez, and Ana M. Gómez-Caravaca. "Use of HPLC-and GC-QTOF to determine hydrophilic and lipophilic phenols in mango fruit (Mangifera indica L.) and its by-products." *Food Research International* 100 (2017): 423–434.

Lunardelli Negreiros de Carvalho, Patrícia, Eliane de Oliveira Silva, Daniela Aparecida Chagas-Paula, Jaine Honorata Hortolan Luiz, and Masaharu Ikegaki. "Importance and implications of the production of phenolic secondary metabolites by endophytic fungi: A mini-review." *Mini Reviews in Medicinal Chemistry* 16, no. 4 (2016): 259–271.

Madhavi Sastry, G., Matvey Adzhigirey, Tyler Day, Ramakrishna Annabhimoju, and Woody Sherman. "Protein and ligand preparation: Parameters, protocols, and influence on virtual screening enrichments." *Journal of Computer-Aided Molecular Design* 27, no. 3 (2013): 221–234.

Maia, Eduardo Habib Bechelane, Letícia Cristina Assis, Tiago Alves De Oliveira, Alisson Marques Da Silva, and Alex Gutterres Taranto. "Structure-based virtual screening: From classical to artificial intelligence." *Frontiers in Chemistry* 8 (2020): 343.

Martínez-Patiño, José Carlos, Beatriz Gullón, Inmaculada Romero, Encarnación Ruiz, Mladen Brnčić, Jana Šic Žlabur, and Eulogio Castro. "Optimization of ultrasound-assisted extraction of biomass from olive trees using response surface methodology." *Ultrasonics Sonochemistry* 51 (2019): 487–495.

Mishra, Amita, Amit Kumar Sharma, Shashank Kumar, Ajit K. Saxena, and Abhay K. Pandey. "Bauhinia variegata leaf extracts exhibit considerable antibacterial, antioxidant, and anticancer activities." *BioMed Research International* 2013 (2013).

Mojerla, Zohreh, and Amirhossein Elhamirad. "Optimization of ultrasound-assisted extraction (UAE) of phenolic compounds from olive cake." *Journal of Food Science and Technology* 55, no. 3 (2018): 977–984.

Muegge, Ingo, and Yvonne C. Martin. "A general and fast scoring function for protein–ligand interactions: A simplified potential approach." *Journal of Medicinal Chemistry* 42, no. 5 (1999): 791–804.

Munir, M. T., Hamid Kheirkhah, Saeid Baroutian, Siew Young Quek, and Brent R. Young. "Subcritical water extraction of bioactive compounds from waste onion skin." *Journal of Cleaner Production* 183 (2018): 487–494.

Mythili, K., C. U. Reddy, D. Chamundeeswari, and P. K. Manna. "Determination of total phenol, alkaloid, flavonoid and tannin in different extracts of Calanthe triplicata." *Journal of Pharmacognsoy and Phytochemistry* 2, no. 2 (2014): 40–44.

Naczk, M., R. Amarowicz, R. Zadernowski, and F. Shahidi. "Antioxidant capacity of phenolics from canola hulls as affected by different solvents." *ACS Symposium Series* (2005). https://doi.org/10.1021/bk-2005-0909.ch006

Nalbantoglu, Sinem. "Metabolomics: Basic principles and strategies." *Molecular Medicine* 10 (2019).

Nelson, Kenrad E., and Carolyn Masters Williams, eds. *Infectious Disease Epidemiology*. Sudbury, MA: Jones & Bartlett Publishers, 2013.

Nipornram, Suriyaporn, Worasit Tochampa, Puntarika Rattanatraiwong, and Riantong Singanusong. "Optimization of low power ultrasound-assisted extraction of phenolic compounds from mandarin (Citrus reticulata Blanco cv. Sainampueng) peel." *Food Chemistry* 241 (2018): 338–345.

Omer, Samia E., Tawasol M. Ibrahim, Omer A. Krar, Amna M. Ali, Alaa A. Makki, Walaa Ibraheem, and Abdulrahim A. Alzain. "Drug repurposing for SARS-CoV-2 main protease: Molecular docking and molecular dynamics investigations." *Biochemistry and Biophysics Reports* 29 (2022): 101225.

Osorio-Tobón, J. Felipe. "Recent advances and comparisons of conventional and alternative extraction techniques of phenolic compounds." *Journal of Food Science and Technology* 57, no. 12 (2020): 4299–4315.

Pandey, Asheesh, Tarun Belwal, K. Chandra Sekar, Indra D. Bhatt, and Ranbeer S. Rawal. "Optimization of ultrasonic-assisted extraction (UAE) of phenolics and antioxidant compounds from rhizomes of Rheum moorcroftianum using response surface methodology (RSM)." *Industrial Crops and Products* 119 (2018): 218–225.

Pimentel-Moral, Sandra, Isabel Borrás-Linares, Jesús Lozano-Sánchez, David Arráez-Román, Antonio Martínez-Férez, and Antonio Segura-Carretero. "Supercritical CO2 extraction of bioactive compounds from Hibiscus sabdariffa." *The Journal of Supercritical Fluids* 147 (2019): 213–221.

Pinelo, Manuel, Beatriz Zornoza, and Anne S. Meyer. "Selective release of phenols from apple skin: Mass transfer kinetics during solvent and enzyme-assisted extraction." *Separation and Purification Technology* 63, no. 3 (2008): 620–627.

Proestos, Charalampos, Konstantina Lytoudi, Olga Konstantina Mavromelanidou, Panagiotis Zoumpoulakis, and Vassileia J. Sinanoglou. "Antioxidant capacity of selected plant extracts and their essential oils." *Antioxidants* 2, no. 1 (2013): 11–22.

Qanash, Husam, Reham Yahya, Marwah M. Bakri, Abdulrahman S. Bazaid, Sultan Qanash, Abdullah F. Shater, and T. M. Abdelghany. "Anticancer, antioxidant, antiviral and antimicrobial activities of Kei Apple (Dovyalis caffra) fruit." *Scientific Reports* 12, no. 1 (2022): 1–15.

Radojković, Marija, Manuela M. Moreira, Cristina Soares, M. Fátima Barroso, Aleksandra Cvetanović, Jaroslava Švarc-Gajić, Simone Morais, and Cristina Delerue-Matos. "Microwave-assisted extraction of phenolic compounds from Morus nigra leaves: Optimization and characterization of the antioxidant activity and phenolic composition." *Journal of Chemical Technology & Biotechnology* 93, no. 6 (2018): 1684–1693.

Robards, Kevin. "Strategies for the determination of bioactive phenols in plants, fruit and vegetables." *Journal of Chromatography A* 1000, no. 1–2 (2003): 657–691.

Routray, Winny, and Valerie Orsat. "MAE of phenolic compounds from blueberry leaves and comparison with other extraction methods." *Industrial Crops and Products* 58 (2014): 36–45.

Roy, Kunal, Supratik Kar, and Rudra Narayan Das. *Understanding the Basics of QSAR for Applications in Pharmaceutical Sciences and Risk Assessment.* Academic Press, Elsevier, Massachusetts. USA, 2015.

Salmaso, Veronica, and Stefano Moro. "Bridging molecular docking to molecular dynamics in exploring ligand-protein recognition process: An overview." *Frontiers in Pharmacology* 9 (2018): 923.

Saqallah, Fadi G., Wafaa M. Hamed, Wamidh H. Talib, Roza Dianita, and Habibah A. Wahab. "Antimicrobial activity and molecular docking screening of bioactive components of Antirrhinum majus (snapdragon) aerial parts." *Heliyon* 8, no. 8 (2022): e10391.

Schenone, Monica, Vlado Dančík, Bridget K. Wagner, and Paul A. Clemons. "Target identification and mechanism of action in chemical biology and drug discovery." *Nature Chemical Biology* 9, no. 4 (2013): 232–240.

Selvamuthukumaran, M., and John Shi. "Recent advances in extraction of antioxidants from plant by-products processing industries." *Food Quality and Safety* 1, no. 1 (2017): 61–81.

Shirzad, Habib, Vahid Niknam, Mehdi Taheri, and Hassan Ebrahimzadeh. "Ultrasound-assisted extraction process of phenolic antioxidants from Olive leaves: A nutraceutical study using RSM and LC—ESI—DAD—MS." *Journal of Food Science and Technology* 54, no. 8 (2017): 2361–2371.

Singh, Rajeshwari, Sumeet Goel, Pascale Bourgeade, Lotfi Aleya, and Devesh Tewari. "Ayurveda Rasayana as antivirals and immunomodulators: Potential applications in COVID-19." *Environmental Science and Pollution Research* 28, no. 40 (2021): 55925–55951.

Singh, Sandeep Kumar, and Arjun Patra. "Evaluation of phenolic composition, antioxidant, anti-inflammatory and anticancer activities of Polygonatum verticillatum (L.)." *Journal of Integrative Medicine* 16, no. 4 (2018): 273–282.

Sliwoski, Gregory, Sandeepkumar Kothiwale, Jens Meiler, and Edward W. Lowe. "Computational methods in drug discovery." *Pharmacological Reviews* 66, no. 1 (2014): 334–395.

Stan, Diana, Ana-Maria Enciu, Andreea Lorena Mateescu, Andreea Cristina Ion, Ariana Cristina Brezeanu, Dana Stan, and Cristiana Tanase. "Natural compounds with antimicrobial and antiviral effect and nanocarriers used for their transportation." *Frontiers in Pharmacology* (2021): 2405.

Sticher, Otto. "Natural product isolation." *Natural Product Reports* 25, no. 3 (2008): 517–554.

Tiwari, Brijesh K. "Ultrasound: A clean, green extraction technology." *TrAC Trends in Analytical Chemistry* 71 (2015): 100–109.

Tsugawa, Hiroshi, Yuki Tsujimoto, Masanori Arita, Takeshi Bamba, and Eiichiro Fukusaki. "GC/MS based metabolomics: Development of a data mining system for metabolite identification by using soft independent modeling of class analogy (SIMCA)." *BMC Bioinformatics* 12, no. 1 (2011): 1–13.

Vichapong, Jitlada, Maliwan Sookserm, Voranuch Srijesdaruk, Prasan Swatsitang, and Supalax Srijaranai. "High performance liquid chromatographic analysis of phenolic compounds and their antioxidant activities in rice varieties." *LWT-Food Science and Technology* 43, no. 9 (2010): 1325–1330.

Wooller, Sarah K., Graeme Benstead-Hume, Xiangrong Chen, Yusuf Ali, and Frances M. G. Pearl. "Bioinformatics in translational drug discovery." *Bioscience Reports* 37, no. 4 (2017).

Xia, Xuhua. "Bioinformatics and drug discovery." *Current Topics in Medicinal Chemistry* 17, no. 15 (2017): 1709–1726.

Xu, Zhihong, Barrett Eichler, Eytan A. Klausner, Jetty Duffy-Matzner, and Weifan Zheng. "Lead/drug discovery from natural resources." *Molecules* 27, no. 23 (2022): 8280.

Yang, Wen-Bo, Jie-Chao Liu, Hui Liu, Chun-Ling Zhang, Zhen-Zhen Lv, and Zhong-Gao Jiao. "Optimization of supercritical fluid extraction of phenolic compounds from peach blossom (Amygdalus Persica) by response surface methodology." *Current Topics in Nutraceutical Research* 17, no. 2 (2019).

Yuan, Haidan, et al. "The traditional medicine and modern medicine from natural products." *Molecules* 21, no. 5 (2016): 559.

Zabidi, Nur Athirah, Nur Akmal Ishak, Muhajir Hamid, and Siti Efliza Ashari. "Subcritical water extraction of antioxidants from Curculigo latifolia root." *Journal of Chemistry* 2019 (2019).

Zakaria, Siti Maisurah, Siti Mazlina Mustapa Kamal, Mohd Razif Harun, Rozita Omar, and Shamsul Izhar Siajam. "Extraction of phenolic compounds from Chlorella sp. microalgae using pressurized hot water: kinetics study." *Biomass Conversion and Biorefinery* (2020): 1–9.

Zannella, Carla, Rosa Giugliano, Annalisa Chianese, Carmine Buonocore, Giovanni Andrea Vitale, Giuseppina Sanna, Federica Sarno et al. "Antiviral activity of Vitis vinifera leaf extract against SARS-CoV-2 and HSV-1." *Viruses* 13, no. 7 (2021): 1263.

Zhang, Yuanyuan, Ping Cai, Guanghui Cheng, and Yongqiang Zhang. "A brief review of phenolic compounds identified from plants: Their extraction, analysis, and biological activity." *Natural Product Communications* 17, no. 1 (2022): 1934578X211069721.

Zoete, Vincent, Aurélien Grosdidier, and Olivier Michielin. "Docking, virtual high throughput screening and in silico fragment-based drug design." *Journal of Cellular and Molecular Medicine* 13, no. 2 (2009): 238–248.

6 The Role of Tissue Engineering in the Treatment of Degenerative Diseases

Hitesh Malhotra, Sweta Kamboj*, Amrit Sarwara*, Rudraksh*, Tanu Devi*, and Rupesh K. Gautam**,†*
*Guru Gobind Singh College of Pharmacy, Yamunanagar, Haryana, India; **Department of Pharmacology, Indore Institute of Pharmacy, IIST Campus, Rau, Indore (M.P.), India
†Corresponding Author: rupeshgautammmu@gmail.com

ABBREVIATIONS

Abbreviation	**Full Form**
AMD	Age-related macular degeneration
CNS	Central nervous system
ECM	Extracellular matrix
HA	Hyaluronic acid
IL-1 beta	Interleukin-1 beta
NSAIDs	Non-steroidal anti-inflammatory drugs
OA	Osteoarthritis
PNS	Peripheral nervous system
RP	Retinal disorders
TE	Tissue engineering
TGF	Tissue growth factor
TNF	Tumour necrosis factor
VEGF	Vascular endothelial growth factor

6.1 INTRODUCTION

Those in attendance at the first NSF-sponsored meeting in 1988 gave the term tissue engineering its first official definition as the "application of the principles and methods of engineering and life sciences toward a fundamental understanding of the structure-function relationship in normal and pathological mammalian tissues and the development of biological substitutes for the repair or regeneration of tissue or organ function" (Trese et al. 2012) Tissue engineering is an interdisciplinary field that applies the

DOI: 10.1201/9781003354437-6

principles of engineering and life sciences toward the development of biological substitutes that restore, maintain, or enhance tissue or organ function, according to Langer and Vacanti, who summarised the early developments in this field in 1993. Currently, tissue or organ transplantation may be replaced with tissue engineering. The generally accepted definition of this field states that it applies the principles and techniques of biomaterials engineering and medicine to analyse the relationship between structure and function in both pathological and healthy human tissue, as well as to design and create biological replacements that enhance, restore, or maintain tissue function (Gonçalves et al. 2021). In the realm of bone tissue engineering, polymeric scaffolds, for example, are a practical substitute for traditional grafts. The tissue-engineered products may have the ability to integrate and produce the anticipated functional tissue upon implantation, or they may be completely functioning at the time of therapy. Biomaterials may occasionally be altered to promote the migration and adhesion of particular cell populations that replace or repair damaged tissue (Chapekar 2000). Organ and tissue injury and loss result in metabolic and structural alterations that can significantly increase morbidity and lower quality of life. The currently used therapies for treating joint tissue loss or disease are ineffective since they rely on metal joint prostheses, which only provide a limited functional replacement. Artificial implants also lack the physiological functions of the tissue. The purpose of TE is to offer biological/physiological alternatives that can replace lost tissue as a result of disease, birth defects, or trauma.

The biological replacement should, in theory, be structurally and morphologically identical to native tissue and be capable of carrying out comparable biological activities. Due to improved biocompatibility, integration into surrounding tissues, and the capacity to remodel to the body's needs, biologically engineered tissue may provide superior long-term performance than artificial implants (Moreira-Teixeira et al. 2011). When cells, biomaterials, and biological cues are coupled, TE is widely described as the reconstruction of the structural and functional properties of mammalian tissues. TE is a very interdisciplinary field that integrates expertise in engineering, cell and molecular biology, materials science, and medicine. Given that osteoarthritis affects the entire joint, applying the TE method as a treatment is considerably more difficult. To prevent future degeneration of the cartilage and the surrounding tissue, the TE package should integrate the restoration of the normal composition and function of the injured articular cartilage (Nesic et al. 2006).

Degenerative retinal diseases are a broad category of illnesses that, if neglected, can cause permanent blindness. Age-related macular degeneration (AMD) and retinitis pigmentosa are two prevalent retinal disorders. Both of these degenerative retinal disorders, despite having distinct aetiologies, are defined by a gradual loss of photoreceptor cells. Wet AMD patients today have access to a wide range of treatment options, such as photodynamic therapy and intraocular injections of anti-vascular endothelial growth factor (VEGF) medications. However, there are now only a few early-stage medication studies and dietary supplements available to patients with atrophic retinal illnesses, such as dry AMD and RP. These treatments aim to slow the progression of the condition. Another potential treatment approach that has gained popularity recently is gene therapy. This is mostly because a clinical experiment that successfully reprogrammed the mutated RPE65 gene in people with Leber congenital amaurosis was successful (Tuli et al. 2003). If this study is a success, it could have significant effects on those who have atrophic macular degeneration. It is thought that the inner retina's survival is a result of its dual blood supply, in which the inner retina is satiated by the retinal circulatory system and the outer retina is fed by the fenestrated chorio capillaries. Several therapeutic strategies, including cell-based therapies, can be supported by this distinct disease pathophysiology (Sun et al. 2021).

Degenerative conditions like osteoarthritis (OA), osteoporosis, rheumatoid arthritis, and other musculoskeletal conditions also have a significant impact on how quickly joints fail after developing osteochondrocyte (OC) lesions. The most prevalent kind of arthritis, OA, is a chronic articular joint disease marked by autologous chondrocyte (AC) deterioration and dysfunction in the affected joint. Around 250 million people worldwide suffer from OA, with 30% of them being over 60. Total joint arthroplasty is the conventional treatment for severe osteoarthritis. One drawback of this procedure is the potential for implant loosening, which could cause articular cartilage injury and degeneration over time. Young patients with sports injuries usually have localised lesions such as osteochondritis dissecans and chondral abnormalities. A chondral defect is one that only affects the cartilage itself and does not extend into the subchondral bone. Because the cartilage has no blood supply, spontaneous healing is only possible in certain circumstances. Osteochondral lesions affect the subchondral bone and mesenchymal chondroprogenitor cells, which migrate to the lesions to heal them. The new cartilage, however, loses the lower friction and elastic qualities since it is made up primarily of type I collagen and increased fibronectin. The scaffold plays a crucial function in tissue engineering by acting as an extracellular matrix (ECM) to give cells a three-dimensional conformation and direction. The chondrogenic phenotype and the ability for re-differentiation are typically lost with subsequent culturing passages in chondrocytes that are grown as a monolayer, such as in Petri dishes and tissue culture flasks.

On the other hand, cells that have been introduced into a structure together with a growth factor can preserve the phenotypic and promote cell growth. Gelatine, collagen, alginate, and some of its derivatives are utilised to create scaffolds in the form of hydrogels and porous structural forms for cartilage tissue engineering. However, this type of hydrogel scaffold still has issues with weak biomechanical and handling qualities. Traditional techniques for creating 3D porous scaffolds include electrospinning and freeze-drying. To create 3D-ordered scaffolds, new solid freeform fabrication methods have been proposed, including photolithographic patterning and stacking, direct writing, and two-photon stereo lithography (Hu 2021). These techniques need expensive robotic control and time-consuming pixel-by-pixel writing, yet they produce highly ordered scaffolds. The development of a trustworthy, affordable scaffolding technique could aid cartilage tissue engineering (Sun et al. 2021). In adult organisms, mature cartilage serves a variety of roles, including articulation capacity in joints and elastic and loading capacity in intervertebral discs. It arises from the mesodermal lineage. Chondrogenic precursors are essential for the development of the two mature skeletal tissues that make up long bones, adult cartilage and bone, throughout embryogenesis. Endochondral ossification is a series of processes started by mesenchymal condensations that result in the development of long bones. Regenerating and replacing human cells, tissues, and even organs that have been harmed by degenerative diseases, trauma, or other causes is the focus of this relatively new branch of medicine. One of the most exciting areas of regenerative medicine is tissue engineering. Even though it is still the most widely used material for tissue replacement, autologous tissue is only available in small amounts. Furthermore, the patient may experience greater morbidity as a result of the tissue harvest. Studies of materials that can be implanted into the human body and are biologically compatible are a part of tissue engineering. Either improving already-used biomaterials or developing novel ones are the two goals of tissue engineering. Stem cells or mature cells can be seeded into the biomaterials that have been created. Since there is a reduced immune reaction in the body, seeding with the patient's own cells appears to be a beneficial strategy to hasten implant integration (Travnickova and Bacakova 2018). The rapidly expanding field of tissue regeneration has tremendous potential for the production of useful tissue substitutes, particularly cartilage, by producing tissue constructions in vitro for eventual implantation in vivo. The fundamental concept is to create a biocompatible, architecturally, and physically robust scaffold that will be supplied with the appropriate cell source to induce cellular differentiation and/or maturation (Thangprasert et al. 2019).

6.2 COMPONENTS OF TISSUE-ENGINEERED PRODUCTS

Due to their differentiation, cell-to-cell communication, synthesis of biomolecules, and ECM creation, cells are essential for tissue regeneration and repair. A designed tissue may function structurally, metabolically, or both. Engineered tissues could contain cells, or biomaterials and/or biomolecules may be used to recruit cells in vivo. Finding the right cells and being able to separate them from the original source is crucial when choosing the cellular component of a designed product (Figure 6.1). Additionally, without introducing any accidental and particular bacterial agents during this expansion phase, as well as without irreversibly affecting the conformation

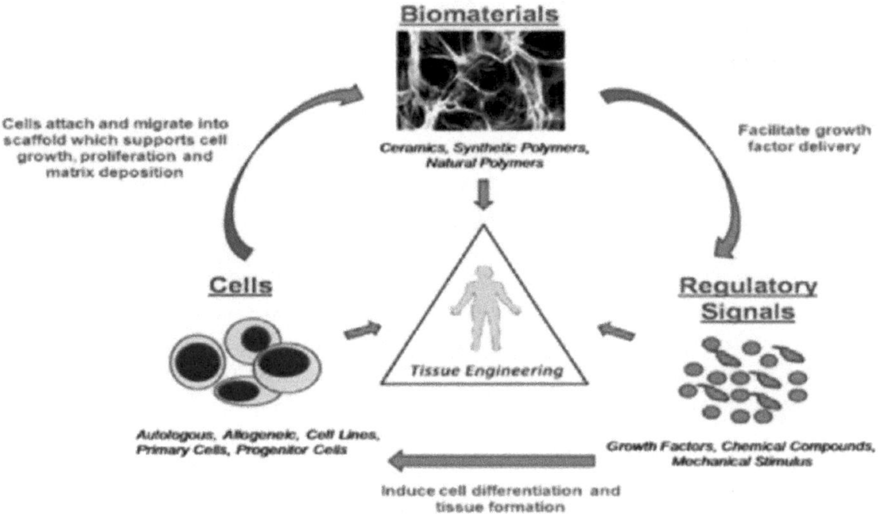

FIGURE 6.1 Components of tissue engineering.

and activity of these cells, the enlargement of these cells sometimes poses therapy failure (Kanakis et al. 2011). The isolation of several adult stem cells, including brain cells, hepatic, and stromal cells, has uncovered a fresh method for producing an endless supply of cells. To control the growth of normal tissue, a thorough comprehension of the elements involved in these cells' differentiation as well as the synchronisation of lineage development is essential. Accordingly, it has been demonstrated that substances, including TGF, inulin, and prednisone, can help mesenchymal stem cells develop into chondrocytes and astrocytic lineages. Researchers are attempting to change the cell surface molecules of allogeneic and xenogeneic cells to lessen their antigenicity because the host immune response to these cells presents a significant obstacle. Human embryonic stem cells, together with embryonic germ cells, have recently used in the therapy (Hauselmann et al. 1994). Until now much focus has not yet been given to these cells' potential for tissue engineering. Developing biomaterials also presents formidable difficulties. The scaffold's composition, architecture, three-dimensional environment, and biocompatibility all have a significant impact on how implanted tissue develops. Additionally, signal peptides like RGD have been included in the substance to successfully copy the intercellular matrix, which promotes cellular motility (Dawson et al. 2008; Hauselmann et al. 1994). The scaffold material's mechanical strength must match the mechanical characteristics of the tissue it is meant to replace or heal. Investigators have also submitted a bid. Also, it is preferred that the biological material decompose in vivo, with the material degradation rate matching the tissue regeneration pace and that the ensuing decomposed by-products are harmless to the host to reduce the long-term biocompatibility problems. Inflammatory reactions to biomaterials have been a significant safety issue. Numerous currently used biomaterials cause inflammatory reactions when implanted (Hu 2021). By creating a barrier to nutrient transfer, the fibrotic capsule created by the inflammatory biomaterials around the transplanted synthetic tissue may further impede tissue remodelling and function.

6.3 TISSUE ENGINEERING'S SIGNIFICANCE IN OSTEOARTHRITIS TREATMENT

One of the most prevalent chronic articular disorders, OA, affects all joint components and ultimately results in pain, persistent morning stiffness, and muscular weakness, all of which contribute to impairment. OA is now recognized as an "organ-level failure" of the whole joint with a diverse as well as complex pathophysiology rather than a "wear and tear" degenerative illness. Growing evidence points to the existence of many OA subtypes that reflect its complex and multifaceted nature. A prevalent trait among patients with obesity or OA is "chronic low-grade inflammation". It has been suggested that a novel attribute of arthritis with a distinctive feature is obesity-induced OA. The localized inflammatory responses inside the articular in obese patients with OA may be indicative of systemic alterations. Clinical signs of OA include swelling, discomfort, and stiffness, which are caused by the development of macrophage-associated synovitis, a new actor in the pathogenesis of OA. Elevated incidence along with the increasing intensity of joint capsule inflammation is associated with the faster course of adiposity-induced inflammatory articular illness, even though the degree of synovitis in OA ranges from minimal indications of inflammation to severe inflammation (Dawson et al. 2008).

6.3.1 Pathogenesis of OA

In the past, OA was only thought of as a degenerative condition brought on by aging, but more recently, it has undergone a classification change to become an inflamed systemic illness with abnormal metabolic implications for the chondrocytes that reside there (Travnickova and Bacakova 2018; Thangprasert et al. 2019). The intercellular matrix (ICM), primarily composed of proteoglycans and collagen, surrounds the chondrocytes that make up articular cartilage. Chondrocytes control ECM synthesis and breakdown to maintain joint homeostasis in healthy joints. Pro-inflammatory cytokines including interleukin-1 beta (IL-1 beta) and tumour necrosis factor (TNF) produce systemic inflammation of all joint tissues, including cartilage, synovial membrane, subchondral bone, and ligaments, in osteoarthritic joints by activating the NF-B signalling pathway (Dawson et al. 2008).

6.3.2 Current Strategies for OA Treatment

6.3.2.1 Pharmacological

Drugs that lessen pain and inflammation are the mainstay of OA therapies. The two most frequently utilised medications are NSAIDs and anti-inflammatory steroids. NSAIDs aid in reducing swelling, lowering the temperature, preventing blood clots, and reducing discomfort. Prolonged use of NSAIDs may result in side effects like kidney disease, heart attack, gastrointestinal ulcers, and bleeding. By inhibiting the cyclooxygenase enzyme, NSAIDs prevent the formation of prostanoids from arachidonic acid, which has anti-inflammatory and antipyretic properties. CSDs are potent anti-inflammatory drugs; however, since they are a form of corticosteroid, they come with a long list of undesirable negative effects, including a higher risk of diabetes, osteoarthritis, and high blood pressure (Kwon et al. 2018).

6.3.2.2 Visco-supplementation

For symptomatic knee OA, knee gel injection using intra-joint injections of lubricin or hyaluronate is frequently employed. The most popular biomaterial for VS is HA. The ECM of cartilage and synovial fluid both heavily contain HA. By promoting the production of intercellular matrix peptides, regulating chemokines and prostaglandins to prevent their breakdown, lowering articular abrasion, and keeping the smoothness and breadth of the cartilage's surfaces, intra-articular injection of HA relieves symptoms. Numerous types of research demonstrated that hyaluronate had a stronger impact on ache alleviation as compared to NSAIDs (Trese et al. 2012; Zylinska et al. 2018). Hydro-gels are desirable scaffolds because they resemble the ECM of diverse tissues structurally. Studies on cartilage regeneration have used hydro-gels more frequently over the last decade. Additionally, it possesses advantageous traits like biocompatibility, biodegradability, and elastic and compressive mechanical qualities (Zylinska et al. 2018; Szczepanczyk et al. 2021). Innovative bioinspired hydrogels have been developed over the past five years for cartilage applications, including hydrogels with polydopamine incorporated that were inspired by mussels.

Hydro-gels have been based on conducting polymers for injection. Since microsurgical procedures using syringes or conduits might lessen the extent of the harm and inflammation brought on by surgery, CPNs are excellent scaffolds for tissue engineering (Corselli et al. 2012). The architecture of parenteral CPNs, which combines microsurgical methods with lyophobic functional CPs, often satisfies the requirements for promoting therapeutic outcomes (Dawson et al. 2008). Under mild physiological conditions, certain sensory or bridge techniques are employed to produce gelation hydrogels. To aid in the repair of damaged structures, shear-thinning CPNs must both have a viscosity that reduces with the extending shear rate and the capacity for self-healing. The separation of the dynamic cross-linking network results in an increase in the fluidity of the CPNs as they go through the injection needle. Because of temporary physical bonding or covalent connections, damaged hydrogels can recover their former condition after injection. Injectable CPNs replicate both mechanical performance (0.01 S/m) and bioelectrical conductivity (Moreira-Teixeira et al. 2011).

6.4 TREATMENT OF ARTICULAR CARTILAGE DEFECTS BY TISSUE ENGINEERING

Periosteal and Perichondral Grafts: The surgery comprises placing a flap of periosteal or perichondral tissue across the location of the cartilage lesion. The 1980s saw the earliest mentions of its use. This procedure can be changed by placing marrow beneath the transplanted graft. The growth sheet (cambium), which is the periosteum's innermost layer, is abundant in progenitor cells and arteries and veins with strong potential, including osteogenic and chondrogenic cells (Cooper and Sefton 2011; Corselli et al. 2012). According to three studies that have been done, the documentation supports the use of periosteal tissue in the therapy of chondral abnormalities. Perichondral grafts have been employed in numerous human and animal therapeutic trials. Rib cartilage served as the source of the substance. In 38% of the cases during the 52-month monitoring period, which was the longest, good outcomes were reported. The two approaches are currently only occasionally employed in medical practice because of the reported success rates (Chen et al. 2018).

6.5 FUTURE PROSPECTS OF OSSEIN TISSUE ENGINEERING

The function and organisation of cartilage have not been successfully restored by any of the several potential cartilage repair techniques that have been identified in long-term investigations. Numerous potential innovative repair methods are now emerging. Cells, biological materials, and beneficial compounds are the main three factors that will generally define the best strategy. Studies on the cellular and molecular level, such as enhanced cell culture, co-culture, cell tagging, gene addition, biochips, and study of protein structures and functions, will give us other hints about potential methods for regenerating joint surfaces. The complicated molecular processes involved in the creation and regulation of the cartilage development trait throughout embryo development may enable the discovery of new cartilage-forming pathways. The potential for developing techniques for cartilage tissue production from embryonic biology research is apparent (Koh et al. 2020).

The future of such cells, the best cell fraction to use, and the ideal growth conditions, however, have not yet been established, and more study is required to identify how they may be executed in the arrangement of articular cartilage. As previously mentioned, growth factors might be crucial for improving cartilage tissue engineering even further. More thorough research is required to prove the usefulness of cytokines in cartilage tissue engineering because it is currently debatable (Chanphai and Tajmir-Riahi 2019). The cell type being used will most likely determine the best growth factor and delivery technique to use. For instance, when MSCs or enlarged primary chondrocytes are employed for cartilage regeneration, other growth factors can be required. Growth factor administration should be optimised to target particular cell types and should have an extended-release profile that protects the proteins from rapid degradation. A further development for cartilage regeneration strategies could be the use of multi-step release rather than single administration methods. More and more biomaterials are indeed being created right now that match the natural environment of cartilage and exhibit high bio-affinity (Frazier et al. 2010).

In situ, polymerised hydrogels, which resemble the natural ICM and can precisely make up uneven faulty locations, are an illustration of these millennial biomaterials. Importantly, the utilisation of in situ gelatine hydrogels in minimally invasive techniques will greatly lessen the load on each patient. Hydrogels that are "smart" and responsive to environmental factors like temperature, pH, or specific biomolecules that might cause swelling or breakdown have been produced (Sims et al. 1996). Dynamic hydrogels have recently received attention because they provide the capacity to carefully regulate the spatial and temporal behaviour of the cells by developing a tissue – an approach that can be paired with the targeted supply of bioactive signals that promote tissue repair. An ongoing area of study that will soon lead to the improvement of cartilage repair techniques is converting a basic understanding of chondrification and hyaline cartilage maintenance further into the development of novel smart materials (Collawn et al. 2012).

6.6 RETINAL TISSUE ENGINEERING

Degenerative retinal diseases are a broad category of illnesses that, if neglected, can cause permanent blindness. Age-related macular degeneration (AMD) and retinitis pigmentosa (RP) are two prevalent retinal disorders. The principal reason for vision loss in people over 60 is a complex multifaceted condition called AMD. It can be categorised as either neovascular (wet) or atrophic (dry). Almost 1 million Americans suffer from RP, a genetic illness. Although there is a lot of variation from patient to patient, visual impairment in these patients typically manifests in the first year of life. Each of these deteriorating retinal disorders, despite having distinct aetiologies, is defined by a gradual loss of photoreceptor cells. Wet AMD patients today have access to a wide range of treatment options, such as photodynamic therapy and intraocular injections of anti–vascular endothelial growth factor (VEGF) medications (De Francesco et al. 2018). However, there are now only a few early-stage medication studies and dietary supplements available to patients with atrophic retinal illnesses, such as dry AMD and RP. These treatments aim to slow the progression of the condition. Another potential treatment approach that has gained popularity recently is gene therapy. This is mostly because a clinical experiment that successfully reprogrammed the mutated RPE65 gene in people with Leber congenital amaurosis was successful (Hauselmann et al. 1994).

If this study is a success, it could have significant effects on those who have atrophic macular degeneration. There is an urgent need to create innovative treatment plans to help the almost 3 million Americans impacted by AMD and RP regain their eyesight. Because of the degeneration of the photoreceptors, vision is lost in both necrotic AMD and RP. As a result of the central nervous system's (CNS) limited capacity to replace these damaged or dead neurons, eyesight loss cannot be reversed. However, inner retinal death is not always a given when there is outer retinal death. Despite severe outer retinal degeneration, recent post-mortem investigations of patients with advanced disease stages have revealed that up to 88% of the inner nuclear layer and 48% of the ganglion cell layer of the retina are still functional. It is thought that the inner retina's vitality is a result of its dual blood supply, in which the inner retina is fed by the retinal circulatory system, while the outer retina is fed by the fenestrated choriocapillaris (Williams 2008).

The microenvironment where the cells develop and grow can have an impact on how long they live and function following transplantation. The idea behind retinal tissue engineering is that usual, strong cells of different sources should be rooted as an unbroken film instead of an injection of a colloidal dispersion. The foundation and "proof of concept" that healthy donor progenitor and stem cells can be transplanted into a damaged retina to aid in visual functional recovery have already been established using subretinal cell delivery through bolus injection. The need for improved cell delivery techniques to improve donor cell survival, integration, and brain connection was stressed by this preclinical research (Figure 6.2). Complete loss of PRs, a defective RPE, and aberrant BM are the hallmarks of advanced AMD. BM is a 2–4 m thick ECM made up of heparan sulphate, chondroitin/dermatan sulphate, laminin, fibronectin, collagen types I and IV, and elastin (Teixeira et al. 2019). The unique form of BM makes it easier for nutrients to go to and from the retina. The BM exhibits more lipid body buildup and collagen cross-linking in the sick condition. The RPE monolayer's tight connections are being disturbed by aging, which further modifies the BM morphology. The adherence and survival of transplanted donor cells are reduced as a result of these aging-related alterations. To aid RPE attachment, several groups tried to resurface the BM. Although laminin, fibronectin, and vitronectin were used to coat the BM, the results did not match those of healthy BM in terms of cell survival and phagocytosis of FITC-labelled bovine photoreceptor outer segments in either the adult or fetal RPE. A better visual function can be saved by transplanting healthy RPE/PR planted in a specially created scaffold that can approximate the BM form and characteristics. The choriocapillaris and the retina need to be able to exchange nutrients and metabolites; therefore, scaffolds must be thin enough to do this (Dolati et al. 2014).

The photoreceptor layer shouldn't physically change after transplantation. The material's low elasticity guards against undesirable outcomes including retinal

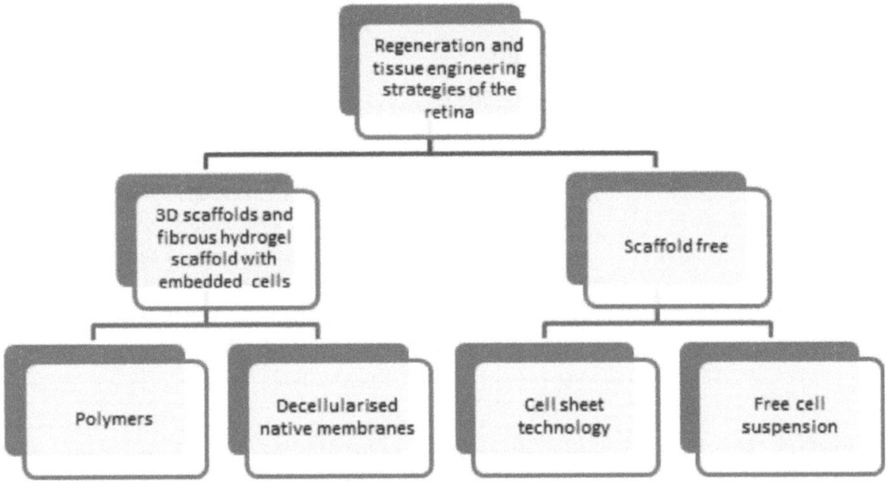

FIGURE 6.2 Approach for retinal tissue engineering.

detachment, retraction, or visual distortion. ECM features and carefully crafted, cutting-edge biomaterials with micro/nanopatterned structures and finely adjusted topographical properties can contain stem and progenitor cell populations effectively and assist in delivering them as a retinal patch into the subretinal space. Scaffolds for retinal tissue engineering have been created using a variety of biomaterials. This includes decellularised tissues, synthetic and natural polymers, hybrid polymers, and thermo-responsive hydrogel polymers (Richards et al. 2017).

6.7 CYTOKINES AND BONE TISSUE ENGINEERING

A deeper comprehension of how these signals interact and relate to one another in healing tissues is necessary to optimise the utilisation of cytokines and signalling molecules in bone tissue engineering. All of these elements have proven beneficial in preclinical models, but translation will be made possible by new knowledge about how their signals are coordinated and when they have an impact on bone regeneration (Table 6.1). BMP-2 is a successful translation example that has received clinical approval for treatment in tibial diaphyseal fractures and spine fusion. Huge dosages of bone morphogenetic protein-2 are nevertheless necessary, and disagreements have surfaced over its efficacy and reports of inflammatory responses and retrograde ejaculation (Lynch et al. 2021). The proliferative action of parathyroid hormone on bone healing could be linked to the stimulation of protein activity according to experimental data. Numerous human studies imply, but do not prove, a proliferative effect on breakage healing. Data interpretation is difficult due to the diversity of human fractures and difficulties with human clinical trial design. The utilisation of these components in a scaffold with cells still presents a challenging task. The huge potential of gene therapy, which was widely anticipated in the 1990s, has not materialised,

TABLE 6.1
Growth Factors and Their Effects

Growth Factor	Tissue	Effects
Bone morphogenetic protein (BMP) 2 and 7	Bone cartilage	Osteoblast differentiation and migration, accelerated bone healing
Fibroblast growth factor 1, 2, and 16	Bone muscles and blood vessels	Proliferation, migration and survival of endothelial cells
Insulin-like growth factor 1	Bone cartilage	Osteoprogenitor cell proliferation and differentiation
PDGF-AA and PDGF-BB	Bone cartilage, blood vessel and muscles	Endothelial cell proliferation, migration and growth

primarily because of safety issues with severe immunological reactions, which have resulted in a few well-known patient fatalities in human studies. Gene therapy requires significant data on the safeness and effectiveness of the expressed target gene as well as for clinical applications (Thangprasert et al. 2019).

6.8 ADVANCEMENTS IN TISSUE ENGINEERING

6.8.1 Using 3D Bioprinting Technology to Regenerate Tissue

Recently, it has been revealed that biodegradable polymeric vascular grafts are produced using digital light processing stereolithography 3D printing technology. Human umbilical vein cells were used to create vascular grafts that were used for operative patching in patients with cardiovascular abnormalities. This finding suggests that 3D bioprinting is extremely effective for the creation of patient-specific medical implants. Additionally, bone regeneration is accomplished by 3D printing. For bone regeneration, printed calcium phosphate scaffolds are frequently employed. In numerous animal trials, the implantation of calcium phosphate scaffold has proven successful. Polydopamine-based techniques for enhancing stem cells' osteogenicity have also been created. Additionally, cartilage regeneration is a possible use for 3D printing. In one study, scaffolds made of nanofibrillated cellulose and alginate were utilised to create 3D-printed ears, and the chondrocyte survival rate after transplantation was 73% to 86%. The size and shape of abnormalities in bone and cartilage tissues might vary depending on the patient, so 3D bioprinting technology may be very helpful for repairing damaged skeletal tissues. The body's largest organ, the skin, serves as a sensory organ, a fluid reservoir, and a barrier against the environment for internal organs. Therefore, skin wound regeneration is essential for both cosmetic and physiologic function restoration (Jeon et al. 2018). Stem cells have been demonstrated to be a successful therapy for the majority of patients in a clinical trial for the treatment of burns, ulcers, and other chronic non-healing wounds. Today, a method of transplanting through artificial skin made of polymers or human skin is frequently utilised in the case of burns or other significant skin wounds. Although commercially accessible, artificial skin substitutes for wound healing have drawbacks such as low viability, a difficult time restoring shape, and significant expenses. It has been observed that skin-derived ECM bio-inks can be used to make up for the typical bio-inks' quick deterioration and significant contraction tendencies. The creation of pre-vascularised skin grafts using a printed mixture of MSCs and endothelial progenitor cells from adipose tissue and ECM significantly speeds up the healing of cuts in animal models (Quintana et al. 2009).

6.8.2 Scaffolds

Scaffolds are synthetic materials used in tissue engineering that act as a prosthetic intercellular matrix to assist cell growth and 3D tissue organisation. The effective use of scaffolds in tissue engineering would depend on their biocompatibility, biodegradability, mechanical and chemical properties, scaffold architecture, and manufacturing techniques. Designing a 3D scaffold for excitable tissues has several challenges, one of which is simulating the electrical milieu to enhance cellular response and establish an electrical connection with the host tissue. To improve the transmission of electrical signals, conductive scaffolds in the type of permeable, fibrous, and hydrogels have thus been widely explored. Due to their remarkable mechanical and electrical qualities, 2D nanomaterials have received a lot of attention among various types of materials (Melchiorri et al. 2016). It is well-recognised that high porosity scaffolds are crucial for regulating cell activity and directing the development of new tissues. A porous scaffold might encourage vascularisation, nutrient transport, and cell adhesion and development, all of which are important for the repair of damaged tissues. As a result, high porosity is preferred for quicker tissue development. Large pores can also encourage the production of fibrosis or scar tissue, which could exacerbate brain regeneration. High porosity also hurts the mechanical qualities of the scaffolds. Unfortunately, there is still debate over the proper porosity and pore size for porous structures. To create porous 3D structures, a variety of techniques are used, including solvent casting, 3D printing, gas foaming, freeze-drying, and phase separation. By mixing a solvent (2D nano-materials solution) and evenly dispersed salt particles (e.g., NaCl) into a polymer solution, solvent casting is an easy and affordable scaffold construction approach. The benefit of this method is that the scaffold that is created will have high porosity (up to 90%), and the pore size can be adjusted (Weiss et al. 2003).

6.8.3 Peripheral Nerve Injury

The PNS is made up of neurons, glial cells, and stromal cells, which are three different types of cells. Peripheral nerves' primary role is to transmit messages from the CNS to the rest of the body. When an injury occurs, the signal transmission mechanism may be partially or completely impaired. This disorder has the potential to have a serious negative influence on a person's motor and sensory function, resulting in discomfort, a lack of sensation, weakened muscles, and total paralysis. Sadly, unlike the CNS, the PNS is not shielded by the blood-brain barrier (BBB) or a strong bone barrier, making it more vulnerable to traumatism and other damage. The frequency of PN injuries is therefore very high, contributing to 1 in 1000 people annually (Inzana et al. 2014). The ability of PNS glial cells (also known as SCs) to form bands of Bungner and stimulate axon regeneration gives the PNS a higher potential for regeneration than CNS nerves, but the healing process is often delayed, and nerve renewal cannot completely restore a significant nerve gap length. The PNS can currently be restored via procedures for rejoining nerve portions, such as the use of prosthetic nerve navigation conduits and the implantation of autografts or allografts between the transected segments. Autografts, which are the most successful of these procedures and are regarded as the benchmark for treating PNS injuries, have the maximum rate of success. However, utilising autografts has certain disadvantages, including morbidities at the donor site, uncomfortable conditions, and a higher risk of infection because of the surgical intervention (Cooper and Sefton 2011). Additionally, there's a chance that the excised nerve region won't regain its full capability.

6.8.4 Hydrogels

A system composed of a web of lipophilic polymeric elements that can react with water without dissolving is known as a hydro-gel. These systems are advantageous for a variety of biological uses, such as medication delivery and tissue regeneration. Their high degree of biocompatibility is one of the main reasons for this. Because hydrogels have a high degree of hydrophilicity, they can closely imitate the structural characteristics of the extracellular matrix and so provide the perfect environment for the development of new cells. The new extracellular matrix can then be secreted by these cells. Additionally, the injured area can be treated using injectable hydrogels using less invasive procedures (Kulseng et al. 1999). Hydro-gels are notorious for having inadequate mechanical strength, which can occasionally present a barrier for researchers when creating systems for tissue engineering applications. Despite these advantages, though, the hydro-stiffness gels have a significant impact on how it interacts with the tissues around them and can modify cell adhesion, differentiation, and proliferation. To make the system as efficient as feasible, this factor needs to be tuned. To optimise the system, additional parameters can be fine-tuned in addition to changing the rigidity and mechanical characteristics of the hydrogel. These include the rate of drug breakdown and the leak kinetics inside the hydrogel. The addition of a second polymer to the network is one way to improve the mechanical strength of a hydro-gel system. When two or even more polymeric systems are present but are not covalently connected, this may take the form of an independent network known as an interpenetrating network. The approach proved successful in fostering and supporting mesenchymal stem cell development, making bone tissue engineering possible (Hendrickson et al. 1994).

6.8.5 3D Scaffold

This is a different choice for creating a tissue engineering system. These scaffolds are designed to mimic the extracellular matrix while additionally offering structural assistance and promoting cell growth. It is important to consider several elements and features when creating a reliable 3D system. These include encouraging the transportation of substances like nutrients and regulatory factors that are essential for cell sustenance and differentiation, deterioration at a rate equal to the rate at which the new cells are grown, and achieving these factors without triggering an inflammatory response. Because the resulting scaffold can be constructed with a great degree of intricacy, 3D printing of scaffolds has grown to be a preferred technique for creating these systems. In the 3D printing process, the scaffold is constructed layer by layer using a solution (known as ink) that comprises a mixture of materials including polymers, biochemicals, and/or living cells. This is an especially challenging method for tissue engineering since the inks employed must be able to mimic the micro-architecture of the extracellular matrix as well as change from a liquid (when placed into the printer as ink) to a solid scaffold after printing. Scaffolds that have been 3D printed give cells a surface on which to grow and regenerate. These scaffolds must have a very porous structure with pores that are the right size to allow the cells to adequately enter it for this to occur. The materials used in 3D printed scaffolds must meet several requirements; in addition to being biocompatible and able to support cell growth, they must also be able to be prepared in a way that allows for 3D printing. Due to this, this type of tissue engineering system is very difficult. Tissue engineering is particularly interested in the application of 3D bioprinting, which involves the utilisation of inks that include cells. Formulas for 3D bioprinting can make use of a variety of approaches. Printing using an inkjet system is the first. Using this method, tiny drops of the bio-ink are applied to a substrate either continuously or "drop-on-demand". The second method relies on extrusion, in which ink is fed into a syringe and driven out through a nozzle to produce a continuous filament devoid of droplets. The link must be extremely viscous while also being capable of flowing out of the needle without the requirement of raised temperature for extrusion-based printing. The third method, often referred to as orifice-free printing or laser-based printing, uses a laser to direct the placement of the ink on the substrate. Bio-inks come in four basic varieties. These are largely categorised according to how they change from being a liquid to a solid or gel. The first method involves printing the ink directly into a cross-linking solution using ionic cross-linking. The second is a bio-ink that is sensitive to temperature changes; it is a liquid inside the syringe but turns into a gel when it touches the platform, which is colder. Bioinks that are photosensitive respond when UV light is applied to them. The final type of common bioink experiences gelation as a result of the shear-thinning pressures it experiences during printing (Teixeira et al. 2019; Sims et al. 1996).

As they surmount the limitations of conventional manufacturing techniques, which are typically based on material removal from a solid block to produce the final structure, additive manufacturing (AM) techniques are proving to have great potential in the fabrication of precision biomaterials (Yeong et al. 2004; Guzzi and Tibbitt 2019). The fact that AM techniques depend on the sequential addition of material to create the 3D structure makes them free-form processes. These cutting-edge processing techniques enable creative design autonomy, the creation of scaffolds with complicated geometries, and the potential for patient-specific fabrications. These form the cornerstone of personalised medicine, in which the treatment option is created to match the patient's medicinal requirements and immune compatibility (Sachlos and Czernuszka 2003). According to the introduction of a trigger or the direct deposition of the substance during the process, AM techniques can be divided into stimulus-triggered AM and deposition-based AM. Due to the possibility that the type of stimulus used during stimulus-triggered AM could affect the final construct's functionality, cells and bioactive molecules are generally added after fabrication in this top-down method. The creation of multi-material scaffolds is not possible with stimulus-triggered AM, despite the high processing rates and high spatial resolutions attained. On the other hand, deposition-based AM allows for the direct fabrication of constructs that are embedded with cells, and by carefully regulating the process parameters and material design limits, cell survival is guaranteed. These methods were developed as top-down strategies (Peltola et al. 2008; Singh and Jonnalagadda 2020).

6.8.6 Nano-Enabled Systems

Nanotechnology is the third option open to scientists for creating tissue engineering constructs. In the past few years, the medical industry has paid a lot of attention to nanotechnology, which is the study of systems and structures that are smaller than one nanometre. Researchers have discovered that the use of nanotechnology (containing components like nanoparticles, nanofibers, and nanowires) can significantly enhance tissue regeneration, targeted drug delivery, and diagnostic capabilities. Nanotechnologies have a high surface-to-volume ratio that promotes enhanced tissue synthesis, making them particularly advantageous for tissue engineering systems (and in particular bone tissue engineering) (Sims et al. 1996). However, to be able to demonstrate the required mechanical strength, bone tissue engineering systems frequently use nano-fibre scaffolds that are sufficiently mechanically strong and have enough porosity throughout, allowing for the infiltration of new cells. Electron spinning is the most promising and extensively researched method for creating nanofibre scaffolds. With this method, nano-fibre scaffolds can be made from a range of substances, such as polymers and biomaterials. According to the needs of the tissue, researchers can also fine-tune specific aspects of the resulting scaffold, such as the fibre diameter and surface morphology. Additionally, nano-fibres can closely resemble the extracellular matrix proteins' size, which ranges from 50 to 500 nanometres (Caterson et al. 2001).

6.8.7 Neurology

There are numerous ways that the central nervous system might be harmed. These include everything from trauma brought on by traumatic incidents like vehicle accidents and sports-related injuries to neurodegenerative illnesses like Alzheimer's and amyotrophic lateral sclerosis. Since the central nervous system has a very limited capacity for self-regulation, the harm brought on by such occurrences has a long-lasting effect on the patients (Marijnissen et al. 2000). This opens up a significant field for research and development of potential tissue engineering remedies. The drawbacks of autologous nerve grafts, such as donor site morbidity and a finite supply of donor's nerves, can be solved via tissue engineering systems. To safeguard the regrowth of the nerve and allow for the transmission of biochemical signals, neural tissue repair scaffolds are necessary, especially in the context of peripheral nervous system repair, because it has a stronger capacity for regeneration than the central nervous system. Biomaterials can offer the necessary physicochemical (like porosity), biomechanical (like stiffness and elasticity), and biological (like biocompatibility) qualities (Solchaga et al. 2002). In terms of brain tissue engineering, the hydro-electroactivity gel improved the neural interface's reactivity and allowed for a close replication of the natural environment. It has been demonstrated that the colloidal hydro-gel has an ideal range (103–107 S/cm) for effective cell proliferation and differentiation. The drug release profile was likewise susceptible to electrical conductivity. Additionally, the hydro-gel was capable of ensuring maximum cell viability. Researchers found that the hydro-properties gel (such as its electrical conductivity and drug dissolution profile) could be changed, allowing further research into the system to modify the resulting hydro-gel to have the desired properties. This technology could act as a reliable platform for the regeneration of many different types of cells and tissues, especially brain systems.

6.8.8 Otolaryngology

The development of the localised flap and grantor tissue transplant techniques have had a significant positive contribution to the field of neck and head surgery, including the restoration of nasal, cochlear, laryngeal, and tracheal tissue. However, there are still difficulties in this area, including poor tissue matching between donors and recipients, a scarcity of donor cells, and transplant rejection. These can be overcome by tissue-engineered systems since they can be created to match the patient's tissue and so prevent rejection.

6.8.9 Ophthalmology

Damage to ocular tissues can result from a wide range of ailments and disorders. These include but are not limited to glaucoma, diabetic retinopathy, trauma or injury, and age-related macular degeneration. The damage to the eye is frequently irreparable, and any vision lost cannot be gained back. Even though these disorders have been the subject of extensive research, many of the available treatments come with side effects such as eye redness and elevated intraocular pressure. Tissue transplants have long been the mainstay of care for many diseased or injured eye tissues, such as the cornea. Allogenic grafts have a history of rejection, and this therapeutic strategy is highly dependent on the accessibility of donor cells, which is rarely easily available (Noth et al. 2002a, 2002b).

6.9 CONCLUSION

The pathogenesis of neurodegenerative diseases and the dearth of regenerative therapeutic approaches suggest that novel, creative therapeutic approaches are required. The use of additive manufacturing methods has grown in importance, demonstrating the enormous potential for creating precise scaffolds that could improve the therapeutic effectiveness and even produce 3D scaffolds that are unique to a given patient.

This could be extremely significant in the area of regenerative medicine and the treatment of neurodegenerative diseases, along with the specific fabrication of scaffolds with precise geometry and structure.

REFERENCES

Caterson EJ, Nesti LJ, Li WJ, Danielson KG, Albert TJ, Vaccaro AR, Tuan RS. Three-dimensional cartilage formation by bone marrow-derived cells seeded in polylactide/alginateamalgam. *J Biomed Mater Res* 2001;57:394–403.

Chanphai P, Tajmir-Riahi HA. Tea polyphenols bind serum albumins: A potential application for polyphenol delivery. *Food Hydrocoll* 2019;89:461–467.

Chapekar MS. Tissue engineering: Challenges and opportunities. *Journal of Biomedical Materials Research: An Official Journal of the Society for Biomaterials, the Japanese Society for Biomaterials, and the Australian Society for Biomaterials and the Korean Society for Biomaterials.* 2000;53(6):617–620.

Chen CC, Yu J, Ng HY, Lee AK, Chen CC, Chen YS, et al. The physicochemical properties of Decellularized extracellular matrix-coated 3D printed poly(epsilon-caprolactone) nerve conduits for promoting Schwann cells proliferation and differentiation. *Materials (Basel).* 2018;11(9).

Collawn SS, Banerjee NS, De La Torre J, Vasconez L, Chow LT. Adipose-derived stromal cells accelerate wound healing in an organotypic raft culture model. *Ann Plast Surg* 2012;68:501–504.

Cooper TP, Sefton MV. Fibronectin coating of collagen modules increases in vivo Huvec survival and vessel formation in SCID mice. *Acta Biomater* 2011;7:1072–1083.

Corselli M, Chen CW, Sun B, Yap S, Rubin JP, Peault B. The tunica adventitia of human arteries and veins as a source of mesenchymal stem cells. *Stem Cells Dev* 2012;21:1299–1308.

Dawson E, Mapili G, Erickson K, Taqvi S, Roy K. Biomaterials for stem cell differentiation. *Adv Drug Deliv Rev* 2008;60:215–228.

De Francesco EM, Sotgia F, Lisanti MP. Cancer stem cells (CSCs): Metabolic strategies for their identification and eradication. *Biochem J* 2018;475:1611–1634.

Dolati F, Yu Y, Zhang Y, De Jesus AM, Sander EA, Ozbolat IT. In vitro evaluation of carbon-nanotube-reinforced bioprintable vascular conduits. *Nanotechnology.* 2014;25(14): 145101.

Frazier RA, Deaville ER, Green RJ, Stringano E, Willoughby I, Plant J, Mueller-Harvey I. Interactions of tea tannins and condensed tannins with proteins. *J Pharm Biomed Anal* 2010;51(2):490–495.

Gonçalves AM, Moreira A, Weber A, Williams GR, Costa PF. Osteochondral tissue engineering: The potential of electrospinning and additive manufacturing. *Pharmaceutics* 2021;13(7):983.

Guzzi EA, Tibbitt MW. Additive manufacturing of precision biomaterials. *Adv Mater* 2019;32:e1901994.

Hauselmann HJ, Fernandes RJ, Mok SS, Schmid TM, Block JA, Aydelotte MB, Kuettner KE, Thonar EJ. Phenotypic stability of bovine articular chondrocytes after long-term culture in alginate beads. *J Cell Sci* 1994;107(Pt 1):17–27.

Hendrickson DA, Nixon AJ, Grande DA, Todhunter RJ, Minor RM, Erb H, Lust G. Chondrocyte-fibrin matrix transplants for resurfacingextensive articular cartilage defects. *J Orthop Res* 1994;12:485–497.

Hu T, Lo AC. Collagen—alginate composite hydrogel: Application in tissue engineering and biomedical sciences. *Polymers* 2021;13(11):1852.

Inzana JA, Olvera D, Fuller SM, Kelly JP, Graeve OA, Schwarz EM, et al. 3D printing of composite calcium phosphate and collagen scaffolds for bone regeneration. *Biomaterials* 2014;35(13):4026–4034.

Jeon J, Lee MS, Yang HS. Differentiated osteoblasts derived decellularized extracellular matrix to promote osteogenic differentiation. *Biomater Res* 2018;22:4.

Kanakis CD, Hasni I, Bourassa P, Tarantilis PA, Polissiou MG, Tajmir-Riahi HA. Milk β-lactoglobulin complexes with tea polyphenols. *Food Chem* 2011;127(3):1046–1055.

Koh RH, Jin Y, Kim J, Hwang NS. Inflammation-modulating hydrogels for osteoarthritis cartilage tissue engineering. *Cells* 2020;9(2):419.

Kulseng B, Skjak-Braek G, Ryan L, Andersson A, King A, Faxvaag A, Espevik T. Transplantation of alginate microcapsules: Generationof antibodies against alginates and encapsulatedporcine islet-like cell clusters. *Transplantation* 1999;67:978–984.

Kwon SG, Kwon YW, Lee TW, Park GT, Kim JH. Recent advances in stem cell therapeutics and tissue engineering strategies. *Biomater Res* 2018;22(1):1–8.

Lynch CR, Kondiah PP, Choonara YE. Advanced strategies for tissue engineering in regenerative medicine: A biofabrication and biopolymer perspective. *Molecules* 2021;26(9):2518.

Marijnissen WJ, van Osch GJ, Aigner J, Verwoerd-Verhoef HL, Verhaar JA. Tissue-engineered cartilage using serially passagedarticular chondrocytes. Chondrocytes in alginate, combinedin vivo with a synthetic (E210) or biologicbiodegradable carrier (DBM). *Biomaterials* 2000;21:571–580.

Melchiorri AJ, Hibino N, Best CA, Yi T, Lee YU, Kraynak CA, et al. 3D-printed biodegradable polymeric vascular grafts. *Adv Healthc Mater* 2016;5(3):319–325.

Moreira-Teixeira LS, Georgi N, Leijten J, Wu L, Karperien M. Cartilage tissue engineering. In Camacho-Hübner O. Nilsson L. Sävendahl (eds) *Cartilage and Bone Development and Its Disorders.* 2011;21:102–115. Basel, Switzerland: Karger Publisher.

Nesic D, Whiteside R, Brittberg M, Wendt D, Martin I, Mainil-Varlet P. Cartilage tissue engineering for degenerative joint disease. *Adv Drug Deliv Rev* 2006;58(2):300–322.

Noth U, Osyczka AM, Tuli R, Hickok NJ, Danielson KG, Tuan RS. Multilineage mesenchymal differentiation potential of humantrabecular bone-derived cells. *J Orthop Res* 2002a;20:1060–1106.

Noth U, Tuli R, Osyczka AM, Danielson KG, Tuan RS. In vitro engineered cartilage constructs produced by press-coatingbiodegradable polymer with human mesenchymal stem cells. *Tissue Eng* 2002b;8:131–144.

Peltola SM, Melchels FP, Grijpma DW, Kellomäki M. A review of rapid prototyping techniques for tissue engineering purposes. *Ann Med* 2008;40:268–280.

Quintana L, Zurnieden NI, Semino CE. Morphogenetic and regulatory mechanisms during developmental chondrogenesis: New paradigms for cartilage tissue engineering. *Tissue Eng Part B: Rev.* 2009;15(1):29–41.

Richards D, Jia J, Yost M, Markwald R, Mei Y. 3D Bioprinting for vascularized tissue fabrication. *Ann Biomed Eng* 2017;45(1):132–147.

Sachlos E, Czernuszka JT. Making tissue engineering scaffolds work. Review: The application of solid freeform fabrication technology to the production of tissue engineering scaffolds. *Eur Cell Mater* 2003;5:29–39, discussion 39–40.

Sims CD, Butler PE, Casanova R, Lee BT, Randolph MA, Lee WP, Vacanti CA, Yaremchuk MJ. Injectable cartilage using polyethyleneoxide polymer substrates. *PlastReconstr Surg* 1996;98:843–850.

Singh M, Jonnalagadda S. Advances in bioprinting using additive manufacturing. *Eur J Pharm Sci* 2020;143:105167.

Solchaga LA, Gao J, Dennis JE, Awadallah A, Lundberg M, Caplan AI, Goldberg VM. Treatment of osteochondral defectswith autologous bone marrow in a hyaluronan-based deliveryvehicle. *Tissue Eng* 2002;8:333–347.

Sun AR, Udduttula A, Li J, Liu Y, Ren PG, Zhang P. Cartilage tissue engineering for obesity-induced osteoarthritis: Physiology, challenges, and future prospects. *J Orthop Translat* 2021;26:3–15.

Szczepanczyk P, Szlachta M, Złocista-Szewczyk N, Chłopek J, Pielichowska K. Recent developments in polyurethane-based materials for bone tissue engineering. *Polymers* 2021;13(6):946.

Teixeira BN, Aprile P, Mendonca RH, Kelly DJ, Thire R. Evaluation of bone marrow stem cell response to PLA scaffolds manufactured by 3D printing and coated with polydopamine and type I collagen. *J Biomed Mater Res B Appl Biomater* 2019;107(1):37–49.

Thangprasert A, Tansakul C, Thuaksubun N, Meesane J. Mimicked hybrid hydrogel based on gelatin/PVA for tissue engineering in subchondral bone interface for osteoarthritis surgery. *Materials Design* 2019;183:108113.

Trávníčková M, Bačáková L. Application of adult mesenchymal stem cells in bone and vascular tissue engineering. *Physiol Res* 2018;67:831–850.

Trese M, Regatieri CV, Young MJ. Advances in retinal tissue engineering. *Materials* 2012;5(1):108–120.

Tuli R, Li WJ, Tuan RS. Current state of cartilage tissue engineering. *Arthritis Res Ther* 2003;5(5):1–4.

Weiss P, Obadia L, Magne D, Bourges X, Rau C, Weitkamp T, et al. Synchrotron X-ray microtomography (on a micron scale) provides threedimensional imaging representation of bone ingrowth in calcium phosphate biomaterials. *Biomaterials* 2003;24(25): 4591–4601.

Williams DF. On the mechanisms of biocompatibility. *Biomaterials* 2008;29(20):2941–2953.

Yeong WY, Chua CK, Leong KF, Chandrasekaran M. Rapid prototyping in tissue engineering: Challenges and potential. *Trends Biotechnol* 2004;22:643–652.

Zylinska B, Silmanowicz P, Sobczyńska-Rak A, Jarosz Ł, Szponder T. Treatment of articular cartilage defects: Focus on tissue engineering. *In Vivo.* 2018;32(6):1289–1300.

7 An Algorithmic Soft Computing Technique for Identifying Lipase-Producing Yeast Using Its Gene Expression Data

Sundaramahalingam M A, Relli Teja, and Sivashanmugam, P†
Chemical and Biochemical Process Engineering Laboratory, Department of Chemical Engineering, National Institute of Technology Tiruchirappalli, Tamilnadu, India
†Corresponding Author: psiva@nitt.edu

ABBREVIATIONS

ANN	Artificial Neural Network
LPY	Lipase-Producing Yeast
NLPY	Non-Lipase-Producing Yeast
GEO	Gene Expression Omnibus
MLFFA	Multilayer Feedforward ANN
MSE	Mean Square Error
MLP	Multilayer Perceptron
GPU	Graphics Processing Unit
TPU	Tensor Processing Unit
CPU	Central Processing Unit

7.1 INTRODUCTION

In nature, lipases are triacylglycerol ester hydrolases with a high ability to catalyze hydrolytic and synthetic processes because of their ability to survive extremes in temperature, pH, and chemical solvents. Moreover, with their chemo, regioselectivity, and enantioselectivity, microbial lipases have received much attention in the industrial sector. Microbes produce extracellular lipases, including bacteria, yeast, and fungi (Sundaramahalingam et al. 2022). Because of benefits such as a more comprehensive substrate range, decreased susceptibility to low dissolved oxygen concentrations and heavy metals, higher product output, rapid growth, and simplicity of genetic manipulation, yeasts have been utilized to produce lipases (Putti Paludo et al. 2018). Lipases

DOI: 10.1201/9781003354437-7

can perform various biochemical reactions such as hydrolysis, transesterification, interesterification, esterification, alcoholysis, and acidolysis (Taskin et al. 2016). Lipases from fungi belonging to the genera *Yarrowia, Penicillium, Aspergillus, Geotrichum, Candida*, and *Rhizomucor* have been studied extensively. Only a few species, such as *Candida antarctica, Geotrichum candidum, Candida cylindracea*, and *Yarrowia lipolytica* secrete lipases (Srimhan et al. 2011). Lipases are employed in wastewater treatment and fine chemical, pharmaceutical, cosmetic, biofuel, and organic compound production. They are also applied in the food, paper, pulp, textile, cosmetics, pharmaceuticals, leather, and detergent industries (Panyachanakul et al. 2020). Chemical catalysts have several drawbacks, including increased sensitivity to free fatty acids, the need for large amounts of water to remove the catalyst from the product, equipment corrosion, energy consumption owing to greater working temperatures, and the possibility of product deterioration (Selvakumar and Sivashanmugam 2019).

Many publicly accessible databases contain a plethora of knowledge about yeast biology. Those databases provide broad information about a yeast's genomic, proteomic, biological, and functional aspects. Some of the databases of yeast are the Saccharomyces Genome Database (SGD), Yeast Proteome Database (YPD), the Munich Information Centre for Protein Sequences (MIPS-GSF), the Kyoto Encyclopedia of Genes and Genomes (KEGG), Gene Expression Omnibus (GEO), and National Centre for Biotechnology Information (NCBI). The essential genes responsible for lipase production are URA3, HIS4, MATA, JMP, SUC, KEX2, RML, LIP2, YITGL3, and YITGL4 (Kohno et al. 2000). TensorFlow is an open-source machine learning framework that quickly constructs models from training data using heterogeneous computing resources such as CPUs, GPUs, and TPUs. TensorFlow has many functions and classes that allow users to create complicated models from the ground up. TensorFlow 2.0 is the most recent version, with significant improvements over the prior version. Because of its ease of use, Python interface, and ability to deploy models on web browsers and mobile devices, TensorFlow has gained widespread appeal among the machine learning community in a short period (Do et al. 2017).

The increase in demand for microbial lipase led to the new study of bioprocess, lipase-producing yeast, and non-lipase-producing yeast from yeast transcriptome data using new data mining and machine learning tools. In recent decades, a surge in interest in machine learning among medical researchers has resulted in many successful data-driven applications ranging from medical image processing and disease diagnosis to decision support and outcome prediction. Most data mining and machine learning techniques are used in biomedical applications (AlAgha et al. 2018). This study uses machine learning tools to develop a bioprocess model that distinguishes between lipase-producing and non-lipase-producing yeast. ANNs are machine learning algorithms initially inspired by the biological nervous system. Support vector machine (SVM) and relevant vector machine (RVM) have emerged as competitive algorithms over the years. It can be applied only to limited volume data sets. So, ANN is the most preferred algorithm for processing large volumes of data. ANN with different shallow models is used in various characterization and classifications. ANN with hybridization of multiple algorithms methodologies also showed improved performance over singularly applied algorithms, offering a pathway in improving characterization and classifications based on supervised machine learning. The main advantage of using ANN is that it does not require any prior assumption of the underlying process and dependency. It also works by offering numerical models capable of establishing relationships between complex nonlinear data problems and can reduce noise in the data (Otchere et al. 2021). The primary processing elements of neural networks are known as neurons. In multilayer perceptron (MLP), the most popular type of ANN, neurons are distributed over several layers: an input layer, an output layer, and one or more hidden layers (Lancashire et al. 2009). The input layer passes data vectors to other layers; the output layer produces an output vector (often representing the classification outcome for the corresponding input vector); and hidden layers take data from an input layer or a previous hidden layer and transform it before passing it to an output layer or another hidden layer. To optimize some error criteria, a learning method is employed to make gradual adjustments to the weights (Pizzi et al. 1995). The identification of lipase utilizing multilayer perceptron ANNs with backpropagation has provided a favourable model for identification (Sundaramahalingam et al. 2022a). MLFFA enables a signal to move from the input, hidden, and output layer in the feedforward phase, and the error signal is back-propagated to modify the weights and biases at the hidden layer automatically until the error is minimized (Chinatambi and Jewaratnam 2023). The BPNN combines forward learning and training of inputs with backpropagation of error data during operation. The weights are then adjusted, and the deviation is updated using gradient descent optimization (Liu 2022). The combination of ANN with MLP makes use of the back-propagation algorithm. It addresses several types of difficulties in handling seismic and well log data that may impede the accuracy of resulting models (Otchere et al. 2021).

By going through the previous discussion, one can conclude that no studies have been reported for identifying high lipase-producing yeast from genomic data. Also, ANN is an essential tool in identifying high lipase-producing yeast. Hence the main objectives of the present study are (i) to develop a model for identifying lipase-producing yeast from genomic datasets. (ii) to use ANN with backpropagation to recognize variance in yeast genetic datasets (iii) to establish the normalization procedure to construct a robust dataset defining the model. In this study, an approach has been made to distinguish lipase-producing yeast (LPY) and non-lipase-producing yeast (NLPY) by using yeast gene expression data, as shown in Figure 7.1.

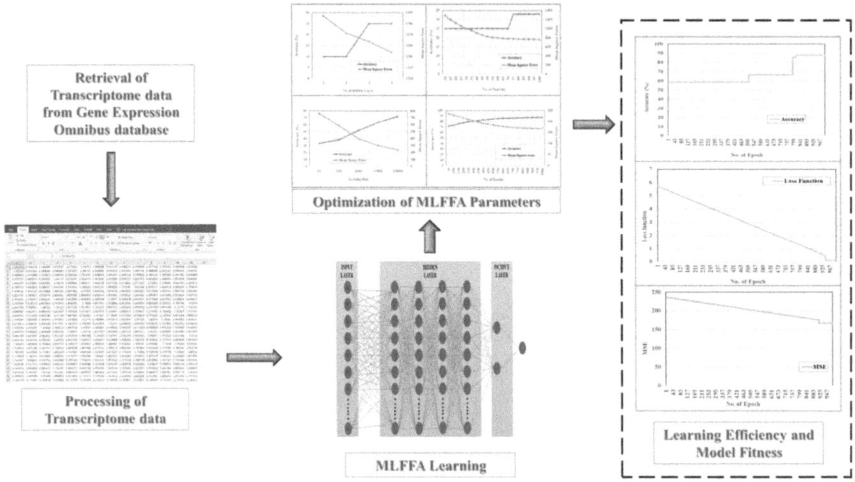

FIGURE 7.1 Overall schematic representation of the experimental process.

7.2 MATERIALS AND METHODS

7.2.1 Collection of Yeast Gene Expression Data

Data required for this study was obtained from GEO. It is currently the world's largest and most comprehensive public gene expression data database (Zhang et al. 2019). The collected yeast gene expression data constitutes 58 genetic datasets, among which 34 are LPY data and 24 are NLPY data. These transcriptome data were acquired as raw data. The 34-LPY transcriptome data, responsible for identifying lipase production, were employed as positive data, whereas the remaining 24 were employed as negative data. The positive data were labelled as L, while the negative data were labelled as NL.

7.2.2 Data Pre-processing

Since data was accumulated from various sources, it may contain noise, inconsistency, and incompleteness. So, the dataset was pre-processed before being fed to the classification model to increase the classification accuracy (Li et al. 2003). Deviations and non-expressed data (NaN) were filtered out and replaced with a null value not affecting the ANN's identification process. Log2 normalization was used to normalize all numeric characteristics in this study. Each data set was placed in its column, with the label appearing in the final row. Data and label data together comprise the gene expression data used for the learning process. This process of arrangement and correction was applied manually for the entire dataset. The entire dataset was compiled into a single comma-separated value file (.CSV format). The data used in this study was structured column-wise rather than row-wise, resulting in a newly modified code for the study.

7.2.3 Python Code Scripting

The Python programming language was used to develop the classification model of the study. Google Collab, an online platform, offered a simple and flexible way to write code and implement the deep neural networks for this study. Google Collab is the online open-source platform for executing the developed Python code in classifying LPY and NLPY. It is a mediant connector between Google Drive (a database to store your data) and GPU (or) TPU, which helps in the faster processing of network algorithms. No additional software is required for its operation; it just needs a Google account. Since it is an online platform, files are easily shared and used anywhere. It requires less computational power than other software, which requires computational RAM for its processing (Vandana et al. 2023). Code for the model had been implemented by incorporating libraries such as NumPy, Pandas, TensorFlow, and scikit learn. The results of the numerical calculations were plotted using Matplotlib (McClarren 2018). TensorFlow 2.0 was utilized for training deep neural networks in this investigation. Prerequisites of adding the activation functions for our suitable data sets were done to incorporate the genetic algorithm with the neural network code. Because the genetic algorithm uses partial derivatives to obtain the general direction in minimizing the loss function, it improved the neural network's accuracy. The code was developed to import the required libraries; import, read, and encode the data to its corresponding variables; shuffle and split data into training and testing data; and define ANN parameters to develop a robust model using the data. It was also made to calculate the model-validating parameters and plot the results. The data and the code used in this study have been uploaded to the public repository (GitHub), and their link is as follows; https://github.com/sundar7mps/Classification-of-Lipase-data-of-GEO.

7.2.4 Model Development and Validation

The model was created by learning the transcriptome data using a Python-coded multilayer feedforward ANN (MLFFA). The learning process was normalized through unsupervised learning by minimizing the mean square error (MSE) and loss function (or) cost function. The model was then validated through mathematical computations. The error in the learning process was rectified by updating the weight and bias value of MLFFA using a back-propagation loop (Siregar and Wanto 2017). An ANN comprises three layers, each with its weight and bias value for processing data and passing it on to the next layer. This study was modelled to learn LPY and NLPY expression data by incorporating four hidden layers and 100 neurons per layer. The training data was fed into the input layer to identify and distinguish between LPY and NLPY. Back-propagation error values in all layers were used as input information for the model layer to normalize the nonlinearity of the data to achieve higher accuracy through the unsupervised learning process. A minimum threshold value had been fixed to maintain the learning process (Oh 1997). The model incorporated a gradient descent optimizer (GDO) to reduce the process error by updating its weight and bias value. These features, as mentioned earlier, were implemented using TensorFlow 2.0.

The prediction accuracy of any model depends upon the training data and the learning algorithm. One algorithm has different accuracies for different sizes of training data. The increase in the training data size increases the model's prediction accuracy. Thus it is essential to fix a correct ratio of training to testing data (Medar et al. 2017). The data set was split into training (80%) and testing (20%). The model was trained at a learning rate of 0.00001 and repeated for 1000 epochs for better learning capability. Log2 normalization was used to normalize the transcriptome data. The change in the threshold value was optimized using the Gradient Descent optimizer. A mathematical function called the "activation function" was defined for the decision process. The weighted inputs of the neuron were used as a parameter in this activation function, which ultimately determines the output value (AlAgha et al. 2018). The activation function used in this study was sigmoidal, a nonlinear function defined as in Eq. 7.1.

$$f(x) = \frac{1}{1 + \exp(-x)} \tag{7.1}$$

Using yeast transcriptome data, this equation simulates a robust model to distinguish LPY and NLPY. The proposed model was validated by the mean square error (MSE), accuracy, and cost function for each epoch.

Weight: The weight matrix influences the output of each neuron. Each neuron's output can be expressed as an Eq. 7.2.

$$y = f(\sum_{i=0}^{n} x(i) * w(ij)) \tag{7.2}$$

Where J = 1, 2, 3, ..., 100
y = output of subsequent layer
f = activation function
x = input vector
w = weight of subsequent neuron

The back-propagation algorithm updated the weights of each layer.

Biases: As a pre-output layer, the neural network's extra matrix was placed before all input layers, and it was added to the matrix to obtain the final output of the layer.

Layer output: Each layer's output is the sum of the input and weight matrices multiplied by the bias matrix. It is calculated using Eq. 7.3

$$\mathrm{Y} = f\left(\sum_{k=0}^{n} y + b\right) \tag{7.3}$$

Y = output of the output layer
b = bias matrix

Accuracy: The accuracy of a classifier is a statistical measure of how well it can distinguish between positive and negative output data occurrences. It was measured using Eq. 7.4

$$Accuracy = \frac{True\ positive + True\ Nagative}{True\ Positive + False\ Native + False\ Positive + True\ Nagative} \tag{7.4}$$

MSE : MSE is the difference between predicted and actual values (Sheta and Hiary 2012). It was analysed using Eq. 7.5

$$MSE = \frac{1}{n}\left(y_i - y_i^{\wedge}\right)^2 \tag{7.5}$$

n = number of samples used to train the model
y_i = predicted value
$y_i^{\wedge}$ = actual value

Cost function or loss function: The difference between the MSE of the computed output and the MSE of the desired output is the cost function (Jafarian et al. 2018).

Normalization: By retaining the least reproducing data, the variations in the genetic data set were standardized using the log2 normalization tool. Eq. 7.6 represents the normalization of the data process mathematically.

$$Normalised\,Value = \frac{x\,value - minimum\,x\,value}{maximum\,x\,value - minimum\,x\,value} \quad (7.6)$$

Gradient descent optimizer: Back-propagation of an artificial neural network failed to capture highly dependent variables in a genetic data set. Using a gradient descent optimizer, the error function's gradient was reduced exponentially with the number of epochs, and the model's large short-term memory captured the highly reproducible data.

Back-propagation reduces the connection strength and bias across layers, minimizes the error along the gradient direction, and determines the network parameters to achieve the minimum error after repeated learning training. The performance of the classification model was evaluated by evaluating metrics: accuracy, mean square error, and cost function or loss function. These evaluating metrics are the functions of model parameters, the number of hidden layers, the number of neurons, and data normalization (Wen et al. 2018).

7.2.5 Optimization of MLFFA Parameters

The number of neurons, hidden layers, learning rate, and epochs in the learning process were optimized to increase the model's efficiency. Hidden layers are vital in increasing accuracy by learning through the MLFFA algorithm (Chen et al. 2019). The hidden layer was varied from 1 to 4 and the neurons were increased from 10 to 100. The learning rate was reduced from 0.1 to 0.00001 to achieve higher learning accuracy. The number of epochs was increased from 50 to 1000. The influence of each parameter was optimized using the characteristic response of the accuracy and error value concerning each condition.

7.3 RESULTS AND DISCUSSION

A suitable model creation and optimization process for an MLFFA model with strong predictive performance should include the modelling software, ANN method, training algorithm, data set partition, data size, input parameters (number of neurons, number of epochs, and learning rate), hidden layer, and performance evaluation.

7.3.1 Effect of Hidden Layers in MLFFA for Classifying LPY and NLPY

The hidden layer is the crucial parameter in the MLFFA model structure. It is reported that a data size larger than 100 or features above 400 requires a higher number of hidden layers for easy learning and efficient prediction. The present study has more than 10,695 features requiring many hidden layers. Figure 7.2 shows that the increase in the hidden layer initially increases the prediction accuracy. The further increase does not affect the classification process's accuracy or MSE. So, the number of the hidden layer was optimized to be 4. The higher number of hidden layers for the vast data shows good prediction capability in algorithmic tools. On the other hand, more hidden layers added insignificantly to the accuracy of the results in cases with small sample sizes (Aunkun et al. 2021).

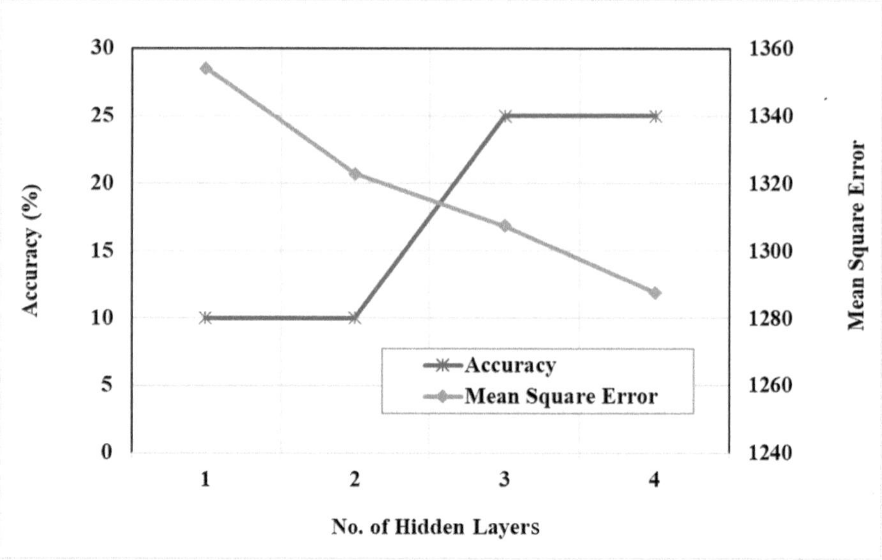

FIGURE 7.2 One-variable analysis of hidden layer in classifying LPY and NLPY.

7.3.2 Effect of Neurons per Layer in MLFFA for Classifying LPY and NLPY

The number of neurons plays a vital role in the learning process of a prediction tool. The neurons increased initially showed no change in the accuracy, but it showed a decrease in the MSE. The further increase in the number of neurons above 70 increased the accuracy above 30% and stabilized the learning process. The increase in neurons above 90 also stabilized the MSE value. From Figure 7.3, it is clear that increasing the number of neurons decreases the error significantly and increases the accuracy simultaneously. The decrease in the error is due to the increased learning efficiency and the ability of the model to classify the given data. It was also found that maintaining the same number of neurons in all hidden layers and input layers increased the model's efficiency (Kalam et al. 2022).

7.3.3 Effect of Learning Rate in MLFFA for Classifying LPY and NLPY

The learning rate plays a significant role in improving classification accuracy and reducing the error rate of MLFFA. The training algorithm hyperparameters: learning rate, epoch, batch size, and optimizer algorithm are the key ways to improve the prediction accuracy of a model network. Increasing the number of hidden layers based on the output, dropout optimization, activation function type, training epoch repetition, and weight initialization drastically improves the learning capability of the model (Sangwan et al. 2021). It is clear from Figure 7.4 that the decrease in the learning rate increased the accuracy to above 70% and reduced the MSE to below

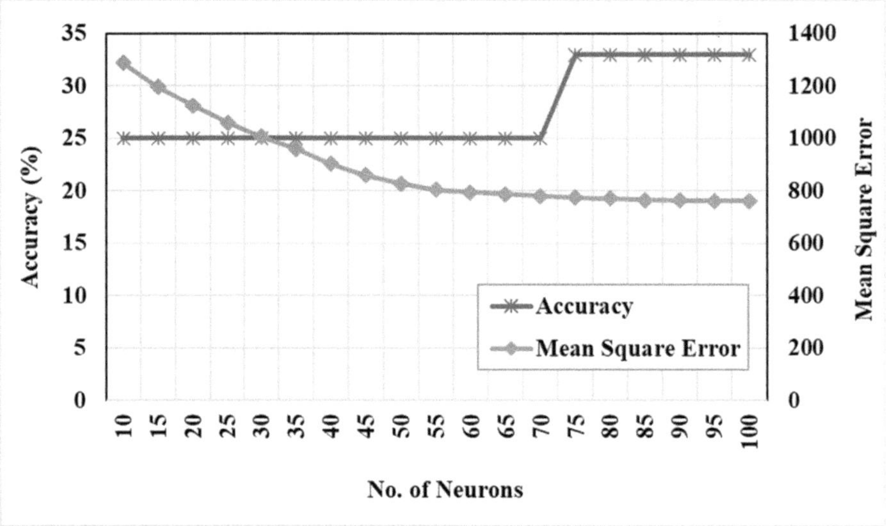

FIGURE 7.3 One-variable analysis of the number of neurons in classifying LPY and NLPY.

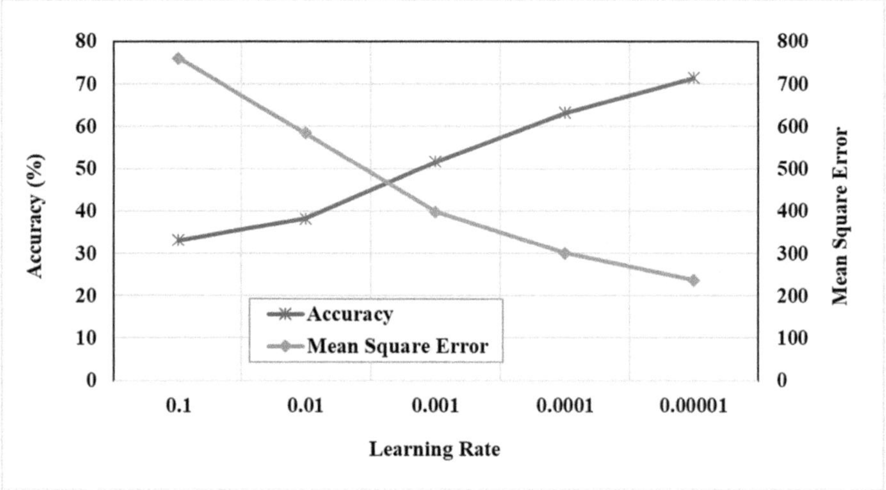

FIGURE 7.4 One-variable analysis of learning rate in classifying LPY and NLPY.

300. The decrease in the learning rate above 0.0001 slightly stabilized the learning efficiency. So, the learning rate of 0.00001 is taken to be an optimum condition.

7.3.4 Effect of Epochs in MLFFA for Classifying LPY and NLPY

The increase in the epoch number increases the learning efficiency and decreases the MSE. With the increase in epoch number from 50 to 850, the accuracy gradually

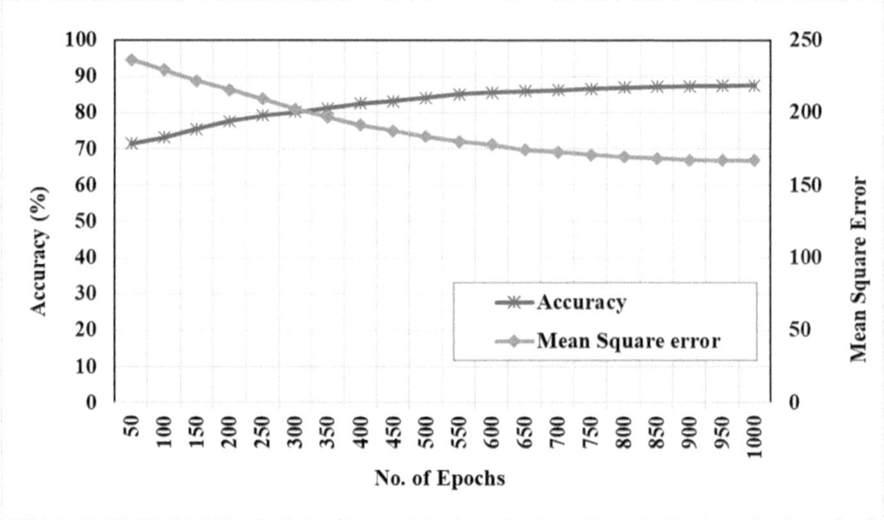

FIGURE 7.5 One-variable analysis of the number of epochs in classifying LPY and NLPY.

increases, making the model more efficient. Moreover, it also minimizes the MSE of the prediction process, as shown in Figure 7.5. Thus, the increased epoch number makes the model learn more efficiently for several defined iterations. The change in epoch number influences the learning efficiency and decreases MSE (Jeffrey et al. 2021).

7.3.5 Optimized Condition for Higher Classification Accuracy

Accuracy and MSE indicate the efficiency of the model. Initially, the accuracy and MSE of the developed model were found to be 0% and 1354.11, respectively. The step-by-step single variable optimization of the process parameters reduced the MSE drastically (167.04) and increased the accuracy to a higher value of about 87.56%. The final optimized value of the parameters is the number of hidden layers (4), the number of neurons per layer (100), the learning rate (0.00001), and the number of epochs (1000).

7.3.6 Learning Characteristics at the Optimized Condition

7.3.6.1 Accuracy

The model's accuracy was initially 0%. After training, model parameters were tweaked to improve accuracy. The number of hidden layers, epochs, learning rate, and number of neurons are all model factors that affect accuracy. In Figure 7.6, the model's accuracy is demonstrated. The maximum accuracy for the classification model (87.77%), distinguishing between LPY and NLPY, was reached by continuous

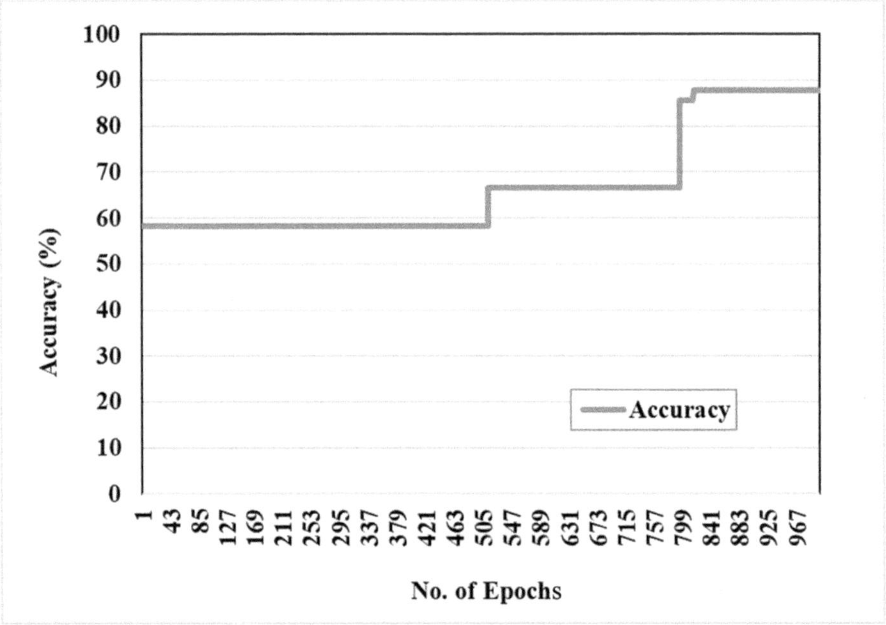

FIGURE 7.6 Accuracy response for the learning process using MLFFA.

learning of the data for 1000 epochs. Model fit for nonlinear gene expression data is shown by high accuracy. Improved control of the parameters and characteristics with the classification process is shown by increased accuracy (Wen et al. 2018). The accuracy value increases with the regression coefficient, indicating that the model's error decreases (Huang and Wang 2018). Back-propagation reduces errors using a gradient descent optimizer, improving the model's efficiency by increasing accuracy. Back-propagation with MLFFA is a superior alternative to the spike-timing-dependent plasticity model for biological data sets. It also overcomes the difficulty of deep network training (Kim et al. 2018).

7.3.6.2 Cost Function

As the number of epochs grows, the loss function (or cost function) exhibits a significant decrease in value. The cost function was found to be 5.72 before training. Increasing the number of epochs to 1000 lowered the cost function to 0.12 after training through the constant learning process. Figure 7.7 depicts the changes in the cost function and their corresponding epochs. The loss function calculates the indirect improvement in the learning process. The improvement in the loss function demonstrates the method's efficiency in detecting the LPY and NLPY utilizing its transcriptome data (Hu et al. 2018). The loss function decreases, indicating that the parameters fit the proposed model well (Gu et al. 2018). The feature extraction for LPY and NLPY identification was done appropriately and precisely. The loss function's stability demonstrates the model's stability with the provided data. It also shows improved

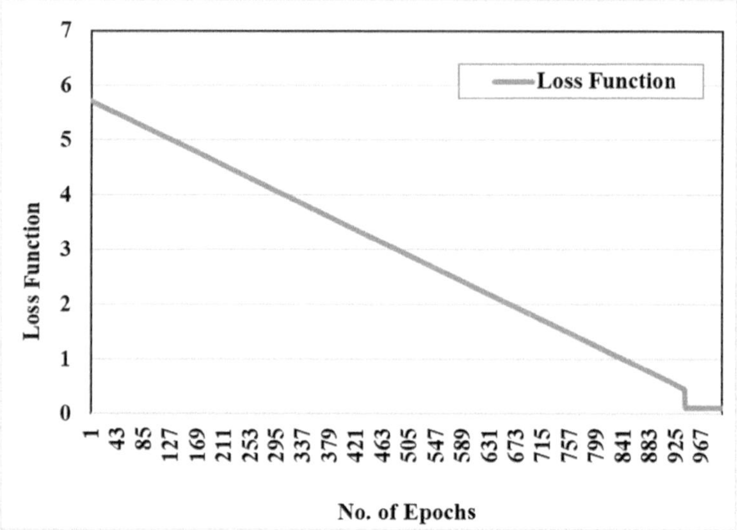

FIGURE 7.7 Loss function response for learning process using MLFFA.

parameter functionality with minor errors (Takase et al. 2018). The trained model has a lower loss function, which means that the model is more accurate, demonstrating the idealistic nature of backpropagation in learning (Qian et al. 2018).

7.3.6.3 Mean Square Error

Before training, the model's MSE was found to be 1290.42. The number of epochs dropped as the number of epochs increased. MSE was standardized to 166.8 after 1000 epochs, indicating robust data for the defined data. The learning process is standardized with the yeast transcriptome data to produce a robust model while eliminating the least reproducing feature. The MSE for the same epoch is shown in Figure 7.8. The plot's consistent deviations show that it has been adjusted from more significant deviations (Ryczko et al. 2018). The drop in MSE value also illustrates the efficacy of the feedback gradient descent optimization process, which increases the weight of the input data to ensure that the parameters fit into the model correctly (Rady 2011). It also maintains data consistency for the input dataset using a robust model with constant parameters. MSE is also used to assess the neural network model's performance. The mean square error has dropped, suggesting that the error between the network output and the target output has decreased, demonstrating that the model is well-fitting to the process (Katić et al. 2018).

7.3.7 Efficiency of MLFFA in Classification

The accuracy of the present study (87.77%) is comparatively lower than any classification study because the number of features used in this study is 10,695 (whole gene expression data of LPY and NLPY) and the availability of similar group data is very

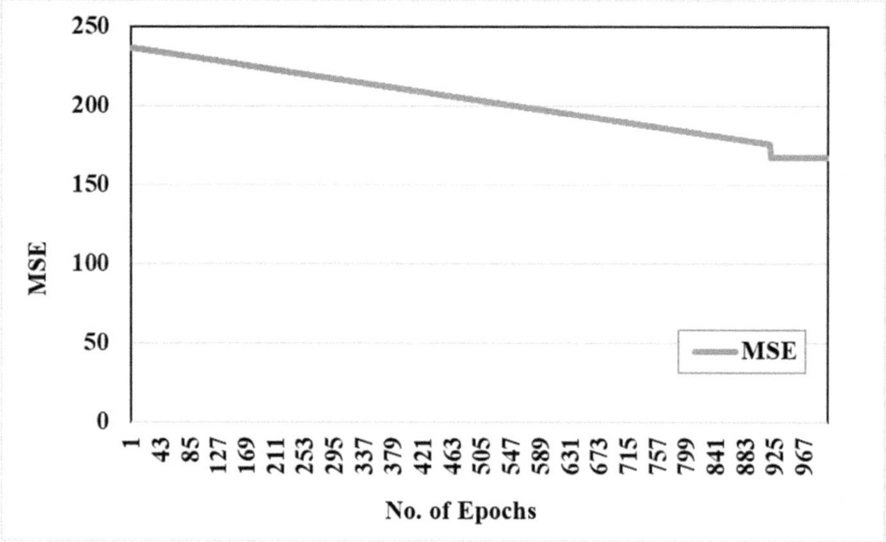

FIGURE 7.8 MSE response for learning process using MLFF.

minimal (58 datasets, among which only 34 have the positive data). So the training of vast amounts of data in the future could increase the model efficiency.

7.4 FUTURE PROSPECTIVES AND LIMITATIONS

A neural network can perform a complex critical problem that can't be solved using linear algorithms. Due to the parallel functioning characteristics of the neural network, it can operate normally even at diminished object parameters. A neural network decides in any situation without the need for reprogramming. It is applicable in any decision-making process. The only shortcoming of ANN usage is that it requires training before any process like classification and detection. A good number of training data sets should be made available for efficient results. It also requires a higher computing time. Despite of its minor disadvantage, it is being applied in all industries, including food, energy, environmental, medicine, and clinical applications. Current researchers focus on improving the data availability for all applications, and they also concentrate on hybrid deep learning networks for maximum model efficiency (Dragović 2022).

7.5 CONCLUSION

This study yielded a novel method for analysing the genomic data set of a yeast sample and classifying LPY and NLPY data using cognitive computing. The ideal approach for an identification tool for LPY, leveraging their transcriptome data, is the hybridization of a genetic dataset with its prediction model developed with an algorithm. The settings of the MLFFA algorithm were tweaked to create a more efficient model. With four hidden layers, 100 neurons per layer, and 1000 epochs, the learning process showed maximum accuracy at a learning rate of 0.0001. The interconnected MLFFA with back-propagation produced a good model fit with the diagnosis process, with an accuracy of 87.77% in prediction. The accuracy, mean square error, and loss function prove that the model fits well with the classification model. A new model for classifying LPY and NLPY has been developed using transcriptome data. Training the model with the vast data extracted from the same analyser could further increase the accuracy of the process in the future. This cognitive solution could also be a key factor for similar classification processes. It could also sort critical genes involved in the desired applications.

7.6 ACKNOWLEDGEMENT

M A Sundaramahalingam acknowledges the Ministry of Human Resource Development (MHRD) India to support a research grant through the Prime Minister's Research Fellows (PMRF) Scheme May 2020 cycle.

REFERENCES

AlAgha, A S, Faris H, Hammo B H, and Ala'M A-Z. 2018. "Identifying β-Thalassemia Carriers Using a Data Mining Approach: The Case of the Gaza Strip, Palestine." *Artificial Intelligence in Medicine* 88:70–83. https://doi.org/10.1016/j.artmed.2018.04.009

Aunkun X, Chang H, Xu Y, Li R, Li X, and Zhao Y. 2021. "Applying Artificial Neural Networks (ANNs) to Solve Solid Waste-Related Issues: A Critical Review." *Waste Management* 124:385–402. https://doi.org/10.1016/j.wasman.2021.02.029

Chen N, Xiong C, Du W, Wang C, Lin X, and Chen Z. 2019. "An Improved Genetic Algorithm Coupling a Backpropagation Neural Network Model (IGA-BPNN) for Water-Level Predictions." *Water* 11(9). https://doi.org/10.3390/w11091795

Chinatamby P, and Jewaratnam J. 2023. "A Performance Comparison Study on PM2. 5 Prediction at Industrial Areas Using Different Training Algorithms of Feedforward-Backpropagation Neural Network (FBNN)." *Chemosphere*:137788. https://doi.org/10.1016/j.chemosphere.2023.137788

Chun L, He P-A, and Jun W. 2003. "Artificial Neural Network Method for Predicting Protein-Coding Genes in the Yeast Genome." *Internet Electronic Journal of Molecular Design* 2:527–538.

Do Q, Son T C, and Chaudri J. 2017. "Classification of Asthma Severity and Medication Using TensorFlow and Multilevel Databases." *Procedia Computer Science* 113:344–351. https://doi.org/10.1016/j.procs.2017.08.343

Dragović S. 2022. "Artificial Neural Network Modeling in Environmental Radioactivity Studies—A Review." *Science of the Total Environment*:157526. https://doi.org/10.1016/j.scitotenv.2022.157526

Gu J, Wang Z, Kuen J, Ma L, Shahroudy A, Shuai B, Liu T, Wang X, Wang G, Cai J, and Chen T. 2018. "Recent Advances in Convolutional Neural Networks." *Pattern Recognition* 77:354–377. https://doi.org/10.1016/j.patcog.2017.10.013

Hu K, Zhang Z, Niu X, Zhang Y, Cao C, Xiao F, and Gao X. 2018. "Retinal Vessel Segmentation of Color Fundus Images Using Multiscale Convolutional Neural Network with an Improved Cross-Entropy Loss Function." *Neurocomputing* 309:179–191. https://doi.org/10.1016/j.neucom.2018.05.011

Huang L, and Wang J. 2018. "Global Crude Oil Price Prediction and Synchronization Based Accuracy Evaluation Using Random Wavelet Neural Network." *Energy* 151:875–888. https://doi.org/10.1016/j.energy.2018.03.099

Jafarian A, Nia S M, Golmankhaneh A K, and Baleanu D. 2018. "On Artificial Neural Networks Approach with New Cost Functions." *Applied Mathematics and Computation* 339:546–555. https://doi.org/10.1016/j.amc.2018.07.053

Jeffrey J A, Kumar S S, Vaidyaa P, Nicho A, Chrish A, and Joshith J. 2022. "Effect of Turning Parameters in Cylindricity and Circularity for O1 Steel Using ANN." *Materials Today: Proceedings* 59:1291–1294. https://doi.org/10.1016/j.matpr.2021.11.518

Kalam S, Yousuf U, Abu-Khamsin S A, Waheed U B, and Khan R A. 2022. "An ANN Model to Predict Oil Recovery from a 5-Spot Waterflood of a Heterogeneous Reservoir." *Journal of Petroleum Science and Engineering* 210:110012. https://doi.org/10.1016/j.petrol.2021.110012

Katić K, Li R, Verhaart J, and Zeiler W. 2018. "Neural Network Based Predictive Control of Personalized Heating Systems." *Energy and Buildings* 174:199–213. https://doi.org/10.1016/j.enbuild.2018.06.033

Kim J, Kim H, Huh S, Lee J, and Choi K. 2018. "Deep Neural Networks with Weighted Spikes." *Neurocomputing* 311:373–386. https://doi.org/10.1016/j.neucom.2018.05.087

Kohno M, Enatsu M, Takee R, and Kugimiya W. 2000. "Thermal Stability of Rhizopus Niveus Lipase Expressed in a Kex2 Mutant Yeast." *Journal of Biotechnology* 81(2–3):141–150. https://doi.org/10.1016/S0168-1656(00)00284-4

Lancashire L J, Lemetre C, and Rkohno Ball G. 2009. "An Introduction to Artificial Neural Networks in Bioinformatics--Application to Complex Microarray and Mass Spectrometry Datasets in Cancer Studies." *Brief Bioinform* 10(3):315–329. https://doi.org/10.1093/bib/bbp012

Liu C. 2022. "Risk Prediction of Digital Transformation of Manufacturing Supply Chain Based on Principal Component Analysis and Backpropagation Artificial Neural Network." *Alexandria Engineering Journal* 61(1):775–784. https://doi.org/10.1016/j.aej.2021.06.010

McClarren R G. 2018. "NumPy and Matplotlib." In *Computational Nuclear Engineering and Radiological Science Using Python*, 53–74. https://doi.org/10.1016/b978-0-12-812253-2.00005-4

Medar R, Rajpurohit V S, and Rashmi B. 2017. "Impact of Training and Testing Data Splits on Accuracy of Time Series Forecasting in Machine Learning." *International Conference on Computing, Communication, Control and Automation (ICCUBEA)*:1–6. https://doi.org/10.1109/ICCUBEA.2017.8463779

Oh S-H. 1997. "Improving the Error Backpropagation Algorithm with a Modified Error Function." *IEEE Transactions on Neural Networks* 8(3):799–803. https://doi.org/10.1109/72.572117

Otchere DA, Ganat TOA, Gholami R, and Ridha S. 2021. "Application of Supervised Machine Learning Paradigms in the Prediction of Petroleum Reservoir Properties: Comparative Analysis of ANN and SVM Models." *Journal of Petroleum Science and Engineering* 200:108182. https://doi.org/10.1016/j.petrol.2020.108182

Panyachanakul T, Lomthong T, Lorliam W, Prajanbarn J, Tokuyama S, Kitpreechavanich V, and Krajangsang S. 2020. "New Insight Into Thermo-Solvent Tolerant Lipase Produced by Streptomyces sp. A3301 for Re-polymerization of Poly (Dl-Lactic Acid)." *Polymer* 204:122812. https://doi.org/10.1016/j.polymer.2020.122812

Pizzi N, Choo L-P, Mansfield J, Jackson M, Halliday W C, Mantsch H H, and Somorjai R L. 1995. "Neural Network Classification of Infrared Spectra of Control and Alzheimer's Diseased Tissue." *Artificial Intelligence in Medicine* 7(1):67–79. https://doi.org/10.1016/0933-3657(94)00027-p

Putti Paludo M, de Oliveira K S D, Trevisol T C, and de Medeiros Burkert J F. 2018. "Isolation of Lipase-Producing Yeasts from Industrial Oily Residues in Different Culture Media." *International Journal of Current Microbiology and Applied Sciences* 7(1):2348–2362. https://doi.org/10.20546/ijcmas.2018.701.283

Qian S, Liu H, Liu C, Wu S, and San Wong H. 2018. "Adaptive Activation Functions in Convolutional Neural Networks." *Neurocomputing* 272:204–212. https://doi.org/10.1016/j.neucom.2017.06.070

Rady H A K. 2011. "Shannon Entropy and Mean Square Errors for Speeding the Convergence of Multilayer Neural Networks: A Comparative Approach." *Egyptian Informatics Journal* 12(3):197–209. https://doi.org/10.1016/j.eij.2011.09.002

Ryczko K, Mills K, Luchak I, Homenick C, and Tamblyn I. 2018. "Convolutional Neural Networks for Atomistic Systems." *Computational Materials Science* 149:134–142. https://doi.org/10.1016/j.commatsci.2018.03.005

Sangwan P, Deshwal D, and Dahiya N. 2021. "Performance of a Language Identification System Using Hybrid Features and ANN Learning Algorithms." *Applied Acoustics* 175:107815. https://doi.org/10.1016/j.apacoust.2020.107815

Selvakumar P, and Sivashanmugam P. 2019. "Ultrasound Assisted Oleaginous Yeast Lipid Extraction and Garbage Lipase Catalyzed Transesterification for Enhanced Biodiesel Production." *Energy Conversion and Management* 179:141–151. https://doi.org/10.1016/j.enconman.2018.10.051

Sheta A F, and Hiary R. 2012. "Modeling Lipase Production Process Using Artificial Neural Networks." *International Conference on Multimedia Computing and Systems.* https://doi.org/10.1109/ICMCS.2012.6320191

Siregar S P, and Wanto A. 2017. "Analysis of Artificial Neural Network Accuracy Using Backpropagation Algorithm in Predicting Process (Forecasting)." *IJISTECH (International Journal of Information System & Technology)* 1(1):34–42. https://doi.org/10.30645/ijistech.v1i1.4

Srimhan P, Kongnum K, Taweerodjanakarn S, and Hongpattarakere T. 2011. "Selection of Lipase Producing Yeasts for Methanol-Tolerant Biocatalyst as Whole Cell Application for Palm-Oil Transesterification." *Enzyme and Microbial Technology* 48(3):293–298. https://doi.org/10.1016/j.enzmictec.2010.12.004

Sundaramahalingam M A, Kabra R, and Singh S. 2022a. "Construction of Feedforward Multilayer Perceptron Model for Diagnosing Leishmaniasis Using Transcriptome Datasets and Cognitive Computing." In Singh S (eds) *Machine Learning and Systems Biology in Genomics and Health.* Springer, Singapore. https://doi.org/10.1007/978-981-16-5993-5_1

Sundaramahalingam M A, Sivashanmugam P, Rajeshbanu J, and Ashokkumar M. 2022. "A Review on Contemporary Approaches in Enhancing the Innate Lipid Content of Yeast Cell." *Chemosphere* 293:133616. https://doi.org/10.1016/j.chemosphere.2022.133616

Takase T, Oyama S, and Kurihara M. 2018. "Effective Neural Network Training with Adaptive Learning Rate Based on Training Loss." *Neural Networks* 101:68–78. https://doi.org/10.1016/j.neunet.2018.01.016

Taskin M, Ucar M H, Unver Y, Kara A A, Ozdemir M, and Ortucu S. 2016. "Lipase Production with Free and Immobilized Cells of Cold-Adapted Yeast Rhodotorula Glutinis HL25." *Biocatalysis and Agricultural Biotechnology* 8:97–103. https://doi.org/10.1016/j.bcab.2016.08.009

Vandana M N, and Chaudhary D. 2023. "A Hybrid Model for Depression Detection Using Deep Learning." *Measurement: Sensors* 25:100587. https://doi.org/10.1016/j.measen.2022.100587

Wen S, Xie X, Yan Z, Huang T, and Zeng Z. 2018. "General Memristor with Applications in Multilayer Neural Networks." *Neural Networks* 103:142–149. https://doi.org/10.1016/j.neunet.2018.03.015

Zhang G, Wang H, Zhu K, Yang Y, Li J, Jiang H, and Liu Z. 2019. "Investigation of Candidate Molecular Biomarkers for Expression Profile Analysis of the Gene Expression Omnibus (GEO) in Acute Lymphocytic Leukemia (ALL)." *Biomedicine & Pharmacotherapy* 120:109530. https://doi.org/10.1016/j.biopha.2019.109530

8 Plant Phenolic Compound Isolation and Its Bioinformatics Approaches to Molecular Mechanisms in Antimicrobial Activities and Resistance

Odangowei Inetiminebi Ogidi,† and*
*Ngozi Georgewill Emaikwu***
*Department of Biochemistry, Faculty of Basic Medical Sciences, Bayelsa Medical University, Yenagoa, Bayelsa State, Nigeria; **Department of Biotechnology, Federal University of Technology, Owerri, Nigeria
†Corresponding Author: ogidiodangowei@gmail.com

ABBREVIATIONS

AB	Antibiotics
ADV	Adeno viruses
AMR	Antimicrobial resistance
ARG	Arginine
BLASTn	Basic local alignment search tool nucleotide
CART	Cardiac arrest risk triage
DMF	N,N dimethylformamide
EBV	Epstein-Barr virus
EC 50	Half maximal effective concentration
EGCGs	(-)-Epigallocatechin-3-gallates
FTIR	Fourier transform infrared spectroscopy
GATK	Genome analysis toolkit
GO	Gene ontology
HCV	Hepatitis C virus
HIV	Human immunodeficiency virus
HPLC	High-performance liquid chromatography

DOI: 10.1201/9781003354437-8

HSV	Herpes simplex virus
IR	Infrared
IRES	Internal ribosome entry site
KEGG	Kyoto Encyclopedia of Genes and Genomes
LC50	Lethal concentration 50
LLE	Liquid-liquid extraction
MAE	Microwave-assisted extraction
MDR	Multidrug resistance
MIC	Minimum inhibitory concentration
ML	Machine learning
MRSA	Methicillin-resistant *Staphylococcus aureus*
NMR	Nuclear magnetic resonance
PAL	Phenylalanine ammonia-lyase
PATRIC	Pathosystems Resource integration Center
RF	Radio frequency
ROS	Reactive oxygen species
SARS-CoV-2	Severe acute respiratory syndrome coronavirus 2
SCM	Set covering machine
SNPs	Single nucleotide polymorphisms
SVM	Support vector machine
TLC	Thin-layer chromatography
UAE	Ultrasound-assisted extraction
UV	Ultraviolet
WGS	Whole genome sequencing

8.1 INTRODUCTION

The bioactive phenolics found in plants are abundant and useful resources. They may be used in a number of different domains, including anti-inflammatory, antioxidant, antiviral, anticancer, and anti-pyretic (Salinas-Moreno et al. 2017). As a result, they have caught the attention of several health specialists, and numerous organisations and health care systems are progressively urging people to consume fruits and vegetables every day (Lin et al. 2016).

With at least one aromatic ring and one or more hydroxyl groups in their structures, phenolics are one of the most prevalent and varied classes of active chemicals in plants (Gharaati et al. 2017). They fall into two different types. The first group includes soluble substances found in the plant cell vacuole, such as flavonoids, quinones, and phenylpropanoids, while the second category includes insoluble substances found in cell walls, such as lignins, condensed tannins, and hydroxycinnamic acid (Pereira et al. 2009).

These organisations participate in a variety of plant processes. Numerous studies have been conducted in an effort to use synthetic sequence processes to synthesise diverse chemicals, such as natural compounds, because of the significance and value of phenolic compounds for human health (Vaou et al. 2022; Cheynier et al. 2013; Ogidi 2023; Enenebeaku et al. 2022a, 2022b; Ogidi and Enenebeaku 2023). They have distinct physical and chemical properties based on the different phenolic structures, which are quite crucial and put the focus on the extraction procedures (Dai and Mumper 2010). Therefore, it is important and advantageous to be familiar with the numerous techniques for phenolic compound extraction, isolation, identification, and quantification.

There is a critical need to discover and create novel chemicals to battle human diseases due to the rising occurrence of life-threatening bacterial and viral illnesses and their propensity to develop resistance to existing treatment methods. Antimicrobial resistance (AMR) is a factor in the failure of antibiotic (AB) therapy and rising death rates in a number of infectious illnesses. The formation of AMR, which in certain strains leads to multidrug resistance (MDR), is related to the improper use of particular AB and excessive use of wide-spectrum AB. Fast and accurate testing of antibiotic susceptibility is required to begin effective therapy as soon as feasible due to the increase of MDR pathogens in clinical settings (CDC 2019). However, particularly in gram-negative bacteria, not all of the molecular processes generating AMR have been discovered or understood (Liu et al. 2020).

Because whole genome sequencing (WGS) has facilitated rapid access to de novo sequenced genomes of pathogens and the collection of sufficiently large datasets of clinical isolates, it is now possible to use advanced bioinformatics approaches (machine learning) to gain new insights into the more complex molecular mechanisms of antimicrobial resistance. By examining several forms of data based on genomes or metabolomics and evaluating many samples at once, these methodologies may gain new insights that were previously unattainable (More et al. 2022).

The subject of biological AMR prediction has advanced quickly in recent years. This chapter therefore discusses phenolic compounds and their classifications, roles of phenolic compounds in human health, phenolic compound extraction, isolation and purification methods, plant phenolic compounds with antibacterial activity, synergistic antibacterial activity, phenolic compounds with antiviral and antifungal activities, bioinformatics approaches of molecular mechanisms in antimicrobial resistance, and future prospectives and limitations.

8.2 PHENOLIC COMPOUNDS

Among the secondary metabolites found in plants, phenolics play a crucial function in plant physiology and structure (Boudet 2007). Phenolic compounds (Figure 8.1) comprise aromatic compounds with at least one phenyl ring and one or more hydroxyl groups, and they have a broad range of structures and functions (-OH-) (Lattanzio et al. 2006). This definition of phenolic compounds is inadequate since it include substances like oestrone, a female sex hormone with terpenoid origins at its core. An origin-based definition is favoured as a result. The molecules that come from the phenylpropanoid metabolism and the shikimate pathway are referred to as plant phenolic compounds. Because of factors related to metabolism, a number of substances—including cinnamic acid, linoleic acid, shikimic acid, and quinic acid—are regarded as phenolic substances even though they do not have an aromatic ring (Albuquerque et al. 2021). Most phenolic compounds are derived from cinnamic acid, which is made from phenylalanine by the branch-point enzyme phenylalanine ammonia-lyase (PAL), which catalyses the transition between the shikimate route and the phenylopropanoid pathway (Bartwal et al. 2013). Plants have been shown to have more than 9000 distinct phenolic structures (Xiao et al. 2011).

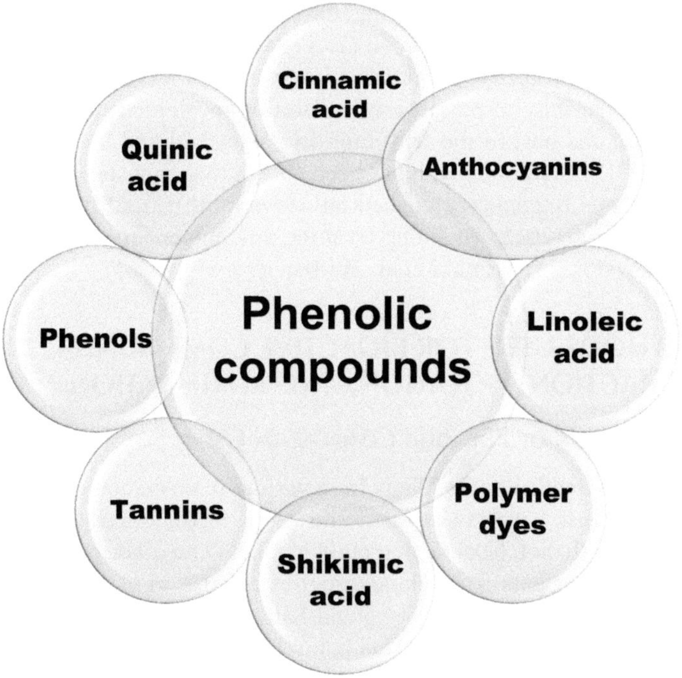

FIGURE 8.1 Phenolic compounds.

8.3 CLASSIFICATION OF PHENOLIC COMPOUNDS

Different phenolic chemicals may be found in plants. They may exist as non-extractable forms, soluble compounds in aqueous acetone, methanol, or water. Phenolic compounds are single-aromatic-ring molecules that are small and simple. The term "phenolic substance" also includes large, complex tannins and their derivative polyphenols (Kumar 2014). Many phenolic compounds may be synthesised from phenylalanine or tyrosine, two amino acids. These amino acids (phenylalanine or tyrosine) are split into cinnamic acids in the phenolic compound biosynthesis route, where they then enter the phenylpropanoid pathways. According to Crozier et al. (2006), the two primary phenolic compound categorisation schemes are as follows: how many carbon atoms are present in the molecule or how many phenolic rings are present (Kumar 2014).

8.4 ROLE OF PHENOLIC COMPOUNDS IN HUMAN HEALTH

The advantages of phenolic compounds for health and their antioxidant power have received a lot of attention recently. Since phenolic compounds in fruit are recognised to have significant therapeutic qualities pertaining to brain health due to their antioxidative activities against beta and neuronal reactive oxygen species (ROS), they are recommended for dietary intervention in Alzheimer's disease. Additionally, it has been observed that anthocyanins have immunostimulatory potential against radiation-induced immunosuppression (Fan et al. 2012).

When the neuroprotective potential of lingonberries was examined, it was shown that the fruit's capacity to preserve cell viability and inhibit the release of lactose dehydrogenase was best in the fruit high in flavan-3-ol and flavonol (Bhullar and Rupasinghe 2015). Additionally, it has been shown that fruit spreads with decreased sugar and various lingonberry concentrations exhibit natural preservation against fungus (Ermis et al. 2015). In a long-term therapy, lingonberry juice reduced blood pressure at low doses (Kivimaki et al. 2013).

8.5 METHODS USED FOR BIOACTIVE COMPOUND EXTRACTION, ISOLATION, AND PURIFICATION

8.5.1 Extraction of Phenolic Compounds Using Solvents

For the goal of extracting antioxidants from various plant components, such as leaves and seeds, scientists have investigated and assessed the effects of various solvent types, such as methanol, hexane, and ethyl alcohol. The efficient extraction of various phenolic components from plants requires the use of many solvents of varied polarity as shown in Figure 8.2 (Wong and Kitts 2006). Scientists have also discovered that highly polar solvents like methanol have powerful antioxidant properties.

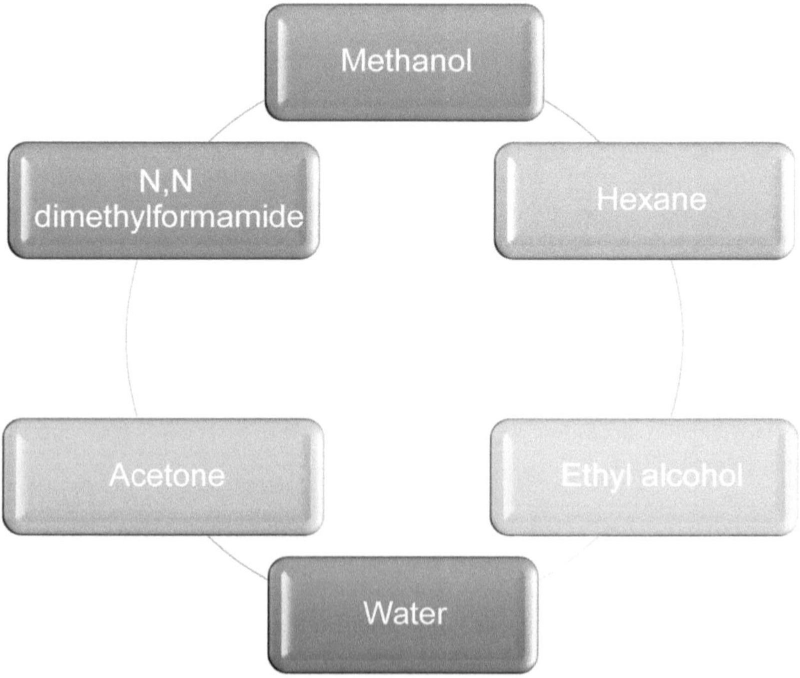

FIGURE 8.2 Solvents for extraction.

In contrast to what was found by Koffi et al. (2010), who found that methanol was more effective than ethanol in extracting a significant quantity of phenolic compounds from walnut fruits, Anokwuru et al. (2011), found that acetone and N,N dimethylformamide (DMF) are very effective at extracting antioxidants (Koffi et al. 2010; Anokwuru et al. 2011).

Ethanolic extracts of Ivorian plants were said to extract higher concentrations/amounts of phenolics than acetone, water, and methanol (Koffi et al. 2010). Dried plant powder was often used by scientists for the dual purposes of extracting bioactive components and neutralising the effect of water. A number of different solvents have been used in the past for phytochemical extraction. Solvents are used to remove biomolecules from plants, with the choice depending on the polarity of the desired solute. The proper dissolution of the solute will occur in a solvent with a polarity similar to that of the solute. Multiple solvents may be used in sequence to decrease the amount of identical compounds in the desired yield.

8.5.2 Liquid-Liquid Extraction

Researchers have looked into and examined the extraction of phenolic compounds from various plant components, including leaves and seeds, using a variety of solvents. They have been able to extract diverse combinations of phenolics from plants using this straightforward and affordable extraction approach, multiple solvent polarity, and variable temperature and pH settings (Jiao et al. 2015).

Phenolic chemicals, which may have simple or complex structures, are found in varying concentrations in plants. Finding an acceptable technique for the extraction of all phenolic compounds will be challenging since there is a chance that these chemicals might interact with other components in plants, such as proteins and carbohydrates (Yu et al. 2005). Using liquid-liquid extraction (LLE) methods, various phenolic compounds may be isolated; further purification is then required. The LLE technique may be used to extract phenolic chemicals by three different extraction methods: Soxhlet extraction, maceration, and hydro-distillation. Key considerations in these extraction methods include the chemical composition and physical properties of the materials being extracted as well as the kind and polarity of the solvents being used, the ratio of these solvents, the length of time, and the temperature required for extraction (Garcia-Salas et al. 2010).

8.5.3 Ultrasound-Assisted Extraction

In several food-processing applications, ultrasound-assisted extraction (UAE) has been employed to draw bioactive chemicals from plant sources (Williams et al. 2004). Plant cell walls are broken down using ultrasound at frequencies higher than 20 kHz, which enhances the solvent's capacity to enter the cells and results in a better extraction yield. UAE can process at a low operating temperature while still producing chemicals with good extract quality. UAE is regarded as one of the simplest extraction methods since it makes use of standard laboratory tools like an ultrasonic bath. In this method, the temperature and extraction time are regulated as the sample is crushed and combined with the appropriate solvent before being put in the ultrasonic bath (Garcia-Salas et al. 2010). The UAE approach has been taken into consideration in comparison to conventional methods since it is straightforward, simple to use, inexpensive, highly effective, uses less organic solvent, and takes less time to extract. It may be used as an efficient and dependable method for a variety of phenolic compounds at large-scale level and industry (Olmo-Garcia et al. 2018).

Temperature, duration, and solvent type may have a significant impact on extraction compositions as well as extraction efficiency when the extraction process is being carried out on a large scale. The industry places a lot of emphasis on the careful analysis of these characteristics in order to get the greatest extraction efficiency. Although it is crucial to note that low consumption of renewable energy sources is also a major factor at the large-scale level and in industry (Garcia-Salas et al. 2010).

8.5.4 Microwave-Assisted Extraction

Researchers are interested in MAE because it may be used to extract bioactive chemicals from a range of plants and natural remnants (Anokwuru et al. 2011). Electromagnetically radiated waves from microwaves have wavelengths between 1 cm and 1 m and occur at frequency between 300 MHz and 300 GHz. Both an electrical and a magnetic field are present in these electromagnetic waves. It is said that they are two perpendicular fields. Microwaves were first used to heat up materials that could partially absorb electromagnetic energy and turn it into heat. The frequency 2450 MHz is often used by commercial microwave equipment, and this equates to an energy output of 600–700 watts (Ballard et al. 2010).

Modern methods are now available to cut down on bioactive chemical loss without lengthening extraction times. As a result, microwave-assisted extraction has shown to be an effective method in a variety of domains, particularly in the field of medicinal plants. Additionally, this method decreased the losses of the isolated biological substances (Kingston and Jessie 1998). MAE has been used as an alternative to conventional methods for the extraction of antioxidants due to the potential for significant reductions in both extraction time and extraction solvent volume (Suzara et al. 2013). In reality, MAE's principal purpose is to heat the solvent in order to extract plant antioxidants with a reduced amount of these solvents (Ballard et al. 2010). The innovative MAE approach developed by Christophoridou et al. (2005) can extract a specific chemical by converting energy into heat (Christophoridou et al. 2005). Reduced solvent consumption, shorter extraction times, and enhanced sensitivity to target molecules are only some of the advantages of MAE that Williams et al. (2004) revealed.

8.6 TECHNIQUES OF ISOLATION AND PURIFICATION OF BIOACTIVE MOLECULES FROM PLANTS

Purifying and isolating bioactive compounds from plants has taken a new turn in recent years (Altemimi et al. 2015; Ogidi 2022). This cutting-edge technique provides for a parallel between the development and availability of numerous complex bioassays and, on the other hand, the supply of precise techniques for isolation, separation, and purification. When on the hunt for bioactive chemicals, it is ideal to find a method that is quick, easy, and accurate in screening the source material for bioactivity such as antioxidant, antibacterial, or cytotoxic activity (Mulinacci et al. 2004).

In vitro techniques are generally favoured over *in vivo* studies since animal experiments are more expensive, time-consuming, and susceptible to ethical disputes. There are several factors to consider when trying to choose the best methodology or process to extract and identify certain bioactive chemicals. This may be because the bioactive phytochemicals have different chemical structures and physicochemical features and because different plant parts (tissues) produce different compounds (Sarajlija et al. 2012). The initial steps in isolating and identifying a bioactive phytochemicals are the selection and collection of plant materials. The penultimate step involves gathering ethnobotanical data to find bioactive chemicals. Extracts may be made using different solvents to separate the bioactive components responsible for the action. Separating and purifying the bioactive components may involve the use of column chromatography techniques. Technologies like high-performance liquid chromatography (HPLC) speed up the purification of the bioactive chemical. Spectroscopic techniques such as ultraviolet-visible, infrared, nuclear magnetic resonance, and mass spectrometry may be used to identify the purified compounds (Popova et al. 2009).

8.6.1 Purification of the Bioactive Molecule

Several bioactive substances have been isolated and purified using paper thin-layer and column chromatography methods. Column chromatography and thin-layer chromatography (TLC) continue to be extensively used because of their convenience, low cost, and vast variety of stationary phases (Zhang et al. 2005). The most effective materials for separating the phytochemicals are silica, alumina, cellulose, and polyamide. Plant materials contain high amounts of complex phytochemicals, making isolation difficult. Therefore, increasing polarity with many mobile phases is advantageous for extremely valuable separations. Conventionally, thin-layer chromatography has been used to analyse the chemical fractions obtained from column chromatography. Thin-layer chromatography and silica gel column chromatography are two examples of analytical techniques that have been used to isolate bioactive substances (Zhang et al. 2005).

8.6.2 Structural Clarification of the Bioactive Molecules

UV-visible, infrared (IR), nuclear magnetic resonance (NMR), and mass spectroscopy data are used to deduce the structure of individual molecules. The fundamental idea behind spectroscopy is to expose an organic molecule to electromagnetic radiation, some of which it absorbs. A spectrum may be created by counting how much electromagnetic energy is absorbed. Specific bonds in a molecule have distinct spectra. These spectra may be used to determine the organic molecule's structure. Ultraviolet (UV), visible (Vis), infrared (IR), radio frequency (RF), and electron beam spectra are the most common spectra used by scientists for structural clarity as shown in Figure 8.3 (Popova et al. 2009).

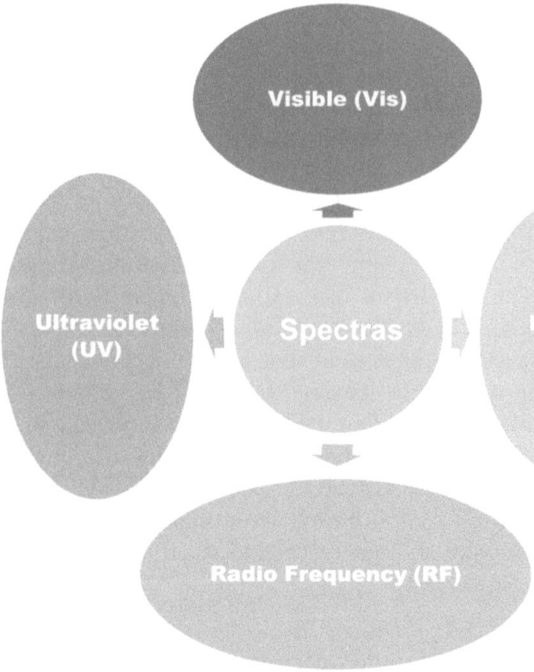

FIGURE 8.3 Spectra used for structural clarity.

8.6.3 UV-Visible Spectroscopy

UV-visible spectroscopy may be utilised for qualitative research and the identification of certain types of compounds in both pure and biological mixtures. Quantitative studies of aromatic compounds are conducted using UV-visible spectroscopy because these compounds are potent chromophores in the UV region. Natural chemicals may be identified with the use of UV-visible spectroscopy (Kemp 1991). The ultraviolet/visible (UV-Vis) spectroscopy has demonstrated that phenolic compounds, such as anthocyanins, tannins, polymer dyes, and phenols, form complexes with iron. It was also shown that spectroscopic UV-Vis approaches are not as discriminating as previously thought and may give insight into the composition of polyphenol concentration. The total phenolic extract (280 nm), flavones (320 nm), phenolic acids (360 nm), and total anthokyanids were all assessed using the UV-Vis spectroscopy (520 nm) (520 nm) (Urbano et al. 2006).

8.6.4 Infrared Spectroscopy

Some infrared wavelengths are absorbed by an organic molecule, whereas others pass through unnoticed when illuminated by infrared light. When a molecule is exposed to infrared light, it undergoes changes in vibration that are linked to infrared absorption. As a result, it is possible to think of infrared spectroscopy as a kind of vibrational spectroscopy. The vibrational frequencies of the various bonds (C-C, C=C, C C, C-O, C=O, O-H, and N-H) vary. These bonds may be detected in organic molecules by looking for an absorption band at a certain frequency in the infrared spectrum. Fourier transform infrared spectroscopy (FTIR) is a high-resolution analytical technique used to identify individual chemical components and provide structural clarity for molecules of interest. Herbal extracts or powders may be quickly and nondestructively fingerprinted using FTIR (Urbano et al. 2006).

8.6.5 Nuclear Magnetic Resonance Spectroscopy

NMR primarily studies the magnetic properties of a number of atomic nuclei, including the hydrogen nucleus, the proton nucleus, the carbon nucleus, and a carbon isotope. By capturing the variations between the different magnetic nuclei and providing a detailed image of their locations inside the molecule, NMR spectroscopy has allowed several researchers to examine molecules (Betancur et al. 2020; Guo et al. 2022). Additionally, it will show which atoms are found in nearby groupings. It is possible to determine how many atoms are present in each of these habitats in the end. Preparative and semi-preparative thin-layer chromatography, liquid chromatography, and column chromatography have all been used to separate phenols in the past; their structures were then determined off-line using nuclear magnetic resonance spectroscopy (Kemp 1991).

8.7 ANTIBACTERIAL ACTIVITY OF POLYPHENOLS

Purified natural products and crude extracts from plants high in polyphenols have been shown to exhibit antibacterial action, according to several study groups as shown in Table 8.1. Flavonoids are classified into subclasses such as flavanols, flavonols, flavones, flavanones, and isoflavones based on distinctions in their backbone structures.

8.7.1 Antibacterial Activity of Flavonols

Due to their various modes of action, flavonols have outstanding efficacy against a variety of gram-negative (*Escherichia coli*, *Prevotella* species, *Fusobacterium nucleatum, and Porphyromonas gingivalis*) and gram-positive (*Staphylococcus aureus* and *Actinomyces naeslundii*) bacteria (Cushrine et al. 2007; Ogidi et al. 2019a). The flavonols quercetin, kaempferol, and myricetin have the strongest antibacterial action (Al-Saif et al. 2014). The inhibition of the DNA gyrase enzyme is the most plausible antibacterial action of quercetin and other flavonols (i.e. in *E. coli*). An *in vitro* study showed that quercetin significantly reduces bacterial membrane potential and cell motility, making it an effective antibacterial agent (Mirzoeva et al. 1997).

Liu et al. (2010) showed that quercetin aglycones had potent antibacterial activity against S. *aureus* and *Staphylococcus haemolyticus*. Quercetin has been shown to be effective against *E. coli* by Lee et al. (2010), while luteolin has been shown to be effective against *Streptococcus pyogenes* by Siriwong et al. (2015). Rhamnetin,

TABLE 8.1
Summary of Antibacterial Activities of Polyphenols

S/N	Polyphenols	Bacteria	References
1	Flavonols	*Escherichia coli, Prevotella* spp., *Fusobacterium nucleatum, Staphylococcus aureus, Actinomyces naeslundii, Porphyromonas gingivalis, Staphylococcus haemolyticus*	Cushine et al. 2007; Ogidi et al. 2019a; Liu et al. 2010; Lee et al. 2010.
2	Flavan-3-ols	*Escherichia coli, Staphylococcus* spp., *Streptococcus mutans, Clostridium perfringens*	Borris 1996; Cui et al. 2012.
3	Flavanones	*Pseudomonas aeruginosa, Salmonella typhimurium, Helicobacter pylori, Staphylococcus aureus, Aeromonas hydrophylia*	Vikram et al. 2011; Baker et al. 2012
4	Isoflavones	*Staphylococcus aureus*	Hatano et al. 2000
5	Phenolic acids	*Escherichia coli, Staphylococcus aureus, Listeria innocua, Salmonella typhimurium, Shigella dysenteriae, Streptococcus pneumonia*	Lou et al. 2011; Sung and Lee 2010
6	Tannins	*Escherichia coli, Corynebacterium diphtheriae, Streptococcus pneumonia, Staphylococcus epidermidis, Staphylococcus aureus, Bacillus subtilis*	Puupponen-Pimia et al. 2001; Krauze-Baranowska et al. 2014.
7	Stilbenes	*Vibrio cholera, Staphylococcus aureus, Enterococci* spp.	Sakagami et al. 2007; Augustine et al. 2014.

myricetin, morin, and quercetin were shown to have strong antibacterial activity against the gram-negative bacterium *Chlamydia pneumonia* in a different study using polyphenol doses ranging from 0.5 to 50 mM (Alvesalo et al. 2006)

8.7.2 Antibacterial Activity of Flavan-3-Ols

Catechin, epicatechin, gallocatechin, epigallocatechin, and their corresponding gallate esters make up the group of flavonoids known as flavan-3-ols. The majority of EGCG's antibacterial effects against *Staphylococcus* spp. are exerted via a variety of mechanisms, including damage to the cell membrane (Cui et al. 2012), a reduction in slime formation (Sudano et al. 2004), and the capacity to neutralise enterotoxin B. (Hisano et al. 2003). Tea (*Camellia sinensis*) catechins and their gallates have been shown to exhibit antibacterial action in research utilising *in vitro* techniques since the 1990s, inhibiting the development of various bacterial species including *Vibrio cholerae, Streptococcus mutans, Clostridium perfringens*, and *E. coli* (Borris 1996).

S. aureus, Serratia marcescens, Pseudomonas aeruginosa, and *Helicobacter pylori* are only some of the microorganisms that have been demonstrated to be vulnerable to tea polyphenols' antibacterial effects in other studies (Radji et al. 2013). Among the several catechins, the most common one, EGCG, has the strongest antibacterial activity against various bacteria, including *S. aureus, S. pyogenes*, coagulase-negative *Staphylococci*, and *Streptococcus mutans* (Betts et al. 2015). Additionally, researchers have shown that flavonoids and other substances work together to combat resistant bacterial strains (Stapleton et al. 2004).

8.7.3 Antibacterial Activity of Flavanones

Numerous studies have shown the antibacterial properties of flavanones, including naringenin, hesperidin, and hesperetin (Tombola et al. 2003). It was discovered that naringenin is effective against *P. aeruginosa* and *Salmonella typhimurium* (Vikram et al. 2011). It has been shown that hesperidin is effective in treating *Aeromonas hydrophylia* and *S. aureus*. Hesperetin and hesperidin have also been found to have action against *H. pylori* in addition to their inhibitory efficacy against *S. aureus* (Bakar et al. 2012).

8.7.4 Antibacterial Activity of Isoflavones

Daidzein is one of the most active isoflavones, and investigations on its antibacterial properties have been published (Dastidar et al. 2004). The most active substance *in vitro* was daidzein (MIC range: 16–128 g/mL), and the most sensitive strain was vancomycin-resistant *Enterococcus faecalis*, among other bacteria. Genistein and daidzein were shown to be effective against various bacteria (Chin et al. 2012). Genistein and other isoflavones have been shown to inhibit *S. aureus* (MRSA strains) at concentrations between 16 and 128 g/mL. (Hatano et al. 2000). The suppression of the bacterial topoisomerase IV enzyme is thought to be the cause of the antibacterial effects (Verdrengh et al. 2004).

8.7.5 Antibacterial Activity of Phenolic Acids

Different strains of *Listeria monocytogenes* have been shown to be susceptible to the bacteriostatic and bactericidal effects of pure phenolic acids like hydroxycinnamic acid (Wen et al. 2003). In addition, gram-positive and gram-negative bacteria, including *E. coli*, have been found to be vulnerable to ferulic, p-coumaric, and caffeic acids (*S. aureus*). Esterified hydroxycinnamic acids, chlorogenic acids have antibacterial (Lou et al. 2011), antiviral (Xie et al. 2013), and antifungal activities in the body (Sung and Lee 2010).

Chlorogenic acid considerably inhibited the development of *E. coli* (O157:H7) and *Listeria innocua* (by >90%) compared to the control. Furthermore, *Salmonella typhimurium*, *Shigella dysenteriae*, *S. pneumoniae*, and *E. coli* are all known to be susceptible to chlorogenic acid's antimicrobial effects (Lou et al. 2011). In contrast, cinnamic acids and chlorogenic acids only inhibit gram-negative bacteria at very high concentrations (500 g well-1), with chlorogenic acid being the least effective inhibitor against *E. coli*. This result was found by Puupponen-Pimia et al. (2001). Researchers have shown that brewed coffee has antimicrobial effects against

Legionella pneumophila with the identified active ingredients being caffeic, chlorogenic, and protocatechuic acids (Dogazaki et al. 2002; Furuhata et al. 2002).

8.7.6 Antibacterial Activity of Tannins

Tannin-rich traditional medicinal herbs have been shown to have antibacterial properties (Lipinska et al. 2014; Ogidi et al. 2022; Ogidi and Julius 2021). Numerous antibacterial actions for condensed tannins (proanthocyanidins) as well as hydrolysable tannins (gallotannins and ellagitannins) have been reported. A number of pathogens, including *P. aeruginosa*, *E. coli*, and other bacteria, have been demonstrated to produce less biofilm when exposed to proanthocyanidin (Leshem et al. 2011). Proanthocyanidins have been shown by Liu et al. (2013a,b) to exhibit inhibitory effect against *E. coli* at low inhibitory concentrations (20–50 g/mL) in the condensed tannins of *Dalea purpurea*.

Hydrolysable tannins are well recognised for their antimicrobial activities (Puupponen-Pimia et al. 2001). Sanguiin H-6 (Ellagitannins), which was examined by Krauze-Baranowska et al. (2014), shown bactericidal efficacy against *Corynebacterium diphtheria, S. pneumoniae, Streptococcus* group A, and *Staphylococcus epidermidis.* Additionally, it inhibited the species of *Moraxella catarrhalis, Clostridium sporogenes, S. aureus*, and *Bacillus subtilis.* Ellagic acid had the same effectiveness against several strains as sanguiin H-6 in the same investigation. However, *Neisseria meningitides* showed an inhibitory effect, whereas *S. pneumoniae* and *S. epidermidis* showed no antimicrobial activity. Additionally, their investigation supported the efficacy of ellagic acid against *H. pylori*, but dimeric sanguiin H-6 failed to demonstrate any antibacterial action.

8.7.8 Antibacterial Activity of Stilbenes

Resveratrol in particular is known to have an anti-carcinogenic impact by inducing several types of cell death in a number of tumour cells (Mohan et al. 2006). Numerous writers have noted the antibacterial effects of stilbenes in addition to their chemo-preventive qualities. In wild-type strains of *Proteus mirabilis*, resveratrol reduced the production of virulence factors and the cholera toxin (Wang et al. 2006). Resveratrol has been shown to exhibit antibacterial efficacy against *Vibrio cholerae* and to reduce the growth of biofilms, according to Augustine et al. (2014). Two resveratrol trimmers (gnemonol B and gnetin E) from the *Gnetum* species were described by Sakagami et al. (2007), and it was discovered that they have potent antibacterial properties against methicillin-resistant *S. aureus* and vancomycin-resistant enterococci. Natural stilbenes that were obtained by Nitta et al. (2002) from the roots of *Cyphostemma bainessi*, and the bark of *Shorea hemsleyana* had significant antibacterial action against the MRSA strain.

8.8 SYNERGISTIC ANTIBACTERIAL ACTIVITY

Phenolic chemicals may logically be coupled with other antibacterial compounds to effectively treat multi-drug-resistant bacteria if precise mechanisms of action are recognised (Zhao et al. 2020; Stan et al. 2021). Many phenolic compounds have previously been shown to have synergistic effects when mixed with commonly used antibiotics (Amin et al. 2015; Hemaiswarya and Doble 2010), as well as essential oil constituents (Lim et al. 2016; Oh and Jeon 2015). Membrane-disrupting substances, such as phenolics, have been linked to several synergistic actions that speed up or facilitate the entrance of intracellular poisons to their targets (Amin et al. 2015; Hemaiswarya and Doble 2010; Oh and Jeon 2015). In addition, strains that use efflux pumps to remove toxins may be attacked in a synergistic manner by first blocking the pumps with one chemical and then providing an intracellular toxin (Tegos and Stermitz 2002; Prasch and Bucar 2015; Oh and Jeon 2015).

Additionally, it has been shown that efflux pump expression is downregulated (Oh and Jeon 2015). The effectiveness of current antibacterial drugs may be enhanced by synergistic effects between additional modes of action, particularly in the fight against drug resistance mechanisms (Lobiul et al. 2023).

8.9 ANTIVIRAL ACTIVITY OF FLAVONOID AND NON-FLAVONOID COMPOUNDS

According to their backbone structure, flavonoids are classified into subclasses including flavonols, flavanols, flavones, flavanones, and other phenolics depending on their antiviral activity as shown in Table 8.2.

8.9.1 Antiviral Activity of Flavonols

The antiviral activity of quercetin has received the greatest attention among flavonols. Quercetin showed dose-dependent antiviral activity in cell cultures against HSV-1, HSV-2, poliovirus type 1, and respiratory syncytial virus (Kang et al. 2004). In cell culture experiments, quercetin was shown to have considerable inhibitory action against the generation of the hepatitis C virus (HCV) at a concentration of 50 M (Gonzalez et al. 2009). According to *in vivo* research, quercetin is effective

TABLE 8.2
Summary of Antiviral Activities of Flavonoids

S/N	Flavonoids	Virus	References
1	Flavonols	HSV-1, HSV-2, polio virus type 1, respiratory syncytial virus, hepatitis C virus (HCV), and influenza A virus	Kang et al. 2004; Cho et al. 2015
2	Flavones	HSV-1, polio virus type 2, HCV, adenovirus (ADV), hepatitis B virus, Epstein-Barr virus (EBV), and HIV-1	Zhang et al. 2014; Williamson and Clifford 2010.
3	Flavan-3-ols	Influenza virus, HCV, and herpes simplex virus	Calland et al. 2012; Chan et al. 2012
4	Flavanones	Semliki forest virus, Sindbis virus, HCV, HIV, HSV-1, and HSV-2	Pohjala et al. 2011; Argenta et al. 2015

against influenza A subtypes (Cho et al. 2015). Recent investigations have also identified quercetin's antiviral properties against a variety of influenza virus types (Wu et al. 2015). Additionally, canine distemper, respiratory syndrome, swine epidemic diarrhoea, and other viruses that are transmitted by arthropods have been found to be resistant to quercetin and its derivatives (Carvalho et al. 2013).

8.9.2 Antiviral Activity of Flavones

In an *in vitro* investigation, apigenin, a key component of plant extracts, was shown to have antiviral action against HSV-1, poliovirus type 2, HCV, as well as adenoviruses (ADVs) and the hepatitis B virus. It was discovered that apigenin inhibits the African swine fever virus, blocks viral IRES (internal ribosome entry site) activity, and interferes with the translation of enterovirus-71 (Zhang et al. 2014).

The largest inhibitory potencies against HCV activity were shown by apigenin and luteolin, which had EC50 values of 7.9 M and 4.3 M, respectively (Liu et al. 2012). Additionally, it was noted that luteolin showed a functional inhibition of non-structural protein-5B polymerase enzymatic action with an IC_{50} of 1.12 Mm (Luo et al. 2000). It was discovered that luteolin significantly inhibited the reactivation of the Epstein-Barr virus (EBV) in cells and had an antiviral impact on HIV-1 reactivation (Williamson and Clifford 2010). By interfering with viral RNA replication, luteolin demonstrated the strongest suppression of all 400 investigated chemicals in the natural compound-based antiviral investigation, according to Xu et al. (2014). Other substances of the flavones family, such as baicalein, inhibited the reproduction of the H5N1 avian influenza virus (Sithisarn et al. 2013; Nayak et al. 2014), exhibited anti-influenza action, and showed promise as potential substitutes for the treatment of Tamiflu-resistant viruses (Chung et al. 2014). It was utilised to treat HIV-1-infected cells that were in the early stages of infection and greatly decreased the protein levels of human cytomegalovirus (Cotin et al. 2012; Kim et al. 2013). From *Marrubium peregrinum* L., Haid et al. (2012) discovered ladanein, which has anti-HCV action at 2.5 M concentration.

8.9.3 Antiviral Activity of Flavan-3-Ols

The antiviral action of flavan-3-ols such as catechin and its derivatives epicatechin, epicatechin gallate (ECG), and EGCG is primarily being researched. Different studies have discovered EGCG to be a fresh entrance inhibitor for HCV (Chan et al. 2012). Different investigations indicated that EGCG had varying IC_{50} (5 M and 21 M), and that it also prevented HCVpp entrance into hepatoma-derived cells (Calland et al. 2012; Chan et al. 2012). EGCG has been found to be effective against the influenza virus, the herpes simplex virus, and as an anti-HCV molecule (Fukazawa et al. 2012). Boceprevir or cyclosporin might be used with EGCG as a synergistic drug for greater effectiveness against HCV replication (Ciesek et al. 2011).

8.9.4 Antiviral Activity of Flavanones

According to research, naringenin, a member of the flavanones class, reduces the cytopathic impact caused by sindbis and semliki forest viruses as well as the reproduction of a neurovirulent strain of sindbis virus (Pohjala et al. 2011). Studies on naringenin's impact on HCV particle secretion, which may prevent the formation of intracellular HCV particles, were also conducted (Goldwasser et al. 2011). Hepatocytes were cultured, and the inhibitory action was shown after naringenin administration at 200 M concentrations. During the virus's intracellular reproduction, hesperetin was shown to have the strongest anti–chikungunya virus (CHIKV) action, with an IC50 of 8.5 M (Ahmadi et al. 2016). Additionally, it has been shown that genistein prevents HIV from infecting resting macrophages and CD4 T cells. Also, it prevented HSV-1 and HSV-2 reproduction by preventing the virus's transcription (Argenta et al. 2015).

8.10 ANTIFUNGAL ACTIVITY OF PHENOLIC COMPOUNDS

Only a small number of the millions of known fungal species are harmful to people, leading to local or systemic fungal infections and more than 150 million severe instances of fungal infections globally. Life-threatening invasive fungal infections are more common in patients with compromised immune systems, whether as a result of illnesses like leukaemia or HIV or medical treatments like chemotherapy or prolonged hospitalisation in critical care units, as in the case of SARS-CoV-2–infected patients (Ogidi et al. 2019b; Kainz et al. 2020; Ogidi et al. 2021a; Koehler et al. 2014).

It has been more difficult to create novel chemicals with antifungal action in recent years because the human cell and the structure and metabolism of fungi are so similar. This makes antifungal medications more hazardous and likely to have side effects. Currently, pyrimidines, allylamines, azoles, polyenes, and echinocandins are the five main types of antifungal medications utilised in clinical settings. These antifungal classes come from plants that contain phenolic chemicals. The modes of action specifically target the metabolism of ergosterol, the key component of the fungal cell membrane and the fungus's analogue of cholesterol. They also affect other eukaryotic cell types, such as human cells. Finding antifungal drugs is difficult since there are not many fungal-specific targets, which promotes the growth of fungi that are resistant to treatment. There are other ways that fungi adopt to resist medication treatment that have been identified in the literature, in addition to inherent antifungal resistance (multi-drug-resistant *Candida auris*) (Zheng and Wang 2019; Ogidi et al. 2019c; Howard et al. 2020; Ogidi et al. 2021b, 2021c).

8.11 BIOINFORMATICS APPROACHES TO MOLECULAR MECHANISMS IN ANTIMICROBIAL RESISTANCE

The development of resistance to antibiotics is a major public health concern across the world. Improving our understanding of the underlying molecular mechanisms is essential. Advances in whole genome sequencing and other high-throughput, unbiased instrumental technologies have made it possible to accumulate massive amounts of data that are amenable to bioinformatic analysis and the identification of novel AMR signatures, allowing for the study of the molecular pathogenicity of infectious diseases. Following is a discussion of some of the most significant bioinformatic techniques created to far for studying AMR processes.

8.11.1 Approach 1: Identification of Known Genomic Signatures of AMR from WGS Data

In order to determine the existence of known ARGs or gene variations, WGS (Illumina sequencing) data analysis is the initial step in predicting the AMR. While some genes are found on mobile genetic material (plasmids) that may be transferred across species, others are indigenous to a particular species or strain. Next, ML models may be trained to predict newly sequenced data by using binary (presence/absence) or real number (abundance) vectors that represent such fixed sets of genes and their mutations.

TypeWriter makes use of BLASTn to match constructed genomic contigs to 24 ARG and 120 mutations connected to resistance in *S. aureus* (Gordon et al. 2014). Assembly of the sequenced and assembled genomes is followed by a comparison to a reference strain of the bacterium, ensuring the highest possible quality control throughout the process. This slows everything down and raises questions about how well the workflow would function with a wide range of isolated strains and other species. PointFinder utilises BLASTn to establish a connection between raw data and a database of 16 ARGs and their mutations (Zankari et al. 2017). This method's primary contribution to the field is its expansion and validation in respect to the three species *E. coli, Campylobacter jejuni*, and *Salmonella enterica*. To determine what lineage a particular isolate belongs to among the 92 lineages with known resistance phenotypes, PhyResSE maps shotgun read sequences to the reference genome of *Mycobacterium tuberculosis* (strain H37Rv) using BWA-MEM (Li 2013), a quicker than BLASTn sequence aligner. The procedure does away with the requirement for the genome assembly stage, but it also calls for the use of FastQC, Qualimap, and the Genome Analysis Toolkit (GATK) in order to ensure the quality of called variations (Andrews 2020).

All of these techniques work with a predetermined panel of ARGs and related mutations. When used in clinical contexts, they can provide precise findings with a high degree of trust. The time it takes to sequence a bacterial genome has decreased to around 24 hours, and it no longer need several days of extra *in vitro* growth, as is necessary for conventional laboratory AMR testing. This could speed up the beginning of efficient AB treatment and enhance patient results. It should be noted that the majority of these techniques were created for a single pathogen (typically *M. tuberculosis* since it is difficult to culture), and it is not yet known if these models will perform similarly on other species with possibly more complicated AMR processes.

8.11.2 Approach 2: Identification of AMR Signatures from Gene Expression Data

Studying changes in the isolate's gene expression after medication treatment is the second strategy for AMR analysis and prediction. Suzuki and colleagues subjected *E. coli* to laboratory-induced evolution under pressure from 11 AB at increasing dosages to produce strains with differing degrees of resistance to these medicines, as measured by their minimum inhibitory concentrations (MICs) (Suzuki et al. 2014). Gene expression analysis allowed them to study the pathogen's dynamic compensating mechanisms (based on microarray). They identified a total of eight genes (acrB, ompF, cyoC, pps, tsx, oppA, folA, and pntB) whose expression levels allowed a linear regression model to establish relationship with experimentally observed MIC with R2 values ranging from 0.54 to 0.75 per drug. Darnell and colleagues analysed the transcriptional response to teixobactin in *E. faecalis* (strain JH2–2) (Darnell et al. 2019). After the AB therapy, RNA-seq was used to analyse the transcriptome at the genome level. Enrichment for up-regulated pathways including peptidoglycan, teichoic acid, and cell wall exopolysaccharide production was found among the 573 differentially expressed genes. Later analysis comparing the expression profile to transcriptional responses of *E. faecalis* to various cell wall-targeting antibiotics revealed the same up-regulated CroRS regulon of 219 genes. CroRS is the shorthand for the cellular two-component response to wall stress. The organism's sensitivity to teixobactin was markedly boosted by the matching deletion mutant (DcroRS). Overall, this method shows a lot of potential for understanding AMR molecular processes.

8.11.3 Approach 3: ARG Agnostic Identification of AMR Mechanisms via Pan-Genome Analysis

The third method of revealing AMR processes is gene agnostic and relies on a comparison of the global genomes of several strains with varying drug susceptibilities. For this study, PanPhlAn examined the genomic content and gene expression patterns of 110 reference and 12 metagenomically discovered *E. coli* strains, including commensal and outbreak-related strains (Scholz et al. 2016).

Through this comparison, genes associated with *E. coli* outbreaks were identified, characterised using the Gene Ontology (GO), and mapped to genomic functional modules found in the KEGG database (Kanehisa and Goto 2000). Mahe and Tournoud (2018) applied this method to multiple *M. tuberculosis* and *S. aureus* strains, but they went further than the previous study by extracting any 31-mers of genomic sequences (including from noncoding regions) that were uniquely associated with certain drug combinations and levels of AB susceptibility (Mahe and Tournoud 2018). Using data from the PATRIC database (Wattam et al. 2014), including lineage-defining SNPs, AMR phenotypic, geographic, and other data. Kavvas et al. (2018) generated a pan-genome of *M. tuberculosis* based on 1595 sequenced strains. Using pairwise association tests and a machine learning technique, they identified 97 epistatic interactions associated with 10 classes of resistance in *M. tuberculosis*, as well as 24 unique genetic indicators of AMR (support vector machine [SVM]). Clusters of mutations in these proteins as a result of AB found by mapping to the known 3D structures of a few proteins involved in AMR (Drown et al. 2019). In addition to compiling k-mers associated with susceptibility or resistance, they employed rule-based ML approaches, such as classification and regression trees (CARTs) and set covering machines (SCMs). Insights into the potential role of certain k-mers in decision-making provided by these rule-based models might contribute to the discovery of previously unknown AMR mechanisms across species.

The pan-genome technique has a lot of potential for therapeutic use while needing a previous significant investment in genomic sequencing and genome wide comparison. The main benefit of this strategy is that it examines whole genomes as opposed to only known AMR-related areas, perhaps revealing additional regulatory or mechanism elements (via mutations in noncoding, possibly regulatory regions). These machine learning algorithms have a hurdle in that the input space is quite big (the whole genome), and the thorough examination of newly discovered areas (lab studies) is required to confirm their significance. This is due to a phenomenon as overfitting of ML models, which occurs when particular genomic areas in samples with identical AMR are associated statistically rather than causally. Additionally, these techniques sometimes need for large strain collections, which would be difficult for diseases that have received little research.

8.11.4 Approach 4: Identification of AMR Mechanisms from Metabolomics Data

Yang and colleagues treated *E. coli* with three ABs and examined the changes in the metabolite profiles as the last strategy, which is orthogonal to those discussed earlier (Yang et al. 2019). They were able to do a flux balance analysis by integrating the organism's known metabolic pathways with experimentally determined bounds of metabolite concentrations after drug treatment. Then, to forecast the lethality of a certain AB, metabolite fluxes and metabolic pathways were incorporated into machine learning models. These models also showed how various ABs influence different metabolic pathways and how the bactericidal activity might be strengthened, for instance, by limiting adenine. Similar methods were utilised by Zampieri et al. (2017) to drive either respiratory or fermentative glucose metabolism in *E. coli* lineages grown under the influence of different combinations of three ABs.

The scientists analysed whole genomes to look for mutations brought about by AB-induced evolution in addition to monitoring variations in metabolite concentrations across lineages. They also assessed the gene expression and protein abundance of the multidrug efflux pump gene acrB. It was shown that *E. coli* uses a variety of methods, including mutations and the development of efflux pumps, to counteract the pressure from various antibiotics. These processes also rely on the carbon supply and the organism's current metabolic state. This finding supports the idea that in terms of genotype-phenotype prediction for AMR, gram-negative bacteria are more difficult to research and understand (Zampieri et al. 2017).

Collectively, this strategy offers a fresh viewpoint on how bacteria react to medications and the effect of ABs. This method offers the groundwork for enhancing medication treatment regimens and maximising combination therapy, despite the fact that it is far from being readily applied to practical practise. Since not all species have had their metabolic pathways as well characterised as the model organism *E. coli*, using this strategy to other dangerous organisms may offer difficulties.

8.12 FUTURE PROSPECTIVES AND LIMITATIONS

The reactions of plant-based antimicrobials and their synergistic effects with antibiotics along with their mechanism of action is based on the development of new and current extraction, isolation, and purification technologies of phenolic compounds

(Candelaria-Duenas et al. 2021). Hence, the application of current techniques which includes using standard procedures in antimicrobial assay and determination of medicinal plants materials for quality control and assurance. For instance, using biotechnological methods in identification and isolation of individual or combined plant based secondary metabolites and their mechanism of action may improve the development of effective antimicrobial agents (Stavropoulou et al. 2022).

Additional studies on the investigations of phytochemical compounds and molecular interactions are required for proper explanation of their antimicrobial activities. Researches on the synergy of plant based isolated phytochemicals can show future information on their synergistic and antagonistic mechanisms of actions. Combined techniques in solving an appropriate problem, which includes identification of composite phytochemical compounds (Stavropoulou et al. 2022), the investigation of the nature of phytochemical reactions, and the categorisation of their mechanisms of action together, should be developed. Furthermore, biomarkers from phytochemical compounds which control the synergistic interactions may be important for determining therapeutic strategies (Wu et al. 2021).

The identification of phenolic compounds in complex mixtures reveal biological effects which can be difficult to carry out. In order to overcome this limitation, pulsed ultrafiltration mass spectrometer was employed for medicinal plant extract screening. These extracts may not be totally safe because of the different compositions of phenolic compounds when administered as antimicrobial agents, hence, the need to evaluate these phenolic compounds and identify their residual formations (Shaaban 2020). Bioassay-guided fractionation limitation also involves low concentrations of isolated fractions, which produces biological effects and for that reason is ignored. It is regarded as a time-intensive, dangerous, and expensive method (Possemiers et al. 2011).

8.13 CONCLUSION

Plant-derived phenolic compounds have a variety of uses as antibacterial, antiviral, and antifungal agents. Consequently, they have the capacity to enhance human health. The merits and drawbacks of different phenolic compound extraction techniques from plants were discussed in this chapter. Their advantages and limitations in terms of isolation, purification, and identification were also discussed. Antimicrobial resistance bioinformatics techniques may be generally divided into two groups: those that investigate the fundamental molecular causes of AMR and those that concentrate on quick and accurate predictions of antimicrobial resistance to be used in clinical settings.

REFERENCES

Ahmadi, A., P. Hassandarvish, R. Lani, et al. 2016. Inhibition of chikungunya virus replication by hesperetin and naringenin. *RSC Adv* 6: 69421–69430.

Albuquerque, B.R., S.A. Heleno, M.B.P.P. Oliveira, L. Barros, and I.C.F.R. Ferreira. 2021. Phenolic compounds: Current industrial applications, limitations and future challenges. *Food Funct* 12: 14–29.

Al-Saif, S.S., N. Abdel-Raouf, H.A. El-Wazanani, and I.A. Aref. 2014. Antibacterial substances from marine algae isolated from Jeddah coast of Red sea, Saudi Arabia. *Saudi J Biol Sci* 21(1): 57–64.

Altemimi, A.W., D.G. Watson, M. Kinsel, and D.A. Lightfoot. 2015. Simultaneous extraction, optimization, and analysis of flavonoids and polyphenols from peach and pumpkin extracts using a TLC-densitometric method. *Chem Cent J* 9: 1–15.

Alvesalo, J., H. Vuorela, P. Tammela, M. Leinonen, P. Saikku, and P. Vuorela. 2006. Inhibitory effect of dietary phenolic compounds on Chlamydia pneumoniae in cell cultures. *Biochem Pharmacol* 71(6): 735–741.

Amin, M.U., M. Khurram, B. Khattak, and J. Khan. 2015. Antibiotic additive and synergistic action of rutin, morin and quercetin against methicillin resistant *Staphylococcus aureus*. *BMC Complement Altern Med* 15: 59.

Andrews, S. 2020. *FastQC A Quality Control Tool for High Throughput Sequence Data*. Available online: www.bioinformatics.babraham.ac.uk/projects/fastqc/ (accessed on 14 January 2022).

Anokwuru, C.P., G.N. Anyasor, O. Ajibaye, O. Fakoya, and P. Okebugwu. 2011. Effect of extraction solvents on phenolic, flavonoid and antioxidant activities of three Nigerian medicinal plants. *Nat Sci* 9: 53–61.

Argenta, D.F., I.T. Silva, V.L. Bassani, L.S. Koester, H.F. Teixeira, and C.M. Simões. 2015. Antiherpes evaluation of soybean isoflavonoids. *Arch Virol* 160(9): 2335–2342.

Augustine, N., A.K. Goel, K.C. Sivakumar, R.A. Kumar, and S. Thomas. 2014. Resveratrol--a potential inhibitor of biofilm formation in Vibrio cholerae. *Phytomedicine* 21(3): 286–289.

Bakar, N.S., N.M. Zin, and D.F. Basri. 2012. Synergy of flavone with vancomycin and oxacillin against vancomycinintermediate Staphyloccus aureus. *Pak J Pharm Sci* 25(3): 633–638.

Ballard, T.S., P. Mallikarjunan, K. Zhou, and S. O'Keefe. 2010. Microwave-assisted extraction of phenolic antioxidant compounds from peanut skins. *Food Chem* 120: 1185–1192.

Bartwal, A., R. Mall, P. Lohani, S.K. Guru, and S. Arora. 2013. Role of secondary metabolites and brassinosteroids in plant eefense against Environmental stresses. *J Plant Growth Regul* 32: 216–232.

Betancur, L.A., A.M. Forero, D.M. Vinchira-Villarraga, et al. 2020. NMR-based metabolic profiling to follow the production of anti-phytopathogenic compounds in the culture of the marine strain Streptomyces sp. PNM-9. *Microbiol Res* 239: 126507.

Betts, J.W., A.S. Sharili, L.M. Phee, and D.W. Wareham. 2015. In vitro activity of epigallocatechin gallate and quercetin alone and in combination *versus* clinical isolates of methicillin-resistant Staphylococcus aureus. *J Nat Prod* 78(8): 2145–2148.

Bhullar, K.S. and H.P.V. Rupasinghe. 2015. Partridgeberry polyphenols protect primary cortical and hippocampal neurons against beta-amyloid toxicity. *Food Res Int* 74: 237–249.

Borris, R.P. 1996. Natural products research: Perspectives from a major pharmaceutical company. *J Ethnopharmacol* 51(1–3): 29–38.

Boudet, A. 2007. Evolution and current status of research in phenolic compounds. *Phytochemistry* 68: 2722–2735.

Calland, N., A. Albecka, S. Belouzard, et al. 2012. (-)-Epigallocatechin-3-gallate is a new inhibitor of hepatitis C virus entry. *Hepatology* 55(3): 720–729.

Candelaria-Dueñas, S., R. Serrano-Parrales, M. Ávila-Romero, et al. 2021. Evaluation of the antimicrobial activity of some components of the essential oils of plants used in the traditional medicine of the tehuacán-cuicatlán Valley, Puebla, México. *Antibiotics* 10: 295.

Carvalho, O.V., C.V. Botelho, C.G. Ferreira, et al. 2013. In vitro inhibition of canine distemper virus by flavonoids and phenolic acids: Implications of structural differences for antiviral design. *Res Vet Sci* 95(2): 717–724.

CDC. 2019. *Antibiotic Resistance Threats in the United States, 2019; U.S. Department of Health and Human Services.* CDC: Atlanta, GA, 2019. Available online: www.cdc.gov/drugresistance/pdf/threats-report/2019-arthreats-report-508.pdf (accessed on 17 February 2020).

Chen, C., H. Qiu, J. Gong, et al. 2012. (-)-Epigallocatechin-3-gallate inhibits the replication cycle of hepatitis C virus. *Arch Virol* 157(7): 1301–1312.

Cheynier, V., G. Comte, K.M. Davies, V. Lattanzio, and S. Martens. 2013. Plant phenolics: Recent advances on their biosynthesis, genetics, and ecophysiology. *Plant Physiol Biochem PPB* 72: 1–20.

Chin, Y.P., K.C. Tsui, M.C. Chen, C.Y. Wang, C.Y. Yang, and Y.L. Lin. 2012. Bactericidal activity of soymilk fermentation broth by *in vitro* and animal models. *J Med Food* 15(6): 520–526.

Cho, W.K., P. Weeratunga, B.H. Lee, et al. 2015. Epimedium koreanum Nakai displays broad spectrum of antiviral activity *in vitro* and *in vivo* by inducing cellular antiviral state. *Viruses* 7(1): 352–377.

Christophoridou, S., P. Dais, L.H. Tseng, and M. Spraul. 2005. Separation and identification of phenolic compounds in olive oil by coupling high-performance liquid chromatography with postcolumn solid-phase extraction to nuclear magnetic resonance spectroscopy (lc-spe-nmr). *J Agric Food Chem* 53: 4667–4679.

Chung, S.T., P.Y. Chien, W.H. Huang, C.W. Yao, and A.R. Lee. 2014. Synthesis and anti-influenza activities of novel baicalein analogs. *Chem Pharm Bull (Tokyo)* 62(5): 415–421.

Ciesek, S., T. von-Hahn, C.C. Colpitts, et al. 2011. The green tea polyphenol, epigallocatechin-3-gallate, inhibits hepatitis C virus entry. *Hepatology* 54(6): 1947–1955.

Cotin, S., C.A. Calliste, M.C. Mazeron, et al. 2012. Eight flavonoids and their potential as inhibitors of human cytomegalovirus replication. *Antiviral Res* 96(2): 181–186.

Crozier, A., I.B. Jaganath, and M.N. Clifford. 2006. Phenols, polyphenols and tannins: An overview. In Alan Crozier, Michael N. Clifford and Hiroshi Ashihara (eds.), *Plant Secondary Metabolites: Occurrence, Structure and Role in the Human Diet*, 1–24. Blackwell Publishing Ltd, Oxford.

Cui, Y., Y.J. Oh, J. Lim, et al. 2012. AFM study of the differential inhibitory effects of the green tea polyphenol (-)-epigallocatechin-3-gallate (EGCG) against Gram-positive and Gram-negative bacteria. *Food Microbiol* 29(1): 80–87.

Cushnie, T.P., V.E. Hamilton, D.G. Chapman, P.W. Taylor, and A.J. Lamb. 2007. Aggregation of Staphylococcus aureus following treatment with the antibacterial flavonol galangin. *J Appl Microbiol* 103(5): 1562–1567.

Dai, J., and R.J. Mumper. 2010. Plant phenolics: Extraction, analysis and their antioxidant and anticancer properties. *Molecules (Basel, Switzerland)* 15(10): 7313–7352.

Darnell, R.L., M.K. Knottenbelt, F.O. Todd Rose, I.R. Monk, T.P. Stinear, and G.M. Cook. 2019. Genomewide profiling of the enterococcus faecalis transcriptional response to teixobactin reveals CroRS as an essential regulator of antimicrobial tolerance. *mSphere* 4: e00228–19.

Dastidar, S.G., A. Manna, K.A. Kumar, et al. 2004. Studies on the antibacterial potentiality of isoflavones. *Int J Antimicrob Agents* 23(1): 99–102.

Dogasaki, C., T. Shindo, K. Furuhata, and M. Fukuyama. 2002. Identification of chemical structure of antibacterial components against Legionella pneumophila in a coffee beverage. *Yakugaku Zasshi* 122(7): 487–494.

Drouin, A., G. Letarte, F. Raymond, M. Marchand, J. Corbeil, and F. Laviolette. 2019. Interpretable genotype-to-phenotype classifiers with performance guarantees. *Sci Rep* 9: 4071.

Enenebeaku, C.K., C.E. Ogukwe, C.O. Nweke, et al. 2022a. Antiplasmodial and in vitro antioxidant potentials of crude aqueous and methanol extracts of *Chasmanthera dependens* (Hochst). *Bull Natl Res Cent (Springer Open)* 46(33): 1–12.

Enenebeaku, U.E., C.E. Duru, E.N. Okotcha, et al. 2022b. Phytochemical analysis and antioxidant evaluation of crude extracts from the roots, stem and leaves of dictyandraarborescens (Welw.). *Trop J Nat Prod Res* 6(1): 62–70.

Ermis, E., C. Hertel, C. Schneider, R. Carle, F. Stintzing, and H. Schmidt. 2015. Characterization of in vitro antifungal activities of small and American cranberry (*Vaccinium oxycoccos* L and *V. macrocarpon* Aiton) and lingonberry (*Vaccinium vitis-idaea* L.) concentrates in sugar reduced fruit spreads. *Int J Food Microbiol* 204: 111–117.

Fan, Z., Z. Wang, L. Zuo, and S. Tian. 2012. Protective effect of anthocyanins from lingonberry on radiation-induced damages. *Int J Environ Res Public Health* 9: 4732–4743.

Fukazawa, H., T. Suzuki, T. Wakita, and Y. Murakami. 2012. A cell-based, microplate colorimetric screen identifies 7,8-benzoflavone and green tea gallate catechins as inhibitors of the hepatitis C virus. *Biol Pharm Bull* 35(8): 1320–1327.

Furuhata, K., C. Dogasaki, M. Hara, and M. Fukuyama. 2002. Inactivation of Legionella pneumophila by phenol compounds contained in coffee. *J Antibact Antifung Agents* 2: 20.

Garcia-Salas, P., A. Morales-Soto, A. Segura-Carretero, and A. Fernández-Gutiérrez. 2010. Phenolic-compound extraction systems for fruit and vegetable samples. *Molecules* 15(12): 8813–8826.

Gharaati, S., H. Kargar, and A.M. Falahati. 2017. Tetrahydropyranylation of alcohols and phenols catalyzed by a new multiwall carbon nanotubes-bound tin(IV) porphyrin. *J Iran Chem Soc* 14(6): 169–1178.

Goldwasser, J., P.Y. Cohen, W. Lin, et al. 2011. Naringenin inhibits the assembly and long-term production of infectious hepatitis C virus particles through a PPAR-mediated mechanism. *J Hepatol* 55(5): 963–971.

Gonzalez, O., V. Fontanes, S. Raychaudhuri, et al. 2009. The heat shock protein inhibitor Quercetin attenuates hepatitis C virus production. *Hepatology* 50(6): 1756–1764.

Gordon, N.C., J.R. Price, K. Cole, et al. 2014. Prediction of Staphylococcus aureus antimicrobial resistance by whole-genome sequencing. *J Clin Microbiol* 52: 1182–1191.

Guo, C., Y. He, Y. Wang, and H. Yung. 2022. NMR-based metabolomic investigation on antimicrobial mechanism of Salmonella on cucumber slices treated with organic acids. *Food Control* 137: 108973.

Haid, S., A. Novodomská, J. Gentzsch, et al. 2012. A plant-derived flavonoid inhibits entry of all HCV genotypes into human hepatocytes. *Molecule* 2: 12.

Hatano, T., Y. Shintani, Y. Aga, S. Shiota, T. Tsuchiya, and T. Yoshida. 2000. Phenolic constituents of licorice. VIII. Structures of glicophenone and glicoisoflavanone, and effects of licorice phenolics on methicillinresistant Staphylococcus aureus. *Chem Pharm Bull (Tokyo)* 48(9): 1286–1292.

Hemaiswarya, S., and M. Doble. 2010. Synergistic interaction of phenylpropanoids with antibiotics against bacteria. *J Med Microbiol* 59: 1469–1476.

Hisano, M., K. Yamaguchi, Y. Inoue, et al. 2003. Inhibitory effect of catechin against the superantigen staphylococcal enterotoxin B (SEB). *Arch Dermatol Res* 295(5): 183–189.

Howard, K.C., E.K. Dennis, D.S. Watt, and S. Garneau-Tsodikova. 2020. A comprehensive overview of the medicinal chemistry of antifungal drugs: Perspectives and promise. *Chem Soc Rev* 49(8): 2426–2480.

Jiao, T., C. Li, X. Zhuang, S. Cao, H. Chen, and S. Zhang. 2015. The new liquid-liquid extraction method for separation of phenolic compounds from coal tar. *Chem Eng J* 266: 148–155.

Kabera, J.N., E. Semana, A.R. Mussa, and X. He. 2014. Plant secondary metabolites: Biosynthesis, classification, function and pharmacological properties. *J Pharm Pharmacol* 2: 377–392.

Kainz, K., M.A. Bauer, F. Madeo, and D. Carmona-Gutierrez. 2020. Fungal infections in humans: The silent crisis. *Microb Cel* 7(6): 143–145.

Kanehisa, M., and S. Goto. 2000. KEGG: Kyoto encyclopedia of genes and genomes. *Nucleic Acids Res* 28: 27–30.

Kang, B.K., J.S. Lee, S.K. Chon, et al. 2004. Development of self-microemulsifying drug delivery systems (SMEDDS) for oral bioavailability enhancement of simvastatin in beagle dogs. *Int J Pharm* 274(1–2): 65–73.

Kavvas, E.S., E. Catoiu, N. Mih, et al. 2018. Machine learning and structural analysis of Mycobacterium tuberculosis pan-genome identifies genetic signatures of antibiotic resistance. *Nat Commun* 9: 1–9.

Kemp, W. 1991. Infrared spectroscopy. In *Organic Spectroscopy*, 19–56. Macmillan Press Ltd.: London.

Kingston, H.M., and L.B. Jessie. 1998. *Introduction to Microwave Sample Preparation.* American Chemical Society: Washington, DC.

Kivimaki, A.S., A. Siltari, P.I. Ehlers, R. Korpela, and H. Vapaatalo. 2013. Lingonberry juice lowers blood pressure of spontaneously hypertensive rats (SHR). *J Funct Foods* 5: 1432–1440.

Koffi, E., T. Sea, Y. Dodehe, and S. Soro. 2010. Effect of solvent type on extraction of polyphenols from twenty three ivorian plants. *J Anim Plant Sci* 5: 550–558.

Köhler, J.R., A. Casadevall, and J. Perfect. 2014. The spectrum of fungi that infects humans. *Cold Spring Harb Perspect Med* 5(1): a019273.

Krauze-Baranowska, M., M. Majdan, R. Hałasa, et al. 2014. The antimicrobial activity of fruits from some cultivar varieties of Rubus idaeus and Rubus occidentalis. *Food Funct* 5(10): 2536–2541.

Kumar, D. 2014. Salicylic acid signaling in disease resistance. *Plant Sci* 228: 127–134.

Lattanzio, V., V.M. Lattanzio, and A. Cardinali. 2006. Role of phenolics in the resistance mechanisms of plants against fungal pathogens and insects. *Phytochem Adv Res* 661: 23–67.

Lee, K.A., S.H. Moon, K.T. Kim, A.F. Mendonca, and H.D. Paik. 2010. Antimicrobial effects of various flavonoids on Escherichia coli O157: H7 cell growth and lipopolysaccharide production. *Food Sci Biotechnol* 19: 257–261.

Leshem, R., I. Maharshak, E. Ben-Jacob, I. Ofek, and I. Kremer. 2011. The effect of non-dialyzable material (NDM) cranberry extract on formation of contact lens biofilm by Staphylococcus epidermidis. *Invest Ophthalmol Vis Sci* 52(7): 4929–4934.

Li, H. 2013. Aligning sequence reads, clone sequences and assembly contigs with BWA-MEM. *arXiv* arXiv: 1303.3997.

Lim, A., N. Subhan, J.A. Jazayeri, G. John, T. Vanniasinkam, and H.K. Obied. 2016. Plant phenols as antibiotic boosters: In vitro interaction of olive leaf phenols with ampicillin. *Phyther Res* 30: 503–509.

Lin, D., M. Xiao, J. Zhao, et al. 2016. An overview of plant phenolic compounds and their importance in human nutrition and management of type 2 diabetes. *Molecules (Basel, Switzerland)* 21(10): 10–15.

Lipińska, L., E. Klewicka, and M. Sójka. 2014. The structure, occurrence and biological activity of ellagitannins: A general review. *Acta Sci Pol Technol Aliment* 13(3): 289–299.

Liu, H., Y. Mou, J. Zhao, et al. 2010. Flavonoids from Halostachys caspica and their antimicrobial and antioxidant activities. *Molecules* 15(11): 7933–7945.

Liu, M., M. Feng, K.Yang, et al. 2020. Transcriptomic and metabolomic analyses reveal antibacterial mechanism of astringent persimmon tannin against methicillin-resistant staphylococcus aureus isolated from pork. *Food Chem* 309: 125692.

Liu, M.M., L. Zhou, P.L. He, et al. 2012. Discovery of flavonoid derivatives as anti-HCV agents *via* pharmacophore search combining molecular docking strategy. *Eur J Med Chem* 52: 33–43.

Liu, R., H. Zhang, M. Yuan, et al. 2013a. Synthesis and biological evaluation of apigenin derivatives as antibacterial and antiproliferative agents. *Molecules* 18(9): 11496–11511.

Liu, X.L., Y.Q. Hao, L. Jin, Z.J. Xu, T.A. McAllister, and Y. Wang. 2013b. Anti-Escherichia coli O157:H7 properties of purple prairie clover and sainfoin condensed tannins. *Molecules* 18(2): 2183–2199.

Lobiuc, A., N.E. Pavăl, I.I. Mangalagiu, et al. 2023. Future antimicrobials: Natural and functionalized phenolics. *Molecules* 28(1114): 1–16.

Lou, Z., H. Wang, S. Zhu, C. Ma, and Z. Wang. 2011. Antibacterial activity and mechanism of action of chlorogenic acid. *J Food Sci* 76(6): M398–M403.

Luo, G., R.K. Hamatake, D.M. Mathis, et al. 2000. De novo initiation of RNA synthesis by the RNA-dependent RNA polymerase (NS5B) of hepatitis C virus. *J Virol* 74(2): 851–863.

Mahe, P., and M. Tournoud. 2018. Predicting bacterial resistance from whole-genome sequences using k-mers and stability selection. *BMC Bioinform* 19: 383.

Mirzoeva, O.K., R.N. Grishanin, and P.C. Calder. 1997. Antimicrobial action of propolis and some of its components: The effects on growth, membrane potential and motility of bacteria. *Microbiol Res* 152(3): 239–246.

Mohan, J., A.A. Gandhi, B.C. Bhavya, et al. 2006. Caspase-2 triggers Bax-Bak-dependent and -independent cell death in colon cancer cells treated with resveratrol. *J Biol Chem* 281(26): 17599–17611.

More, G.K., J. Vervoort, P.A. Steenkamp, and G. Prinsloo. 2022. Metabolomic profile of medicinal plants with anti-RVFV activity. *Heliyon* 8: e08936.

Mulinacci, N., D. Prucher, M. Peruzzi, et al. 2004. Commercial and laboratory extracts from artichoke leaves: Estimation of caffeoyl esters and flavonoidic compounds content. *J Pharm Biomed Anal* 34: 349–357.

Nayak, M.K., A.S. Agrawal, S. Bose, et al. 2014. Antiviral activity of baicalin against influenza virus H1N1-pdm09 is due to modulation of NS1-mediated cellular innate immune responses. *J Antimicrob Chemother* 69(5): 1298–1310.

Nitta, T., T. Arai, H. Takamatsu, et al. 2002. Antibacterial activity of extracts prepared from tropical and subtropical plants on methicillin-resistant *Staphylococcus aureus. J Health Sci* 48: 273–276.

Ogidi, O.I. 2022. Phytochemicals of Bioactive compounds of Brassica Juncea (Brown Mustard) Seeds. In Ozturk, M. and G.B. Ameenah (eds) *Medicinal and Aromatic Plants of the World.* Encylopedia of Life Support Systems (EOLSS). United Nations Educational, Scientific and Cultural Organization, Abu Dhabi.

Ogidi, O.I. 2023. Sustainable utilization of important medicinal plants in Africa. In Izah, SC and M. C. Ogwu (eds) *Sustainable Utilization and Conservation of Africa's Biological Resources and Environment, Sustainable Development and Biodiversity.* Bugis, Singapore: Springer Nature Singapore Pte Ltd, Germany.

Ogidi, O.I., M.N. Ayebabogha, P.U. Eze, O. Omu, and C.E. Okafor. 2021b. Determination of phytoconstituents and antimicrobial activities of aqueous and methanol extracts of neem (*Azadirachta indica*) leaves. *Int J Pharmacogn Chem* 2(2): 60–67.

Ogidi, O.I., P. Chukwudi, A.I. Ibe, P.U. Eze, and T.N. Canus. 2021c. Preliminary phytochemical profile and antimicrobial potentials of white-green African garden egg (*solanum macrocarpon*) fruits obtained from Yenagoa. *ASIO J Pharm Herbal Medi Res* 7(2): 1–5.

Ogidi, O.I. and U.E. Enenebeaku. 2023. Medicinal potentials of Aloe vera (*Aloe barbadensis* Miller): Technologies for the production of therapeutics. In Izah, SC and M. C. Ogwu (eds) *Sustainable Utilization and Conservation of Africa's Biological Resources and Environment, Sustainable Development and Biodiversity*. Bugis, Singapore: Springer Nature Singapore Pte Ltd, Germany.

Ogidi, O.I., N.G. Esie, and O.G. Dike. 2019b. Phytochemical, proximate and mineral compositions of *Bryophyllum Pinnatum* (Never die) medicinal plant. *J Pharmacogn Phytochem* 8(1): 629–635.

Ogidi, O.I., D.G. George, and N.G. Esie. 2019a. Ethnopharmacological properties of *Vernonia amygdalina* (Bitter Leave) Medicinal plant. *J Medi Plants Stud* 7(2): 175–181.

Ogidi, O.I., and J.C. Julius. 2021. Assessment of ethno-pharmacological compounds and antimicrobial efficacy of white onion (*Allium cepa*) bulb extracts against pathogenic microbial isolates. *PhytoChem BioSub J* 15(2): 167–174.

Ogidi, O.I., C.C. Okore, U.M. Akpan, M.N. Ayebabogha, and C.J. Onukwufo. 2021a. Evaluation of antimicrobial activity and bioactive phytochemical properties of mango (*Mangifera Indica*) stem-bark extracts. *Int J Pharmacogn* 8(5): 189–195.

Ogidi, O.I., O. Omu, and P.A. Ezeagba. 2019c. Ethno pharmacologically active components of *Brassica Juncea* (Brown Mustard) seeds. *Int J Pharm Res Dev* 1(1): 9–13.

Ogidi, O.I., P.S. Tobia, D.N. Ijere, et al. 2022. Investigation of bioactive compounds and antimicrobial sensitivity of pawpaw (*carica papaya*) leave extracts against morbific microorganisms. *J Appl Pharm Res* 10(1): 21–28.

Oh, E., and B. Jeon. 2015. Synergistic anti-campylobacter jejuni activity of fluoroquinolone and macrolide antibiotics with phenolic compounds. *Front Microbiol* 6: 1129.

Olmo-García, L., A. Bajoub, S. Benlamaalam, et al. 2018. Establishing the phenolic composition of *Olea europaea* L. leaves from cultivars grown in morocco as a crucial step towards their subsequent exploitation. *Molecules (Basel, Switzerland)* 23: 10.

Pereira, D., P. Valento, J. Pereira, and P. Andrade. 2009. Phenolics: From chemistry to biology. *Molecules* 14(6): 2202–2211.

Pohjala, L., A. Utt, M. Varjak, et al. 2011. Inhibitors of alphavirus entry and replication identified with a stable Chikungunya replicon cell line and virus-based assays. *PLoS ONE* 6(12): e28923.

Popova, I.E., C. Hall, and A. Kubátová. 2009. Determination of lignans in flaxseed using liquid chromatography with time-of-flight mass spectrometry. *J Chromatogr A* 1216: 217–229.

Possemiers, S., S. Bolca, W. Verstraete, and A. Heyerick. 2011. The intestinal microbiome: A separate organ inside the body with themetabolic potential to influence the bioactivity of botanicals. *Fitoterapia* 82: 53–66.

Prasch, S., and F. Bucar. 2015. Plant derived inhibitors of bacterial efflux pumps: An update. *Phytochem Rev* 14: 961–974.

Puupponen-Pimiä, R., L. Nohynek, C. Meier, et al. 2001. Antimicrobial properties of phenolic compounds from berries. *J Appl Microbiol* 90(4): 494–507.

Radji, M., R.A. Agustama, B. Elya, and C.R. Tjampakasari. 2013. Antimicrobial activity of green tea extract against isolates of methicillin-resistant Staphylococcus aureus and multi-drug resistant Pseudomonas aeruginosa. *Asian Pac J Trop Biomed* 3(8): 663–667.

Sakagami, Y., A. Sawabe, S. Komemushi, et al. 2007. Antibacterial activity of stilbene oligomers against vancomycin-resistant Enterococci (VRE) and methicillin-resistant Staphylococcus aureus (MRSA) and their synergism with antibiotics. *Biocontrol Sci* 12(1): 7–14.

Salinas-Moreno, Y., C. García-Salinas, J.K. Ramírez-Díaz, and I. La Alemán-de Torre. 2017. Phenolic compounds in maize grains and its nixtamalized products. In M. Soto-Hernández, M. Palma-Tenango, and M.D.R. Garcia-Mateos (eds.), *Importance and Applications. Phenolic Compounds—Natural Sources*. IntechOpen, London.

Sarajlija, H., N. Čkelj, D. Novotni, et al. 2012. Preparation of flaxseed for lignan determination by gas chromatography-mass spectrometry method. *Czech J Food Sci* 30: 45–52.

Scholz, M., D.V. Ward, E. Pasolli, et al. 2016. Strain-level microbial epidemiology and population genomics from shotgun metagenomics. *Nat Methods* 13: 435–438.

Shaaban, H.A. 2020. Essential oil as antimicrobial agents: Efficacy, stability, and safety issues for food application. In *Essential Oils-Bioactive Compounds, New Perspectives and Applications*, 1–33. IntechOpen, London.

Siriwong, S., K. Thumanu, T. Hengpratom, and G. Eumkeb. 2015. Synergy and mode of action of ceftazidime plus quercetin or luteolin on streptococcus pyogenes. *Evid Based Complement Alternat Med* 2015759459.

Sithisarn, P., M. Michaelis, M. Schubert-Zsilavecz, and J. Cinatl Jr. 2013. Differential antiviral and anti-inflammatory mechanisms of the flavonoids biochanin A and baicalein in H5N1 influenza A virusinfected cells. *Antiviral Res* 97(1): 41–48.

Stan, D., A.M. Enciu, A.L. Mateescu, et al. 2021. Natural compounds with antimicrobial and antiviral effect and nanocarriers used for their transportation. *Front Pharmacol* 12(723233): 1–25.

Stapleton, P.D., S. Shah, S., J.C. Anderson, Y. Hara, J.M. Hamilton-Miller, and P.W. Taylor. 2004. Modulation of β-lactam resistance in Staphylococcus aureus by catechins and gallates. *Int J Antimicrob Agents* 23(5): 462–467.

Stavropoulou, E., C.C. Voidarou, G. Rozos, et al. 2022. Antimicrobial evaluation of various honey types against carbapenemase-producing gram-negative clinical isolates. *Antibiotics* 11: 422.

Sudano-Roccaro, A., A.R. Blanco, F. Giuliano, D. Rusciano, and V. Enea. 2004. Epigallocatechin-gallate enhances the activity of tetracycline in staphylococci by inhibiting its efflux from bacterial cells. *Antimicrob Agents Chemother* 48(6): 1968–1973.

Sung, W.S., and D.G. Lee. 2010. Antifungal action of chlorogenic acid against pathogenic fungi, mediated by membrane disruption. *Pure Appl Chem* 82: 219–226.

Suzara, S., D.A. Costa, Y. Gariepyb, S.C.S. Rochaa, and V. Raghavanb. 2013. Spilanthol extraction using microwave: Calibration curve for gas chromatography. *Chem Eng Trans* 32: 1783–1788.

Suzuki, S., T. Horinouchi, and C. Furusawa. 2014. Prediction of antibiotic resistance by gene expression profiles. *Nat Commun* 5: 1–12.

Tegos, G., and F. Stermitz. 2002. Multidrug pump inhibitors uncover remarkable activity of plant antimicrobials. *Antimicrob Agents Chemother* 46: 3133–3141.

Tombola, F., S. Campello, L. De Luca, et al. 2003. Plant polyphenols inhibit VacA, a toxin secreted by the gastric pathogen Helicobacter pylori. *FEBS Lett* 543(1–3): 184–189.

Urbano, M., M.D. Luque de Castro, P.M. Pérez, J. García-Olmo, and M.A. Gómez-Nieto. 2006. Ultraviolet—visible spectroscopy and pattern recognition methods for differentiation and classification of wines. *Food Chem* 97: 166–175.

Vaou, N., E. Stavropoulou, C. Voidarou, et al. 2022. Interactions between medical plant-derived bioactive compounds: Focus on antimicrobial combination effects. *Antibiotics* 11(1014): 1–23.

Verdrengh, M., L.V. Collins, P. Bergin, and A. Tarkowski. 2004. Phytoestrogen genistein as an anti-staphylococcal agent. *Microbes Infect* 6(1): 86–92.

Vikram, A., P.R. Jesudhasan, G.K. Jayaprakasha, S.D. Pillai, A. Jayaraman, and B.S. Patil. 2011. Citrus flavonoid represses Salmonella pathogenicity island 1 and motility in S. Typhimurium LT2. *Int J Food Microbiol* 145(1): 28–36.

Wang, W.B., H.C. Lai, P.R. Hsueh, R.Y. Chiou, S.B. Lin, and S.J. Liaw. 2006. Inhibition of swarming and virulence factor expression in Proteus mirabilis by resveratrol. *J Med Microbiol* 55(Pt 10): 1313–1321.

Wattam, A.R., D. Abraham, O. Dalay, et al. 2014. PATRIC, the bacterial bioinformatics database and analysis resource. *Nucleic Acids Res* 42: D581–D591.

Wen, A., P. Delaquis, K. Stanich, and P. Toivonen. 2003. Antilisterial activity of selected phenolic acids. *Food Microbiol* 20: 305–311.

Williams, O.J., G.S.V. Raghavan, V. Orsat, and J. Dai. 2004. Microwave-assisted extraction of capsaicinoids from capsicum fruit. *J Food Biochem* 28: 113–122.

Williamson, G., and M.N. Clifford. 2010. Colonic metabolites of berry polyphenols: The missing link to biological activity? *Br J Nutr* 104(Suppl. 3): S48–S66.

Wong, P.Y.Y., and D.D. Kitts. 2006. Studies on the dual antioxidant and antibacterial properties of parsley (petroselinum crispum) and cilantro (coriandrum sativum) extracts. *Food Chem* 97: 505–515.

Wu, P., X. Tang, R. Jian, et al. 2021. Chemical composition, antimicrobial and insecticidal activities of essential oils of discarded perfume lemon and leaves (Citrus Limon (L.) Burm. F.) as possible sources of functional botanical agents. *Front Chem* 9: 370.

Wu, W., R. Li, X. Li, et al. 2015. Quercetin as an antiviral agent inhibits influenza A virus (IAV) entry. *Virus* 8(1): 6.

Xiao, Z.P., Z.Y. Peng, M.J. Peng, W.B. Yan, Y.Z. Ouyang, and H.L. Zhu. 2011. Flavonoids health benefits and their molecular mechanism. *Mini-Rev Med Chem* 11: 169–177.

Xie, Y., B. Huang, K. Yu, F. Shi, T. Liu, and W. Xu. 2013. Caffeic acid derivatives: A new type of influenza neuraminidase inhibitors. *Bioorg Med Chem Lett* 23(12): 3556–3560.

Xu, L., W. Su, J. Jin, et al. 2014. Identification of luteolin as enterovirus 71 and coxsackievirus A16 inhibitors through reporter viruses and cell viability-based screening. *Viruses* 6(7): 2778–2795.

Yang, J.H., S.N. Wright, M. Hamblin, et al. 2019. A white-box machine learning approach for revealing antibiotic mechanisms of action. *Cell* 177: 1649–1661.e9.

Yi, S., W. Wang, F. Bai, et al. 2014. Antimicrobial effect and membrane-active mechanism of tea polyphenols against Serratia marcescens. *World J Microbiol Biotechnol* 30(2): 451–460.

Yu, J., M. Ahmedna, and I. Goktepe. 2005. Effects of processing methods and extraction solvents on concentration and antioxidant activity of peanut skin phenolics. *Food Chem* 90(1–2): 199–206.

Zampieri, M., T. Enke, V. Chubukov, V. Ricci, L. Piddock, and U. Sauer. 2017. Metabolic constraints on the evolution of antibiotic resistance. *Mol Syst Biol* 13.

Zankari, E., R. Allesøe, K.G. Joensen, L.M. Cavaco, O. Lund, and F.M. Aarestrup. 2017. PointFinder: A novel web tool for WGS-based detection of antimicrobial resistance associated with chromosomal point mutations in bacterial pathogens. *J Antimicrob Chemother* 72: 2764–2768.

Zhang, W., H. Qiao, Y. Lv, et al. 2014. Apigenin inhibits enterovirus-71 infection by disrupting viral RNA association with trans-acting factors. *PLoS ONE* 9(10): e110429.

Zhang, Z., X. Pang, D. Xuewu, Z. Ji, and Y. Jiang. 2005. Role of peroxidase in anthocyanin degradation in litchi fruit pericarp. *Food Chem* 90: 47–52.

Zhao, X., L. Chen, J. Wu, Y. He, and H.Yang. 2020. Elucidating antimicrobial mechanism of nisin and grape seed extract against Listeria monocytogenes in broth and on shrimp through NMR-based metabolomics approach. *Int J Food Microbiol* 319: 108494.

Zheng, Y.Z., and S. Wang. 2019. Advances in antifungal drug measurement by liquid chromatography-mass spectrometry. *Clinica Chim Acta Int J Clin Chem* 491: 132–145.

9 Computational Evaluation of Peanut Skin Bioactive Compounds for Cancer Treatment

Somya Hari,†, Abirla Murugan**, and Meenambiga Setti Sudharsan***
*Vels Institute of Science, Technology, and Advanced Studies; **University of Pavia
†Corresponding Author: sowmya.se@velsuniv.ac.in

9.1 INTRODUCTION

The peanut, taxonomically known as *Arachis hypogaea*, is a legume crop with edible seeds. They have been taken as food for many years. They have been reported to be used as a food mostly in the Indian subcontinent, East and West Asia, Africa, and North America. They are a rich source of proteins, antioxidants, vitamin B, minerals like iron, magnesium, etc. The research studies have reported that peanut and their parts have several health benefits (Arya et al., 2016; Rohimah et al., 2021). Among the parts, its skin, which is a seed coat over the edible part, has various biomolecules with specific functions (Çiftçi and Suna, 2022). They have an abundant number of antioxidants and dietary fibres (Akhtar et al., 2014; Chukwumah et al., 2009). About 3 percent of a peanut seed is made up of the skin, which is high in phenolic compounds and antioxidants. (Larrauri et al., 2016; Elsorady and Ali, 2018). They are rich in monosaturated and polyunsaturated fatty acids. Peanuts are a fantastic supply of plant-based protein because they contain between 22% and 30% of their total calories as protein. Antioxidants aid in defending the body against oxidative stress, which is a factor in many cancers and other illnesses (Wang et al., 2007). Peanut skins also contain the powerful compound known as resveratrol (Medina-Bolivar et al., 2007). Resveratrol has been demonstrated to help improve stamina, decrease inflammation, and reduce the risk of getting heart disease. (Udenigwe et al., 2008). Like resveratrol, there are other phyto sterols and flavonoids that show antioxidant and anti-cancer properties, which are available in peanuts (Nepote et al., 2005; Prabasheela et al., 2015; Huang et al., 2010; Mohammadhosseinpour et al., 2023). Though peanut skin is a by-product from industries, they can be processed and the available compounds can be extracted and studied for various uses (Zhao et al., 2012; Zhu et al., 2016). Apart from peanut skin, its various parts like pods have also been reported to have medicinal values (Taha et al., 2012; Syed et al., 2021).

 DOI: 10.1201/9781003354437-9

In human cells, the Chromobox protein homolog 3 (CBX3) encodes the heterochromatin protein 1 γ (HP1γ), a DNA-binding subunit of heterochromatin. Here in this approach the molecular docking was performed with the protein CBX3, which has been reported to be expressed highly in cancer cells and promotes proliferation of cancer cells (Zhong et al., 2019; Chen et al., 2018). Among various malignant cancers, lung cancer was among them (Ettinger et al., 2010). About 85% of cancer patients diagnosed with lung cancer are reported to be caused by non–small cell lung cancer (NSLC) (Gridelli et al., 2015; Chen et al., 2014). NSLC is highly instigated by genetic alterations and by the adverse effects of smoking (Herbst et al., 2018). The protein HP1γ has also been stated to enhance the proliferation of lung cancer cells (Alam et al., 2018).

This work involved gas chromatography–mass spectrum (GC-MS) analysis of peanut skin to detect the unknown compounds. Then the detected compounds were screened for their pharmacokinetic properties, and the selected compounds were docked against the receptor molecule.

9.1.1 Taxonomic Information

Kingdom: Plantae
Unranked: Angiosperms
  Eudicots
  Rosids
Order: Fabales
Family: Fabaceae
Genus: Arachis
Species: A. hypogaea

Parts:

- Shell—outer covering, in contact with dirt
- Cotyledons (two)—main edible part
- Seed coat—brown paper-like covering of the edible part
- Radicle—embryonic root at the bottom of the cotyledon, which can be snapped off
- Plumule—embryonic shoot emerging from the top of the radicle

9.2 REVIEW OF THE LITERATURE

Peanuts have been used for various research purposes. Apart from its common properties, it has some novelties to be explored. From examination of the earlier literary work, the medicinal values of peanut and its parts have been studied and the gap of work was analysed and experimented with.

Black peanut skin (BPS) contains anthocyanins with physicochemical stability and the capacity to inhibit digestive enzymes was assessed earlier. The in vitro cell research conducted in this work shows that anthocyanins from BPS demonstrated a strong anti-adipogenesis potential in 3T3-L1 cells by inhibiting the expression of the major adipogenic transcription factors and associated genes. This study emphasizes the possibility that anthocyanins, a natural food colorant with multiple functions, can be found in abundance in black peanut shell. Anthocyanins have greater heat stability, according to the findings (Peng et al., 2019).

Studies on induced hyperglycaemia using in vivo and in vitro techniques are assessed using peanut skin extract made from polyphenol-rich peanut skins (Haruna et al., 2023). The impact of the peanut skin extract on cell viability after exposure to elevated glucose concentrations was investigated using HepG2 (human hepatocellular liver carcinoma) cell lines. The impact of peanut skin extract on sublingual glucose tolerance was examined in vivo. A protective effect against hyperglycaemia-induced cell death was demonstrated by peanut skin extract, which effectively attenuated the decline in cell viability in high glucose-treated HepG2 cells. The peanut skin extract treatment with the glucose reference led to a noticeably lower peak blood glucose response, suggesting that it was successful in reducing the glycaemic response, but there was no change in the glycaemic response area in any treatments using the tolerance test. According to this research, peanut skin phenolic extract has an anti-diabetic effect and is a valuable food ingredient (Christman et al., 2019).

Screening of antioxidant and anti-inflammatory properties of peanut skin. The nitric oxide assay was performed, and the phenolic content was estimated. The peanut skin extraction was made with two solvents (50% acetone, 90% ethanol). The procyanidin was analysed by HPLC. The anti-inflammatory property screening assay was performed with RAW 264.7 cells. The inhibition of COX-2 expression was observed in RAW 264.7 cells (Wanida et al., 2013).

The comparison of the antioxidant properties of the phenolic extracts were studied (Yu et al., 2007). The cytotoxicity activity various carcinoma cell lines have been studied with roasted peanut phenolic extracts. In the peanut parts that were investigated, both the extractable polyphenols (EPPs) and the non-extractable polyphenols (NEPPs) were identified (Taha et al., 2012). The results showed that NEPP was higher than EPP and that the skin had the greatest phenolic content. The antioxidant properties of phenolic compounds and their effects on the oxidative stability of flaxseed oil were also studied (Taha et al., 2012).

The various extractions using different solvents have been carried out with a microwave-assisted procedure to bring out the antioxidant content from the peanut skin extracts. This experiment has employed the polar solvents for extraction processes. The cytotoxicity activity of various carcinoma cell lines has been studied with roasted peanut phenolic extracts. (Tameshia et al., 2010).

The various extracts of peanut skins were compared. Different concentrations of ethanol were used as the solvent during the extraction process (0%, 30%, 50%, 70%, and 96% v/v in purified water). This experiment shows that the antioxidants are available in better quantity in the polar solvent than the non-polar. In this work the peanut skin particle size, the relation solvent-solid for the extraction, extraction contact time, and extraction stages have been analysed. (Nepote et al., 2005).

The effective activity of resveratrol, a compound which has been associated with reducing cancer risk and cardiovascular diseases, has studied. In this work ethanol extract of peanut was purified and analysed. From the extract, the resveratrol compound was isolated from peanuts and red wine and quantitatively analysed. The effectiveness of the compound from both extracts was comparatively analysed (Sanders et al., 2000).

The significant difference in roasted and unroasted peanut skins has been discussed. The free radical scavenging activity was performed for both the roasted and unroasted skin extracts. The phenol content, scavenging activity, and flavonoids are higher in the roasted skin extract. The extract of 80% ethanol had the largest concentration of total phenols and the greatest capacity to scavenge free radicals. In this work the antioxidant activity of the peanut roasted skin extracts were performed with sunflower oil (Sanders et al., 2000).

9.3 MATERIALS AND METHODS

9.3.1 GC-MS Analysis

GC-MS is coupled and used to detect the unknown compounds present in the sample. A total of 2.5 g of the dried peanut skin extract was mixed with 5 mL of ethanol solution and stored in a Falcon tube. The analysis was outsourced from Agilent Technologies, Chennai, by 3 October 2019. Individual compounds from the mixture resulted. The percentages of each compound present are indicated. Finally, GC-MS gives a quantitative analysis of the extracted sample (Leunissen et al., 1996).

9.3.2 Preparation of the Target Protein

CBX3 is the selected protein for the docking study. It was selected based on how this protein is expressed and regulated in NSLC patients. Using the ID 3TZD, protein was acquired from the Protein Data Bank. The three-dimensional structure of CBX3, a protein involved in lung cancer, was downloaded from PDB (PDB ID-3TZD). The protein was prepared by removing the non-bonded atoms, water molecules, using PymoL. The protein was found to have A and T chains, the water molecules were removed, and the protein was prepared by adding Kollman charges.

9.3.3 Ligand Preparation

The compounds characterized from GCMS were chosen as the ligand for docking. The structures of each compound were obtained from PubChem. The compounds were processed for Lipinski filters for the drug property using a free software package, SWISSADME. The compound that satisfies the Lipinski rule was chosen for docking studies. The pharmacokinetic properties of the ligands were predicted from the software SWISSADME. As the need for pharmacokinetic screening was essential and it was the preliminary step to study the drug molecule interaction with the receptor, it was necessary to test the drug-likeliness properties of these compounds from the peanut skin.

9.3.4 Molecular Docking by Arguslab

Each ligand was interacted with the receptor separately at the given active site, and the grid point size was calculated by Arguslab software itself (Kandasamy et al., 2012; Achutha et al., 2021). The interactions were visualized using the software Biovia Discovery Studio.

9.3.5 Molecular Docking Visualization

Ligand interaction was visualized using Discovery Studio Visualizer 3.1. This software package deals with many aspects of molecular docking like molecular modelling, antibody modelling, ligand-receptor interactions, and protein-protein interactions. It generates two-dimensional and three-dimensional structures to visualize and analyse the ligand-protein interaction patterns between them. The ligand-protein interactions were analysed for the bonding, arrangements, etc.

9.4 RESULTS

The GC-MS analysis of the ethanol extract from peanut skin was revealed the presence of 29 compounds. Some work has reported that sterols extracted from peanuts and their parts have a strong anti-cancer property (Soriano-Hernandez et al., 2015). The compounds have been isolated and screened for various therapeutic activities. The compounds from various parts of the peanut are qualitatively analysed by GC-MS and HPLC (Oldoni et al., 2016). The revealed compounds have many medicinal properties. The phytosterols present in the extract such as campsterol, stigmasterol, and siloxanes have potential antioxidant and anti-cancer properties (Awad and Fink, 2000; Awad et al., 2000). The presence of sesquiterpene indicates it has anti-microbial properties too. The bioactive compounds obtained from GC-MS analysis from peanut skin ethanol extract is given in Table 9.1. The expression of

TABLE 9.1
Biologically Active Chemical Compounds of Ethanol Extraction of Peanut Skin.

S. No	Biological Compounds	Molecular Formula	Structure
1	Azulene	$C_{10}H_8$	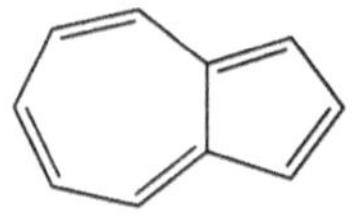 Azulene
2	Di-epi-alpha-cedrene	$C_{15}H_{24}$	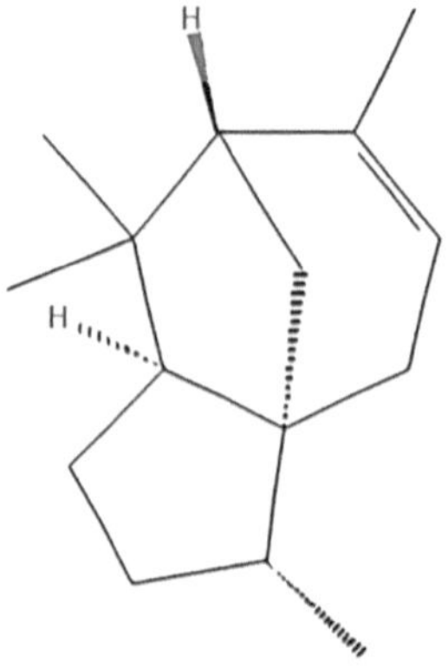 Di-epi-.alpha-cedrene

S. No	Biological Compounds	Molecular Formula	Structure
3	Benzene,1-(1,5-dimethyl-4-hexenyl)-4-methyl-	$C_{15}H_{22}$	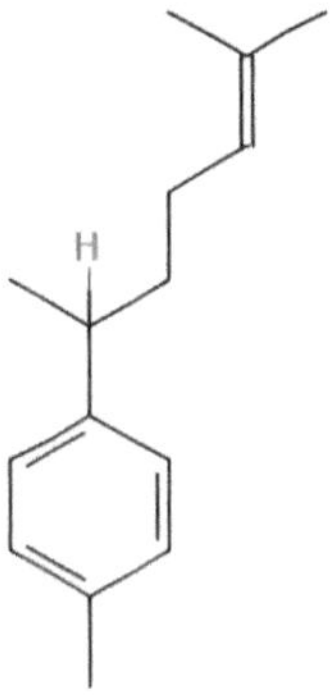 Benzene,1-(1,5-dimethyl-4-hexenyl)-4-methyl-
4	Beta-panasinsene	$C_{15}H_{24}$	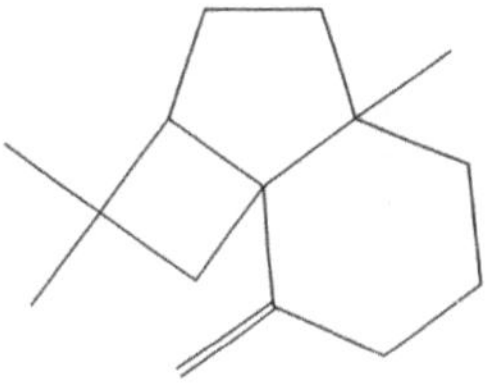 Beta-panasinsene
5	Isoledene	$C_{15}H_{24}$	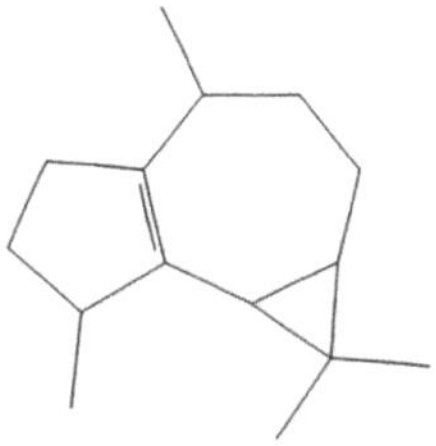 Isoledene
6	1,3-Cyclohexadiene,5-(1,5-dimethyl-4-hexenyl)-2-methyl-,[S-(R*,S*)]-	$C_{15}H_{24}$	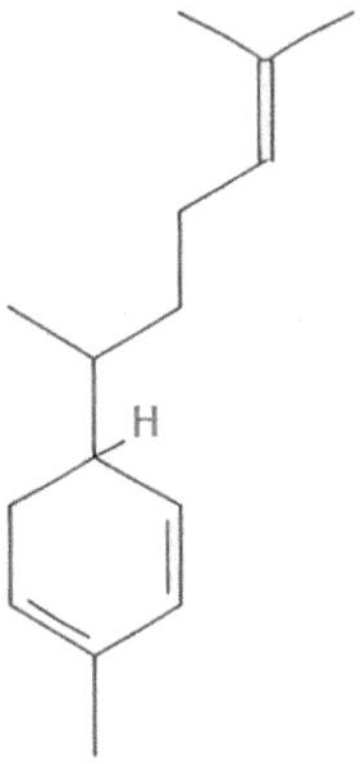 1,3-Cyclohexadiene, 5-(1,5-dimethyl-4-hexenyl)-2-methyl-,[S-(R*,S*)]-

(*Continued*)

TABLE 9.1 (*Continued*)
Biologically Active Chemical Compounds of Ethanol Extraction of Peanut Skin.

S. No	Biological Compounds	Molecular Formula	Structure
7	Beta-bisabolene	$C_{15}H_{24}$	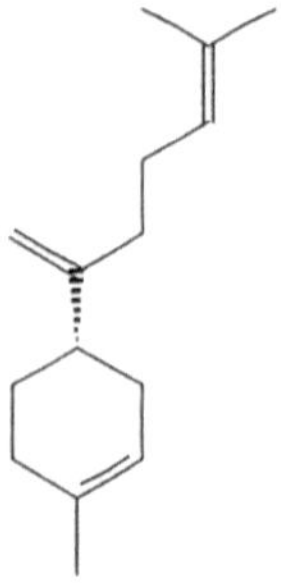 Beta-bisabolene
8	Alpha-farnesene	$C_{15}H_{24}$	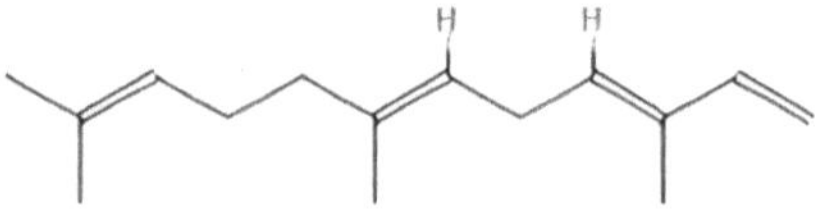 Alpha-farnasene
9	Phenol,2,4-bis (1,1-dimethylethyl)	$C_{14}H_{22}O$	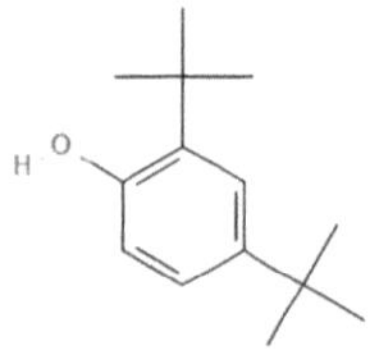 Phenol,2,4-bis(1,1-dimethylethyl)-
10	Cyclohexene,3-(1,5-dimethyl -4-hexenyl)-6-methylene-, [S-(R*,S*)]-	$C_{15}H_{24}$	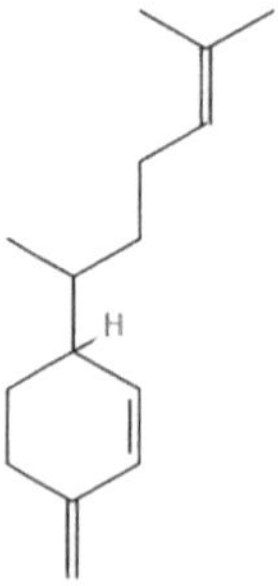 Cyclohexene,3-(1,5-dimethyl-4-hexenyl) -6-methylene-,[S-(R*,S*)]-
11	Diethyl phthalate	$C_{12}H_{14}O_4$	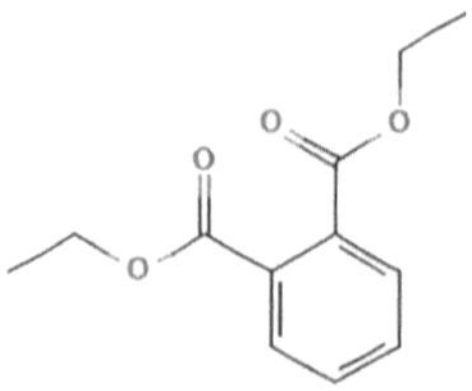 Diethyl phthalate

S. No	Biological Compounds	Molecular Formula	Structure
12	Cis-Z-,alpha-biabolene epoxide	$C_{15}H_{24}O$	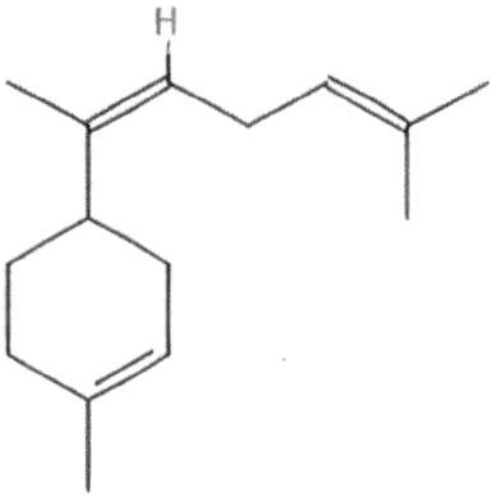 Cis-Z-,alpha-biabolene epoxide
13	Formic acid,3,7, 11-trimethyl-1,6, 10-dodecatrien-3-yl-ester	$C_{16}H_{26}O_2$	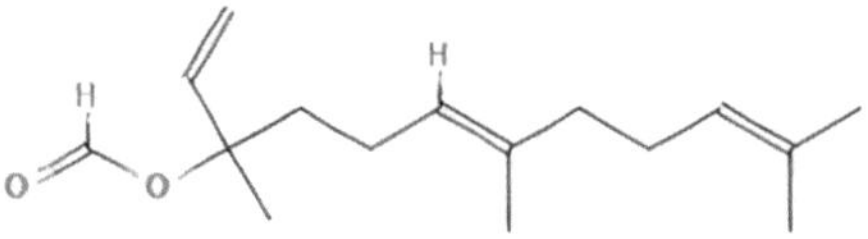 Formic acid,3,7,11-trimethyl-1,6, 10-dodecatrien-3-yl-ester
14	Phthalic acid, butyl undecyl ester	$C_{23}H_{36}O_4$	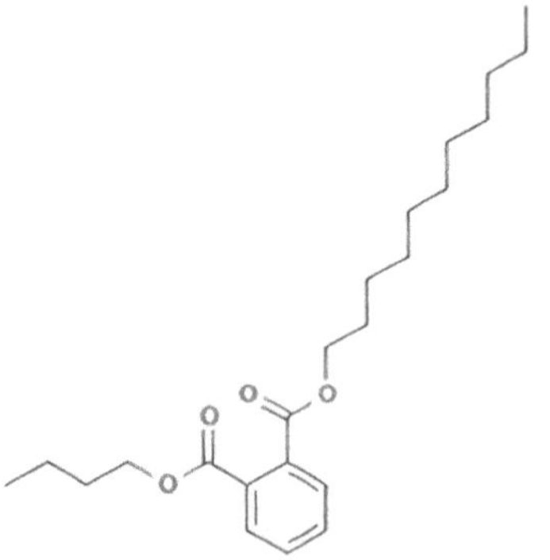 Phthalic acid, butyl undecyl ester
15	Hexadecanoic acid, ethyl ester	$C_{18}H_{36}O_2$	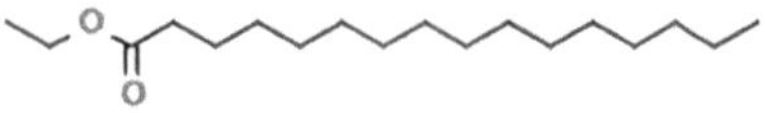 Hexadecanoic acid, ethyl ester
16	9,12-Octadecadienoic acid, ethyl ester	$C_{20}H_{38}O_2$	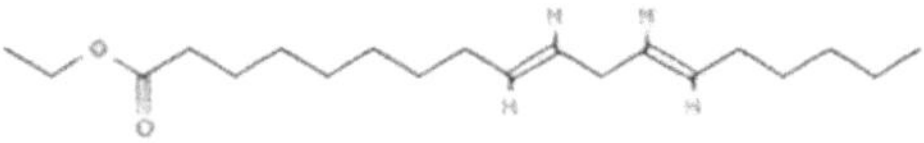 9,12-Octadecadienoic acid, ethyl ester
17	Ethyl oleate	$C_{20}H_{40}O_2$	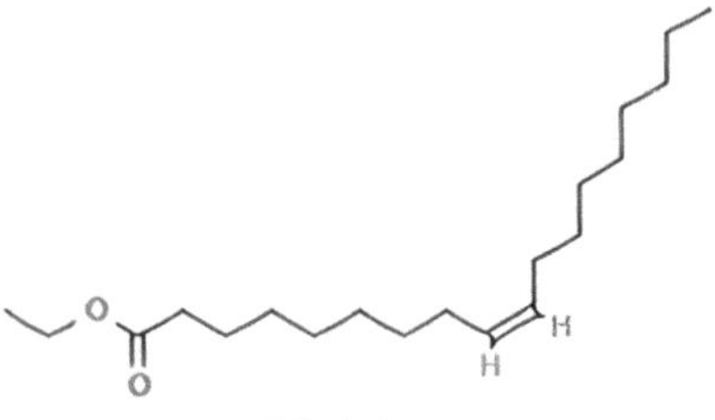 Ethyl oleate

(*Continued*)

TABLE 9.1 (*Continued*)
Biologically Active Chemical Compounds of Ethanol Extraction of Peanut Skin.

S. No	Biological Compounds	Molecular Formula	Structure
18	Octadecadienoic acid, ethyl ester	$C_{20}H_{40}O_2$	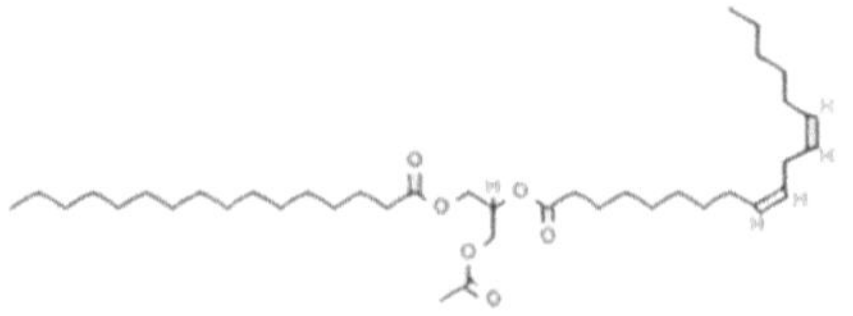 Octadecadienoic acid, ethyl ester
19	Oleic acid	$C_{18}H_{34}O_2$	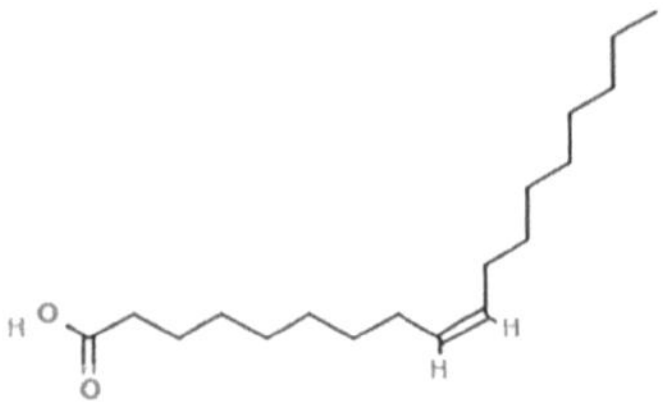 Oleic acid
20	Ethanol, 2-(9, 12-octadecadienyloxy)-,(Z,Z)-	$C_{20}H_{38}O_2$	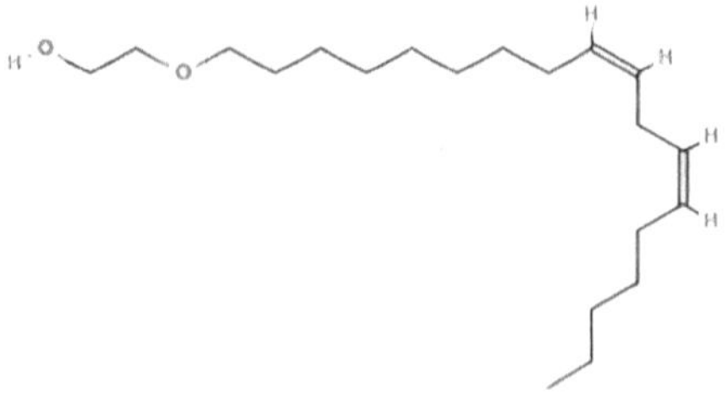 Ethanol, 2-(9,12-octadecadienyloxy)-,(Z,Z)-
21	9-Octadecenoicacid(Z),-2-hydroxy-1-(hydroxymethyl) ethyl ester	$C_{21}H_{40}O_4$	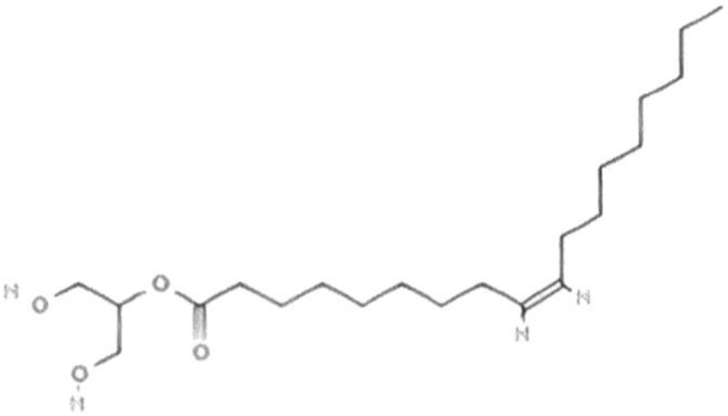 9-Octadecenoicacid(Z),-2-hydroxy -1-(hydroxymethyl)ethyl ester
22	7-Methyl-Z-tetradecen -1-ol acetate	$C_{17}H_{32}O_2$	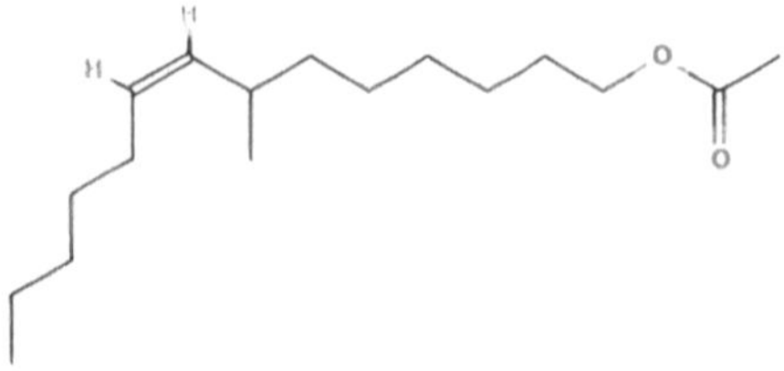 7-Methyl-Z-tetradecen-1-ol acetate

S. No	Biological Compounds	Molecular Formula	Structure
23	Octadecanal,2 -bromo-	$C_{18}H_{35}BrO$	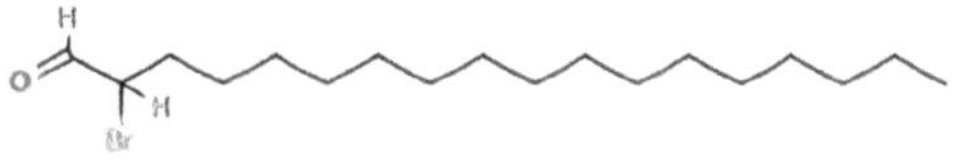 Octadecanal,2-bromo-
24	Octasiloxane 1,1,3,3,5,5, 7,7,9,9,11,11,13,13,15, 15-hexadecamethyl-	$C_{16}H_{50}O_7Si_8$	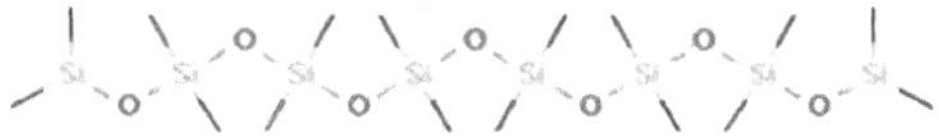 Octasiloxane 1,1,3,3,5,5,7,7,9,9,11,11,13, 13,15,15-hexadecamethyl-
25	Campsterol	$C_{28}H_{48}O$	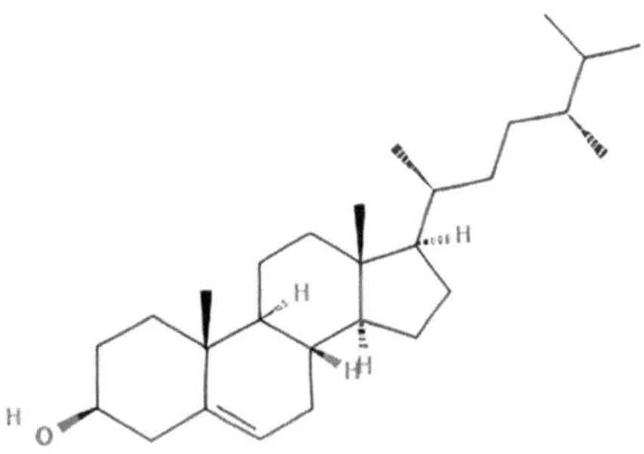 Campsterol
26	Stigmasterol	$C_{29}H_{48}O$	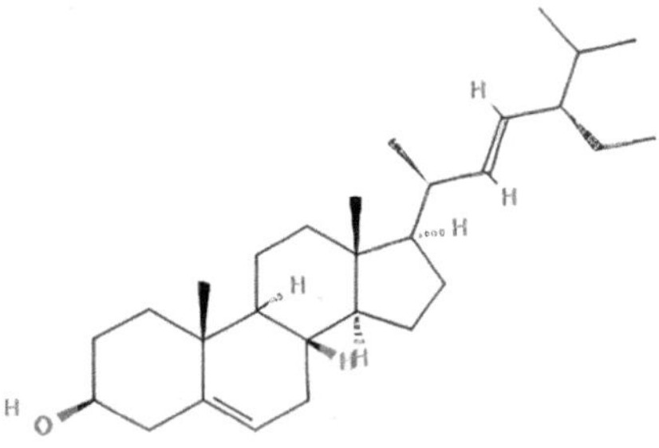 Stigmasterol
27	Gamma-sitosterol	$C_{29}H_{50}O$	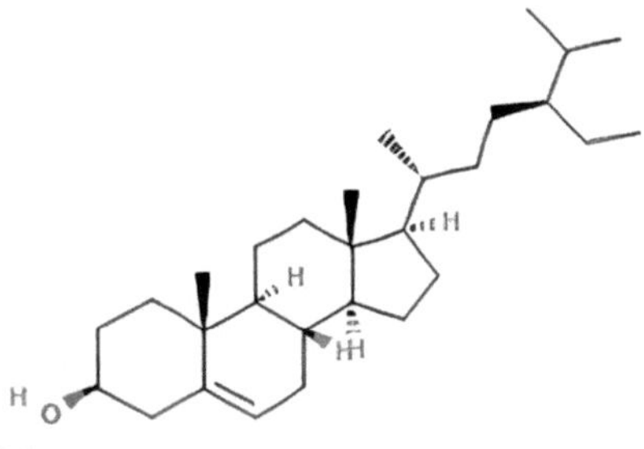 Gamma-sitosterol

(*Continued*)

TABLE 9.1 (*Continued*)
Biologically Active Chemical Compounds of Ethanol Extraction of Peanut Skin.

S. No	Biological Compounds	Molecular Formula	Structure
28	Spirost-8-en-11-one, 3-hydroxy-,(3.beta.,5. alpha.,14.beta.,20. beta.,22.beta.,25R)	$C_{27}H_{40}O_4$	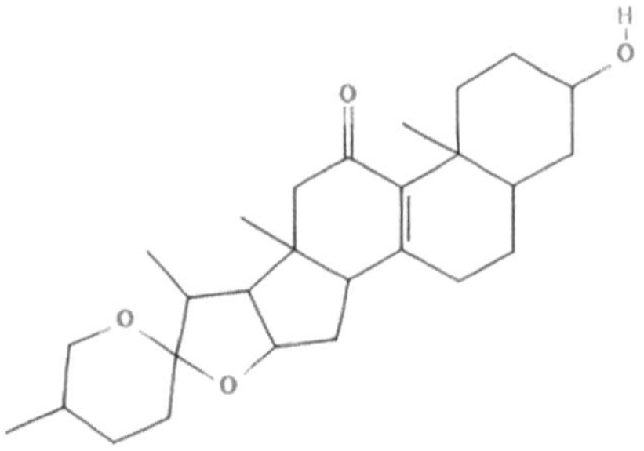 Spirost-8-en-11-one,3-hydroxy-, (3.beta.,5.alpha.,14.beta.,20.beta., 22.beta.,25R)
29	Heptasiloxane,1,1,3,3,5, 5,7,7,9,9,11,11,13, 13-tetradecamethyl	$C_{14}H_{44}O_6Si_7$	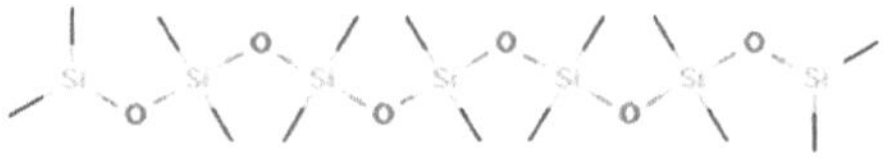 Heptasilox ane,1,1,3,3,5,5,7,7,9,9,11,11,13,13-tetradecamethyl

Note: The figures were adapted from the database PubChem.

CBX3 protein in the NSLC (Chang et al., 2018) and other type of cancers has been already reported (Lin et al., 2020b).

9.4.1 Description of the Compounds

From the GC-MS analysis various bioactive compounds like terpenes, sterols, and siloxanes resulted (Table 9.1). The description of these compounds is as follows:

- Azulene (Table 9.1, Row 1), an organic compound, is an isomer of naphthalene. It consists of two terpenoids, vetivazulene and guaiazulene. The chemical formula is $C_{10}H_8$ and the molecular weight is 128.17 g/mol. IUPAC name: azulene.
- Di-epi-alpha-cedrene (Table 9.1, Row 2) is a sesquiterpene with molecular formula $C_{15}H_{24}$ and molar mass of 204.2 g/mol. IUPAC name: 2,6,6,8-tetramethyltricyclo[5.3.1.0^{1,5}]undec-9-ene.
- Benzene,1-(1,5-dimethyl-4-hexenyl)-4-methyl (Table 9.1, Row 3) is also known as alpha-curcumene with the molecular formula $C_{15}H_{22}$ and a molar mass of 202.2 g/mol. IUPAC name: 1-methyl-4-(6-methylhept-5-en-2-yl) benzene.

- Beta-panasinsene (Table 9.1, Row 4) is an organic compound found in tea and ginseng oil. Its molar mass is 204.3 g/mol, and it contains zero hydrogen bond donors as well as acceptors. The molecular formula of the compound is $C_{15}H_{24}$. IUPAC name: 2,2,4*a*-trimethyl-8-methylidene-2*a*,3,4,5,6,7-hexahydro-1*H*-cyclobuta[i]indene.
- Isoledene (Table 9.1, Row 5) is an aromatic volatile compound with zero hydrogen acceptors and donors. The molecular mass of the compound is 204.3 g/mol. The molecular formula of the compound is $C_{15}H_{24.}$ IUPAC name: 1,1,4,7-tetramethyl-1*a*,2,3,4,5,6,7,7*b*-octahydrocyclopropa [e]azulene.
- 1,3-Cyclohexadiene,5-(1,5-dimethyl-4-hexenyl)-2-methyl-,[S-(R*·S*)] (Table 9.1, Row 6) is known as zingiberene, a constituent of ginger and anise. Its molar mass is 204.35 g/mol, and the molecular formula is $C_{15}H_{24.}$ IUPAC name: 2-methyl-5-(6-methylhept-5-en-2-yl)cyclohexa-1,3-diene.
- Beta-bisabolene (Table 9.1, Row 7) is found in many foods. Its molar mass is 204.35 g/mol, and the molecular formula is $C_{15}H_{24.}$ IUPAC name: (4S)-1-methyl-4-(6-methylhepta-1,5-dien-2-yl)cyclohexene.
- Alpha-farnesene (Table 9.1, Row 8) is a constituent of apple and found in the outer covering of some fruits, and it has zero hydrogen acceptors and donors. The molecular mass of the compound is 204.3 g/mol. The molecular formula of the compound is $C_{15}H_{24}$. IUPAC name: (3E,6E)-3,7,11-trimethyldodeca-1,3,6,10-tetraene.
- Phenol,2,4-bis(1,1-dimethylethyl) (Table 9.1, Row 9) is a compound reported to have antioxidant properties. The molecular mass of the compound is 206.2 g/mol. The molecular formula of the compound is $C_{15}H_{22}O$. IUPAC name: 2,4-ditert-butyl-6-(1-phenylethyl) phenol.
- Cyclohexene,3-(1,5-dimethyl-4-hexenyl)-6-methylene-,[S-(R*·S*)] (Table 9.1, Row 10) is an organic compound with zero hydrogen acceptors and donors. Its molar mass is 204.3 g/mol. The molecular formula of the compound is $C_{15}H_{24.}$ IUPAC name: 3-(6-methylhept-5-en-2-yl)-6-methylidenecyclohexene.
- Diethyl phthalate (Table 9.1, Row 11) is an organic molecule also known as o-benzenedicarboxylic acid diethyl ester. Its molecular mass is 222.1 g/mol and the molecular formula is $C_{12}H_{14}O_4$. IUPAC name: diethyl benzene-1,2-dicarboxylate.
- Cis-Z-,alpha-biabolene epoxide (Table 9.1, Row 12) is *cis* isomer z form of alpha-biabolene epoxide with a molecular formula of $C_{15}H_{24}O$ and molecular mass of 222.3 g/mol. IUPAC name: 1-methyl-4-[(2Z)-6-methylhepta-2,5-dien-2-yl]cyclohexene.
- Formic acid,3,7,11-trimethyl-1,6,10-dodecatrien-3-yl-ester (Table 9.1, Row 13) is a cyclic compound with molecular mass 250.3 g/mol. The molecular formula of this compound is $C_{16}H_{26}O_2$. IUPAC name: [(6E)-3,7,11-trimethyldodeca-1,6,10-trien-3-yl] formate.
- Phthalic acid, butyl undecyl ester (Table 9.1, Row 14) is a compound that has four hydrogen acceptors and zero hydrogen donors. The molecular formula of this compound is $C_{23}H_{36}O_4$ and the molar mass is 376.3 g/mol. IUPAC name: 1-O-butyl 2-O-undecyl benzene-1,2-dicarboxylate.

- Hexadecanoic acid, ethyl ester (Table 9.1, Row 15) is a straight chain ester of palmitic acid with molar mass 284.3 g/mol. The molecular formula of this compound is $C_{18}H_{36}O_2$. IUPAC name: ethyl hexadecanoate.
- 9,12-Octadecadienoic acid, ethyl ester (Table 9.1, Row 16) is a straight chain compound found in plant extracts with antioxidant properties. The molar mass of this compound is 308.3 g/mol. The molecular formula of this compound is $C_{20}H_{38}O_{2.}$ IUPAC name: ethyl (9E,12E)-octadeca-9,12-dienoate.
- Ethyl oleate (Table 9.1, Row 17) is a long chain fatty acid which is naturally found in trees like neem and camphor. The molar mass is 310.3 g/mol. The molecular formula of this compound is $C_{20}H_{40}O_2$. IUPAC name: ethyl (Z)-octadec-9-enoate.
- Octadecadienoic acid, ethyl ester (Table 9.1, Row 18) is a straight chain compound present in the seeds of many plants with anti-inflammatory properties. The molar mass is 312.3 g/mol. The molecular formula of this compound is $C_{20}H_{40}O_2$. IUPAC name: (1-acetyloxy-3-hexadecanoyloxypropan-2-yl) (9Z,12Z)-octadeca-9,12-dienoate.
- Oleic acid (Table 9.1, Row 19) is monounsaturated omega-9 fatty acid with molar mass 282.3 g/mol. The molecular formula of this compound is $C_{18}H_{34}O_2$. IUPAC name: (Z)-octadec-9-enoic acid.
- Ethanol, 2-(9,12-octadecadienyloxy)-,(Z,Z) (Table 9.1, Row 20) is an aliphatic compound have found to be present in flower extracts with a molar mass of 310.3 g/mol. The molecular formula of this compound is $C_{18}H_{34}O_2$. IUPAC name: 2-[(9Z,12Z)-octadeca-9,12-dienoxy] ethanol.
- 9-Octadecenoicacid(Z),-2-hydroxy-1-(hydroxymethyl)ethyl ester (Table 9.1, Row 21) is a straight chain aliphatic compound with molar mass of 310.5 g/mol. This compound was also found in bush weed. The molecular formula of this compound is $C_{21}H_{40}O_{4.}$ IUPAC name: 1,3-dihydroxypropan-2-yl (Z)-octadec-9-enoate.
- 7-Methyl-Z-tetradecen-1-ol acetate (Table 9.1, Row 22) is a straight chain aliphatic compound with molar mass of 268.4 g/mol. This compound is also found in the leaf extracts of several plants. The molar mass of this compound is $C_{17}H_{32}O_2$. IUPAC name: [(Z)-7-methyltetradec-8-enyl] acetate.
- Octadecanal,2-bromo (Table 9.1, Row 23) is a long chain aldehyde with molar mass 347.4 g/mol. The molecular formula for this compound is $C_{18}H_{35}BrO$. IUPAC name: 2-bromooctadecanal. This compound was also considered to be present in the plant extracts.
- Octasiloxane 1,1,3,3,5,5,7,7,9,9,11,11,13,13,15,15-hexadecamethyl (Table 9.1, Row 24) is a bulky silane compound with molecular mass 578.2 g/mol. The molecular formula for this compound is $C_{16}H_{50}O_7Si_8$. IUPAC name: 1,1,3,3,5,5,7,7,9,9,11,11,13,13,15,15-hexadecamethyloctasiloxane.
- Campesterol (Table 9.1, Row 25) is a phytosterol, and its structure is like that of cholesterol. The molar mass of this compound is 400.68 g/mol. The molecular formula of campestrol is $C_{28}H_{48}O$. IUPAC name: (2R,3R,4S,5S,6R)-2-[[(3S,8S,9S,10R,13R,14S,17R)-17-[(2R,5R)-5,6-dimethylheptan-2-yl]-10,13-dimethyl-2,3,4,7,8,9,11,12,14,15,16,17-dodecahydro-1H-cyclopenta[a]phenanthren-3-yl]oxy]-6-(hydroxymethyl)oxane-3,4,5-triol.

- Stigmasterol (Table 9.1, Row 26) is an unsaturated triterpene molecule which is also a phytosterol. The molar mass of the compound is 412.27 g/mol. The molecular formula is $C_{29}H_{48}O$. IUPAC name: (3S,8S,9S,10R,13R,14S,17R)-17[(E,2R,5S)-5-ethyl-6methylhept-3-en-2-yl]-10,13-dimethyl-2,3,4,7,8,9,11,12,14,15,16,17-dodecahydro-1H-cyclopenta[a]phenanthren-3-ol.
- Gamma.-sitosterol (Table 9.1, Row 27) is a stereoisomer of beta-sitosterol found in plants with anti-inflammatory properties. The molar mass is 414.4 g/mol. The molecular formula for this compound is $C_{29}H_{50}O$. IUPAC name: (3S,8S,9S,10R,13R,14S,17R)-17-[(2R,5S)-5-ethyl-6-methylheptan-2-yl]-10,13-dimethyl-2,3,4,7,8,9,11,12,14,15,16,17-dodecahydro-1H-cyclopenta[a] phenanthren-3-ol; hydrate.
- Spirost-8-en-11-one,3-hydroxy-,(3.beta.,5.alpha.,14.beta.,20.beta.,22.beta.,25R) (Table 9.1, Row 28) is a secondary metabolite that consists of a spiro ring with molar mass 428.4 g/mol. The molecular formula for this compound is $C_{27}H_{40}O_4$. IUPAC name: 16-hydroxy-5',7,9,13-tetramethylspiro[5-oxapentacyclo[10.8.0.02,9.04,8.013,18]icos-1(12)-ene-6,2'-oxane]-11-one.
- Heptasiloxane,1,1,3,3,5,5,7,7,9,9,11,11,13,13-tetradecamethyl (Table 9.1, Row 29) is a is a bulky silane compound with molecular mass 503.07 g/mol. The molecular formula for this compound is $C_{14}H_{44}O_6Si_7$. This compound was also found in plant leaf extracts. IUPAC name: 1,1,1,3,3,5,5,7,7,9, 9,11,11,13-tetradecamethylheptasiloxane.

Table 9.1 shows the presence of phytosterols that are rich in anti-cancer benefits (Shahzad et al., 2017). Among these compounds only 11 were eligible for docking, which satisfies the Lipinski rule. The rule comprises five sub-rules: molecular weight less than 500, log P value (<+5.6), less than five hydrogen donors, ten hydrogen bond acceptors, and a molar refractivity range of 40–130. Based on these criteria the compounds, were screened and chosen to dock against the receptor. Table 9.2 represents the Lipinski properties of the eligible compounds. The expression of CBX3 protein in NSLC has been reported (Chang et al., 2018). According to this report the chosen ligands are docked against the active site of the receptor. Table 9.3 and 9.4 showed the drug-likeliness properties and the docking interactions, respectively.

The eligible compounds are docked with the receptor of interest. Molecular docking was performed using the Argus lab tool. The reference ligand was entrectinib, a drug used in cancer treatment (Figure 9.2). This drug has high potential in treating NCLC. Its docking score was −7.23 Kcal/mol. The binding energy of every ligand against the receptor, hydrogen bond interactions, and van der Waals interactions are listed in Table 9.3. The interaction between the receptor and the ligand beta-bisabolene was much stronger than the others. The compound beta-bisabolene, which is a significant phytocomponent, has several anti-cancer properties (Yeo et al., 2016; Sruthikrishna and Shrikumar, 2022). The compound beta-panasinsene interacted with the receptor and resulted in a score of −12.92 Kcal/mol; this compound was also reported to have anti-cancer properties (Sharma et al., 2022).

From Table 9.3 the blood-brain barrier (BBB) permeation determines the distribution of the drug compound into the central nervous system, and BBB can be selectively permeable for drug compounds. Here the compounds azulene, 7-methyl-Z-tetradecen-1-ol acetate, diethyl phthalate, and formic acid,3,7,

TABLE 9.2
Lipinski Properties of the Bioactive Compounds from Peanut Skin

S. No	Compound Name	Molecular Weight (<500 Da)	Log P (<+5.6)	H-bond Donor (<5)	H-bond Acceptor (<10)	Molar Refractivity 40–130
1	Azulene	128	2.45	0	0	43.41
2	Di-epi-alpha-cedrene	220	3.83	0	1	75.85
3	Alpha-farnasene	204	4.12	0	1	73.38
4	7-Methyl-tetradecen-1-ol acetate	268	4.79	0	2	91.81
5	Beta-bisabolene	204	0	0	3.85	74.19
6	Beta-panasinsene	204	0	0	3.96	75.11
7	Diethyl phthalate	222	0	4	2.21	55.57
8	Formic acid 3,7,11-trimethyl-1,6,10-dodecatrien-3-yl ester	250	0	2	4.11	82.18
9	Hexadecanoic acid, ethyl ester	284	0	2	5.29	99.66
10	Isoledene	204	0	0	3.96	75.11
11	Oleic acid	284	1	2	4.73	96.86

11-trimethyl-1,6,10-dodecatrien-3-yl-ester were predicted to be permeable into the BBB. The gastrointestinal (GI) absorption of the compounds hexadecanoic acid ethyl ester, oleic acid, diethyl phthalate, and formic acid,3,7,11-trimethyl-1,6,10-dodecatrien-3-yl-ester were high; this indicates that these compounds have higher permeability into the surface of the GI tract when taken as drug. The metabolism properties of the compounds were predicted. The skin permeation coefficient Log K_p indicates the rate of permeation through the outermost layer of the epidermal skin. The predicted Log K_p values were appreciable.

The CBX3 protein has been reported to be expressed in human carcinogenesis; this protein can act as a novel drug target for cancer therapeutics (Zhang et al., 2018). Based on the literature, this protein was chosen as a receptor in which a suitable ligand could interact with it to block its expression. The phenolic compounds of peanut can control the proliferation of tumour cells, as they possess anti-proliferative activity (Saenglee et al., 2016; Mohammadhosseinpour et al., 2022).

From this table the binding energy of the interacted ligands can be seen. These binding energy values were compared with the reference inhibitor ligand entrectinib. The ligand beta-bisabolene tops the table with very least binding energy, and the interaction of this ligand with the receptor was depicted in Figure 9.6. The second place was attained by the ligand beta-panasinsene with a binding energy of −12.92 Kcal/mol, and its interaction was shown in Figure 9.8. The binding energies of the ligands are first rate when compared to the binding energy of the reference ligand (−7.23 Kcal/mol). The interaction of the bioactive components from the peanut skin extract may have the effect of preventing the protein CBX3 from being involved in the development of NCLC cells. The few pharmacokinetic possessions of those ligands depict their drug properties (Table 9.4). The two- and three-dimensional interaction of the ligands with the receptor is given in Figures 9.1–9.12.

TABLE 9.3
Pharmacokinetics of the Bioactive Compounds from the Peanut Skin Ethanol Extract

S. No	Compounds	Water Solubility (Log S)	Gastrointestinal Absorption	Blood-Brain-Barrier Permeation	P-glycoprotein Substrate	CYP1A2 Inhibitor	CYP2C19 Inhibitor	CYP2C9 Inhibitor	CYP2D6 Inhibitor	CYP3A4 Inhibitor	Skin Permeation ($LogK_p$ cm/s)
1	Azulene	−3.39	low	yes	no	yes	no	no	no	no	−4.81
2	Di-epi-.alpha-cedrene	−4.02	low	no	no	no	yes	yes	no	no	−4.27
3	Alpha-farnasene	−4.57	low	no	no	yes	no	yes	no	no	−3.20
4	7-Methyl-Z-tetradecen -1-ol acetate	−4.54	low	yes	no	no	no	yes	no	no	−3.55
5	Beta-bisabolene	−4.89	low	no	no	no	no	yes	no	no	−2.98
6	Beta-panasinsene	−4.35	low	no	no	no	yes	yes	no	no	−3.89
7	Diethyl phthalate	−2.62	high	yes	no	yes	no	no	no	no	−5.94
8	Formic acid,3,7,11-trimethyl-1,6,10-dodecatrien-3-yl-ester	−4.06	high	yes	no	no	yes	yes	no	no	−4.16
9	Hexadecanoic acid, ethyl ester	−5.51	high	no	no	yes	no	no	no	no	−2.44
10	Isoledene	−3.67	low	no	no	no	yes	yes	no	no	−4.66
11	Oleic acid	−5.41	high	no	no	yes	no	yes	no	no	−2.60

TABLE 9.4
The Binding Energy of Every Ligand Against the Receptor, Hydrogen Bond Interactions, and van der Waals Interactions

S. No	Compounds	Docking Score (Kcal/mol)	Hydrogen Bond Interactions	No. of Hydrogen Bonds	van der Waals Interactions	Total Polar and Non-Polar Bonding
1	Azulene	−11.126Kcal/mol	-	0	VAL31, LYS52, PHE26	VAL31, LYS52, PHE26, PHE54, PHE30, TRP51 (Figure 9.1)
2	Di-epi-.alpha-cedrene	−11.36 Kcal/mol	-	0	VAL31, LYS52, GLY28, GLU29, ALA82, ARG83, GLU62, THR60	VAL31, LYS52, GLY28, GLU29, ALA82, ARG83, GLU62, THR60, PHE26, TRP51, PHE54 (Figure 9.2)
3	Alpha-farnasene	−12.234 Kcal/mol	-	0	ARG83, GLY28, GLU29, GLU62, GLN27	ARG83, GLY28, GLU29, GLU62, GLN27, PHE54, PHE30, ALA86, PHE26, TRP51 (Figure 9.3)
4	7-Methyl-Z-tetradecen-1-ol acetate	−12.053 Kcal/mol	THR60, SER85	2	ALA82, ARG83, TYR25, PHE26, VAL31	ALA82, ARG83, TYR25, PHE26, VAL31, THR60, SER85, PHE54, PHE30 (Figure 9.4)
5	Beta-bisabolene	−13.50 Kcal/mol	-	0	TYR25, LYS52, VAL32	TYR25, LYS52, VAL32, PHE26, PHE30, PHE54, TRP51, VAL31 (Figure 9.5)
6	Beta-panasinsene	−12.92 Kcal/mol	-	0	ASP58, VAL31	PHE26, PHE30, PHE54, TRP51, ASP58, VAL31 (Figure 9.6)
7	Diethyl phthalate	−12.11 Kcal/mol	THR60	1	ALA86, GLY87, GLU62, ASP58, ARG83	THR60, ALA86, GLY87, GLU62, ASP58, ARG83, PHE26, PHE30, PHE54, TRP51 (Figure 9.7)
8	Formic acid,3,7, 11-trimethyl-1,6, 10-dodecatrien-3 -yl-ester	−12.67 Kcal/mol	ALA86	1	THR60, ASP58, ALA82, ARG83, GLY87, PHE26, VAL31	THR60, ASP58, ALA82, ARG83, GLY87, PHE26, VAL31, ALA86 (Figure 9.8)

9	Hexadecanoic acid, ethyl ester	−12.03Kcal/mol	ALA86, SER85	1	ARG83, GLY28, TRP51, PHE26, GLU62, THR60	ALA86, SER85, ARG83, GLY28, TRP51, PHE26, GLU62, THR60, PHE30, TYR25 (Figure 9.9)
10	Isoledene	−12.65Kcal/mol	-	0	VAL31, ASP58, TYR25	VAL31, ASP58, TYR25, PHE26, PHE30, TRP51 (Figure 9.10)
11	Oleic acid	−12.63 Kcal/mol	GLY87	1	LYS52, ARG83, GLN27, PHE26, VAL31, TYR25, ALA82, GLU62, GLY28, SER85	GLY87, LYS52, ARG83, GLN27, PHE26, VAL31, TYR25, ALA82, GLU62, GLY28, SER85, PHE54, PHE30, TRP51 (Figure 9.11)
12	Enrectinib (reference ligand)	−7.23 Kcal/mol	ASN59 GLU33	2	LYS50	LEU36, PHE48, LYS 34, TRP61, ARG39, ASN59, GLU33, LYS50, ASP56 (Figure 9.12)

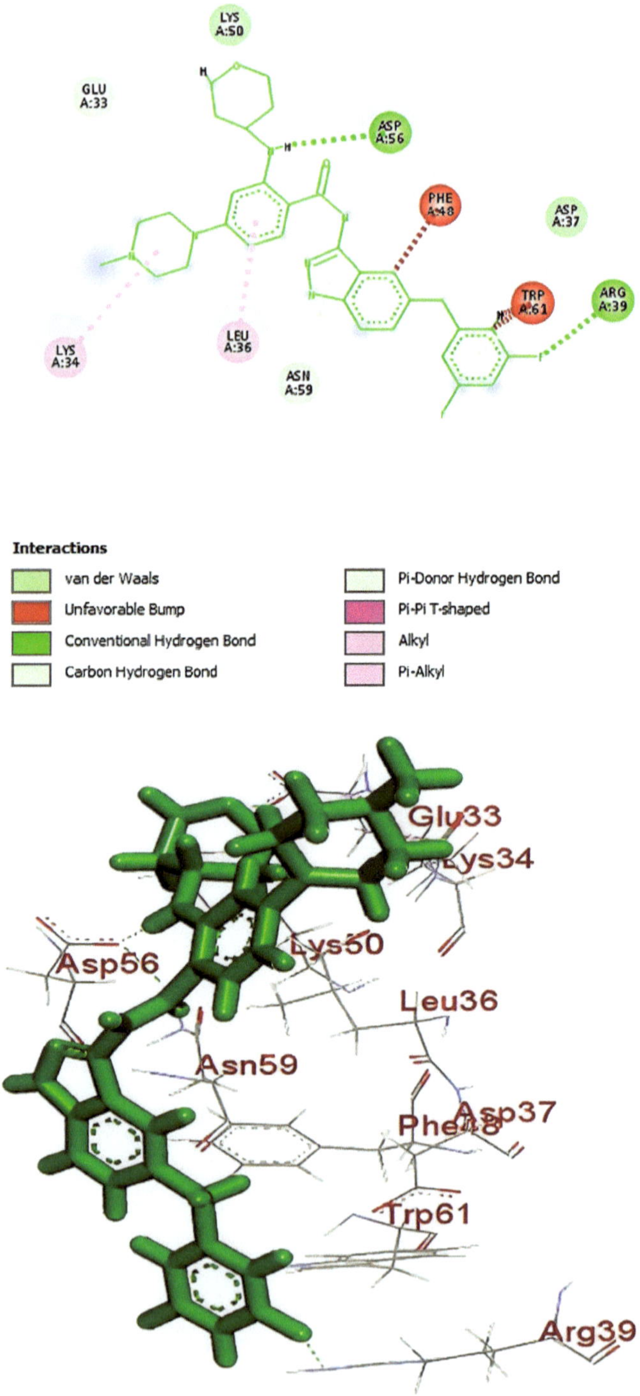

FIGURE 9.1 Two-dimensional and three-dimensional binding analysis of entrectinib with 3TZD and its interactions.

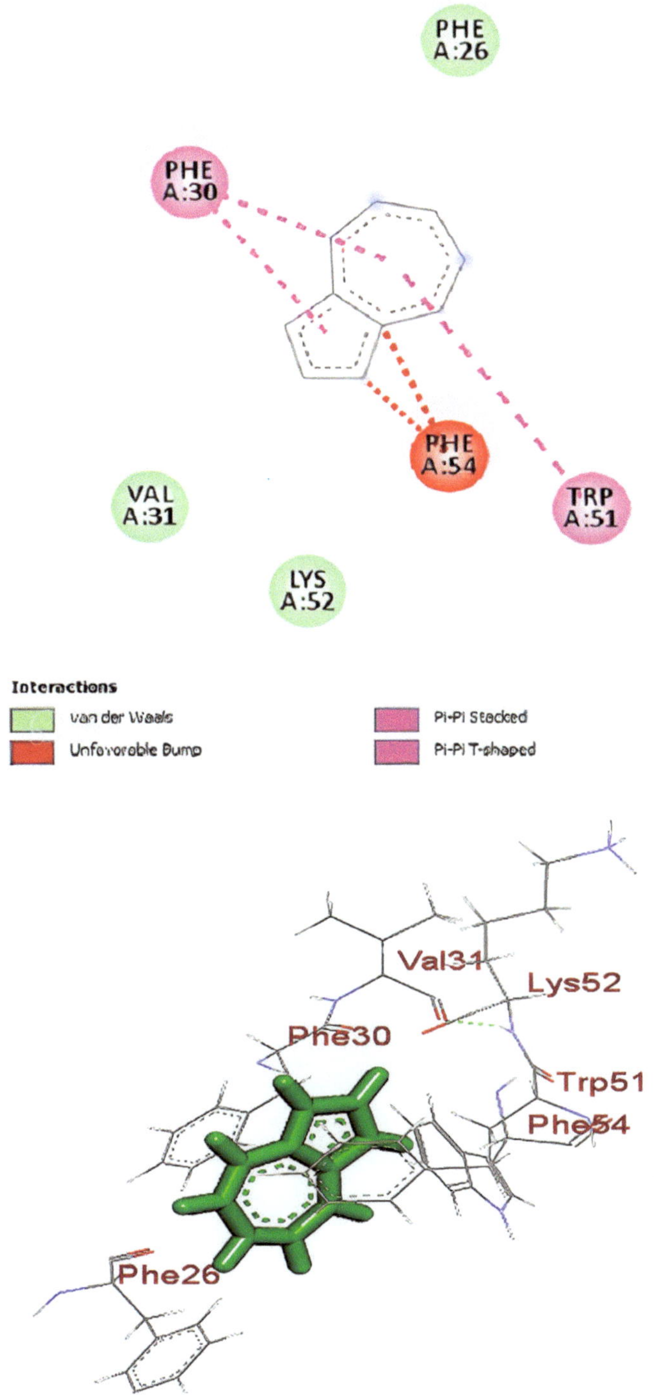

FIGURE 9.2 Two-dimensional and three-dimensional binding analysis of azulene with 3TZD and its interactions.

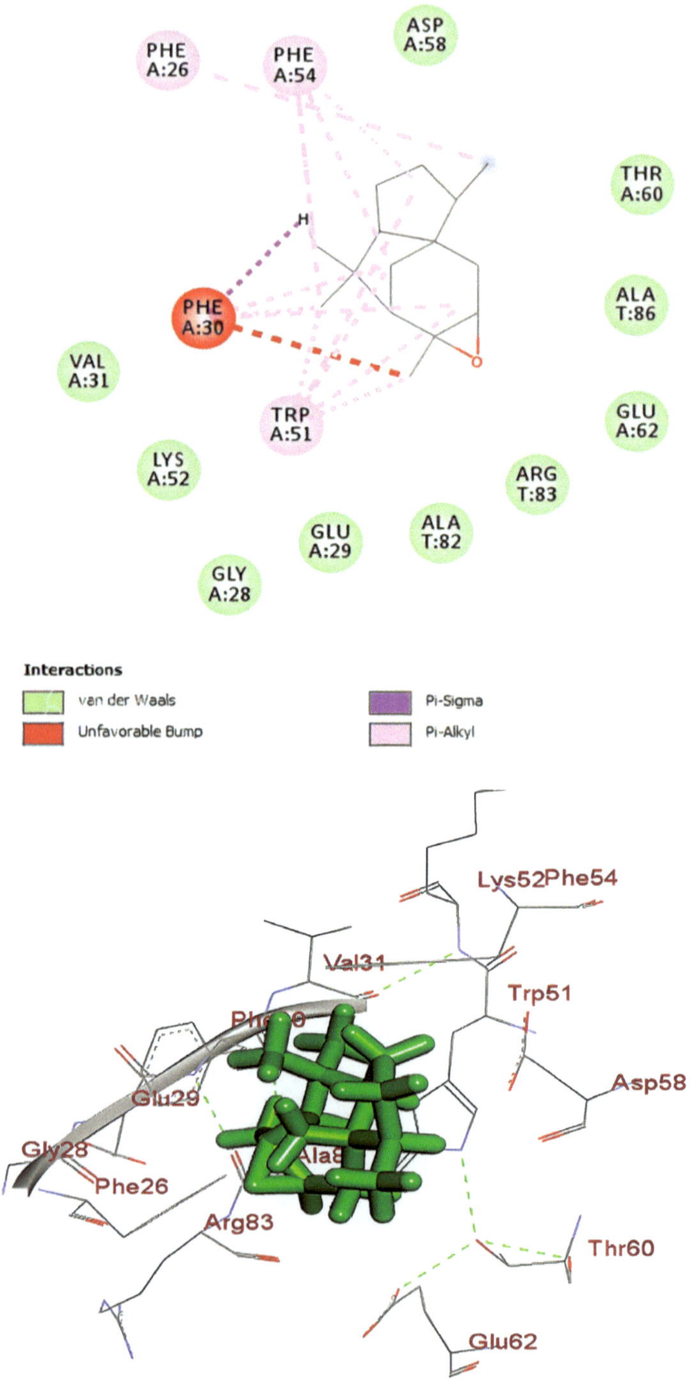

FIGURE 9.3 Two-dimensional and three-dimensional binding analysis of di-epi-alpha-cedrene with 3TZD and its interactions.

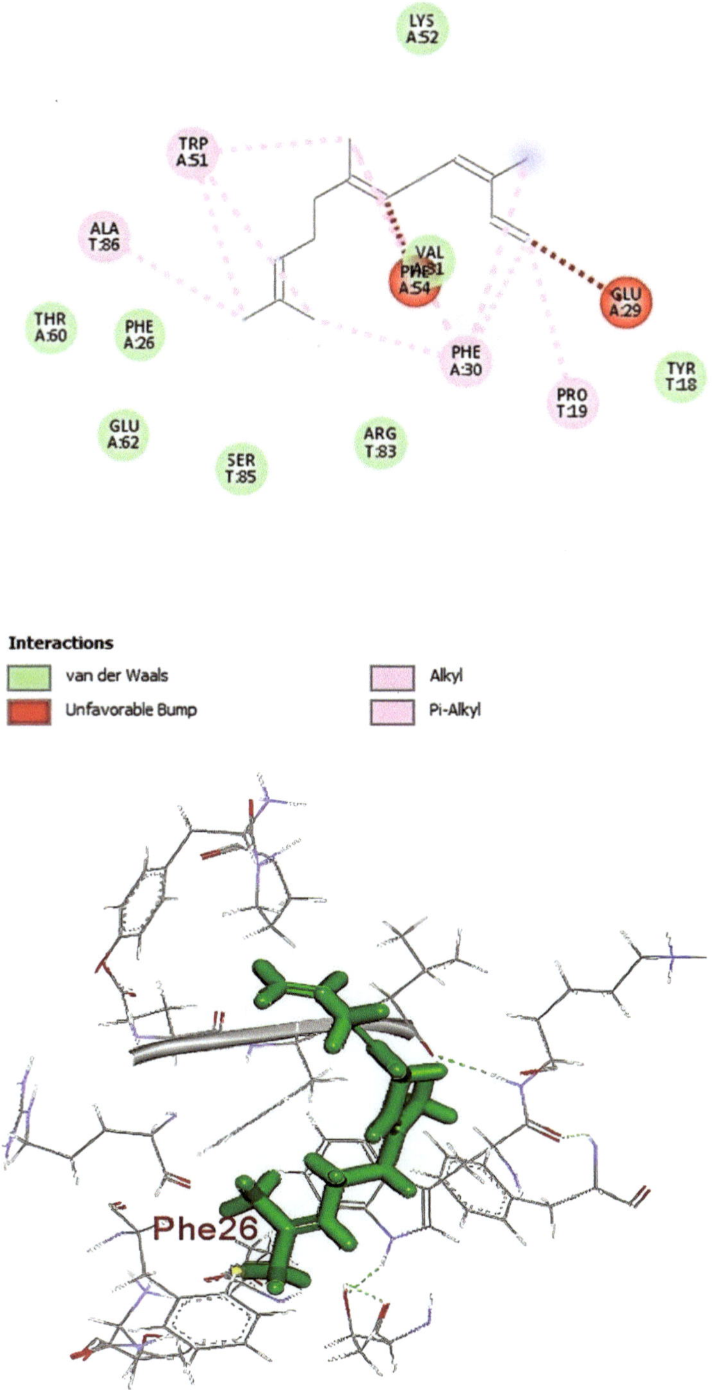

FIGURE 9.4 Two-dimensional and three-dimensional binding analysis of alpha-farnasene with 3TZD and its interactions.

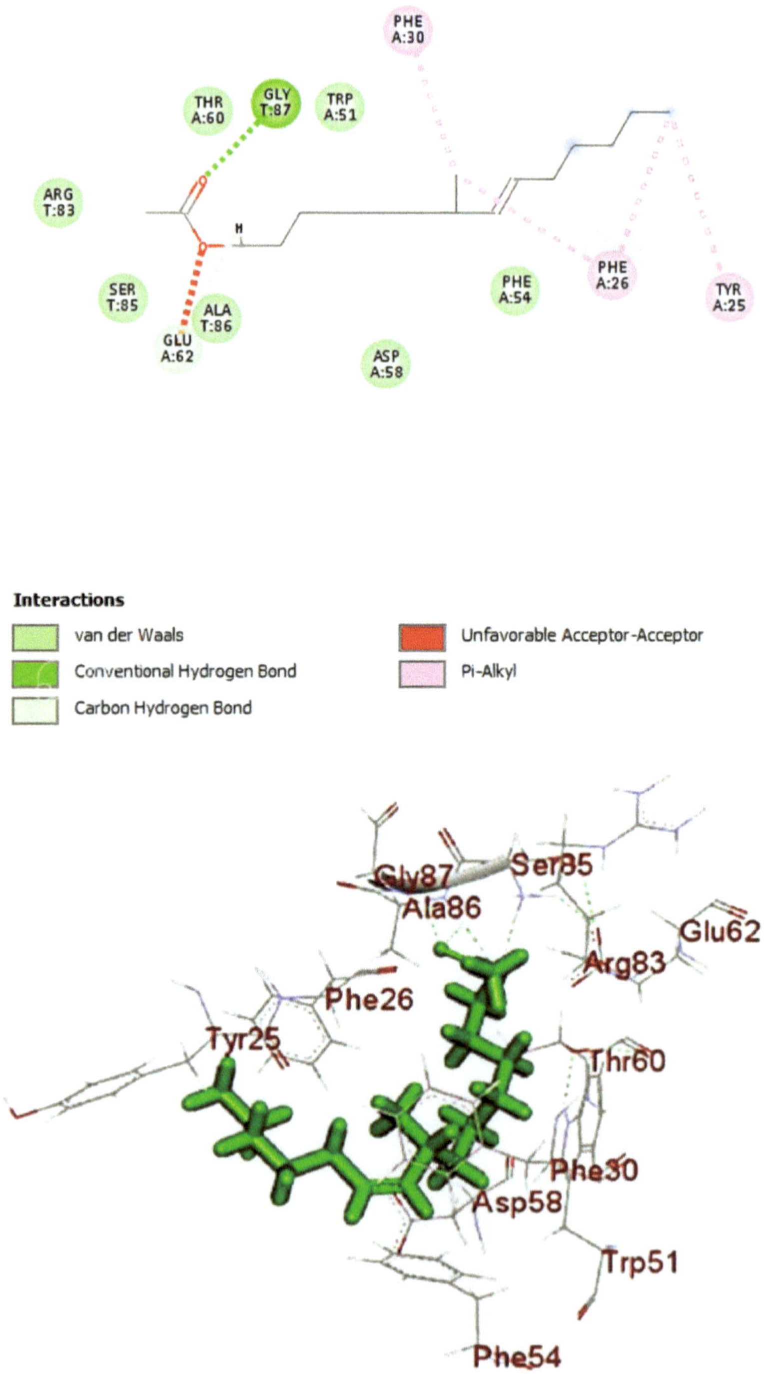

FIGURE 9.5 Two-dimensional and three-dimensional binding analysis of 7-methyl-Z-tetradecen-1-ol acetate with 3TZD and its interactions.

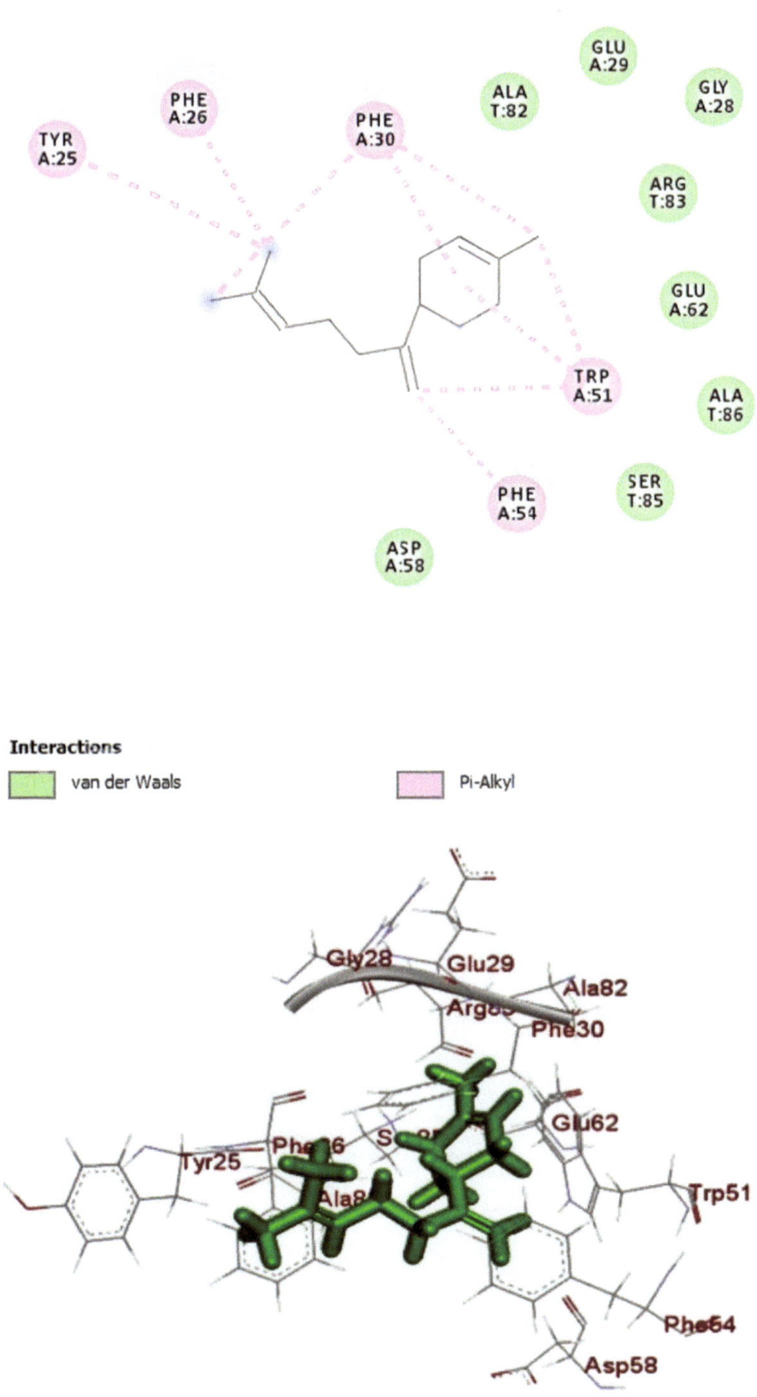

FIGURE 9.6 Two-dimensional and three-dimensional binding analysis of beta-bisabolene with 3TZD and its interactions.

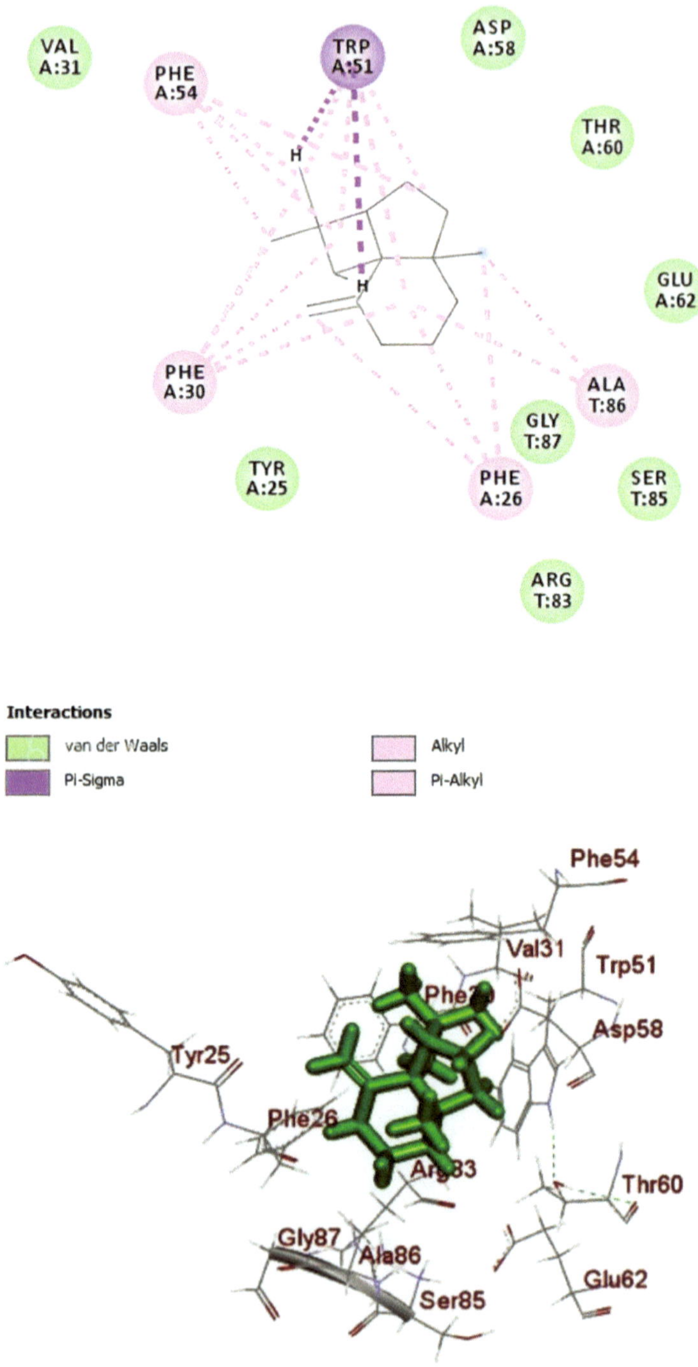

FIGURE 9.7 Two-dimensional and three-dimensional binding analysis of beta-panasinsene with 3TZD and its interactions.

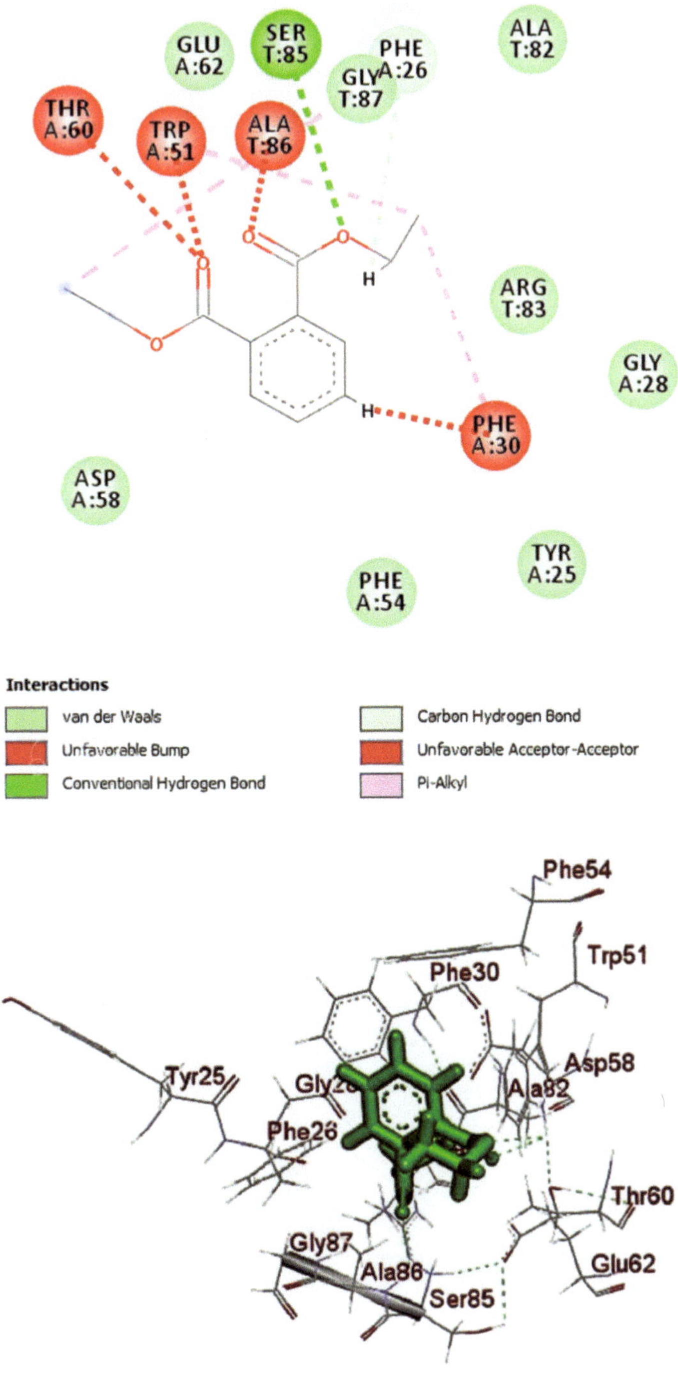

FIGURE 9.8 Two-dimensional and three-dimensional binding analysis of diethyl phthalate with 3TZD and its interactions.

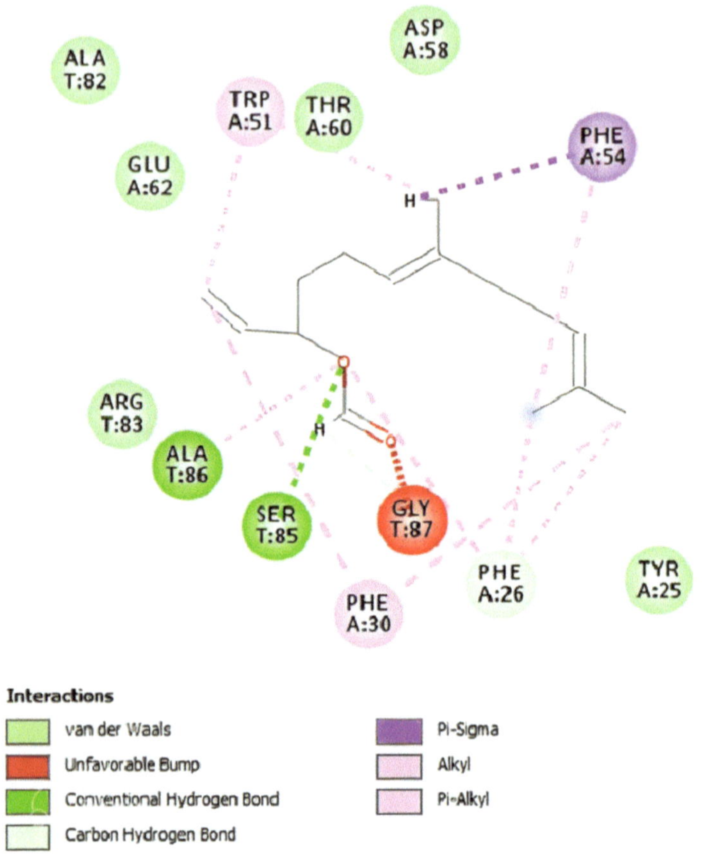

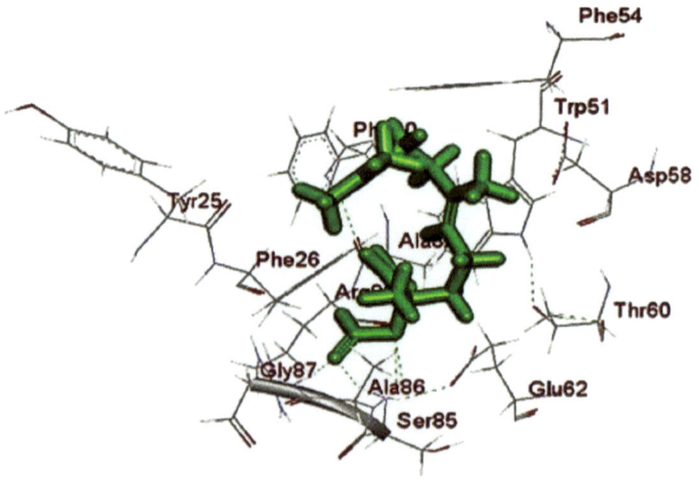

FIGURE 9.9 Two-dimensional and three-dimensional binding analysis of formic acid,3,7,11-trimethyl-1,6,10-dodecatrien-3-yl-ester with 3TZD and its interactions.

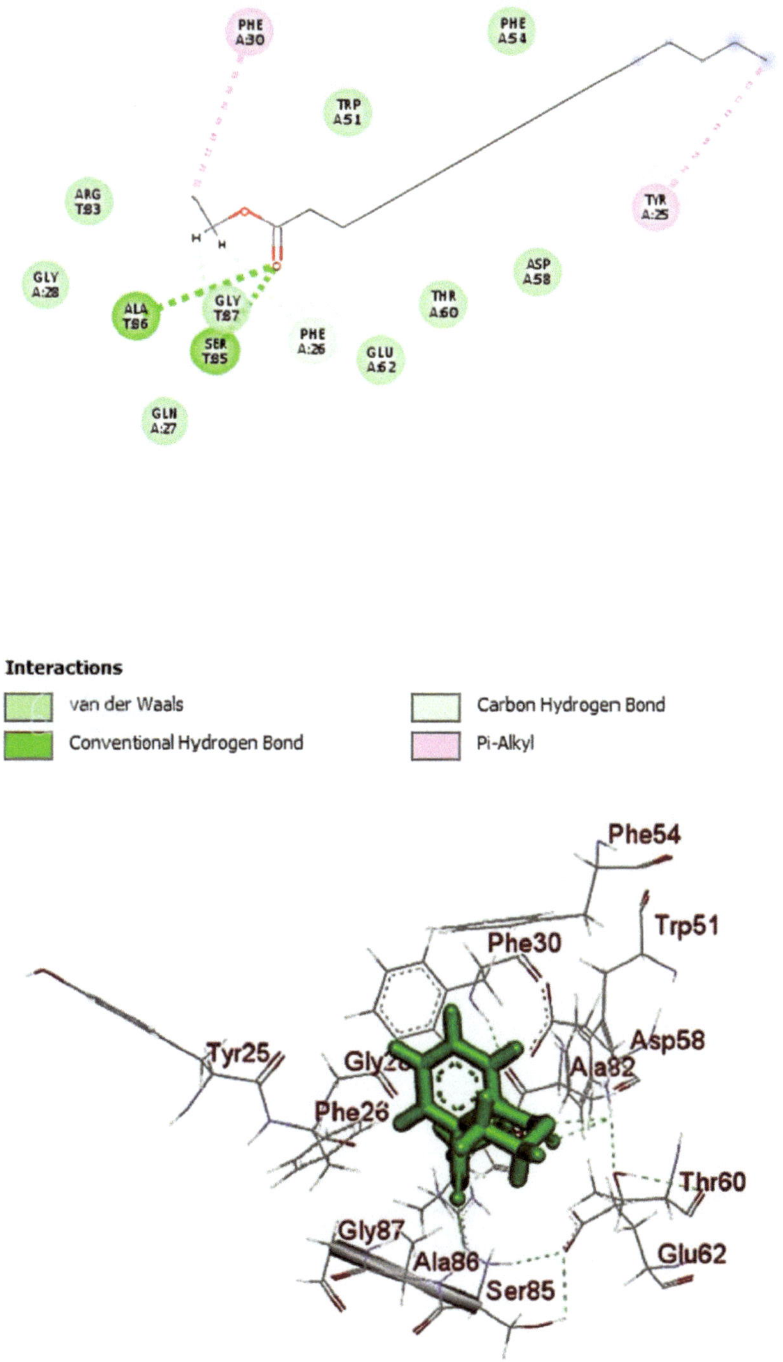

FIGURE 9.10 Two-dimensional and three-dimensional binding analysis of hexadecanoic acid, ethyl ester with 3TZD and its interactions.

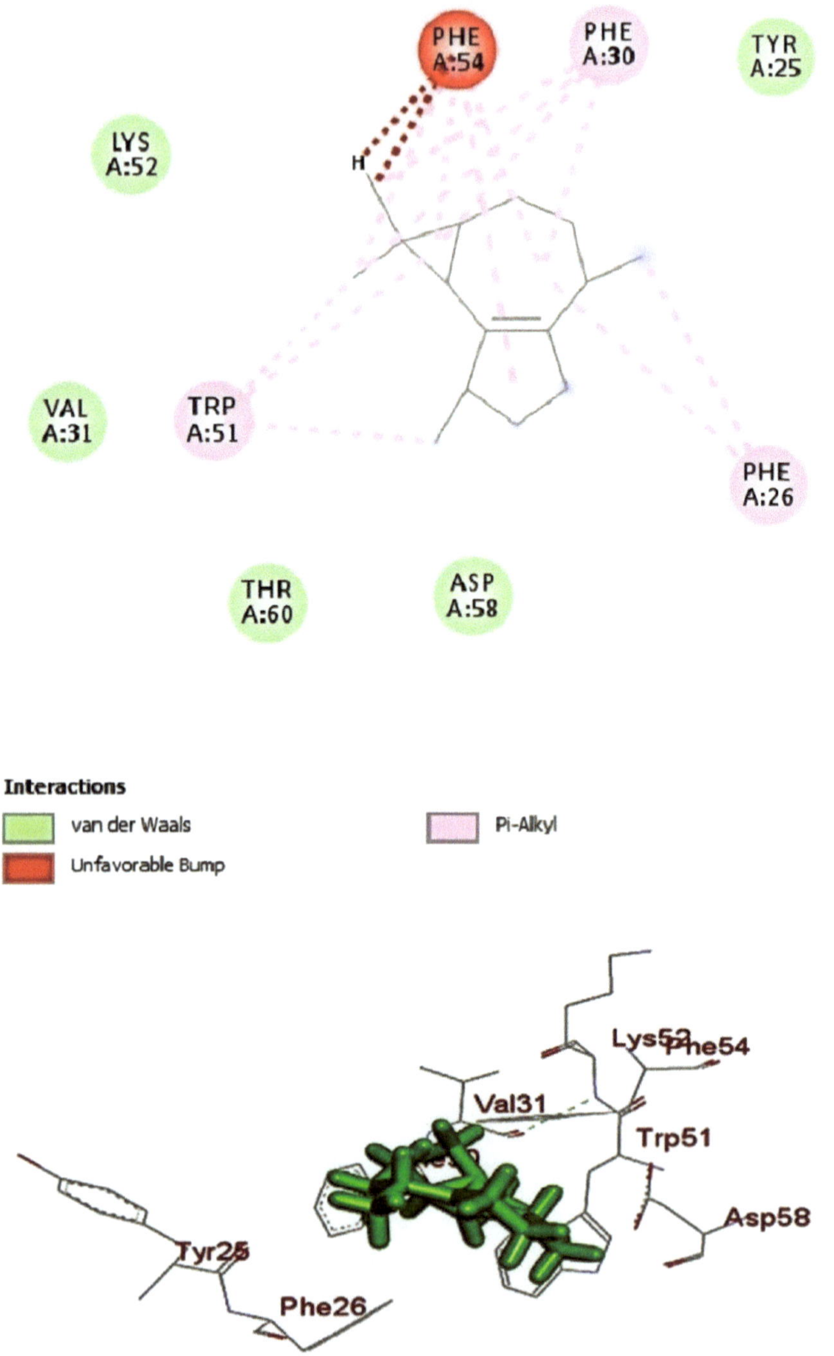

FIGURE 9.11 Two-dimensional and three-dimensional binding analysis of isoledene with 3TZD and its interactions.

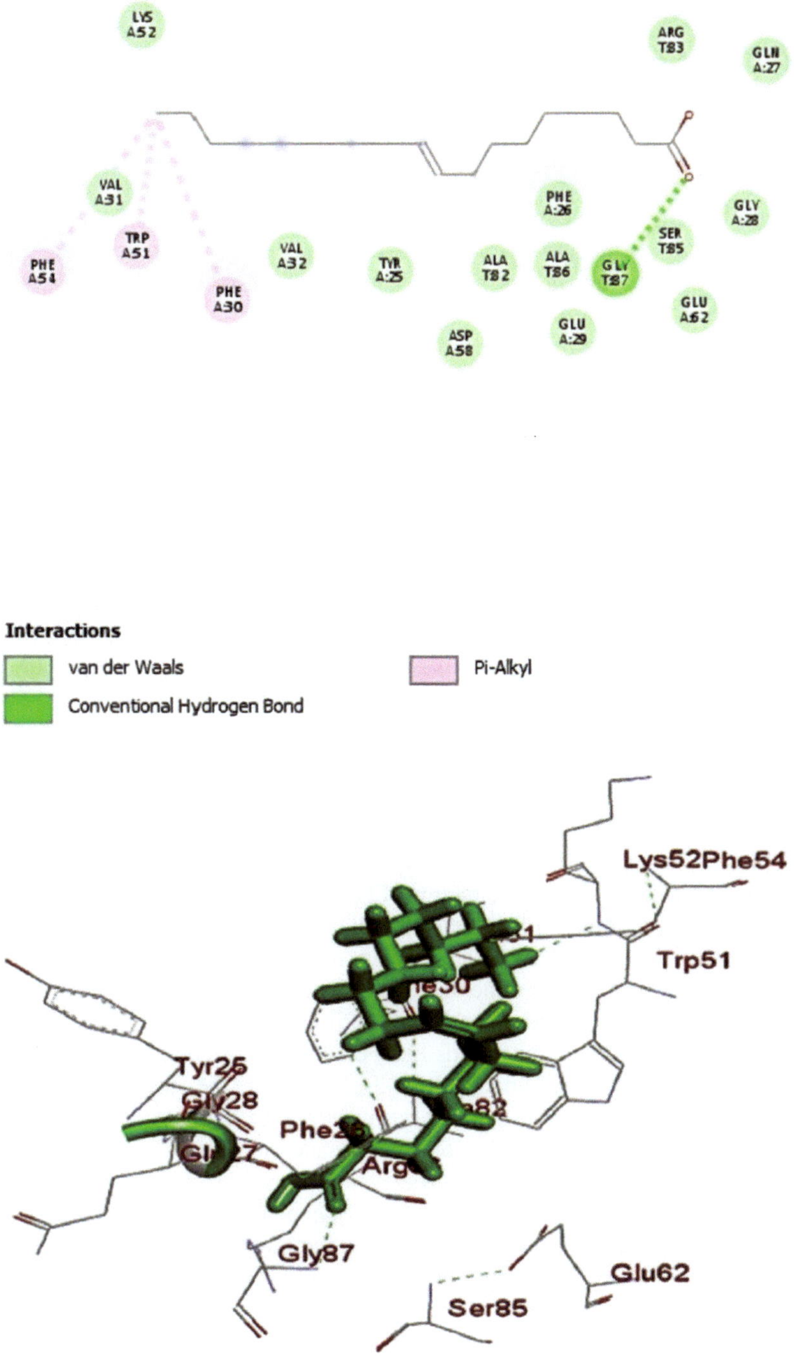

FIGURE 9.12 Two-dimensional and three-dimensional binding analysis of oleic acid with 3TZD and its interactions.

9.5 FUTURE PERSPECTIVES AND LIMITATIONS

At present, researchers are investigating the bioactive compounds from peanuts to test their properties in managing several illnesses. Though peanuts are an allergen, they have benefits. Peanuts can provide leads to screening of several potential anti-cancer drugs. Further, this work can be applied to in vitro studies to test anti-cancer properties of peanut skin with distinct types of cancer cell lines. Various parts of the peanut plant can be explored for their applications. This may lead to the screening of many novel bioactive compounds from the peanut. However, there are a few limitations in this work in that many compounds with medicinal properties present in the extract have not complied with the pharmacokinetic rules. As the hydrogen bond between the ligand and receptor determines the ligand-binding capacity, from the resulted interactions, few compounds lack hydrogen bonding with the receptor.

9.6 CONCLUSION

Currently cancer has increased among the human populations and the need for its prevention is greater than before. Studies on treating or preventing the various types of cancers are on the line. The currently available and approved drugs to treat cancer have their own positive and negative impacts. This makes cancer researchers work on drug candidates to cure cancer. The compound entrectinib was one of the proposed drugs for chemotherapies in treating various cancers. So, we have chosen this compound as a reference ligand for this docking study.

The compounds obtained from GC-MS analysis were screened for Lipinski properties, and the compounds that complied with the rules were chosen for molecular docking. Through in silico approaches by molecular docking, the anti-cancer property of the peanut skin extract was productively studied. From the results, the ligand beta-bisabolene gave the best interaction and docking score of −13.501 kcal/mol. This shows that there was an interaction of beta-bisabolene with the receptor that was better than the interaction of the reference ligand entrectinib with the receptor. The literature has shown that beta-bisabolene has antioxidant and anti-cancer properties. From this work we can determine that the in silico analysis has shown that the bioactive compounds from the peanut skin extract possess anti-cancer properties, and we have also suggested that compounds like beta-bisabolene, beta-panasinsene, formic acid,3,7,11-trimethyl-1,6,10-dodecatrien-3-yl-ester, and the other compounds can be likely drug candidates. However, further studies are needed to research the effectiveness of the peanut skin against various disease and disorders.

The bioinformatic approaches nowadays have been producing promising results and have laid a suitable prediction step before we phase into in vitro studies. Among various bioinformatic applications, molecular docking has been widely used to predict drug interactions. This work may have created an approach for upcoming in silico approaches on studies involving the peanut.

9.7 ACKNOWLEDGEMENT

The management of Vels Institute of Science, Technology, and Advanced Studies is gratefully acknowledged by the authors for their assistance in conducting the study.

9.8 CONFLICT OF INTEREST

Authors declare that there is no conflict of interest.

REFERENCES

Achutha, A. S., V. L. Pushpa, and K. B. Manoj. "Comparative molecular docking studies of phytochemicals as Jak2 inhibitors using Autodock and ArgusLab." *Materials Today: Proceedings* 41 (2021): 711–716.

Akhtar, Shamim, Nauman Khalid, Iftikhar Ahmed, Armghan Shahzad, and Hafiz Ansar Rasul Suleria. "Physicochemical characteristics, functional properties, and nutritional benefits of peanut oil: A review." *Critical Reviews in Food Science and Nutrition* 54, no. 12 (2014): 1562–1575.

Alam, Hunain, Na Li, Shilpa S. Dhar, Sarah J. Wu, Jie Lv, Kaifu Chen, Elsa R. Flores, Laura Baseler, and Min Gyu Lee. "HP1γ promotes lung adenocarcinoma by downregulating the transcription-repressive regulators NCOR2 and ZBTB7A protumorigenic function of HP1γ for lung adenocarcinoma." *Cancer Research* 78, no. 14 (2018): 3834–3848.

Arya, Shalini S., Akshata R. Salve, and Salve Chauhan. "Peanuts as functional food: A review." *Journal of Food Science and Technology* 53 (2016): 31–41.

Awad, Atif B., Karen C. Chan, Arthur C. Downie, and Carol S. Fink. "Peanuts as a source of β-sitosterol, a sterol with anticancer properties." *Nutrition and Cancer* 36, no. 2 (2000): 238–241.

Awad, Atif B., and Carol S. Fink. "Phytosterols as anticancer dietary components: Evidence and mechanism of action." *The Journal of Nutrition* 130, no. 9 (2000): 2127–2130.

Ballard, Tameshia S., Parameswarakumar Mallikarjunan, Kequan Zhou, and Sean O'Keefe. "Microwave-assisted extraction of phenolic antioxidant compounds from peanut skins." *Food Chemistry* 120, no. 4 (2010): 1185–1192.

Chang, Shih-Chieh, Yi-Chun Lai, Yen-Chung Chen, Nai-Kuan Wang, Wei-Shu Wang, and Jiun-I. Lai. "CBX3/heterochromatin protein 1 gamma is significantly upregulated in patients with non—small cell lung cancer." *Asia-Pacific Journal of Clinical Oncology* 14, no. 5 (2018): e283–e288.

Chen, Lian-Yu, Chien-Shan Cheng, Chao Qu, Peng Wang, Hao Chen, Zhi-Qiang Meng, and Zhen Chen. "Overexpression of CBX3 in pancreatic adenocarcinoma promotes cell cycle transition-associated tumor progression." *International Journal of Molecular Sciences* 19, no. 6 (2018): 1768.

Chen, Zhao, Christine M. Fillmore, Peter S. Hammerman, Carla F. Kim, and Kwok-Kin Wong. "Non-small-cell lung cancers: A heterogeneous set of diseases." *Nature Reviews Cancer* 14, no. 8 (2014): 535–546.

Christman, Lindsey M., Lisa L. Dean, Jonathan C. Allen, Sofia Feng Godinez, and Ondulla T. Toomer. "Peanut skin phenolic extract attenuates hyperglycemic responses in vivo and in vitro." *PLoS ONE* 14, no. 3 (2019): e0214591.

Chukwumah, Yvonne, Lloyd T. Walker, and Martha Verghese. "Peanut skin color: A biomarker for total polyphenolic content and antioxidative capacities of peanut cultivars." *International Journal of Molecular Sciences* 10, no. 11 (2009): 4941–4952.

Çiftçi, S., and G. Ü. L. E. N. Suna. "Functional components of peanuts (Arachis Hypogaea L.) and health benefits: A review." *Future Foods* (2022): 100140.

Elsorady, M. E. I., and S. E. Ali. "Antioxidant activity of roasted and unroasted peanut skin extracts." *International Food Research Journal* 25, no. 1 (2018): 43–50.

Ettinger, David S., Wallace Akerley, Gerold Bepler, Matthew G. Blum, Andrew Chang, Richard T. Cheney, Lucian R. Chirieac et al. "Non—small cell lung cancer." *Journal of the National Comprehensive Cancer Network* 8, no. 7 (2010): 740–801.

Gridelli, Cesare, Antonio Rossi, David P. Carbone, Juliana Guarize, Niki Karachaliou, Tony Mok, Francesco Petrella, Lorenzo Spaggiari, and Rafael Rosell. "Non-small-cell lung cancer." *Nature Reviews Disease Primers* 1, no. 1 (2015): 1–16.

Haruna, Suleiman A., Huanhuan Li, Wenya Wei, Wenhui Geng, Xiaofeng Luo, Muhammad Zareef, Selorm Yao-Say Solomon Adade, Ngouana Moffo A. Ivane, Adamu Isa, and Quansheng Chen. "Simultaneous quantification of total flavonoids and phenolic content in raw peanut seeds via NIR spectroscopy coupled with integrated algorithms." *Spectrochimica Acta Part A: Molecular and Biomolecular Spectroscopy* 285 (2023): 121854.

Herbst, Roy S., Daniel Morgensztern, and Chris Boshoff. "The biology and management of non-small cell lung cancer." *Nature* 553, no. 7689 (2018): 446–454.

Huang, Cheng-Po, Lo-Chun Au, Robin Y.-Y. Chiou, Ping-Chen Chung, Su-Yu Chen, Wei-Chien Tang, Chao-Lin Chang, Woei-Horng Fang, and Shwu-Bin Lin. "Arachidin-1, a peanut stilbenoid, induces programmed cell death in human leukemia HL-60 cells." *Journal of Agricultural and Food Chemistry* 58, no. 23 (2010): 12123–12129.

Kandasamy, Saravanakumar, Sunil Kumar Sahu, and Kathiresan Kandasamy. "In Silico studies on fungal metabolite against skin cancer protein (4, 5-Diarylisoxazole HSP90 Chaperone)." *International Scholarly Research Notices* 2012 (2012).

Larrauri, Mariana, Maria P. Zunino, Julio A. Zygadlo, Nelson R. Grosso, and Valeria Nepote. "Chemical characterization and antioxidant properties of fractions separated from extract of peanut skin derived from different industrial processes." *Industrial Crops and Products* 94 (2016): 964–971.

Leunissen, Mary, Valerie J. Davidson, and Yukio Kakuda. "Analysis of volatile flavor components in roasted peanuts using supercritical fluid extraction and gas chromatography–mass spectrometry." *Journal of Agricultural and Food Chemistry* 44, no. 9 (1996): 2694–2699.

Lewis, Wanida E., Gabriel K. Harris, Timothy H. Sanders, Brittany L. White, and Lisa L. Dean. "Antioxidant and anti-inflammatory effects of peanut skin extracts." *Food and Nutrition Sciences* 4, no. 8A (2013): 22–32.

Lin, Hexin, Jiabian Lian, Lu Xia, Guoxian Guan, and Jun You. "CBX3 promotes gastric cancer progression and affects factors related to immunotherapeutic responses." *Cancer Management and Research* 12 (2020a): 10113.

Lin, Hexin, Xin Zhao, Lu Xia, Jiabian Lian, and Jun You. "Clinicopathological and prognostic significance of CBX3 expression in human cancer: A systematic review and meta-analysis." *Disease Markers* 2020 (2020b).

Medina-Bolivar, Fabricio, Jose Condori, Agnes M. Rimando, John Hubstenberger, Kristen Shelton, Sean F. O'Keefe, Selester Bennett, and Maureen C. Dolan. "Production and secretion of resveratrol in hairy root cultures of peanut." *Phytochemistry* 68, no. 14 (2007): 1992–2003.

Mohammadhosseinpour, Sepideh, Linh-Chi Ho, Lingling Fang, Jianfeng Xu, and Fabricio Medina-Bolivar. "Arachidin-1, a prenylated stilbenoid from peanut, induces apoptosis in triple-negative breast cancer cells." *International Journal of Molecular Sciences* 23, no. 3 (2022): 1139.

Mohammadhosseinpour, Sepideh, Alexx Weaver, Meenakshi Sudhakaran, Linh-Chi Ho, Tra Le, Andrea I. Doseff, and Fabricio Medina-Bolivar. "Arachidin-1, a prenylated stilbenoid from peanut, enhances the anticancer effects of paclitaxel in triple-negative breast cancer cells." *Cancers* 15, no. 2 (2023): 399.

Nepote, Valeria, Nelson R. Grosso, and Carlos A. Guzman. "Optimization of extraction of phenolic antioxidants from peanut skins." *Journal of the Science of Food and Agriculture* 85, no. 1 (2005): 33–38.

Oldoni, Tatiane L. C., Priscilla S. Melo, Adna P. Massarioli, Ivani A. M. Moreno, Rosângela M. N. Bezerra, Pedro L. Rosalen, Gil V. J. da Silva, Andréa M. Nascimento, and Severino M. Alencar. "Bioassay-guided isolation of proanthocyanidins with antioxidant activity from peanut (Arachis hypogaea) skin by combination of chromatography techniques." *Food Chemistry* 192 (2016): 306–312.

Peng, Jinming, Yan Jia, Xia Du, Yue Wang, Zimu Yang, and Kaikai Li. "Study of physicochemical stability of anthocyanin extracts from black peanut skin and their digestion enzyme and adipogenesis inhibitory activities." *LWT* 107 (2019): 107–116.

Prabasheela, B., R. Venkateshwari, S. Nivetha, P. MohanaPriya, T. Jayashree, R. Vimala, and K. Karthik. "Phytochemical analysis and antioxidant activity of Arachishypogaea." *Journal of Chemical and Pharmaceutical Research* 7, no. 10 (2015): 116–121.

Rohimah, Azizah, Budi Setiawan, Eny Palupi, Ahmad Sulaeman, and Ekowati Handharyani. "Comparison of peanut and black oncom biscuit: Nutritional characteristics and aflatoxin evaluation with the potential health benefits." *Annals of Agricultural Sciences* 66, no. 1 (2021): 87–92.

Saenglee, Somprasong, Sanun Jogloy, Aran Patanothai, and Thanaset Senawong. "Cytotoxic effects of peanut phenolic compounds possessing histone deacetylase inhibitory activity on human colon cancer cell lines." *Turkish Journal of Biology* 40, no. 6 (2016): 1258–1271.

Sanders, Timothy H., Robert W. McMichael, and Keith W. Hendrix. "Occurrence of resveratrol in edible peanuts." *Journal of Agricultural and Food Chemistry* 48, no. 4 (2000): 1243–1246.

Shahzad, Naiyer, Wajahatullah Khan, M. D. Shadab, Asgar Ali, Sundeep Singh Saluja, Sadhana Sharma, Faisal A. Al-Allaf et al. "Phytosterols as a natural anticancer agent: Current status and future perspective." *Biomedicine & Pharmacotherapy* 88 (2017): 786–794.

Sharma, Mansi, Kamaljit Grewal, Rupali Jandrotia, Daizy Rani Batish, Harminder Pal Singh, and Ravinder Kumar Kohli. "Essential oils as anticancer agents: Potential role in malignancies, drug delivery mechanisms, and immune system enhancement." *Biomedicine & Pharmacotherapy* 146 (2022): 112514.

Soriano-Hernandez, Alejandro D., Daniela G. Madrigal-Perez, Hector R. Galvan-Salazar, Alejandro Arreola-Cruz, Lorena Briseño-Gomez, José Guzmán-Esquivel, Oxana Dobrovinskaya et al. "The protective effect of peanut, walnut, and almond consumption on the development of breast cancer." *Gynecologic and Obstetric Investigation* 80, no. 2 (2015): 89–92.

Sruthikrishna, P. K., and Sapna Shrikumar. "GC-MS analysis of phytocomponents in the ethylacetate extract of Mesua ferrea Linn. leaves." *Asian Journal of Pharmaceutical Analysis* 12, no. 2 (2022): 121–126.

Syed, Faiza, Sania Arif, Iftikhar Ahmed, and Nauman Khalid. "Groundnut (peanut)(Arachis hypogaea)." *Oilseeds: Health Attributes and Food Applications* (2021): 93–122.

Taha, Fakhriya S., Suzanne M. Wagdy, and Fatma A. Singer. "Comparison between antioxidant activities of phenolic extracts from different parts of peanut." *Life Sciences Journal* 9, no. 2 (2012): 207–215.

Udenigwe, Chibuike C., Vanu R. Ramprasath, Rotimi E. Aluko, and Peter J. H. Jones. "Potential of resveratrol in anticancer and anti-inflammatory therapy." *Nutrition Reviews* 66, no. 8 (2008): 445–454.

Wang, Jing, Xiaoping Yuan, Zhengyu Jin, Yuan Tian, and Huanlu Song. "Free radical and reactive oxygen species scavenging activities of peanut skins extract." *Food Chemistry* 104, no. 1 (2007): 242–250.

Yeo, Syn Kok, Ahmed Y. Ali, Olivia A. Hayward, Daniel Turnham, Troy Jackson, Ifor D. Bowen, and Richard Clarkson. "β-Bisabolene, a sesquiterpene from the essential oil extract of opoponax (Commiphora guidottii), exhibits cytotoxicity in breast cancer cell lines." *Phytotherapy Research* 30, no. 3 (2016): 418–425.

Yu, Jianmei, Mohamed Ahmedna, and Ipek Goktepe. "Peanut skin phenolics: Extraction, identification, antioxidant activity, and potential applications." *ACS Symposium Series* 956 (2007).

Zhang, HuaYong, WeiChao Chen, XiaoYan Fu, Xuan Su, and AnKui Yang. "CBX3 promotes tumor proliferation by regulating G1/S phase via p21 downregulation and associates with poor prognosis in tongue squamous cell carcinoma." *Gene* 654 (2018): 49–56.

Zhao, Xiaoyan, Jun Chen, and Fangling Du. "Potential use of peanut by-products in food processing: A review." *Journal of Food Science and Technology* 49 (2012): 521–529.

Zhong, Xiaoping, Anna Kan, Wancong Zhang, Jianda Zhou, Huayong Zhang, Jiasheng Chen, and Shijie Tang. "CBX3/HP1γ promotes tumor proliferation and predicts poor survival in hepatocellular carcinoma." *Aging (Albany NY)* 11, no. 15 (2019): 5483.

Zhu, Minghui, Xin Wen, Jinhong Zhao, Fang Liu, Yuanying Ni, Liyan Ma, and Jingming Li. "Effect of industrial chemical refining on the physicochemical properties and the bioactive minor components of peanut oil." *Journal of the American Oil Chemists' Society* 93, no. 2 (2016): 285–294.

10 Bioinformatics Tools for the Discovery of Potential Anti-Diabetic Drugs from Lichens

Madhushree M.V. Rao, Likith M**, Gayathri D S***, Ravikumar H****, and Hariprasad T P N****,†*
*Defence Institute of Advanced Technology (Deemed to be University), Girinagar, Pune, India; **Department of Biotechnology, Dayananda Sagar College of Engineering, Bangalore, Karnataka, India; ***Department of Zoology, BGS Science Academy, Chikkaballapura, Karnataka, India; ****Department of Life Science, Bangalore University, Bangalore, Karnataka, India
†Corresponding Author: hariprasad.tpn@gmail.com

ABBREVIATIONS

ADMET	Absorption, distribution, metabolism, excretion, and toxicity
BBB	Blood-brain barrier
CAM	Complementary and alternative medicine
CASTp	Compound Atlas of Surface Topography of proteins
CVD	Cardiovascular diseases
Da	Dalton
HBA	Hydrogen bond acceptor
HBD	Hydrogen bond receiver
HIA	Human intestinal absorption
HIV	Human immunodeficiency virus
IR	Insulin receptor
PDB	Protein data bank
RCSB	Research Collaboratory for Structural Bioinformatics
SDF	Structural data format
SMILES	Simplified molecular input line entry system
WHO	World Health Organization

DOI: 10.1201/9781003354437-10

10.1 INTRODUCTION

Diabetes is a progressive metabolic condition exemplified by hyperglycemia, which is triggered by either a total absence of insulin (type 1), inadequate insulin or insulin that cannot be used efficiently (type 2) (Baharvand-Ahmadi et al. 2016). The global incidence of diabetes was corroborated at 463 million in 2019 and is projected to afflict up to 700 million by 2045 (IDF 2021). As of 2021, India ranks second on the global ranking for the highest prevalence of diabetes, with over 74 million individuals (IDF 2021). Despite efforts to cure the disease through pharmacological (oral hypoglycemic agents, insulin) and non-pharmacological intervention (diet, exercise, etc), diabetes still remains a silent epidemic (Chaudhury et al. 2017). Antidiabetic medications currently combat the underlying pathologies by either modulating or inhibiting a protein that plays a cardinal role in diabetes. However, their detrimental effects are inevitable like insulin resistance, renal toxicity, increased risk of heart disease, hypoglycemic coma and so on (Vo et al. 2016).

The complexity of diabetes ensures prolonged commitment and adherence to the treatment coupled with the involvement of multidimensional healthcare facilities, making it a socio-economic burden (Prasopthum et al. 2022). Further, compliance with keeping a healthy weight, exercising regularly and abiding by a healthy diet has a great impact on the quality of life, and the efficacy of conventional treatment serves as a major dilemma to human health (Choudhury et al. 2018). Besides, for a developing country like India, where more than half (53.1%) of people are undiagnosed and the mortality rate due to epidemiological transition, diabetes is perplexing and costly affair (Pradeepa and Mohan 2021; Das et al. 2022).

New initiatives by several researchers have focused on exploring natural sources as a promising alternative (Sharma et al. 2020). Complementary and alternative medicine (CAM) is presumed to be easy to access and is synonymous with safety and effectiveness due to personal or cultural beliefs or recommendations by family and friends (Low et al. 2016). These factors, in addition to the inability to obtain medication, poor living conditions, and inadequacy of conventional medicines, have compelled patients to use CAM like natural remedies, yoga and self-care techniques, or to turn to traditional approaches as it is associated with patient ideology and is less authoritarian (Kim et al. 2011). CAMs are 1.6 times more popular among diabetic patients than non-diabetics (Candar et al. 2018).

As a result, lichens were proposed as a natural medicinal therapy to impede diabetes and their analogous comorbidities by enhancing glycemic regulation in order to increase quality of life. Lichens are a symbiotic amalgamation of a mycobiont, a fungal partner with a primary role in protection and absorption of nutrients and a photobiont such as green algae, cyanobacteria or both, assigned the role of synthesizing organic nutrients (Shahid et al. 2020). They have been known since antiquity as a reservoir of secondary metabolites which are churned out predominantly by one of the three pathways: the acetate-polymalonate pathway: aliphatic substances like zeorin compounds, polyhydric alcohols, aromatic substances like depsides, benzyl esters, diphenylene oxide derivatives, depsones, depsidones, dibenzofurans, tridepsides, usnic acids and derivatives, anthraquinones, naphthaquinones, xanthone; the mevalonic acid pathway: steroids, triterpenes; and the shikimic acid pathway: pulvinic acid derivatives and terphenylquinones (Wa et al. 2021; Adenubi et al. 2022). About 350 different secondary lichen metabolites, which are all of fungal ancestry, have been identified to retain varied biological activities including anti-HIV properties (Neamati et al. 1997), antioxidant, antiproliferative and cytotoxic, analgesic (Hidalgo et al. 1994), antipyretic, antimycobacterial, anti-inflammatory and antiviral (Ranković et al. 2007; Huneck 1999; Halama and Van Haluwin 2004) properties.

The other application of lichens is in the domain of regulation of circadian clocks through their biosynthesized secondary metabolites (Srimani et al. 2022). It is highly praised in the field of nanotechnology for the fabrication of green synthesized nanomaterials as a result of its low cost and biocompatible attributes displaying a wide spectrum of enhanced biological activities. Additionally, its reducible activity to assemble different nanomaterials has applications in the biomedical and biotechnological sectors (Hamida et al. 2021). Silver nanoparticles produced by *Pseudevernia furfuracea* and *Lobaria pulmonaria* exhibited excellent anti-bacterial properties against six different bacterial strains, and various lichens are used for the fabrication of nanoparticles including *Usnea longissi, Cetraria islandica, Parmelia perlata, Parmotrema tinctorum, Acroscyphus sphaerophoroides Lev, Sticta nylanderiana, Ramalina fraxinea,* etc. (Goga et al. 2021). Lichens act as excellent bio-indicators, as the external environment can affect their growth and development. Since every change in the climate is likely to have an impact on the growth and development of lichens, they are used to monitor global changes. They are employed to measure air quality and radioactive contamination, seeing as they can collect and hold pollutants like heavy metals (Aptroot et al. 2021; Anderson et al. 2022; Sujetoviene and Cesynaite 2021).

Lichens and their metabolites have been exploited for their biopharmaceutical application as an anti-diabetic agent, with many exploratory studies supporting the claim (Cui et al. 2012; Karthik et al. 2011; Thadhani and Karunaratne 2017; Salin Raj et al. 2014). This paradigm shift is mainly attributed to the rich and diverse bioactive phytochemicals present in these compounds, which could have additive and synergistic effects in purging diabetes and its complications (Sharma et al. 2020). Lichens phytoconstituents, methyl β-orcinolcarboxylate, zeorin and methylorsellinate derived from *Cladonia* sp. demonstrated better anti-diabetic potential by inhibiting α-glucosidase when compared to standard acarbose (Karunaratne et al. 2014). Similar results were exemplified by psoromic acid, vulpinic acid, and usnic acid metabolites (Gulçin et al. 2018). Salazinic acid, sekikaic acid and usnic acid showed affirmative results for their α- and β-glucosidase inhibition (Verma et al. 2012). Antarctic lichens *Stereocaulon alpinum, Umbilicaria antarctica* and *Lecidella carpathica* exhibited satisfactory inhibition of the protein tyrosine phosphatise activity, attributing this potential to the presence of their metabolites like lobaric acid, methyl orsellinate, gyrophoric acid, lecanoric acid, hopane-6α,22-diol, brialmontin 1 and atraric acid (Seo et al. 2009a, 2009b; Seo et al. 2011). The lichen metabolite erythrin, when evaluated against 14 diabetic target proteins, illustrated potential anti-diabetic activity (Rao and Hariprasad 2021).

A path towards successful new drug development involves the investigation of several prospectives, including possessing a state of knowledge about the protein, scrutinizing the protein-compound interactions and depicting the drug-likeness characteristics of the newly identified compound, preferably leading in the direction of cost-effective development of alternate therapy at a faster pace complying with the growing demands (Damián-Medina et al. 2020). To facilitate this, computational methods like molecular docking and virtual screening were enforced. Docking enables us to ascertain the ligand's efficacy by understanding the protein-ligand relationship (Rathore et al. 2016). Additionally, drug likeness prediction aids in compound screening, minimizing time and money waste. Taken together, an *in silico* analysis of lichen metabolites was conducted to assess their potential as anti-diabetic drugs. Molecular docking simulation and *in silico* drug-likeness prediction and toxicity studies of three lichen metabolites: calcyin, stictic acid and physodic acid, were performed along with three standard anti-diabetic drugs: metformin, repaglinide and sitagliptin, against 12 proteins known to play important roles in diabetes to optimise them as effective management therapy.

10.2 MATERIALS AND METHODS

10.2.1 Selection and Preparation of Protein Targets

Twelve proteins (1FM9, 1IR3, 1XU7, 2HWQ, 2Q5S, 2QMJ, 2ZJ3, 3C45, 3CTT, 3L2M, 4A5S, 4Y14) known to play a pivotal role in diabetes were selected from the literature and were assessed as targeted diabetic receptor proteins by molecular docking simulations. X-ray crystallographic structures of the 12 proteins (three-dimensional) were retrieved from the Protein Data Bank (www.pdb.org) and saved as .pdb files (Table 10.1). The preparatory step of the proteins entailed removal of water molecules, incorporating polar hydrogen atoms and merging of nonpolar hydrogen atoms. The proteins were then transformed from PDB to PDBQT format while keeping the other parameters at the default setting.

10.2.2 Preparation of Ligands

The 3D structures of the ligands enrolled for the docking simulation were retrieved from PubChem (/https://pubchem.ncbi.nlm.nih.gov/) in structural data format (.SDF) and converted to protein data bank (.PDB) format by Open Babel online converter. Ligands then later were checked for torsion and were converted into

TABLE 10.1
The 12 Selected Therapeutic Proteins of Diabetes Used for Molecular Docking

Sl. No.	Protein	Protein Name
1	1FM9	Heterodimer of the human RXR ALPHA and PPAR GAMMA ligand binding domains bound with 9-cis retinoic acid and GI262570 and coactivator peptides
2	1IR3	Phosphorylated insulin receptor tyrosine kinase in a complex with peptide substrate and ATP analogue
3	1XU7	Tetrameric 11B-HSD1
4	2HWQ	Peroxisome proliferator-activated receptor agonists
5	2Q5S	PPARGAMMA bound to a partial agonist NTZDPA
6	2QMJ	N-terminal subunit of human maltase-glucoamylase in a complex with acarbose
7	2ZJ3	Isomerase domain of human glucose:fructose-6-phosphate amidotransferase
8	3C45	Human dipeptidyl peptidase IV/CD26 in a complex with a fluoroolefin inhibitor
9	3CTT	N-terminal human maltase-glucoamylase with casuarina
10	3L2M	Pig pancreatic alpha-amylase with alphacyclodextrin
11	4A5S	Human DPP4 in a complex with a novel heterocyclic DPP4 inhibitor
12	4Y14	Tyrosine phosphatase 1B complexed with inhibitor (PTP1B:CPT157633)

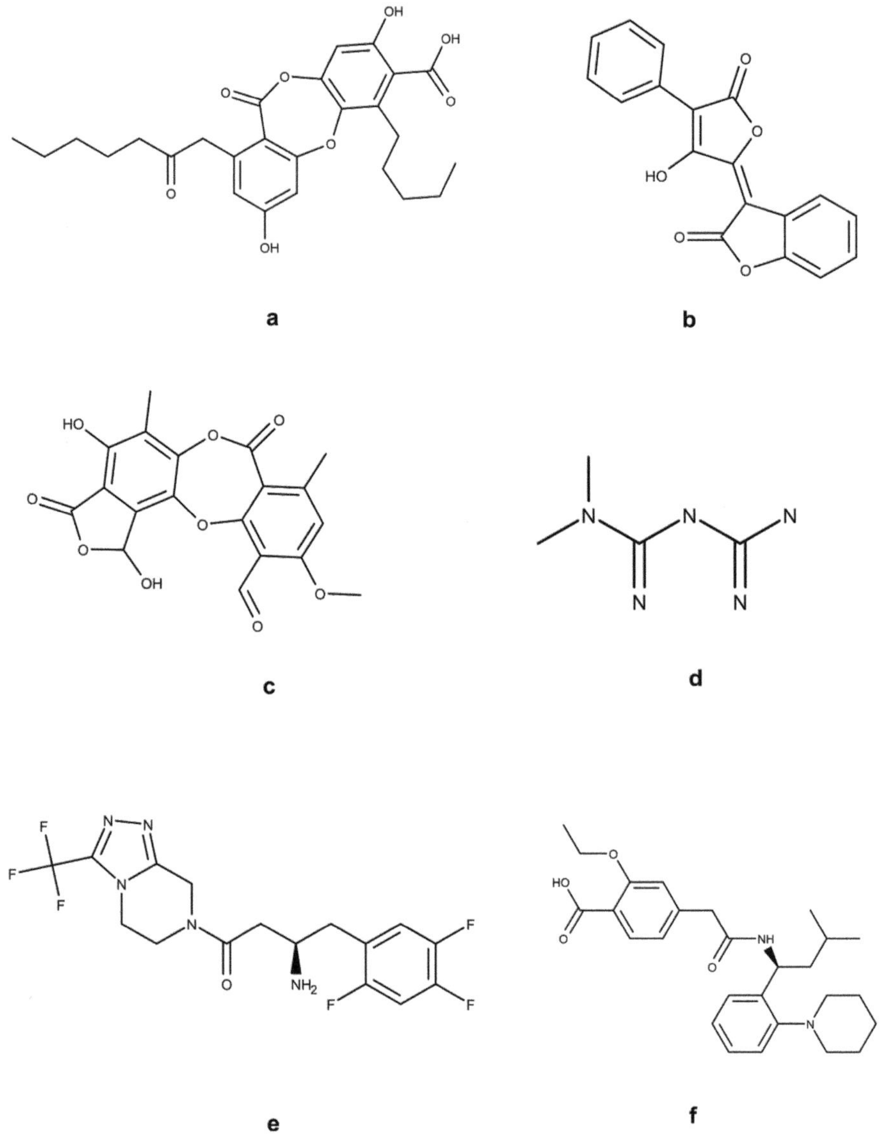

FIGURE 10.1 Two-dimensional structure of the ligands. a. Physodic acid, b. calycin, c. stictic acid, d. metformin, e. sitagliptin, f. repaglinide.

(Physodic acid, calycin and stictic acid are the putative anti-diabetic compounds in this study; Metformin, sitagliptin and repaglinide are standard antidiabetic drugs.)

PDBQT format. The structure of all three screened lichen metabolites, physodic acid, calycin and stictic acid, along with three standard anti-diabetic drugs, metformin (PubChem CID:4091), sitagliptin (PubChem CID: 4369359) and repaglinide (PubChem CID:65981), are represented in Figure 10.1.

10.2.3 Active Site Prediction

Protein active site prediction plays a predominant role in the protein and ligand interface. As a result the online server CASTp, i.e., Compound Atlas of Surface Topography of proteins (http://cast.engr.uic.edu) was used to forecast the active site of proteins. The PDB IDs of all 12 proteins were submitted to castP and the binding pocket was recorded. The first binding pocket was considered as the most suitable active site for docking trials (Table 10.2).

TABLE 10.2
Amino Acids of the Receptors Interacting with the Ligands

Receptors	Calycin	Physodic Acid	Stictic Acid
1FM9	CYS285, HIS323, HIS449, ILE281, ILE326, ILE456, LEU453, PHE282, PHE360, PHE363, SER289, TYR473	CYS285, GLN286, GLY361, HIS323, HIS449, ILE281, ILE326, LEU330, LEU353, LEU356, LEU453, LEU465, LEU469, MET364, PHE282, PHE360, PHE363, SER289, TYR327, TYR473	ARG288, CYS285, GLN286, HIS323, HIS449, ILE326, LEU330, LEU453, LEU465, LEU469, LYS367, MET364, PHE282, SER289
1IR3	ALA1028, ASP1150, GLU1047, GLU1077, GLY1082, GLY1149, LEU1002, LEU1078, LYS1030, MET1076, MET1079, MET1139, VAL1010, VAL1060	ALA1028, ASP1083, ASP1150, GLU1047, GLY1003, GLY1005, GLY1082, LEU1002, LYS1030, MET1051, MET1076, MET1079, MET1139, PHE1151, SER1086, VAL1010	ALA1028, ASN1137, ASP1150, GLU1077, GLY1003, GLY1082, LEU1002, MET1076, MET1079, MET1139, VAL1010
1XU7	ALA65, ARG66, ASN119, GLY41, GLY45, GLY91, HIS120, ILE121, ILE46, LYS44, MET93, THR92	ALA223, ALA65, ASN119, GLY216, GLY41, GLY47, HIS120, ILE121, ILE218, ILE46, LEU215, LEU217, SER169, SER170, THR220, THR222, TYR183, VAL168	ALA223, ALA226, ASN119, GLY216, ILE121, ILE218, LEU215, LEU217, LYS187, SER169, SER170, THR124, THR222, TYR183, VAL168
2HWQ	CYS285, GLN286, HIS323, HIS449, LEU330, LEU469, LYS367, MET334, MET364, PHE282, PHE363, SER289, TYR327, TYR473	ALA278, ALA292, ARG288, CYS285, GLU343, HIS449, ILE326, ILE341, LEU330, LEU333, LEU340, LYS367, MET334, MET364, PHE282, PHE360, PHE363, SER289, SER342, TYR327	ALA292, ARG288, ILE326, ILE341, LEU330, SER289, SER342, VAL339
2Q5S	ASN424, ASP380, GLU378, GLU427, HIS425, PRO426, SER428	ALA231, ALA235, ARG234, ASP380, GLU378, LEU379, LYS230, LYS240, THR238, THR241, THR242	ASN424, GLU378, GLU427, HIS425, LEU423, PRO426, SER428

Receptors	Calycin	Physodic Acid	Stictic Acid
2QMJ	ARG526, ASP203, ASP327, ASP443, ASP542, HIS600, PHE450, THR204, TRP406, TRP441, TYR299	ALA576, ARG526, ASP203, ASP327, ASP443, ASP542, ASP571, HIS600, ILE364, MET444, PHE575, THR204, THR205, TRP406, TRP441, TRP539, TYR299	ALA576, ARG526, ASP203, GLN603, GLY602, MET444, PHE575, TRP406, TYR299, TYR605
2ZJ3	ALA472, CYS373, GLN421, GLU560, LEU419, LEU673, LYS675, SER376, SER420, SER422, SER473, THR425, VAL471	ALA426, ALA674, ASP427, CYS373, GLN421, GLU680, GLY374, LEU673, LYS675, SER376, SER422, SER473, SER676, THR375, THR425, VAL471, VAL677	ALA674, GLN421, GLU560, LEU673, LYS675, SER376, SER420, SER473, THR425, VAL471, VAL677
3C45	ARG125, ARG669, GLU205, GLU206, PHE357, SER209, SER630, TYR547, TYR631, TYR662, TYR666, VAL656, VAL711	ARG125, ARG429, CYS551, GLN553, GLY549, HIS740, PHE357, PRO550, SER552, SER630, TRP659, TYR456, TYR547, TYR585, TYR631, TYR662, TYR666, VAL656	ARG358, ARG669, GLU206, GLY549, PHE357, PRO550, SER552, TYR547, TYR666
3CTT	ALA746, ARG315, ASN356, ASN357, GLN359, GLY358, LEU319, LEU745, THR742, THR743, TYR321	ALA746, ARG315, ASN356, ASN357, ASN741, GLN359, GLY358, HIS355, LEU745, LYS749, THR742, THR743, TYR321	ARG315, ASN314, ASN357, GLN318, GLN359, LEU319, THR742, THR743, TYR321
3L2M	GLN161, GLY147, GLY164, ILE148, LEU162, SER145, TYR151, VAL163	ALA198, ASP197, GLU233, HIS101, HIS201, ILE235, LEU162, LEU165, LYS200, SER199, TYR151, TYR62, VAL163, VAL234	ASP300, GLN63, GLY104, LEU165, TRP58, TRP59, TYR62, VAL163,
4A5S	ARG631, ARG87, ASN672, GLU167, GLU168, HIS702, PHE319, SER592, TYR593, TYR624, TYR628, VAL618, VAL673	ARG87, ASN672, ASP507, ASP671, GLU167, GLY590, GLY594, GLY703, HIS702, LYS516, SER592, TRP163, TRP589, TRP591, TYR509, VAL508	GLY590, GLY594, GLY703, HIS702, SER592, TRP589, TRP591, TYR509, VAL508
4Y14	ALA217, ARG221, ASP181, ASP48, GLN262, GLY220, ILE219, PHE182, SER216, TYR46, VAL49	ALA217, ARG221, ARG47, ASP181, ASP48, GLN262, GLN266, GLY220, ILE219, PHE182, SER216, TYR46	ALA217, ARG221, ASP181, GLN262, ILE219, LYS120, PHE182, SER216, TYR46, VAL49

10.2.4 Molecular Docking Analysis

Molecular docking simulations are of paramount importantance, as they depict the affinity between the target proteins and the compounds by assigning a binding energy for the interaction. The best docking poses were the ones with minimum binding energy and are projected as the most stable conformations for interacting with the active site of the proteins. Autodockvina 1.1.2. was adopted to annotate the binding mode between the compounds and 12 established therapeutic targets. The MGLTools 1.5.6 (http://mgltools.scripps.edu) package was employed to generate the docking input files. The grid map spacing was set as 0.375A° and co-ordinates, dimensions were recorded and default parameters were exercised. The best-scoring geometry and interaction were chosen and visually examined using Biovia Discovery Studio 2021 visualizer.

10.2.5 Drug Likeness Prediction

Pharmacological check points like molecular properties and drug likeness for all the test compounds including three anti-diabetic drugs were obtained using Molsoft prediction server (http://molsoft. com/mprop/), which uses Lipinski's rule of five (Ro5) as the basis of selection. Information regarding their canonical SMILES was gathered from PubChem and applied as input data for obtaining information pertaining to their molecular weight, total number of hydrogen bond acceptors and donors, partition coefficient values, polar surface area, dissolution factor and drug likeness.

10.2.6 ADMET Analysis

ADMET parameters of natural products upon consumption were evaluated by AdmetSAR (http://lmmd.ecust.edu.cn/admetsar2/), a platform used to predict the pharmacokinetic and pharmacodynamic properties of compounds and showed if the drug complies with Lipinski's Rule. Blood-brain barrier (BBB) penetration, human intestinal absorption (HIA), Caco-2 permeability, carcinogen toxicity, mutagenicity and other conditions were forecasted. The SMILES for the ligands were retrieved from PubChem, and the AdmetSAR program was used to check for toxicity.

10.3 RESULTS

10.3.1 Molecular Docking

Virtual screening of compounds to estimate their putative binding affinity with the therapeutic target forms an integral part of structure-based drug design process, further contributing to the advancement of the compound as a lead drug and also minimizing the compound failure at experimental testing substantially. Molecular docking renders a better understanding about a compound's affinity for target proteins. In the present study, Autodock Vina was used to carry out the docking simulations and Discovery Studio was used to visualize the docked structures and binding site analysis. The selected compounds were docked, and their binding energies (kcal/mol) are presented in Table 10.3 and Figure 10.2. The test compounds exhibited favorable energies ranging from (–5.4 to −8.4 kcal/mol) for physodic acid, (–7.2 to −8.9 kcal/mol) for calycin and (–6.8 to −8.8 kcal/mol) for stictic acid. The highest binding energy was observed by calycin against 2QMJ (–8.9 kcal/mol). These results were compared with the standard drugs sitagliptin (–7.3 to −9.0 kcal/mol), metformin (–4.8 to –5.8 kcal/mol) and repaglinide (–6.5 to −8.1 kcal/mol). Calycin

TABLE 10.3
Energy of the Ligands (kcal/mol) Against the Selected Receptors of Diabetes

Receptors	Physodic Acid	Calycin	Stictic Acid	Sitagliptin	Metformin	Repaglinide
1FM9	−7.7	−7.6	−7.9	−7.7	−5.3	−6.9
1IR3	−7	−8.4	−7.2	−7.4	−5	−6.7
1XU7	−7	−8.1	−8	−7.7	−5.2	−6.6
2HWQ	−8	−8.7	−8.5	−8.6	−4.8	−7.5
2Q5S	−8.4	−8.2	−8.7	−8.8	−5.3	−7.6
2QMJ	−8	−8.9	−8.5	−9	−5.3	−7.5
2ZJ3	−5.4	−7.2	−7.1	−7.3	−5.1	−6.6
3C45	−6.8	−8.8	−8.2	−8.5	−5.4	−7.4
3CTT	−7.2	−8.5	−8.5	−8.5	−5.3	−8.1
3L2M	−7	−8.1	−8.8	−8.2	−5.6	−7.6
4A5S	−6.8	−8.6	−8.2	−8.2	−5.8	−7.6
4Y14	−5.8	−7.2	−6.8	−7.4	−5	−6.5

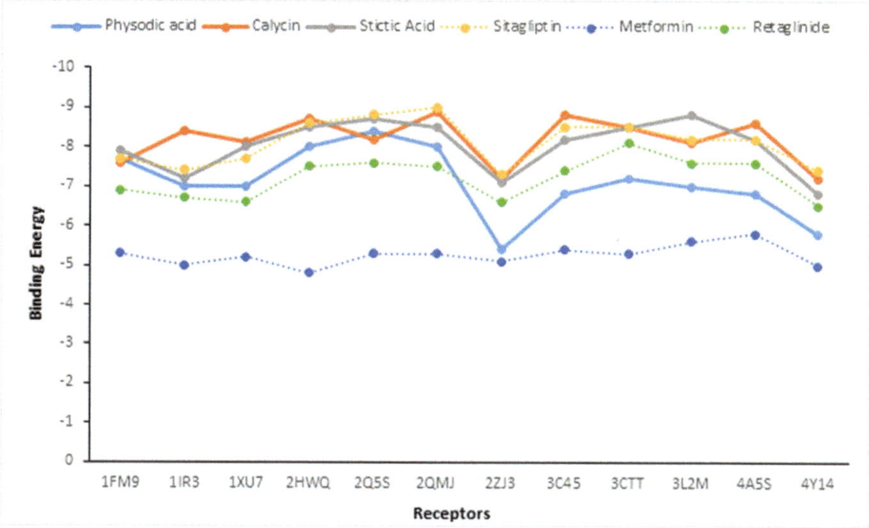

FIGURE 10.2 Binding energies of the three putative and three standard antidiabetic ligands upon interaction with the 12 therapeutic proteins of diabetes.

and stictic acid fared better when compared to the standard drugs metformin and repaglinide and had comparable results to sitagliptin. Physodic acid yielded underwhelming results in comparison to sitagliptin but presented on an equal energy level with repaglinide, inferring that our test compounds garnered desirable results. Top four docking poses are presented for physodic acid (Figure 10.3), calycin (Figure 10.4) and stictic acid (Figure 10.5).

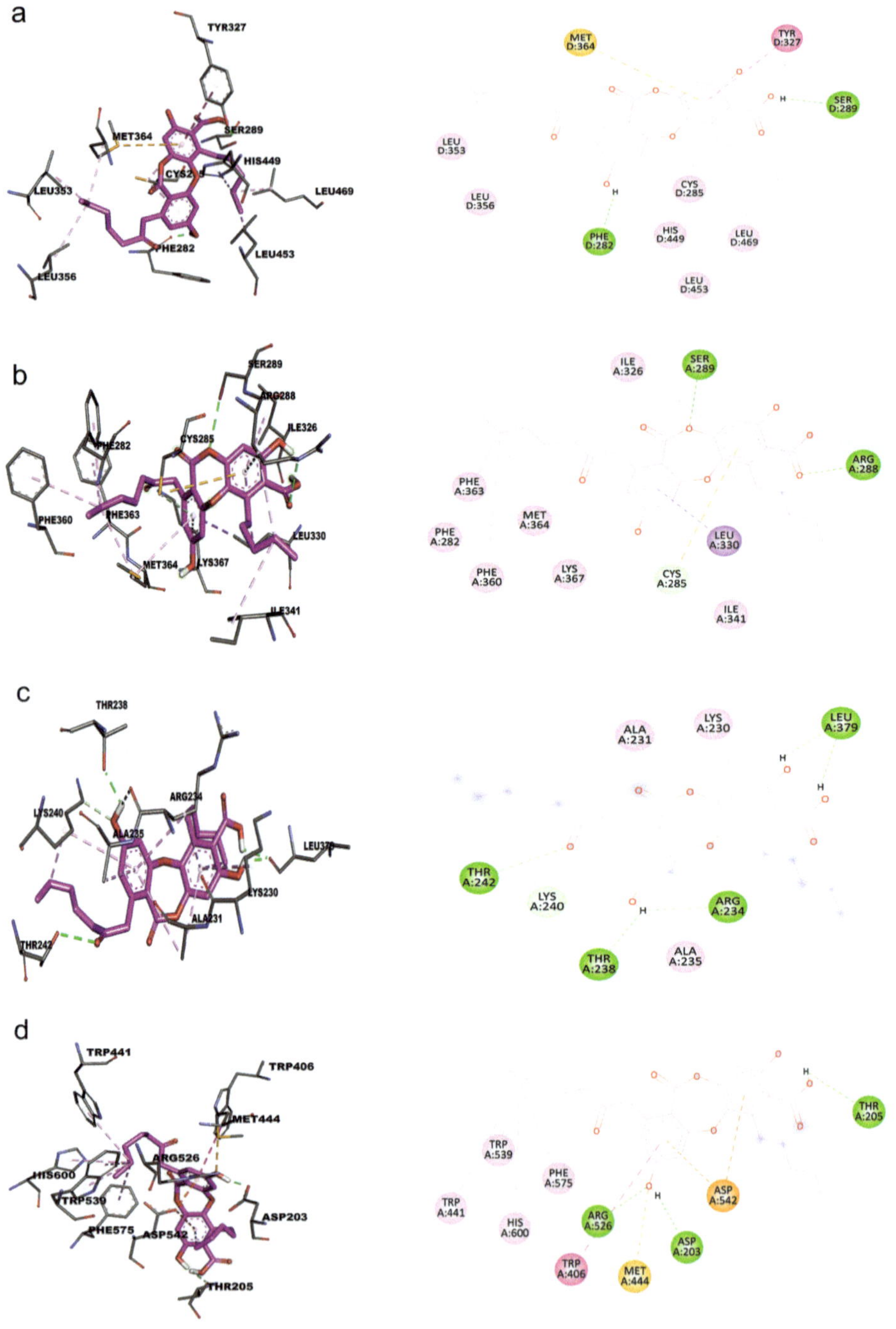

FIGURE 10.3 Three- and two-dimensional molecular docking interactions of physodic acid against the therapeutic proteins of diabetes. a. 1FM9, b. 2HWQ, c. 2Q5S, d. 2QMJ (only the top four interactions are presented).

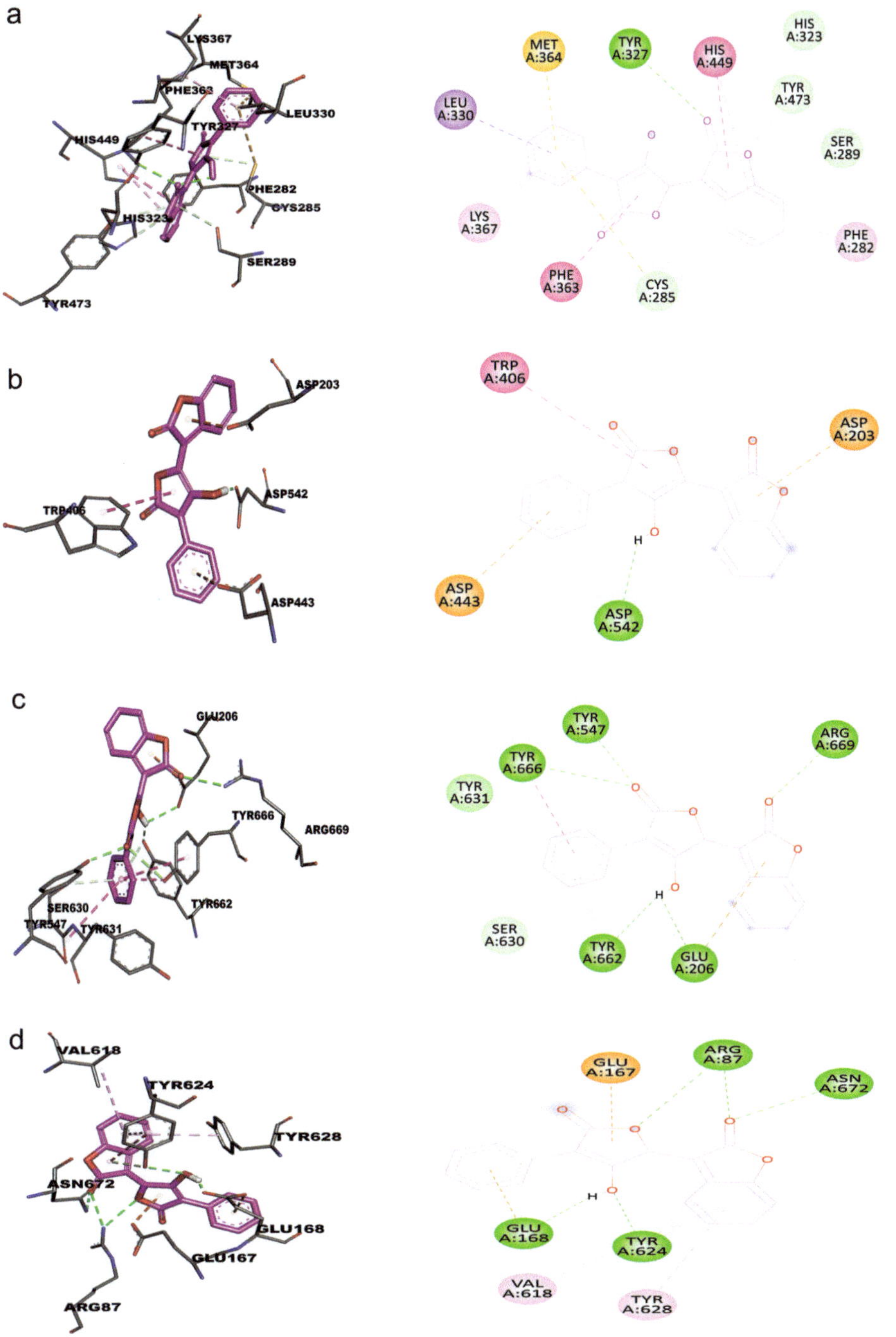

FIGURE 10.4 Three- and two-dimensional molecular docking interactions of calycin against the therapeutic proteins of diabetes. a. 2HWQ, b. 2QMJ, c. 3C45, d. 4A5S (only the top four interactions are presented).

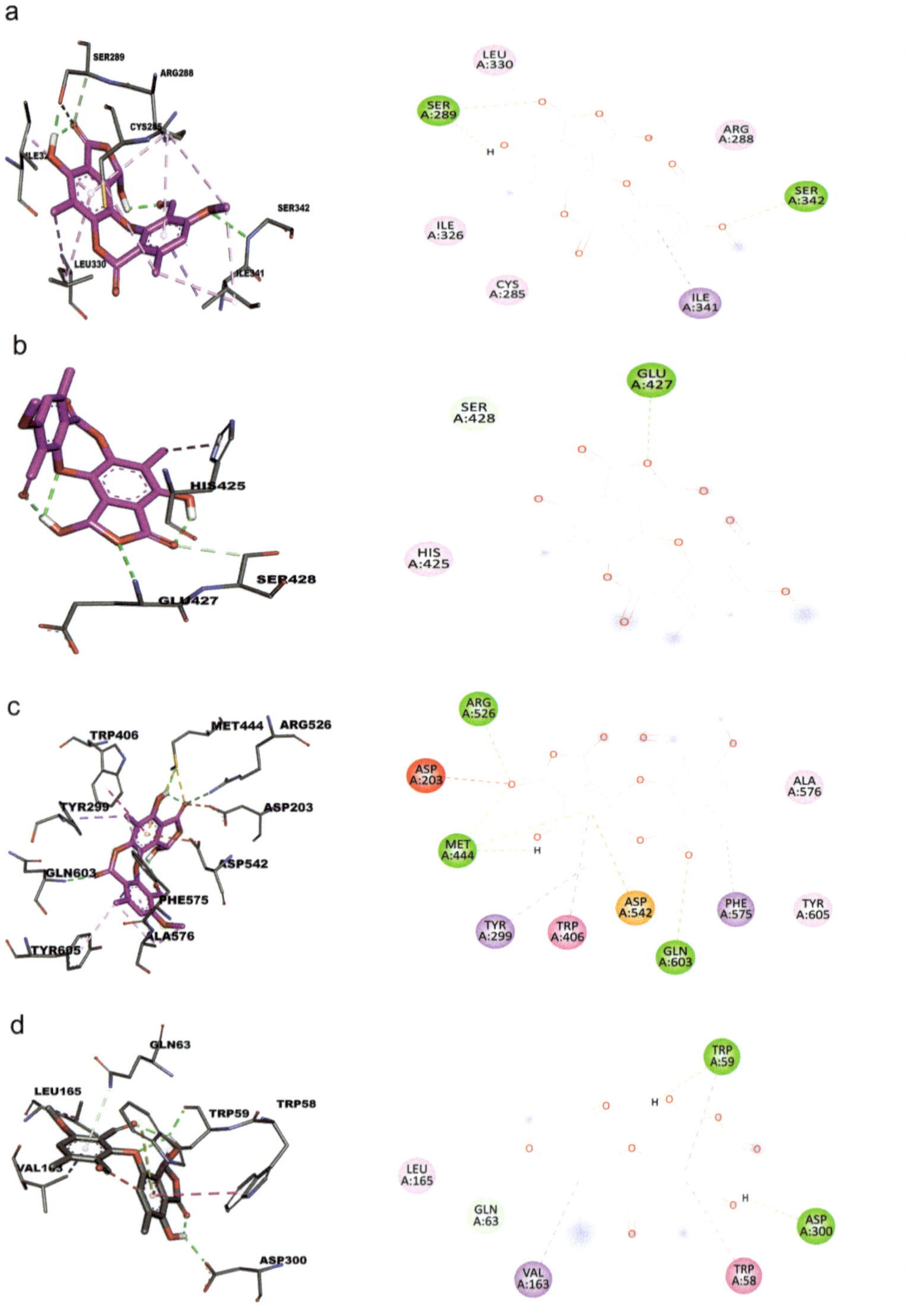

FIGURE 10.5 Three- and two-dimensional molecular docking interactions of stictic acid against the therapeutic proteins of diabetes. a. 2HWQ, b. 2Q5S, c. 2QMJ, d. 3L2M (only the top four interactions are presented).

10.3.2 Drug-Likeness Prediction

To understand if a compound possess a drug-like property, a theoretical demonstration of pharmacological properties was cumulated by the bioinformatics tool molsoft which respects Lipinski's Ro5. The Ro5 states that a considered drug molecule should have properties including molecular weight ≤500 Da, number of hydrogen bond donors <5, hydrogen bond acceptors ≤10 and the water-octanol coefficient ratio <5. It was seen that all the test compounds as well as the three standard drugs abide by Lipinski's rule pertaining to molecular weight, total number of hydrogen bond acceptors and donors, polar surface area and dissolution factor, with one violation made by the test compound physodic acid and standard drug repaglinide (log p of 6.35 and 5.20, respectively) where the cut-off was (<5); additionally, Molsoft gives information regarding drug likeness which interprets the ability of a particular molecule to be a drug or non-drug. The values for all the parameters are presented in Table 10.4 and Figure 10.6

10.3.3 ADMET

Detection of compounds with desirable pharmacokinetics and toxicological parameters advances their selection and development as an oral drug, minimizing the trials deemed necessary. The admetSAR server was adopted to calibrate these independent ADMET variables associated with cell permeation, bioavailability and toxicity. Both HIA and Caco-2 alter the penetration of oral drugs through the intestinal barrier, and all compounds exhibited a positive result for HIA permeability, whereas only stictic acid and calycin demonstrated affirmative results for Caco-2, implying gradual oral bio-accessibility influence. Carcinogenicity was not observed in any compounds, whereas mutagenicity was observed with stictic acid from the *in silico* prediction (Table 10.5).

TABLE 10.4
Molecular Properties of the Ligands Including the Standard Drugs

Molecules	Molecular Weight	Number of HBA	Number of HBD	MolLogP	MolLogS moles/L	MolPSA (A^2)	MolVol (A^3)	Drug Likeness Score
Physodic acid	470.19	8	3	6.35	−5.52	103.40	493.75	0.00
Calycin	306.05	5	1	2.40	−3.14	59.18	318.17	−0.31
Stictic Acid	386.06	9	2	2.27	−2.25	103.88	372.54	−0.36
Sitagliptin	407.12	4	2	1.34	−1.74	61.67	329.55	0.52
Metformin	129.10	2	5	−1.00	−0.54	69.77	119.98	−0.82
Repaglinide	452.27	4	2	5.20	−4.60	62.84	478.12	0.85

HBA: Hydrogen bond acceptors, HBD: Hydrogen bond donors.

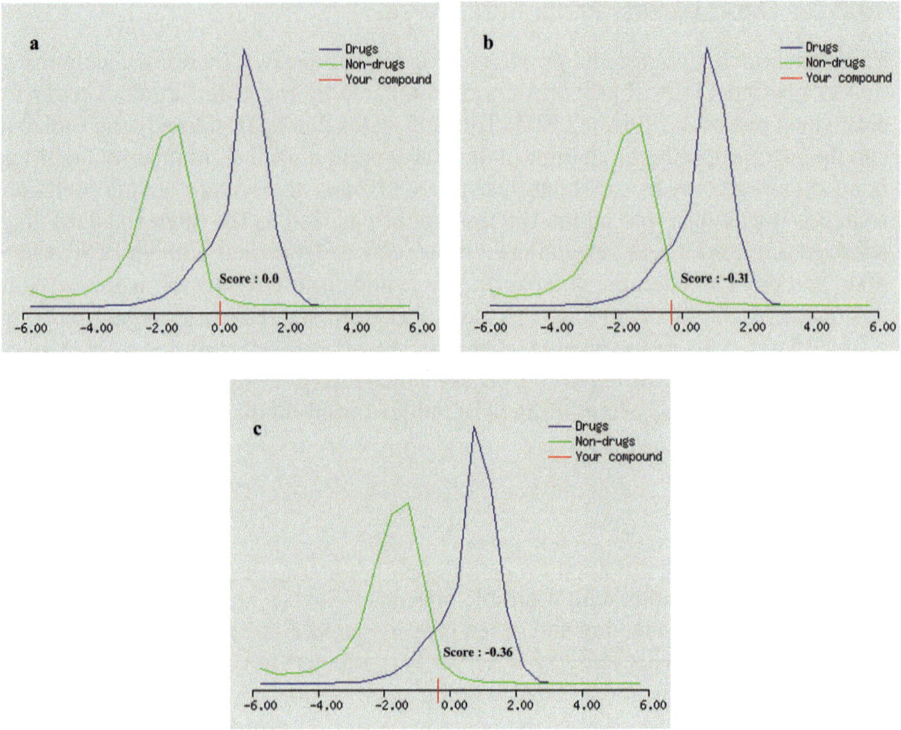

FIGURE 10.6 Drug likeliness scores of the ligands. a. Physodic acid, b. Calycin, c. Stictic acid.

TABLE 10.5
Toxicological and Pharmacokinetic Properties of the Ligands and Standard Drugs

	HIA		Caco-2		BBB		Carcinogenicity		Ames Mutagenesis	
Molecules	*V*	*P*	*V*	*P*	*V*	*P*	*V*	*P*	*V*	*P*
Physodic Acid	+	0.9700	–	0.7048	+	0.8701	–	0.9429	–	0.9300
Calycin	+	0.9843	+	0.6202	–	0.3704	–	0.7888	–	0.6700
Stictic Acid	+	0.9745	+	0.6414	+	0.8207	–	0.9286	+	0.5700
Sitagliptin	+	0.9733	–	0.6132	+	0.9821	–	0.8429	–	0.6800
Metformin	+	0.9687	–	0.9372	+	0.9807	–	0.5600	–	0.6600
Repaglinide	+	0.9862	–	0.7491	+	0.9449	–	0.7429	–	0.8200

V: value, P: probability, HIA: human intestinal absorption, BBB: blood brain barrier.

10.4 DISCUSSION

Diabetes, often considered as a silent epidemic, is an endocrine disorder elicited by the malfunctioning of insulin secretion, action or both, plaguing around 9.3% of the world populace (IDF 2021). The current available anti-diabetic drugs are known to have detrimental effects, thereby driving the momentum to investigate newer, safer and more effective alternatives in remedying the situation (Trinh and Le 2014). Of late, attention has been focused on natural compounds as they are effective. Natural compounds such as lichens are a plethora of therapeutic moieties, having served us as an ancillary guide with their diverse ability to encumber several etiologies (Hawksworth 2015). But to propel these bioactive compounds as marketable drugs, explication of their mode of action, drug characteristics and incidence of toxicity is deemed necessary. Computational biology, a new systematic concept, has provided a holistic understanding of natural compounds by evincing their effectiveness and biosafety, legitimizing them as a future lead drug in ameliorating the disorder, thereby saving resources and time (Rathore et al. 2016). In the current study, metabolites derived from lichens were tested as a promising anti-diabetic therapy by evaluating their modulating potential against 12 proteins from documented therapeutic targets known to mediate carbohydrate metabolism. Impeding these proteins implicated a substandard flux of glucose in the blood and thus can be explored as a pharmacotherapy. Docking analysis provided the insights regarding the protein-ligand interaction, substantiating the effectiveness of the compound. *In silico* drug likeness and toxicity profile help us in understanding the drug characterstics of the compound.

The absolute binding energy values ranged from −5.2 kcal/mol to −8.9 kcal/mol for all compounds, and the top four docking poses were chosen and presented for physodic acid (Figure 10.3), calycin (Figure 10.4) and stictic acid (Figure 10.5). All compounds performed well, though there were some fluctuations in this range, which could be attributed to the amino acid composition of each protein. Good docking results reflect that the selected protein is amenable to modification by inhibiting or activating by interaction, i.e., ligands forming bonds with receptor residues.

The binding capability of each compound was displayed on a line graph (Figure 10.2). Following this chart, the calycin line remained at the top level, followed by the stictic acid line in the center and the physodic acid line at the bottom. The best ligand for binding the receptors, according to this evidence, was calycin. Almost all of the values on this line are more than −8.0 kcal/mol in absolute value. The calycin line is therefore at the top for this reason. Following the stictic acid line, which interacted with eight receptors with energies of over −8.0 kcal/mol, the physodic acid line is in last place on the chart because the majority of its interactions were with energies between −5.4 kcal/mol and −7.7 kcal/mol.

Discovery Studio software was utilized for analyzing the docking phenomenon by emphasizing prominent binding sites. All of the test compounds were discovered to make bonds with the insulin receptor's (IR) critical substrate recognition sites at Asn 1137, Ser 1006, Glu 1077, Met 1079, Asp 1083, Lys

1030 and Asp 1150, suggesting that the insulin signaling cascade has likely been initiated (Ganugapati et al. 2012). It may be possible to maintain glucose homeostasis by interacting with functional PPARg residues at Arg 288, His 323, Ser 342, His 449 and Tyr 473 (Bharti et al. 2013). The interconversion of glucocorticoids, cortisone and cortisol could be hampered by test compounds bound inside the binding site pocket of Asn 119, Leu 217, Thr 220 and Thr 222 and 11β-HSD receptors, which would ultimately result in the impedance of insulin production (Damián-Medina et al. 2020). The compounds can display a DPP-IV suppressive effect by engaging with the residues Glu-205, Glu 206, Ser 630, Tyr 631 and Tyr 662, which allows the activity of the glucose-regulating incretin hormones (GLP-1), which regulates blood sugar and stimulates insulin (Rozano et al. 2017).

The PTP1B receptor, which negatively regulates insulin biosynthesis, has key residues such as Ser 216, Ala 217, Ile 219 and Arg 221 that test compounds interacted well with, suggesting that the receptor may be attenuated, facilitating the development of an effective anti-diabetic medication (Damián-Medina et al. 2020). Test compounds interacting with critical binding-site regions Gln 111, Phe 62, Ile 217, Asn 112 and Trp 186 of mono-ADP ribosyltransferase-sirtuin-6 (SIRT6) receptor controls glucose uptake by the cells and could alter it, paving the path for an anti-diabetic medication (Singh et al. 2019). The results illustrate that the test compounds are well bound within the binding site pocket of glucosidase at His 600, Asp 443, Ala 536 and Ala 285, with a nearly identical binding pattern (Lee et al. 2014), speculating compounds may retain a postprandial glucose-suppressing operation.

Numerous drug candidates fail in clinical trials due to inadequate pharmacokinetic properties, which necessitates acquiring preliminary insights by employing *in silico* techniques, thereby streamlining the drug discovery process and conserving resources (Rathore et al. 2016). When a compound exerts a substantial biological activity, achieving optimal physicochemical along with ADMET properties becomes an imperative measure, as they play a vital role in establishing the efficacy and safety of the compound (Singh and Singh 2010). In the present study, compounds were screened for their drug likeness and ADMET characteristics using Molsoft and the admetSAR online server. The molecular weight helps in the optimization of drug action by manipulating the absorption parameter of the compound; hence, a compound with less molecular weight (≤500 Da) is a preferable target to reach. All our test ligands were well within the limits. Biological membrane absorption or permeability factor is governed by number of HBA (≤10) and HBD (≤5). Lipinski's rule of five was followed by the proposed compounds, thereby illustrating satisfactory absorption. The capability of compounds to maneuver through cell membrane depends on its lipophilicity, which is denoted by Log p. Thus, it can be suggested that the compounds obeying rule of five (<5) could have improved cell permeability upon reaching a specific target (Leo et al. 1971). Physodic acid and repaglinide both showed slight deviations from the suggested limit. The surface contributing to oxygen and nitrogen, including the hydrogens bound to these atoms, is exemplified by the molecular polar surface. PSA greater than 140 angstroms correlates to deficient permeation. The potency of the oral dosage relies on the drug's innate ability to dissolve in GI tract fluids (Ertl 2008). Candidates with aqueous solubility log S >−6 were perceived to be well-dissolved drugs (Singh and Singh 2010). All candidates exhibited PSA of less than 140 angstroms and log S >−6, highlighting their drug-like characteristics.

Incidentally, the migration through the intestinal epithelial barrier, which dictates the rate and magnitude of human absorption and eventually influences its bioavailability, is one of the consequential challenges facing an oral drug. The admetSAR online server was deployed to audit the pharmacokinetics and toxicological features of compounds. The value of human intestinal absorption nearer to 1 is seen to reflect superior absorption through the intestine (Elekofehinti et al. 2018). Ames mutagenicity assessment divulges plausible teratogenicity and genotoxicity at the incipient stage of drug discovery (Shah et al. 2019). All candidates except for stictic acid demonstrated a negative result, making it an unfit drug candidate. Similarly, the toxicological node capturing the predominant risk for human health was carcinogenicity, which contributes to the withdrawal of many medications from the market (Murugesan et al. 2020). No carcinogenic property was observed in the candidates. All in all, the selected candidates can be considered as possible potent anti-diabetic drugs.

10.5 FUTURE PROSPECTS AND LIMITATIONS

Diabetes, a metabolic disease with alarming blood glucose level as a pathognomonic sign, is spreading like a wildfire. The chronic metabolic disequilibrium attributed with this ailment places a tremendous burden on healthcare; therefore, comprehending the pathophysiology of this disease will aid in the mitigation of repercussions such as cardiovascular disease (CVD), diabetic retinopathy, nephropathy and neuropathy (Gan et al. 2020). Furthermore, diabetes can be averted or impeded through dietary modifications; thus, the World Health Organization (WHO) is advocating the use of natural resources for the treatment of diabetes mellitus (Tran et al. 2020).

Given the prospective of lichens as natural phyto-pharmaceuticals, it is required to investigate the bioactive compounds that are still unreported for the application as an anti-diabetic medication. Despite their extensive range of biological activities, lichens have long been disregarded for their extensive application in the pharmaceutical industry due to their slow development and restricted synthesis of compounds in nature or in axenic cultures (Verma and Behera 2019). Furthermore, lichen compounds are particularly sensitive to pH, stability, light absorption, etc., which affects their bioactivity. More research is necessary to establish, enhance and scale up innovative technologies of industrial and national value (Varol 2019).

The lichen tissue culture techniques which can endorse symbiont growth harvesting secondary metabolites in abundance within a short period of time must be strengthened, delivering a steady, reliable source for valuable products. Understanding the gene chemistry and the use of gene technologies in pathways involved in the secondary metabolism will offer foundations for the synthesis of commercially viable lichen compounds (Verma and Behera 2019). The application of contemporary recombinant techniques to construct transgenic cultures and control the regulation of biosynthetic pathways and cell cultures can be usable for large-scale production secondary metabolites. Additional, bioinformatics tools can potentially be used to streamline the procedure to a larger extent (Zambare and Christopher 2012).

There is a critical need to isolate lichen compounds and understand their underlying mechanisms. Lichens are an unexplored source of industrially important biological moieties, and their potency has yet to be completely studied and harnessed. Bioactive chemicals obtained from lichens are to be explored for biopharmaceutical applications for the betterment of human life.

10.6 CONCLUSION

Diabetes is a systemic condition, and understanding its etiology can aid in the prevention of its micro and macro complications. The current anti-diabetic medications have catastrophic effects, necessitating the investigation of a novel, natural compound. In this regard, an effort has been made to design a drug which could help in combating the situation, employing various *in silico* techniques. The three screened lichen metabolites underwent docking simulation to evaluate their affinity towards the target proteins, where calycin and physodic acid emerged as suitable candidates. Further, for a compound to become a successful oral drug, possessing optimal physicochemical as well as ADMET properties is a quintessential prerequisite. In this study, ADMET and Molsoft servers were deployed, which revealed that the compounds calycin and physodic acid had the innate ability to be manifested as a potent anti-diabetic drug along with docking studies.

REFERENCES

Adenubi, O. T., I. M. Famuyide, L. J. McGaw and J. N. Eloff. 2022. Lichens: An update on their ethnopharmacological uses and potential as sources of drug leads. *J Ethnopharmacol* 298: 115657.

Anderson, J., N. Lévesque, F. Caron, P. Beckett and G. A. Spiers. 2022. A review on the use of lichens as a biomonitoring tool for environmental radioactivity. *J Environ Radioact* 243: 106797.

Aptroot, A., N. J. Stapper, A. Košuthová and K. C. van Herk. 2021. Lichens as an indicator of climate and global change. In *Climate Change; Observed Impacts on Planet Earth*, ed. T. M. Letcher, 483–497. Amsterdam: Elsevier.

Baharvand-Ahmadi, B., M. Bahmani, P. Tajeddini, N. Naghdi and M. Rafieian-Kopaei. 2016. An ethno-medicinal study of medicinal plants used for the treatment of diabetes. *J Nephropathol* 5(1): 44–50.

Bharti, S. K., A. Kumar, N. K. Sharma, O. Prakash, S. K. Jaiswal, S. Krishnan, A. K. Gupta and A. Kumar. 2013. Tocopherol from seeds of *Cucurbita pepo* against diabetes: Validation by *in vivo* experiments supported by computational docking. *J Formos Med Assoc* 112(11): 676–690.

Candar, A., H. Demirci, A. K. Baran and Y. Akpınar. 2018. The association between quality of life and complementary and alternative medicine use in patients with diabetes mellitus. *Complement Ther Clin Pract* 31: 1–6.

Chaudhury, A., C. Duvoor, V. S. Reddy Dendi, et al. 2017. Clinical review of antidiabetic drugs: Implications for type 2 diabetes mellitus management. *Front Endocrinol* 8: 6. https://doi.org/10.3389/fendo.2017.00006

Choudhury, H., M. Pandey, C. K. Hua, et al. 2018. An update on natural compounds in the remedy of diabetes mellitus: A systematic review. *J Trad Complement Med* 8(3): 361–376.

Cui, Y., J. H. Yim, D. S. Lee, Y. C. Kim and H. Oh. 2012. New diterpene furanoids from the Antarctic lichen Huea sp. *Bioorg Med Chem Lett* 22(24): 7393–7396.

Damián-Medina, K., Y. Salinas-Moreno, D. Milenkovic, et al. 2020. In silico analysis of antidiabetic potential of phenolic compounds from blue corn (*Zea mays* L.) and black bean (*Phaseolus vulgaris* L.). *Heliyon* 6(3): e03632. www.cell.com/heliyon/pdf/S2405-8440(20)30477-1.pdf

Das, A. K., B. Saboo, A. Maheswari, et al. 2022. Health care delivery model in India with relevance to diabetes care. *Heliyon* 8(10): e10904. www.cell.com/heliyon/pdf/S2405-8440(22)02192-2.pdf

Elekofehinti, O. O., O. C. Ejelonu, J. P. Kamdem, et al. 2018. Discovery of potential visfatin activators using in silico docking and ADME predictions as therapy for type 2 diabetes. *Beni-Suef Univ J Basic Appl Sci* 7(2): 241–249.

Ertl, P. 2008. Polar surface area. In. *Molecular Drug Properties: Measurement and Prediction*, ed. R. Manhold, 111–126. Weinheim, Germany: Wiley-VCH, Verlag GmbH & Co. KGa.

Gan, Q., J. Wang, J. Hu, G. Lou, H. Xiong, C. Peng, S. Zheng and Q. Huang. 2020. The role of diosgenin in diabetes and diabetic complications. *J Steroid Biochem Mol Biol* 198: 105575.

Ganugapati, J., A. Baldwa and S. Lalani. 2012. Molecular docking studies of banana flower flavonoids as insulin receptor tyrosine kinase activators as a cure for diabetes mellitus. *Bioinformation* 8(5): 216–220.

Goga, M., M. Baláž, N. Daneu, J. Elečko, L. Tkáčiková, M. Marcinčinová and M. Bačkor. 2021. Biological activity of selected lichens and lichen-based Ag nanoparticles prepared by a green solid-state mechanochemical approach. *Mater Sci Eng C* 119: 111640. https://doi.org/10.1016/j.msec.2020.111640

Gulçin, İ., P. Taslimi, A. Aygün, et al. 2018. Antidiabetic and antiparasitic potentials: Inhibition effects of some natural antioxidant compounds on α-glycosidase, α-amylase and human glutathione S-transferase enzymes. *Int J Biol Macromol* 119: 741–746.

Halama, P. and C. Van Haluwin. 2004. Antifungal activity of lichen extracts and lichenic acids. *BioControl* 49(1): 95–107.

Hamida, R. S., M. A. Ali, N. E. Abdelmeguid, M. I. Al-Zaban, L. Baz and M. M. Bin-Meferij. 2021. Lichens—a potential source for nanoparticles fabrication: A review on nanoparticles biosynthesis and their prospective applications. *J Fungi* 7(4): 291.

Hawksworth, D. L. 2015. *Lichen Secondary Metabolites: Bioactive Properties and Pharmaceutical Potential*. Ed. B. Ranković. Basel, Switzerland: Springer International.

Hidalgo, M. E., E. Fernandez, W. Quilhot and E. Lissi. 1994. Antioxidant activity of depsides and depsidones. *Phytochemistry* 37(6): 1585–1587.

Huneck, S. 1999. The significance of lichens and their metabolites. *Naturwissenschaften* 86(12): 559–570.

International Diabetes Foundation (IDF). 2021. https://idf.org/ accessed on 6th April 2021.

Karthik, S., K. C. Nandini, P. T. R. Kekuda, K. S. Vinayaka and S. Mukunda. 2011. Total phenol content, insecticidal and amylase inhibitory efficacy of *Heterodermia leucomela* (L). *Ann Biol Res* 2(4): 38–43.

Karunaratne, V., V. M. Thadhani, S. N. Khan and M. I. Choudhary. 2014. Potent α-glucosidase inhibitors from the lichen Cladonia species from Sri Lanka. *J Natl Sci Found SRI* 42(1): 95–98.

Kim, H. J., K. H. Chun, D. J. Kim, et al. 2011. Utilization patterns and cost of complementary and alternative medicine compared to conventional medicine in patients with type 2 diabetes mellitus. *Diabetes Res Clin Prac* 93(1): 115–122.

Lee, S. H., S. M. Kang, S. C. Ko, S. H. Moon, B. T. Jeon, D. H. Lee and Y. J. Jeon. 2014. Octaphlorethol A: A potent α-glucosidase inhibitor isolated from *Ishige foliacea* shows an anti-hyperglycemic effect in mice with streptozotocin-induced diabetes. *Food Funct* 5(10): 2602–2608.

Leo, A., C. Hansch and D. Elkins. 1971. Partition coefficients and their uses. *Chem Rev* 71(6): 525–616.

Low, L. L., S. F. Tong and W. Y. Low. 2016. Selection of treatment strategies among patients with type 2 diabetes mellitus in Malaysia: A grounded theory approach. *PLoS ONE* 11(1): e0147127. https://journals.plos.org/plosone/article/file?id=10.1371/journal.pone.0147127&type=printable

Murugesan, S., M. R. Venkateswaran, S. Jayabal and S. Periyasamy. 2020. Evaluation of the antioxidant and anti-arthritic potential of *Zingiber officinale* Rosc. by *in vitro* and *in silico* analysis. *S Afr J Bot* 130: 45–53.

Neamati, N., H. Hong, A. Mazumder, et al. 1997. Depsides and depsidones as inhibitors of HIV-1 integrase: Discovery of novel inhibitors through 3D database searching. *J Med Chem* 40(6): 942–951.

Pradeepa, R. and V. Mohan. 2021. Epidemiology of type 2 diabetes in India. *Indian J Ophthalmol* 69(11): 2932–2938.

Prasopthum, A., T. Insawek and P. Pouyfung. 2022. Herbal medicine use in Thai patients with type 2 diabetes mellitus and its association with glycemic control: A cross-sectional evaluation. *Heliyon*: e10790. www.cell.com/action/showPdf?pii=S2405-8440%2822%2902078-3

Rankovic, B., M. Misic and S. Sukdolak. 2007. Evaluation of antimicrobial activity of the lichens *Lasallia pustulata, Parmelia sulcata, Umbilicaria crustulosa* and *Umbilicaria cylindrica. Microbiology* 76(6): 723–727.

Rao, M. M. and T. P. N. Hariprasad. 2021. *In silico* analysis of a potential antidiabetic phytochemical erythrin against therapeutic targets of diabetes. *In Silico Pharmacol* 9(1): 1–12.

Rathore, P. K., V. Arathy, V. S. Attimarad, P. Kumar and S. Roy. 2016. In-silico analysis of gymnemagenin from *Gymnema sylvestre* (Retz.) R. Br. with targets related to diabetes. *J Theor Biol* 391: 95–101.

Rozano, L., A. Zawawi, M. Redha, M. A. Ahmad and I. B. Jaganath. 2017. Computational analysis of *Gynurabicolor* bioactive compounds as dipeptidyl peptidase-IV inhibitor. *Adv Bioinformatics*. https://downloads.hindawi.com/archive/2017/5124165.pdf

Salin Raj, P., A. Prathapan, J. Sebastian, et al. 2014. *Parmotrema tinctorum* exhibits antioxidant, antiglycation and inhibitory activities against aldose reductase and carbohydrate digestive enzymes: An in vitro study. *Nat Prod Res* 28(18): 1480–1484.

Seo, C., Y. H. Choi, J. S. Ahn, J. H. Yim, H. K. Lee and H. Oh. 2009b. PTP1B inhibitory effects of tridepside and related metabolites isolated from the Antarctic lichen *Umbilicaria antarctica*. *J Enzyme Inhib Med Chem* 24(5): 1133–1137.

Seo, C., J. HanYim, H. Kum Lee and H. Oh. 2011. PTP1B inhibitory secondary metabolites from the Antarctic lichen *Lecidella carpathica*. *Mycology* 2(1): 18–23.

Seo, C., J. H. Sohn, J. S. Ahn, Y. H. Yim, H. K. Lee and H. Oh. 2009a. Protein tyrosine phosphatase 1B inhibitory effects of depsidone and pseudodepsidone metabolites from the Antarctic lichen *Stereocaulon alpinum*. *Bioorg Med Chem Lett* 19(10): 2801–2803.

Shah, M. A., W. Reanmongkol, N. Radenahmad, R. Khalil, Z. Ul-Haq and P. Panichayupakaranant. 2019. Anti-hyperglycemic and anti-hyperlipidemic effects of rhinacanthins-rich extract from Rhinacanthus nasutus leaves in nicotinamide-streptozotocin induced diabetic rats. *Biomed Pharmacother* 113: 108702. www.sciencedirect.com/science/article/pii/S0753332218373116?via%3Dihub

Shahid, M., A. Rasool, F. Anjum and M. T. Rehman. 2020. Biomedical perspectives of lichen-derived products. In *Lichen-Derived Products: Extraction and Applications*, ed. M. Yusuf, 263–276. Beverly, MA: Wiley, Scrivener Publishing.

Sharma, P., T. Joshi, T. Joshi, S. Chandra and S. Tamta. 2020. *In silico* screening of potential antidiabetic phytochemicals from *Phyllanthus emblica* against therapeutic targets of type 2 diabetes. *J Ethnopharmacol* 248: 112268. www.sciencedirect.com/science/article/abs/pii/S0378874119305914?via%3Dihub

Singh, P., V. K. Singh and A. K. Singh. 2019. Molecular docking analysis of candidate compounds derived from medicinal plants with type 2 diabetes mellitus targets. *Bioinformation* 15(3): 179–188.

Singh, Y. P. and R. A. Singh. 2010. Insilico studies of organosulfur-functional active compounds in garlic. *Biofactors* 36(4): 297–311.

Srimani, S., C. X. Schmidt, M. P. Gómez-Serranillos, H. Oster and P. K. Divakar. 2022. Modulation of cellular circadian rhythms by secondary metabolites of lichens. *Front Cell Neurosci* 16: 907308. https://doi.org/10.3389/fncel.2022.907308

Sujetovienė, G. and J. Česynaitė. 2021. Assessment of air pollution at the indoor environment of a shooting range using lichens as biomonitors. *J Toxicol Environ Health, Part A* 84(7): 273–278.

Thadhani, V. M. and V. Karunaratne. 2017. Potential of lichen compounds as antidiabetic agents with antioxidative properties: A review. *Oxid Med Cell Longev*: 2079697. https://downloads.hindawi.com/journals/omcl/2017/2079697.pdf

Tran, N., B. Pham and L. Le. 2020. Bioactive compounds in anti-diabetic plants: From herbal medicine to modern drug discovery. *Biology* 9(9): 252. www.ncbi.nlm.nih.gov/pmc/articles/PMC7563488/

Trinh, Q. and L. Le. 2014. An investigation of antidiabetic activities of bioactive compounds in Euphorbia hirta Linn using molecular docking and pharmacophore. *Med Chem Res* 23(4): 2033–2045.

Varol, M. 2019. Lichens as a promising source of unique and functional small molecules for human health and well-being. In *Studies in Natural Products Chemistry*, ed. Atta-ur-Rahman, 60, 425–458. Amsterdam: Elsevier.

Verma, N. and B. C. Behera. 2019. Future directions in the study of pharmaceutical potential of lichens. In *Lichen Secondary Metabolites: Bioactive Properties and Pharmaceutical Potential*, ed. B. Ranković, 237–260. Cham, Switzerland: Springer.

Verma, N., B. C. Behera and B. O. Sharma. 2012. Glucosidase inhibitory and radical scavenging properties of lichen metabolites salazinic acid, sekikaic acid and usnic acid. *Hacettepe J Biol Chem* 40(1): 7–21.

Vo, T. H. N., N. Tran, D. Nguyen and L. Le. 2016. An in silico study on antidiabetic activity of bioactive compounds in *Euphorbia thymifolia* Linn. *SpringerPlus* 5(1): 1–13.
Wa, E., M. O. Elnahas and G. M. Daba. 2021. Lichentherapy: Highlights on the pharmaceutical potentials of lichens. *J Microbiol Biotechnol* 6(1). https://medwinpublishers.com/OAJMB/lichentherapy-highlights-on-the-pharmaceutical-potentials-of-lichens.pdf
Zambare, V. P. and L. P. Christopher. 2012. Biopharmaceutical potential of lichens. *Pharm Biol* 50(6): 778–798.

11 *In Silico* Analysis of Lapachol and Nickel Lapachol Against Tumor Proteins

Insights into the Molecular Interactions and Drug Likeliness

Likith M, Madhushree M.V. Rao**, Gayathri D S***, Ravikumar H****, and Hariprasad T P N****,†*

Department of Biotechnology, Dayananda Sagar College of Engineering, Bangalore, Karnataka, India; **Defence Institute of Advanced Technology (Deemed to be University), Girinagar, Pune, India; ***Department of Zoology, BGS Science Academy, Chikkaballapura, Karnataka, India; ****Department of Life Science, Bangalore University, Bangalore, Karnataka, India

†Corresponding Author: hariprasad.tpn@gmail.com

ABBREVIATIONS

ADMET	Absorption, distribution, metabolism, excretion, and toxicity
BBB	Blood-brain barrier
CASTp	Compound Atlas of Surface Topography of proteins
HBA	Hydrogen bond acceptor
HBD	Hydrogen bond receiver
HIA	Human intestinal absorption
PDB	Protein Data Bank
RCSB	Research Collaboratory for Structural Bioinformatics
ROS	Reactive oxygen species
IAR	The International Agency for Research on Cancer
SDF	Structural data format
SMILES	Simplified molecular input line entry system
WHO	World Health Organization

DOI: 10.1201/9781003354437-11

11.1 INTRODUCTION

Cancer is a multi-stage complex disease, characterized by abnormal and uncontrollable cell growth. The progression of tumors involves several mutations that activate oncogenes and deactivate tumor suppressor genes, which control cell cycle and cell death via apoptosis. (Schmandt and Mills 1993; Knudson 1993). The mortality rate of cancer was estimated to be about 10 million in 2020 (IARC 2020). The most cancer deaths (millions) were lung (1.80), colon and rectum (0.9), liver (0.8), stomach (0.76), and breast (0.68) in 2022, and approximately 0.4 million children develop cancer annually (WHO 2022). A resolution "Cancer prevention and control in the context of an integrated approach (WHA70.12)" was passed by the World Health Assembly in 2017 to reduce premature mortality in cancer (WHO 2022). Chemotherapy is the frontline defense against cancer, but the chemotherapeutic agents lack specific toxicity, cause a lot of side effects, and also many tumors are developing resistance (Yarbro 1992). The overall 5-year survival rate from cancer has been reported at about 65%, whereas the survival rate is 84% for localized cancer and only 35% for metastatic ones (Siegel et al. 2019).

Cancer therapy involves various combined approaches such as chemotherapy, radiotherapy, hormonal therapy, targeted therapy, stem cell transplantation and surgery. Chemotherapy is the frontline defense against cancer, but common chemotherapeutic agents like carboplatin, cisplatin, etc., have side effects ranging from hair loss and appetite loss to organ damage like nerve and kidney, etc. (American Cancer Society 2022); hence promising compounds are to be synthesized to improve the treatment. One of the approaches to treating cancer is to direct the drug molecules to specifically targeted cells/tissues, thereby enhancing the efficiency of the drug while minimizing side effects (Kumar et al. 2013; Ruoslahti et al. 2010). Therefore, research has to be focused on deriving new drugs by finding the active principles from natural products which intervene with the processes of tumorigenesis (Hardman et al. 1996). To turn an active principal compound into a drug, the intrinsic molecular mechanisms of cancer development and progression have to be well studied.

Plants are an extensive resource for anticancer agents, and the natural products from them have been used in traditional medicine (Newman et al. 2003). The rich biodiversity spots offer great possibilities and are a prospectus in identifying new drugs (Mans et al. 2000). This biodiversity provides wide chemical diversity for newer drugs (Kinghorn et al. 2003). From 1940 to 2014, 49% of the drugs were either botanicals or their derivatives. From 1946 to 2019, about 11% of the anticancer drugs were unaltered and about 20% were derivatives of natural products. (Newman and Cragg 2016).

Quinones and their derivatives have an incredible variety of biological functions (Bolton et al. 2000; El-Najjar et al. 2011). They may act as vitamins, antioxidants, antibacterial, antiallergic and anticancer agents (Tseng et al. 2013). They can be cytotoxic by various mechanisms including redox cycles, break in DNA strands, alkylation of DNA and proteins, intercalation and free radicals (Tseng et al. 2013). Some of the quinone-based compounds used as anticancer agents are doxorubicin, mitoxantrone and mitomycin C (Bolton and Dunlap 2017; Cardoso et al. 2014).

Naphthoquinones are compounds present in a variety of plants and also in bacteria and fungi (Epifano et al. 2014) like juglone (K vitamins) and plumbagin. These naphthoquinone compounds are advantageous in the treatment of cancer due to their cytotoxic effects, which are exerted by oxidative stress and nucleophilic alkylation

(Bolton et al. 2000). Naphthoquinone derivatives too are important as cytotoxic, antiviral, antibacterial, insecticidal, antipyretic, antiprotozoal, antifungal and anti-inflammatory agents (Grolig and Wagner 2005; Rani et al. 2022; Ieque et al. 2021)

Among the naphthoquinones, three compounds, lapachol and α and β-lapachone, are reported to have efficient anticancer effects. Lapachol was isolated by E. Paterno in 1882 for the first time from *Tabebuia impetiginosa* (Thomson 1971). *T. impetiginosa* belongs to the class Bignoniaceae, which is commonly called Tpé Roxo' in South America (Fetrow and Åvila 1999). Lapachol, the active principal ingredient, was isolated from its stem and seeds and has been medicinally used by the locals for centuries. It has been also isolated from other families like Sapotaceae, Leguminosae, Verbenaceae, Scrophulariaceae, Proteaceae and Malvaceae (Oliveira 2000; Hussain et al. 2007). It has been reported that lapachol exhibits anti-inflammatory, anticancer, antimicrobial, antimalarial, antiparasitic, analgesic, antiviral, antipsoriatic, antioxidant, antileishmanial, fungicidal, pesticidal, termiticidal, molluscicidal and many more properties (Hussain et al. 2007; Oliveira et al. 2002; Castellanos et al. 2009; Almeida et al. 1990; Guerra et al. 2000; Andrade-Neto et al. 2004; Almeida 2009; Carvalho et al. 1988; Grazziotin et al. 1992). Bioprospecting lapachol from endophytic fungi is also being explored (Srinivas et al. 2022)

As early as 1968, lapachol was tested for *in vivo* antitumor activity on mouse models and the activity was found to be significant (Rao et al. 1968). *In vivo* evaluation of lapachol on HeLa cells at maximum non-toxic concentrations was found to induce alterations in the protein profile (DeWhite et al. 2004; Linardi et al. 1975). Lapachol acts on the electron transport in the respiratory chain by inhibiting succinate oxidase as shown in *Plasmodium knowlesi* (Pardee et al. 2002; Yoshito and Nobuhiro 2002), inhibits matrix metalloproteinase in fibrosarcoma cells (Kim and Kim 2021), inhibits cytochromes b and c (Hussain et al. 2007) and also inhibits glycolysis by PKM2 inhibition (Shankar Babu et al. 2018). A lapachol-loaded nanoemulsion was found to enhance the antitumor activity in breast cancer models (Miranda et al. 2021). Lapachol derived from methanolic extracts of *Kigelia africana* root showed cytotoxic effects on human prostate, cervical and mouse fibroblast cell lines (Atolani et al. 2021), and glycosides synthesized from lapachol showed antiproliferative activity (Ottoni et al. 2021).

Lapachol derivatives modified for better efficiency have been studied. Synthesized derivative 4 showed anticancer activity against cell lines of breast and liver cancer (Zhang et al. 2016) and analogues 5 and 6 against lung, renal, melanoma, breast, ovarian and prostate cancers (Vargas et al. 2007). The patent applications filed regarding the anticancer properties of lapachol in the past 20 years shows its competence to be a prospective anticancer compound (Hussain and Green 2017).

Although lapachol was also reported to be a candidate for modification to study its pharmacokinetic profile, as it was found to be significantly less toxic, it still possesses some detrimental effects (Subramanian et al. 1998). Such modifications can benefit associated inertness/oxidation reactivity, substitutional hydrophilicity/hydrophobicity and systematic/target biocompatibility suitable to treatment conditions (Mital and Ziora 2018; Thota et al. 2018; Galanski et al. 2005). Metal-bearing scaffolds tone down the toxicity and significantly increase the efficacy in cancer therapy and allow further binding to the intercellular target molecules and also can be used as DNA-targeted metallodrugs (Meier-Menches et al. 2018; Coverdale et al. 2018; Foltinova et al. 2008, Senol et al. 2021).

Lapachol metal complexes have shown to be effective on various cancers. Lapachol is stable with nickel (Farfan et al. 2009), copper, iron, zinc, cobalt (Sawhney et al. 1983; Martinez et al. 2005), bismuth, antimony (de Oliveira et al. 2011), ruthenium (Oliveira et al. 2021), calcium, barium and lead (Bhatia and Vohra 1982).

It has been discovered that numerous nickel complexes are effective for use in a variety of therapeutic procedures. Preparation and structural characterization of Ni(II) with lapacholate anion was first reported by (Hernández-Molina et al. 2007). The cytotoxic characteristics of the Ni(II) complex of lapachol were investigated against cervical, hepatocellular and colorectal adenocarcinoma cells, which showed significant inhibition at a low concentration (Tabrizi et al. 2017). Chelation with nickel showed shrinking tumors and was found to reduce pain in cancers such as the prostate, liver, breast, kidney, colon, lung and cervix (Lee 2006; Lee et al. 2005; Zhu et al. 2015; Heng et al. 2020; Gond et al. 2022). The radiosensitization of a nickel lapachol was effective in killing Chinese hamster ovary (CHO) cells and amplifying DNA breaks in hypoxia, which are assumed to be caused by the naphthoquinone ligand rather than the metal's reduction (Skov et al. 1993). When hypoxic mammalian cells were also treated with nickel–lapachol, they became more sensitive to the harmful effects of cisplatin, establishing the chemosensitizing role of Ni complex lapachol. It has been proposed that the interaction takes place at the DNA level (Skov et al. 1988). Nickel complexes have shown anticancer activity against OVCAR 3 cells (Dheodware et al. 2021), lung cancer (Diyali et al. 2022), gastric cancer cells (Saremi et al. 2021), prostrate cell lines (Qu et al. 2022) and Ehrlich ascites carcinoma cells (Qurban et al. 2022).

The human genome contains about 6000 to 8000 potential pharmacological targets with fewer than 400 proven drug proteins, and cancer has a plethora of potential targets (Chen et al. 2016; Drews 2000; Lazo and Sharlow 2016). There are several cancer molecules where corresponding targets are unidentified, and few targets are undruggable due to their ineffective active sites (Takarabe et al. 2012; Lazo and Sharlow 2016). To use the known or new potential cancer drugs, the characterization of binding sites for drug interaction and target bioinformatic approaches becomes critical (Cui et al. 2020). Computational methods such as network-based and ML-based models are mainly employed to understand the interactions between receptors and drugs. Molecular docking is a structure-based protocol to study binding affinities and drug-receptor interactions (Ferreira et al. 2015). Flexible or rigid docking can be employed depending on the flexibility of the ligands (Dias and De Azevedo 2008; Halperin et al. 2002). Various software such as AutoDock, DOCK, Discovery Studio, FlexX, Glide, Sybyl, etc., can be employed for molecular docking (Cui et al. 2020). They evaluate the binding free energy to determine the compounds which can bind to targets effectively (Huang et al. 2010)

The efficacy of the new drug molecules or known putative drug molecules relies on *in silico* tools to simplify the process. (Huang et al. 2002). Computational docking is a direct and rational approach for drug discovery; it can be used to establish *in silico* models of ligand-receptor interactions at the atomic level that can be further used to validate in *in vivo* assays, which can reduce time and cost (Meng et al. 2011). Molecular similarity searching tools are ligand-based approaches based on the idea that "molecules tend to perform similar biological effects due to the high structural similarity" (Zhavoronkov et al. 2019).

The drug discovery methods which are ligand based depend upon the structure of the potent ligand and are known as an indirective protocols. These approaches can be used for novel ligands and to improve drug pharmacokinetics such as ADMET properties (Cui et al. 2020).

Taken together, lapachol is an established anticancerous substance, but its metal derivatives are far less ventured. Despite nickel lapachol complexes' efforts as a potential anticancerous moiety, more research in the field is required to validate this. Therefore, the present study is comprehensive *in silico* study using computation approaches to understand the molecular interactions and assess the potential of lapachol and nickel-chelated lapachol as anticancer molecules targeting 50 different tumor proteins involved in the carcinogenesis of various cancers.

11.2 MATERIALS AND METHODS

11.2.1 Preparation of Receptors

The Protein Data Bank (www.pdb.org) was consulted for the three dimensional X-ray crystallographic protein structures relevant for molecular docking investigations. A total of 50 proteins involved in tumerogenesis were selected (Table 11.1) for the study. The PDB files were cleaned of water molecules and unnecessary heteroatoms and were modelled for any missing regions using SWISS-MODEL (https://swissmodel.expasy.org/).

TABLE 11.1
Selected Receptors Involved in Various Cancers for Molecular Docking

Sl. No	Receptors	Name of the Receptor
1	1AXC	Human PCNA
2	1IKN	IKAPPA BALPHA/NF-KAPPAB COMPLEX
3	1JDH	Crystal structure of BETA-CATENIN AND HTCF-4
4	1BGW	Topoisomerase residues 410–1202
5	1BXL	Structure of BCL-XL/BAK PEPTIDE COMPLEX, NMR, MINIMIZED
6	1D3Y	Structure of the DNA TOPOISOMERASE VI A subunit
7	1D5R	Crystal structure of the PTEN tumor suppressor
8	1F16	Pro-apoptotic protein BAX
9	1FI6	REPS1 EH domain
10	1G5J	BCL-XL
11	1G5M	Human BCL-2, isoform 1
12	1GJH	Human BCL-2, isoform 2
13	1I4O	Crystal structure of the XIAP/CASPASE-7 COMPLEX
14	1K4T	Human DNA topoisomerase I (70 KDA)
15	1KZ7	DH/PH fragment of murine DBS
16	1MOX	Human epidermal growth factor receptor

(Continued)

TABLE 11.1 (*Continued*)
Selected Receptors Involved in Various Cancers for Molecular Docking

Sl. No	Receptors	Name of the Receptor
17	1MRK	Crystal structures active center geometry and depurine mechanism of two ribosome-inactivating proteins
18	1OIS	Yeast DNA topoisomerase I, N-terminal fragment
19	1P4O	Structure of APO unactivated IGF-1R kinase domain at 1.5A resolution
20	1TGR	Crystal structure of mini-IGF-1(2)
21	1ZXM	Human topo IIA ATPASE/AMP-PNP
22	2A2R	Crystal structure of glutathione transferase PI
23	2AR9	Crystal structure of a dimeric caspase-9
24	2AX6	Crystal structure of the androgen receptor ligand binding
25	2AXI	HDM2 in complex with a beta-hairpin
26	2J5F	Crystal structure of EGFR kinase domain
27	2R7G	Structure of the retinoblastoma protein pocket domain
28	2ROC	Solution structure of MCL-1 complexed with PUMA
29	2VOF	Structure of mouse A1 bound to the PUMA BH3-domain
30	2W3L	Crystal structure of chimeric Bcl2-XL and phenyl
31	2W96	Crystal structure of CDK4 in complex with a D-type cyclin
32	2X39	Structure of 4-AMINO-N-(4-CHLOROBENZYL)-1-(7H-PYRROLO(2,3-D)
33	2X70	Crystal structure of MHC class I HLA-A2.1
34	3B2T	Structure of phosphotransferase
35	3HHM	Crystal structure of P110ALPHA H1047R mutant
36	3M89	Structure of TUBZ-GTP-G-S
37	3MJG	Structure of a platelet-derived growth factor receptor complex
38	3MJK	Structure of a growth factor precursor
39	3POZ	EGFR kinase domain complexed with TAK-285
40	3PPO	Structure of the substrate-binding protein
41	3QX3	Human topoisomerase IIBETA in complex with DNA and ETOPOSIDE
42	4GIZ	Crystal structure of full-length human papillomavirus oncoprotein E6
43	4HRL	Structural basis for eliciting a cytotoxic effect in HER2-
44	4QNQ	Crystal structure analysis of full-length BCL-XL
45	4YK3	Crystal structure of the BID domain of BEPE
46	5AGX	BCL-2 ALPHA BETA-1 linear complex
47	5JSB	Crystal structure of MCL1-inhibitor complex
48	5JUY	Active human poptosome with procaspase-9
49	BCL-2	Solution structure of the antiapoptotic protein BCL-2
50	HER-2	*Legionella pneumophila* NTPDASE1 crystal form III (closed)

11.2.2 Preparation of Ligands

The structure of ligands, lapachol and nickel lapachol (Figure 11.1) for docking were taken from PubChem (/https://pubchem.ncbi.nlm.nih.gov/) in SDF, which was then energy minimized using force-field mmff94 and transformed to PDB via Open Babel.

11.2.3 Molecular Docking

The proteins were transformed into Autodock file format PDBQT files by eliminating water molecules, adding polar hydrogen atoms and charges, merging nonpolar hydrogen atoms and using MGL tools; then the ligands were torsion-tested and transformed converted to PDBQT format. The grid parameter file (gpf) was generated from the grid menu, and the grid box was configured with 0.375 Å spacing to cover the target receptors. Selecting the receptor as rigid and the ligand as flexible, the Lamarckian genetic algorithm was used as a search algorithm with random seeding to generate 100 ligand poses, and a docking parameter file (dpf) was created. Autogrid4 was run to produce grid maps, followed by Autodock4 to dock, and different poses of ligands were then analyzed for their binding energies and were visualized to study interactions via Discovery Studio Client v20.1.0.19295.

11.2.4 Drug Likeness Prediction

The MolSoft program (https://molsoft.com/mprop/) was used to forecast a molecule's drug likeness. Molecular weight, total number of hydrogen bond acceptors and donors and logP values were employed to compute the overall score according to

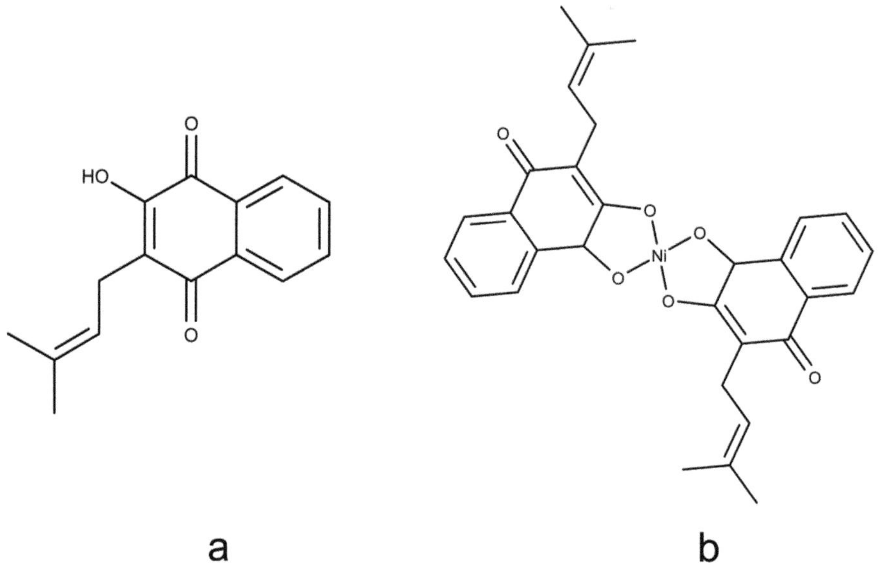

FIGURE 11.1 Two-dimensional structure of the ligands. a. Lapachol, b. nickel lapachol.

Lipinski's rule of five (Ro5). PubChem server's canonical SMILES data was utilized as the input for Molsoft's prediction. Calculations were made to determine other data, like polar surface area, dissolving factor and drug likeness.

11.2.5 Absorption, Distribution, Metabolism, Excretion and Toxicity Analysis

AdmetSAR (http://lmmd.ecust.edu.cn/admetsar2/) was utilized to anticipate the ADMET profiles of lapachol and nickel lapachol. Projected results included human intestinal absorption, blood-brain barrier penetration, CaCo-2 permeability, carcinogen toxicity and mutagenicity. The ligands' SMILES were acquired from PubChem and later submitted to the AdmetSAR tool.

11.3 RESULTS AND DISCUSSION

11.3.1 Molecular Docking Analysis and Molecular Interactions

To determine the binding affinities, both the ligands were docked with 50 receptors. The binding energies of nickel lapachol ranged from –7.27 to –10.32 kcal/mol, whereas those of lapachol ranged from –4.64 to –7.87 kcal/mol, as shown in Table 11.2. Figure 11.2 demonstrates the clear distinction between the energies. This difference indicates that nickel lapachol has a higher affinity for all receptors than lapachol.

TABLE 11.2
The Binding Affinity of the Ligands Against the Receptors Involved in Various Cancers

		Ligands	
Sl. No	Receptors	Lapachol	Nickel Lapachol
1	1AXC	–6.33	–8.32
2	1IKN	–6.69	–9.23
3	1JDH	–5.9	–8.2
4	1BGW	–6.61	–9.43
5	1BXL	–5.67	–8.7
6	1D3Y	–5.79	–7.91
7	1D5R	–6.82	–8.95
8	1F16	–6.98	–9.02
9	1FI6	–5.81	–8.08
10	1G5J	–6.47	–8.78
11	1G5M	–6.47	–8.66
12	1GJH	–6.81	–8.33
13	1I4O	–6.09	–8.18
14	1K4T	–6.54	–9.17
15	1KZ7	–7.08	–8.48

Sl. No	Receptors	Ligands	
		Lapachol	Nickel Lapachol
16	1MOX	−6.77	−8.95
17	1MRK	−7.09	−8.74
18	1OIS	−6.53	−9.76
19	1P4O	−6.73	−10.25
20	1TGR	−6.27	−7.91
21	1ZXM	−7.22	−9.49
22	2A2R	−6.62	−9.17
23	2AR9	−6.43	−8.55
24	2AX6	−7.36	−8.51
25	2AXI	−5.97	−8.71
26	2J5F	−6.51	−8.75
27	2R7G	−6.51	−8.81
28	2ROC	−5.32	−8.16
29	2VOF	−6.51	−8.51
30	2W3L	−5.44	−8.68
31	2W96	−7.12	−8.83
32	2X39	−6.33	−9
33	2X70	−6.83	−9.58
34	3B2T	−6.1	−8.57
35	3HHM	−7.87	−10.23
36	3M89	−6.98	−9.12
37	3MJG	−5.29	−7.45
38	3MJK	−6.97	−9.36
39	3POZ	−7.28	−10.32
40	3PPO	−7.27	−8.76
41	3QX3	−6.98	−8.8
42	4GIZ	−7.17	−9.69
43	4HRL	−5.65	−7.84
44	4QNQ	−5.89	−8.96
45	4YK3	−4.99	−7.49
46	5AGX	−5.82	−8.32
47	5JSB	−5.43	−7.64
48	5JUY	−7.52	−10.05
49	BCL−2	−6.36	−8.7
50	HER−2	−6.82	−9.66

The molecular interactions between ligands and receptors were explored with the aid of Discovery Studio Visualizer. Figure 11.3 displays the interactions between lapachol and the top six receptors (3HHM, 5JUY, 2AX6, 3POZ, 3PPO and 1ZXM), which have greater binding energies. Figure 11.4 depicts the interactions of nickel lapachol with the top six receptors (3POZ, 1P4O, 3HHM, 5JUY, 1OIS and 4GIZ), with high binding energies producing more conventional hydrogen bonds. For each receptor, a list of interacting residues is presented in Table 11.3.

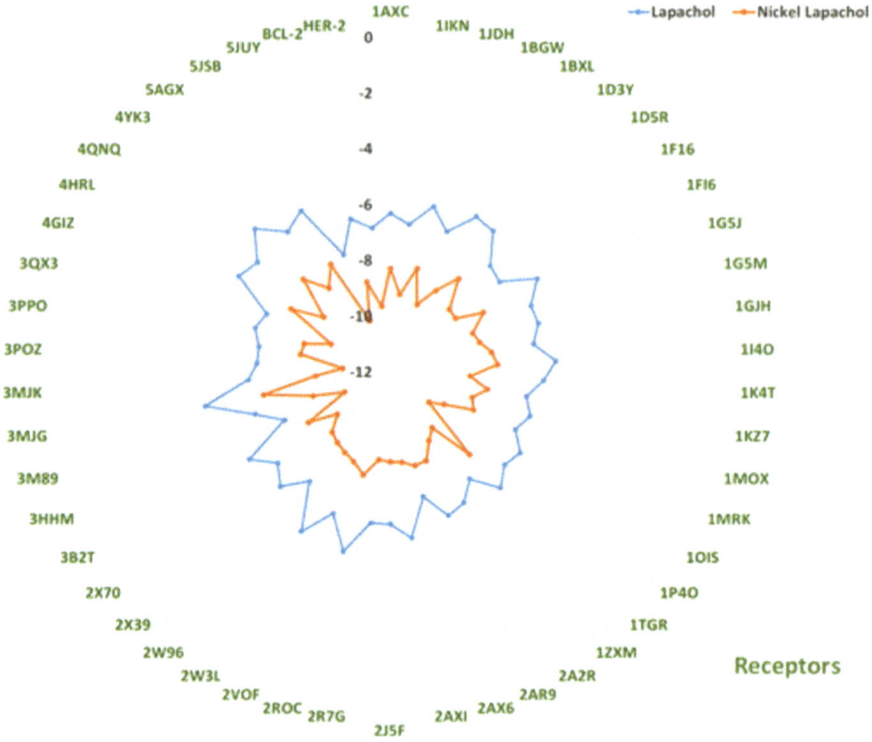

FIGURE 11.2 Radar graph showing the binding energies of the ligands, lapachol (blue) and nickel lapachol (orange) upon interaction with the various cancer proteins (green).

The amino acids of the ligands involved in the interaction with the receptor 3HHM against lapachol are ASP288, ALA758, ARG662, PRO168, PRO757, GLN661, VAL166, TYR167, LEU752, TYR698 and HIS701 (Figure 11.3c) and with 5JUY are TYR594, LEU1247, MET592, ALA584 and LEU56 (Figure 11.3f). The top interactions with nickel lapachol were GLY1125, GLU1020, MET1024, VAL1023, HIS1103 and ASP1105 against IP4O (Figure 11.4b) and LEU844, ASN842, CYS797, ALA722, PHE723, VAL726, LYS745, LEU788, ALA743, LEU777, MET766 and ASP855 against 3POZ (Figure 11.4d).

11.3.2 Drug-Likeness Prediction

"Lipinski's rule of five," which states that the "molecular weight should be less than or equal to 500 Da, the number of hydrogen bond donors should be less than 5 and the number of hydrogen bond acceptors should be less than or equal to 10," was implemented to the bioinformatics tool Molsolf to ascertain whether a compound has drug-relevant properties. It is recommended that the water-octanol coefficient

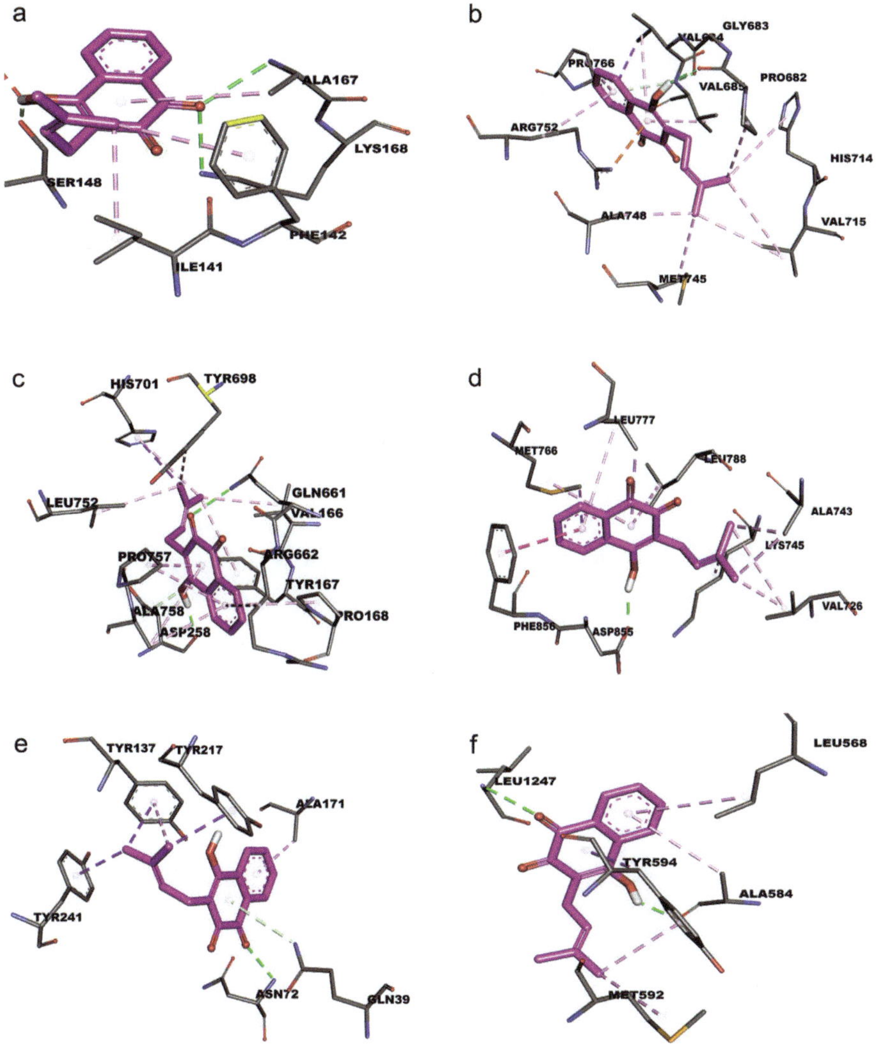

FIGURE 11.3 Molecular docking interactions of lapachol against various cancer proteins. a. 1ZXM, b. 2AX6, c. 3HHM, d. 3POZ, e. 3PPO, f. 5JUY (only the top six interactions are presented); green dashed lines—conventional hydrogen bonds, light pink dashed lines—alkyl bonds and dark pink dashed line—pi-pi stacked bonds.

ratio be under 5. If a compound only breaches one filter requirement, it is considered to fulfil the drug-like standard. While nickel lapachol violates the requirements for both Log P ≤5 and molecular weight >500, lapachol complies with the rules without any deviations. Lapachol and nickel lapachol had drug-likeness scores of 0.19 and 0.04, respectively, as shown in Table 11.4 and Figure 11.5.

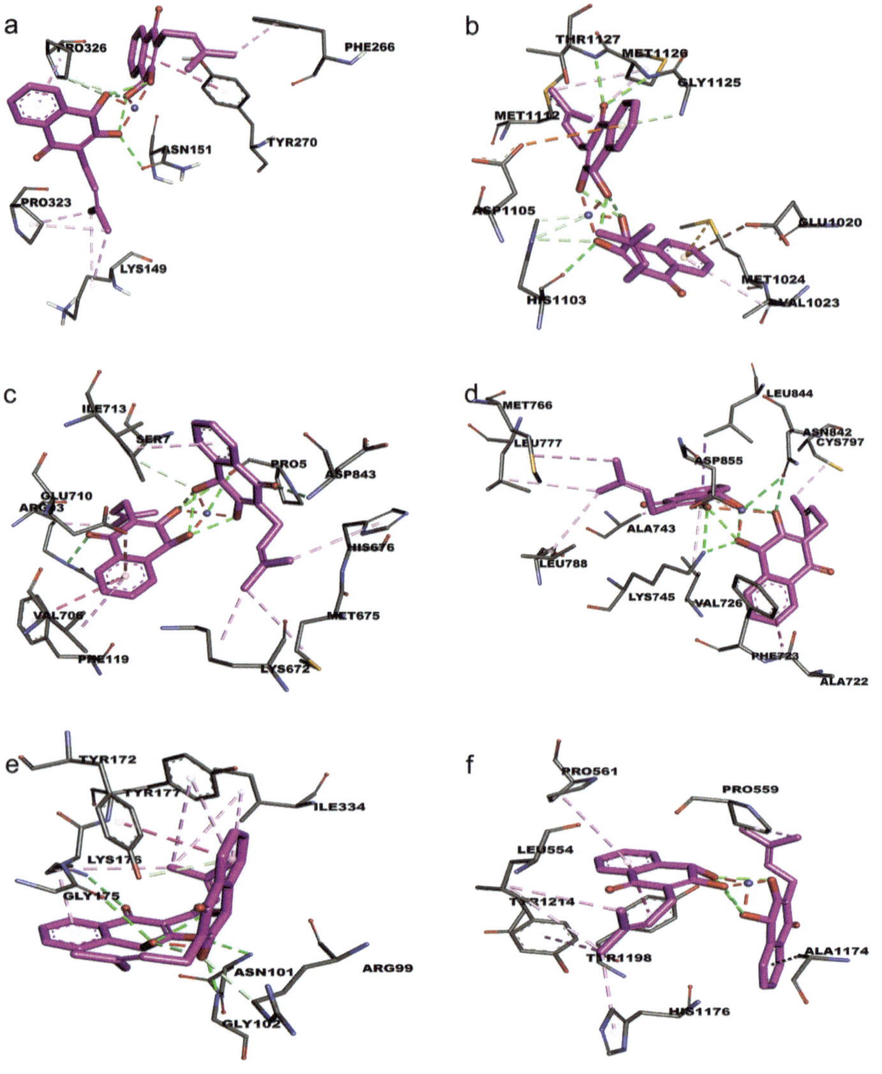

FIGURE 11.4 Molecular docking interactions of nickel lapachol against various cancer proteins. a. 101S, b. 1P4O, c. 3HHM, d. 3POZ, e. 4G1Z, f. 5JUY (only the top six interactions are presented); green dashed lines—conventional hydrogen bonds, light pink dashed lines—alkyl bonds and dark pink dashed line—pi-pi stacked bonds.

11.3.3 ADMET

The ADMET profiles of the drugs' pharmacokinetics, pharmacodynamics and toxicological aspects were established by the admetSAR server (Table 11.5). Both compounds demonstrated considerable human intestinal absorption and Caco-2 values that were favorable. No compounds were reported to be mutagenic or carcinogenic.

TABLE 11.3
Key Interacting Residues of the Ligands with Various Selected Cancer Receptors

Receptor	Lapachol	Nickel Lapachol
1AXC	ALA26, ASP122, GLU124, GLU25, HIS44, LEU121, MET40, SER39, VAL123	ALA208, ALA252, HIS44, ILE255, LEU47, LYS254, MET40, PRO234, PRO253, SER43, SER46, VAL45
1IKN	ALA188, ALA192, ARG187, ARG274, ARG30, ASN186, ASP277, GLN220, GLY31, SER276, THR191	ARG108, ASN115, CYS105, GLN114, HIS111, ILE110, PHE113, SER112, TYR100
1JDH	GLN601, GLU567, HIS544, ILE610, LEU602, PRO606, SER605, THR547, TYR604, VAL570	ASP372, ASP412, ASP413, GLN375, GLN407, LEU408, PRO373, SER374, SER411, THR371, THR404, VAL378, VAL416
1BGW	GLY875, HIS867, ILE877, PHE870, PRO868, THR874, THR876, TRP869, TRP873	ARG907, ASN757, ASN829, GLN704, GLN744, GLN751, GLY748, ILE747, ILE759, LEU749, LEU761, LYS701, PHE700, THR745, TYR760
1BXL	ALA93, ARG100, GLU96, GLY138, PHE97, TYR101, TYR195, VAL141	ALA104, ALA142, ARG100, GLN111, LEU108, LEU112, LEU130, PHE105, PHE146, PHE97, TYR101, VAL126
1D3Y	ARG231, ARG235, GLU238, GLU239, HIS136, LYS234, THR182	ASN185, ASP93, GLU156, GLU157, LEU184, LEU90, LYS183, THR182
1D5R	ASP187, GLU99, LEU181, LEU182, LEU186, LEU98, LYS102, PRO103, TYR178, TYR188	ASP187, GLN97, GLU99, LEU100, LEU181, LEU98, LYS102, PRO103, TYR188
1F16	ASP84, ILE80, LEU120, LEU181, LEU185, LYS119, PHE116, PRO88, TYR115, VAL83, VAL91	ALA35, ALA42, ARG37, ASP48, GLN28, GLN32, GLU44, GLY36, GLY39, GLY40, LEU125, LEU45, MET38, PRO43, PRO51, VAL50
1FI6	GLN19, LYS42, PHE20, PHE39, PHE40, PHE74, SER43	LYS42, LYS81, PHE20, PHE39, PHE40, PHE74, SER43, TYR15, VAL77, VAL78
1G5J	ASP15, ASP33, GLU11, GLU35, GLU36, THR39, VAL14, VAL34	ASN37, ASP33, GLU35, GLU36, LEU21, SER18, SER29, TRP28, TYR26, VAL34
1G5M	ARG98, HIS20, HIS94, ILE14, LEU97, LYS17, TYR18, TYR21	ALA131, ARG183, GLU135, HIS184, PHE138, THR187, TYR180, VAL134, VAL142
1GJH	ASN11, AS*P10, GLN190, GLY194, HIS186, ILE189, TRP195, TYR9	ALA4, ASP191, ASP196, GLN190, GLY194, GLY5, HIS186, HIS3, ILE189, TRP195, TYR9
1I4O	ARG237, GLN243, GLN276, GLU274, HIS272, PHE273, SER234, SER275, TRP232, TRP240	ARG187, ASN148, GLU147, GLU216, ILE159, LYS160, PHE221, PRO227, THR163, TYR223, VAL292
1K4T	ARG210, ARG434, GLU213, GLU438, GLY214, ILE435, LYS216, LYS439, PRO212, TYR211	ARG376, GLU232, GLU255, GLY359, LYS262, PHE259, PHE309, PRO229, PRO357, PRO358, TYR231

(*Continued*)

TABLE 11.3 (*Continued*)
Key Interacting Residues of the Ligands with Various Selected Cancer Receptors

Receptor	Lapachol	Nickel Lapachol
1KZ7	ARG633, ARG634, ASN638, CYS704, GLU781, ILE705, LEU640, LEU778, LEU779, LEU783, PRO708, SER786, TYR785, VAL636, VAL711	ALA817, ALA886, ASN810, CYS729, GLN730, GLU736, GLU884, HIS814, LEU766, LYS732, PRO733, PRO887, SER812, TYR889, VAL769, VAL809
1MOX	ALA265, ARG231, ARG84, CYS224, CYS227, CYS236, GLU60, LEU225, LYS4, THR266, VAL226	ASP279, CYS240, GLY281, HIS280, LEU243, LEU245, MET244, MET253, PRO242, SER262, SER282, TYR246
1MRK	ARG163, ASN110, GLU160, GLU189, GLY109, ILE155, ILE71, TRP192, TYR111, TYR70	ALA86, ASN110, ASN245, GLU85, GLY109, ILE155, ILE71, SER87, TYR111, TYR70
1OIS	ASN151, ILE154, PHE155, PRO325, PRO326, PRO328, TYR270, VAL153	ASN151, ASP269, HIS150, LYS149, PHE266, PRO323, PRO325, PRO326, PRO328, TRP333, TYR270, VAL324
1P4O	ASN1110, ASP1123, GLY1122, GLY1125, HIS1103, MET1126, PHE1124, THR1127	ARG1104, ARG1109, ASN1110, ASP1105, ASP1123, GLY1122, GLY1125, HIS1103, MET1024, MET1112, MET1126, SER979, THR1127, VAL1023, VAL1102
1TGR	ASP43, CYS37, CYS38, CYS42, CYS6, GLU9, ILE33, LEU10, LEU44, LEU47, SER41	ALA30, GLU3, GLY7, LEU10, LYS27, LYS31, PHE25, THR4, VAL11, VAL34
1ZXM	ALA167, ARG162, ASN150, ASN163, GLY161, GLY164, GLY166, ILE141, LYS168, PHE142, SER148, SER149, THR147, TYR165	ALA318, GLN309, GLN310, GLN60, ILE311, LYS321, MET61, PHE308, SER312, SER320, THR319, TRP62, TYR72
2A2R	ALA121, ASN110, GLN125, GLY114, LEU106, LEU122, LYS102, SER105, TYR118	ARG13, ASN204, CYS101, GLN51, GLN64, GLY12, ILE104, LEU52, PHE8, TYR108, TYR7, VAL10
2AR9	LYS398, MET400, PHE348, PHE351, THR347, TYR397, VAL352	ALA286, ARG180, ARG355, GLN285, HIS237, PRO357, SER287, SER353, THR179, THR181, TRP354, VAL352
2AX6	ALA765, ARG752, GLN711, GLY683, HIS714, PHE764, PRO682, PRO766, TYR763, VAL684, VAL685, VAL715	ALA748, ARG752, ASN756, GLU681, GLY683, LEU805, PHE804, PRO682, PRO766, PRO801, TRP751, TYR763, VAL684, VAL685
2AXI	GLY58, HIS96, ILE103, ILE61, ILE99, LEU54, LEU57, LEU82, PHE86, PHE91, TYR100, VAL93	GLN59, GLN72, GLY58, HIS73, ILE103, ILE61, ILE99, LEU54, LEU57, LEU82, MET62, PHE55, PHE86, PHE91, VAL93
2J5F	ASP1003, GLU1004, GLY729, LEU1001, LEU730, LEU792, LYS728, MET1002, MET1007, PRO741, VAL1010, VAL742	ASP1003, LEU1001, LEU792, LYS728, MET1002, PHE795, PRO741, PRO794, PRO990, SER991, VAL1010
2R7G	GLN689, ILE573, LEU647, LYS577, LYS652, SER576, SER648, TYR651, TYR655, TYR692	ARG467, GLU464, GLU533, LEU476, LEU649, LYS530, LYS537, MET460, SER534, TYR529
2ROC	ARG284, ARG291, ASP153, GLU152, GLY292, LEU155, LEU287, VAL288	ASN241, ASP304, GLN303, GLY243, HIS301, PHE299, PHE300, TRP242, VAL197, VAL302

Receptor	Lapachol	Nickel Lapachol
2VOF	ALA25, CYS34, GLN18, GLN38, HIS15, LEU12, LEU37, PRO30, TYR16, TYR19, VAL23	ALA25, ALA29, CYS34, GLN18, GLN38, GLU27, HIS15, PRO24, PRO30, TYR19, VAL23
2W3L	ALA108, ALA59, ARG105, ARG66, ASP62, GLY104, PHE63, TYR161, TYR67, VAL107	ASP130, ASP31, GLU124, GLU29, MET125, PRO127, TRP30, TYR28, VAL121
2W96	ALA187, CYS68, CYS73, GLN183, GLU69, GLU74, GLU75, HIS158, LYS72, PHE78, PRO79	ALA39, ASN198, ASN83, GLU35, GLU36, ILE196, PHE195, PRO199, PRO200, PRO40, SER197, VAL42
2X39	ARG176, ASN233, ASP284, GLU230, GLU433, LYS285, TYR177, TYR231	ASP293, ASP440, GLU236, GLU279, GLY159, GLY161, LEU158, LYS160, MET282, PHE238, PHE239, PHE439, PHE443, THR292, TYR438
2X70	ARG97, ASP77, LEU81, LYS146, THR143, THR73, TRP147, TYR116, TYR123, TYR84, VAL152	ALA69, ARG97, GLN155, GLU63, HIS70, LEU156, LYS66, MET45, MET5, PHE9, THR163, TRP167, TYR159, TYR171, TYR7, VAL67
3B2T	ALA726, ASP723, ILE707, LYS724, MET722, PRO705, PRO725, THR698, TRP694, TYR704	ALA523, ASP521, GLU465, GLU467, GLU525, GLY558, LEU468, LEU519, LEU528, LEU560, LYS520, THR524, THR555, TYR466
3HHM	ALA758, ARG662, ASP258, GLN661, HIS701, LEU752, PRO168, PRO757, TYR167, TYR698, VAL166	ARG93, ASP843, GLN75, GLU710, GLU76, GLY122, GLY842, HIS676, ILE713, LYS672, MET675, PHE119, PRO5, SER6, SER673, SER7, THR74, VAL706, VAL845,
3M89	ASN282, ASP356, ASP382, GLU360, GLY381, ILE363, LYS355, PHE354, PHE380, THR359, VAL345, VAL357	ALA132, ARG137, GLN133, GLY136, GLY144, LEU135, PHE139, PHE151, PHE177, PRO179, THR140, VAL146
3MJG	ARG27, CYS43, GLU24, ILE25, LEU38, PRO42, TRP40, VAL39	ARG68, CYS43, GLU45, LEU91, PRO41, VAL22, VAL44, VAL46, VAL70
3MJK	ALA94, ASN134, CYS132, CYS133, CYS179, CYS96, GLN37, ILE38, PRO93, SER36, VAL95	ASN134, CYS132, CYS133, CYS179, GLN37, HIS39, ILE38, PRO93, SER136, THR135, VAL95
3POZ	ALA743, ARG776, ASP855, ILE744, LEU777, LEU788, LEU858, LYS745, MET766, PHE856, THR790, VAL726	ALA722, ALA743, ARG841, ASN842, ASP855, CYS797, GLY721, GLY724, LEU777, LEU788, LEU844, LYS745, PHE723, SER720, THR790, THR854, VAL726,
3PPO	ALA171, ASN135, ASN72, ASP169, GLN39, SER71, THR136, THR94, TYR137, TYR217, TYR241, TYR91	ASN170, ASN68, ASP169, ASP220, ASP282, GLN198, GLY200, ILE199, LEU201, MET41, SER40, THR42, TYR217
3QX3	ALA869, ARG945, ASN795, ASN867, ASN882, GLN742, GLU870, GLY737, GLY793, GLY868, LYS739, PHE738, SER794	ASN790, ASN798, GLN801, GLN805, GLU1198, GLY804, GLY807, ILE803, LYS909, PHE791, PHE806, PRO802, THR980

(Continued)

TABLE 11.3 (*Continued*)
Key Interacting Residues of the Ligands with Various Selected Cancer Receptors

Receptor	Lapachol	Nickel Lapachol
4GIZ	ARG99, ASN333, ASP96, ILE330, ILE334, TYR100, TYR172, TYR177	ARG99, ASN101, ASN174, ASN333, ASP96, GLY175, ILE334, LYS176, TYR172, TYR177
4HRL	ARG110, ASP109, ASP77, ASP79, GLY47, PHE76, TYR46, TYR78	ALA75, ARG110, ASP109, ASP72, ASP77, ASP79, GLY47, HIS43, PHE76, THR49, TYR78
4QNQ	ALA93, ARG100, GLU96, LEU194, PHE191, PHE97, TYR101, TYR195, VAL141	ALA104, ALA142, ARG139, GLU129, GLY138, LEU108, LEU130, PHE105, PHE146, PHE97, TYR101, VAL126
4YK3	ASP236, GLU192, GLY191, PRO188, SER189, SER195, SER240, THR239, THR243	ARG211, ARG221, ASN212, GLY210, LEU208, LEU213, LYS207, THR203
5AGX	ARG109, ARG26, GLN25, GLU152, GLY155, LYS22, PHE104, PHE112, SER105, TYR108, VAL156, VAL159	ARG129, ASP111, GLN118, GLU136, GLU152, LEU119, LEU137, MET115, PHE104, PHE112, PHE153, VAL133
5JSB	ARG201, ARG207, ARG214, ASP195, LEU210, LYS197, MET199, PRO198, SER202, THR196	ARG310, ASN260, GLN309, GLU317, GLY314, LYS308, PHE318, TRP261, TRP305
5JUY	ALA584, ASN590, ASP589, GLU587, GLU596, LEU1247, LEU593, LEU595, LYS581, LYS585, MET592, TYR594	ALA1174, ARG557, ARG612, GLN1211, GLY1149, GLY1177, GLY1178, GLY1196, HIS1176, HIS553, LEU554, LYS1200, PHE1213, PRO1167, PRO559, PRO561, SER1169, TYR1198, TYR1214,
BCL-2	ARG204, GLU197, GLY200, LEU92, PRO201, THR93, VAL196, VAL89	ALA41, ARG38, ASN37, GLU11, GLU36, GLU40, GLU43, GLU48, GLY44, HIS91, PRO42, SER47, THR39
HER-2	ASN179, ASN292, GLN178, GLN217, ILE219, LYS180, PRO197, SER181, THR173, TRP164, VAL177, VAL182	ASN168, ASN179, ASN218, ASN289, GLN178, GLN217, ILE219, LYS180, PRO197, SER181, THR173, TRP164, VAL177, VAL182

TABLE 11.4
Molecular Properties of the Ligands

Molecules	Molecular Weight	Number of HBA	Number of HBD	MolLogP	MolLogS moles/L	MolPSA (A^2)	MolVol (A^3)	Drug Likeness Score
Lapachol	242.09	3	1	2.99	−3.22	41.52	282.63	0.19
Nickel lapachol	542.12	6	2	6.33	−5.60	82.54	552.06	0.04

HBA: Hydrogen bond acceptors, HBD: Hydrogen bond donors.

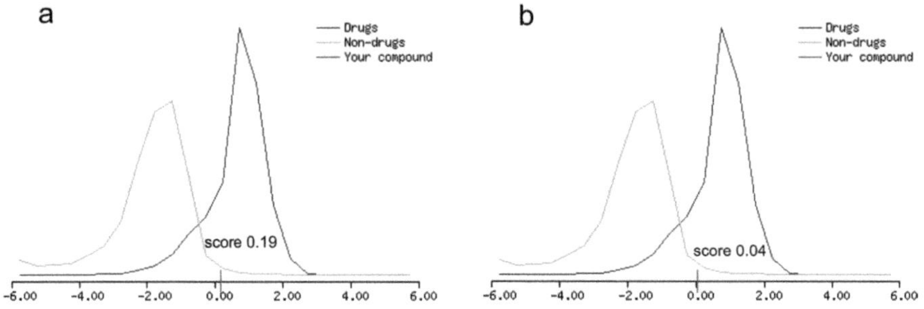

FIGURE 11.5 Drug likeliness scores of the ligands. a. Lapachol, b. Nickel lapachol.

TABLE 11.5
Toxicological and Pharmacokinetic Properties of the Ligands

	HIA		Caco-2		BBB		Carcinogenicity		Ames Mutagenesis	
Molecules	V	P	V	P	V	P	V	P	V	P
Lapachol	+	1.000	+	0.8998	+	0.5750	–	0.8928	–	0.7200
Nickel lapachol	+	0.9898	+	0.8398	+	0.6000	–	0.9100	–	0.6500

V: value, P: probability, HIA: human intestinal absorption, BBB: blood-brain barrier.

In this study, we docked lapachol and nickel lapachol with the 50 receptors that are important in cancer and studied their binding affinities and their interactions. The molecular docking analysis revealed that nickel lapachol has a high affinity in binding to all selected receptors and helps in better inhibition when compared to lapachol. Analyzing the key interactions, more hydrogens bonds were observed with high affinity in the case of nickel lapachol. The *in silico* binding of lapachol to the receptor 1ZJH showed a binding energy (–9.34 kcal/mol) forming hydrogen bonds with ASN69, GLY467, ASN43 and ILE468 (Shankar Babu et al. 2018) and interacts with the PKM2 receptor (–6.8 kcal/mol) sharing hydrogen bonds with PHE26, LEU353 and TYR390 (Mustofa et al. 2020). Lapachol also inhibits glycolysis by interacting with CYP450R (–7.5 kcal/mol), bonding with PRO533, TYR604, GLN606, ASN635 and ASP639; the binding of lapachol to PKM2 and CYP450R causes glycolysis inhibition and oxidative stress releasing ROS (Mustofa et al. 2020). The objective of the Molsoft investigation was to comprehend the drug-likeness potential of nickel lapachol and lapachol. Drug likeness is an important consideration before selecting a compound for further analysis as a putative drug molecule (Keller et al. 2006; Ursu et al. 2011). Compounds within the “drug-like” range may lead to drug discovery (Leeson and Springthorpe 2007). Drug likeness may be affected by parameters such as permeability, solubility, metabolic stability and transporter effects (Bickerton et al. 2012). Compounds with a lower molecular weight (<500 Da) offer a more favorable target reach, but nickel lapachol showed a higher value, pointing to a challenge in transportation. Both compounds had acceptable values for the number of HBA and HBD, indicating excellent drug permeability. Nickel lapachol displayed a significantly higher value, with a 1.33 deviation from the established limit for log p (≤5), which measures cell membrane permeability. Given that the log s values for both compounds were within −6, they both have an effective dissolution potential. AdmetSAR was applied to predict pharmacokinetic and toxicological characteristics like BBB (Cblood/Cbrain), intestinal absorption in humans, binding of plasma protein and carcinogenic and mutagenic properties. Quantitative estimation of drug-likeness QED values can range from 0 to 1, where 0 indicates unfavorable of all the Ro5 of Lipinski, while 1 indicates all are favorable (Bickerton et al. 2012). It can be seen that a value for human intestinal absorption that is closer to 1 indicates better absorption through the intestine. Compounds were also non-mutagenic and non-carcinogenic. Lapachol and nickel lapachol can therefore be seen as potentially effective treatments for cancer.

11.4 FUTURE SCOPE

The second most common cause of death globally is cancer, with 10 million deaths and about 19 million new cases in 2021, which may run in families or develop spontaneously (Kumavath et al. 2021). Computational and non-computational techniques are employed in cancer diagnosis. Imaging, fluorescence in situ hybridization (FISH), tumor markers and cytologic and histological methods are among the non-computational methods (Valand et al. 2022). For the majority of non-computational cancer screening techniques, the sensitivity and specificity values fall between 70–80% and 60–70%, respectively, thereby propelling the advancement of bioinformatics tools to identify tumors. These technologies can significantly increase the specificity and accuracy in screening cancers (Schiffman et al. 2015). Insights from molecular docking studies are extremely valuable in understanding stability and release, facilitating the fabrication of the desired formulation, standardizing the conventional use, limiting failure rates in clinical trials and aiding comprehension of disease dynamics in the pursuit of developing novel drug candidates (Yadav et al. 2018).

The field of bioinformatics is rapidly evolving, with a predominant focus on health to develop new medical tools that are accessible to researchers, medical professionals and patients. As a result, bioinformatics is gaining more momentum in decoding critical diseases like cancer. The current healthcare system and management will only get better with further developments in the fields of genomics, proteomics, artificial intelligence and personalized medicine that are aiming at a massive rise in biological research (Qazi and Raza 2021)

11.5 CONCLUSION

The molecular interaction of lapachol and nickel lapachol was studied against 50 various cancer proteins. The binding energies of nickel lapachol ranged from −7.27 to −10.32 kcal/mol, whereas those of lapachol ranged from −4.64 to −7.87 kcal/mol. 3HHM, 5JUY and 3POZ receptors were closely associated with both ligands and were among the top six interactions. Both ligands were found to be non-carcinogenic and non-mutagenic. Lapachol and nickel lapachol showed drug-likeness scores of

0.19 and 0.04, respectively, concluding that both ligands show properties to be putative natural products against various tumors, and among the two ligands, nickel lapachol was found to have a significant role in interacting with tumor proteins, with a possibility of being a putative potential anticancer molecule.

REFERENCES

Almeida, E. R. 2009. Preclinical and clinical studies of lapachol and beta-lapachone. *Open Nat Prod J* 2:42–47.

Almeida, E. R., A. A. Silva-Filho, E. R. Santos and C. A. C. Lopes. 1990. Antiinflammatory action of lapachol. *J Ethnopharmacol* 29(2):239–241.

American Cancer Society. 2022. www.cancer.org/treatment/treatments-and-side-effects/treatment-types/chemotherapy.html (accessed October 2022).

Andrade-Neto, V. F., M. O. F. Goulart, J. F. Silva-Filho, et al. 2004. Antimalarial activity of phenazines from lapachol, B-lapachone and its derivatives against *Plasmodium falciparum in vitro* and *Plasmodium berghei in vivo*. *Bioorg Med Chem Lett* 14:1145–1149.

Atolani, O., G. A. Olatunji and O. S. Adeyemi. 2021. Cytotoxicity of lapachol and derivatized analogues from *Kigelia africana* (Lam.) Benth. on Cancer cell lines. *Arab J Sci Eng* 46:5307–5312.

Bhatia, B. M. L. and N. Vohra. 1982. Kinetic studies of the nonisothermal decomposition of metal chelates of lapachol with calcium (II), barium (II), and lead (II). *Thermochim Acta* 53:361–364.

Bickerton, G. R., G. V. Paolini, J. Besnard, S. Muresan and A. L. Hopkins. 2012. Quantifying the chemical beauty of drugs. *Nat Chem* 4(2):90–98.

Bolton, J. L. and T. Dunlap. 2017. Formation and biological targets of quinones: Cytotoxic versus cytoprotective effects. *Chem Res Toxicol* 30:13–37.

Bolton, J. L., M. A. Trush, T. M. Penning, G. Dryhurst and T. J. Monks. 2000. Role of quinones in toxicology. *Chem Res Toxicol* 13:135–160.

Cardoso, M. F. C., P. C. Rodrigues, M. E. I. M. Oliveira, et al. 2014. Synthesis and evaluation of the cytotoxic activity of 1,2-furanonaphthoquinones tethered to 1,2,3–1H-triazoles in myeloid and lymphoid leukemia cell lines. *Eur J Med Chem* 84:708–717.

Carvalho, L. H., E. M. Rocha, D. S. Raslan, et al. 1988. *In vitro* activity of natural and synthetic naphthoquinones against erythrocytic stages of *Plasmodium falciparum*. *Braz J Med Biol Res* 21:485–487.

Castellanos, J. R. G., J. M. Prieto and M. Heinrich. 2009. Red Lapacho (*Tabebuia impetiginosa*)-A global ethnopharmacological commodity? *J Ethnopharmacol* 121:1–13.

Chen, X., C. C. Yan, X. Zhang, et al. 2016. Drug-target interaction prediction: Databases, web servers and computational models. *Briefings Bioinf* 17:696–712.

Coverdale, J. P., I. Romero-Canelón, C. Sanchez-Cano, et al. 2018. Asymmetric transfer hydrogenation by synthetic catalysts in cancer cells. *Nat Chem* 10:347–354.

Cui, W., A. Aouidate, S. Wang, Q. Yu, Y. Li and S. Yuan. 2020. Discovering anti-cancer drugs via computational methods. *Front Pharmacol* 11:733.

Deodware, S. A., A. Ubale, N. Karajagi, U. B. Barache, et al. 2021. Synthesis, characterization and molecular docking studies of nickel(II) complexes derived from 4-amino-5-mercapto-3-methyl-1,2,4-triazole: In vitro antimicrobial and anticancer activities. *Res Sq* 1–16. https://doi.org/10.21203/rs.3.rs-471368/v1

de Oliveira, L. G., M. M. Silva, F. C. S. de Paula, et al. 2011. Antimony(V) and bismuth(V) complexes of lapachol: Synthesis, crystal structure and cytotoxic activity. *Molecules* 16:10314–10323.

De White, N. V., A. O. M. Stoppani and M. A. Dubin. 2004. 2-Phenyl-betalapachone can affect mitochondrial function by redox cycling mediated oxidation. *Arch Biochem Biophys* 432(2):129–135.

Dias, R. and W. F. De Azevedo Jr. 2008. Molecular docking algorithms. *Curr Drug Targets* 9:1040–1047.

Diyali, S., A. K. Mohanty, S. Sarkar, M. F. Hossain, B. Bhowmik and B. Biswas. 2022. A mononuclear Nickel (II) complex: Synthesis, X-ray structure, spectroscopic characterization and anti-tumor activity. *Adv Chem Res* 1(1):22–30.

Drews, J. 2000. Drug discovery: A historical perspective. *Science* 287:1960–1964.

El-Najjar, N., H. Gali-Muhtasib, R. A. Ketola, P. Vuorela, A. Urtti and H. Vuorela. 2011. The chemical and biological activities of quinones: Overview and implications in analytical detection. *Phytochem Rev* 10:353–370.

Epifano, E., S. Genovese, S. Fiorito, V. Mathieu and R. Kiss. 2014. Lapachol and its congeners as anticancer agents: A review. *Phytochem Rev* 13:37–49.

Farfan, R. A., J. A. Espindola, M. A. Martinez, et al. 2009. Synthesis and crystal structure of a new lapacholate complex with nickel(II), [Ni(Lap)2(DMF)(H2O)]. *J Coord Chem* 62:3738–3744.

Ferreira, L. G., R. N. Dos Santos, G. Oliva and A. D. Andricopulo. 2015. Molecular docking and structure-based drug design strategies. *Molecules* 20:13384–13421.

Fetrow, C. W. and J. R. Avila. 1999. *Professional's Handbook of Complementary and Alternative Medicines*. 491–493. Spring House, Pennsylvania, USA: Springhouse Corporation.

Foltinova, V., S. L. Sindlerova, V. Horvath, et al. 2008. Mechanisms of effects of platinum(II) and platinum(IV) complexes. Comparison of cisplatin and oxaliplatin with satraplatin and LA-12, new Pt(IV)-based drugs. A minireview. *Scr Med* 81:105–116.

Galanski, M., M. A. Jakupec and B. K. Keppler. 2005. Update of the preclinical situation of anticancer platinum complexes: Novel design strategies and innovative analytical approaches. *Curr Med Chem* 12:2075–2094.

Gond, M. K., S. K. Pandey, R. Singh, M. K. Bharty, et al. 2022. In vitro and in silico anticancer activities of Mn (ii), Co (ii), and Ni (ii) complexes: Synthesis, characterization, crystal structures, and DFT studies. *New J Chem* 46(23):11056–11070.

Grazziotin, J. D., E. E. Schapoval, C. G. Chaves, et al. 1992. Phytochemical and analgesic investigation of *Tabebuia chrysotricha*. *J Ethnopharmacol* 36:249–251.

Grolig, J. and R. Wagner. 2005. Naphthoquinones. In *Ullmann's Encyclopedia of Industrial Chemistry*. Weinheim: Wiley-VCH.

Guerra, M. O., A. S. B. Mazoni, M. A. F. Brandao and V. M. Peters. 2000. Toxicology of lapachol in rats: Embryolethality. *Braz J Biol* 61:171–174.

Halperin, I., B. Ma, H. Wolfson and R. Nussinov. 2002. Principles of docking: An overview of search algorithms and a guide to scoring functions. *Proteins* 47:409–443.

Hardman, J. G., L. E. Limbird, P. B. Molinoff, R. W. Ruddon and A. G. Gilman. 1996. The pharmacological basis of therapeutics. *Library of Congress Cataloging*:1225–1287.

Heng, M. P., K. S. Sim and K. W. Tan. 2020. Nickel and zinc complexes of testosterone N4-substituted thiosemicarbazone: Selective cytotoxicity towards human colorectal carcinoma cell line HCT 116 and their cell death mechanisms. *J Inorg Biochem* 208:111097

Hernández-Molina, R., I. Kalinina, P. Esparza, M. Sokolov, J. Gonzalez-Platas, A. Estévez-Braun and E. Pérez-Sacau. 2007. Complexes of Co (II), Ni (II) and Cu (II) with lapachol. *Polyhedron* 26(17):4860–4864.

Huang, C. C., C. V. Smith, M. S. Glickman, W. R. Jacobs and J. C. Sacchettini 2002. Crystal structures of mycolic acid cyclopropane synthases from *Mycobacterium tuberculosis*. *J Biol Chem* 277(13):11559–11569.

Huang, S. Y., S. Z. Grinter and X. Zou. 2010. Scoring functions and their evaluation methods for protein-ligand docking: Recent advances and future directions. *Phys Chem Chem Phys* 12:12899–12908.

Hussain, H. and I. R. Green. 2017. Lapachol and lapachone analogs: A journey of two decades of patent research (1997–2016). *Expert Opin Ther Pat* 27(10):1111–1121.

Hussain, H., K. Krohn, V. U. Ahmad, G. A. Miana and I. R. Green. 2007. Lapachol: An overview. *Arkivoc* ii:145–171.

Ieque, A. L., H. C. D. Carvalho, V. P. Baldin, N. C. D. S. Santos, et al. 2021. Antituberculosis activities of lapachol and β-lapachone in combination with other drugs in Acidic pH. *Microb Drug Resist* 27(7):924–932.

International Agency for Research on Cancer, IARC. 2020. https://gco.iarc.fr/today/data/factsheets/cancers/39-All-cancers-fact-sheet.pdf (accessed September 2022)

Keller, T. H., A. Pichota and Z. Yin. 2006. A practical view of 'druggability'. *Curr Opin Chem Biol* 10:357–361.

Kim, J. and M. Kim. 2021. Effect of lapachol on the inhibition of matrix metalloproteinase related to the invasion of human fibrosarcoma cells. *Curr Mol Pharmacol* 14(4):620–626.

Kinghorn, A. D., N. R. Farnsworth, D. D. Soejarto, et al. 2003. Novel strategies for the discovery of plant-derived anticancer agents. *Pharm Biol* 41:53–67.

Knudson, A. G. 1993. Antioncogenes and human cancer. *Proc Natl Acad Sci USA*. 90:10914–10921.

Kumar, A., X. Zhang and X. J. Liang. 2013. Gold nanoparticles: Emerging paradigm for targeted drug delivery system. *Biotechnol Adv* 31:593–606.

Kumavath, R., S. Paul, H. Pavithran, M. K. Paul, P. Ghosh, D. Barh and V. Azevedo. 2021. Emergence of cardiac glycosides as potential drugs: Current and future scope for cancer therapeutics. *Biomolecules* 11(9):1275. https://doi.org/10.3390/biom11091275

Lazo, J. S. and E. R. Sharlaow. 2016. Drugging undruggable molecular cancer targets. *Annu Rev Pharmacol Toxicol* 56:23–40.

Lee, J. H., J. Cheong and Y. H. Parkym Choi. 2005. Down-regulation of cyclooxygenase-2 and telomerase activity by beta-lapachone inhuman prostate carcinoma. *Pharmacol Res* 51(6):553–560.

Lee, J. I. 2006. B-Lapachone induces growth inhibition and apoptosis in bladder cancer cells by modulation of bcl-2 family and activation of caspases. *Exp Oncol* 28(1):30–35.

Leeson, P. D. and B. Springthorpe. 2007. The influence of drug-like concepts on decision-making in medicinal chemistry. *Nature Rev Drug Discov* 6:881–890.

Linardi, M., F. da Consolacao, M. M. de Oliveira and M. R. P. Sapaio. 1975. A lapachol derivative against mouse leukemia P-388. *J Med Chem* 18:1159–1164.

Mans, D. R. A., A. B. da Rocha and G. Schwartsmann. 2000. Anti-cancerdrug discovery and development in Brazil: Targeted plant collection as a rational strategy to acquire candidate anti-cancer compounds. *Oncologist* 5:185–198.

Martinez, M. A., M. C. L. de Jimenez, E. E. Castellano, et al. 2005. Two isostructural complexes of Co (II) and Zn (II) with lapacholate, dimethylformamide and water. *J Arg Chem Soc* 93:185–193.

Meier-Menches, S. M., C. Gerner, W. Berger, C. G. Hartinger and B. K. Keppler. 2018. Structure—activity relationships for ruthenium and osmium anticancer agents—towards clinical development. *Chem Soc Rev* 47:909–928.

Meng, X. Y., H. X. Zhang, M. Mezei and M. Cui. 2011. Molecular docking: A powerful approach for structure-based drug discovery. *Curr Comput Aided Drug Des* 7:146–157.

Miranda, S. E. M., J. de Alcântara Lemos, R. S. Fernandes, J. de Oliveira Silva, et al. 2021. Enhanced antitumor efficacy of lapachol-loaded nanoemulsion in breast cancer tumor model. *Biomed Pharmacother* 133:110936.

Mital, M. and Z. Ziora. 2018. Biological applications of Ru(II) polypyridyl complexes. *Coord Chem Rev* 375:434–458.

Mustofa, H. N., H. L. Wiraswati, S. Ekawardhani, P. I. Fianza and S. Windria 2020. Anticancer activities of saponins and quinones group through oxidative stress and glycolysis inhibition via *in Silico* studies. *Biomed Pharmacol J* 13(2):999–1010.

Newman, D. J. and G. M. Cragg. 2016. Natural products as sources of new drugs from 1981 to 2014. *J Nat Prod* 79:629–661.

Newman, D. J., G. M. Cragg and K. M. Snader. 2003. Natural products as sources of new drugs over the period 1981–2002. *J Nat Prod* 66:1022–1037.

Oliveira, K. M., J. Honorato, F. C. Demidoff, M. S. Schultz, et al. 2021. Lapachol in the design of a new ruthenium (II)-diphosphine complex as a promising anticancer metallodrug. *J. Inorg. Biochem* 214:111289.

Oliveira, M. F. 2000. *Contribuição ao Conhecimento Químico das Espécies Tabebuia serratifolia Nichols e Tabebuia rosa Bertol.* Doctoral thesis, Curso de Pós-Graduação em Química Orgânica. Universidade Federal do Ceará, Fortaleza.

Oliveira, M. F., T. L. G. Lemos, M. C. D. Mattos, et al. 2002. New enamine derivatives of lapachol and biological activity. *An Acad Bras Cie* 74:211–221.

Ottoni, F. M., L. B. Marques, J. M. Ribeiro, L. L. Franco, et al. 2021. Synthesis of lapachol-based glycosides and glycosyl triazoles with antiproliferative activity against several cancer cell lines. *Res Sq*:1–36.

Pardee, A. B., L. Y. Zhi and C. J. Li. 2002. Cancer therapy with betalapachone. *Curr Cancer Drug Targets* 2(3):227–242.

Qazi, S. and K. Raza. 2021. Translational bioinformatics in healthcare: Past, present, and future. In *Translational Bioinformatics in Healthcare and Medicine*, ed. K. Raza and N. Dey, 13, 1–12. Cambridge, United States: Academic Press, Elsevier.

Qu, J. J., L. L. Shi, Y. B. Wang, J. Yan, et al. 2022. The novel function of unsymmetrical chiral CCN pincer nickel complexes as chemotherapeutic agents targeting prostate cancer cells. *Molecules* 27:3106.

Qurban, J., S. D. Al-Qahtani, A. Alsoliemy, A. Alharbi, et al. 2022. Tailoring of new Ni (II) and UO2 (II)—hydrazide complexes: characterization, studies in-vitro and in-silico as well as the Hartree-Fock modeling. *J Saudi Chem Soc* 26(3):101477.

Rani, R., K. Sethi, S. Kumar, R. S. Varma and R. Kumar. 2022. Natural naphthoquinones and their derivatives as potential drug molecules against trypanosome parasites. *Chem Biol Drug Des* 100(6):786–817.

Rao, K. V., T. J. McBride and J. J. Oleson. 1968. Recognition and evaluation of lapachol as an antitumor agent. *Cancer Res* 28:1952–1954.

Ruoslahti, E., S. N. Bhatia and M. J. Sailor. 2010. Targeting of drugs and nanoparticles to tumors. *J Cell Biol* 188:759–768.

Saremi, L. H., K. D. Noshahr, A. Ebrahimi, A. Khalegian, K. Abdi and M. Lagzian. 2021. Multi-stage screening to predict the specific anticancer activity of Ni(II) mixed-ligand complex on gastric cancer cells; biological activity, FTIR spectrum, DNA binding behavior and simulation studies. *Spectrochim Acta A Mol Biomol Spectrosc* 251:119377.

Sawhney, S. S., S. D. Matta, R. Jain, et al. 1983. Investigation on the interaction of 2-hydroxy-3-(3-methyl-2-butenyl)-1,4-naphthoquinone (lapachol) with copper(II) and iron(II). *Thermochim Acta* 70:367–371.

Schiffman, J. D., P. G. Fisher and P. Gibbs. 2015. Early detection of cancer: Past, present, and future. *Am Soc Clin Oncol Educ Book* 35(1):57–65.

Schmandt, R. and G. B. Mills. 1993. Genomic components of carcinogenesis. *Clin Chem* 39:2375–2385.

Şenol, A., E. A. Akanbong, M. Sudagidan and A. K. Devrim. 2021. DNA-metal interaction and the biological activities of metal complexes: an overview in the light of recent literature. *Rev Roum Chim* 66(8–9):701–711.

Shankar Babu, M., S. Mahanta, A. J. Lakhter, T. Hato, S. Paul and S. R. Naidu. 2018. Lapachol inhibits glycolysis in cancer cells by targeting pyruvate kinase M2. *PLoS ONE* 13(2):e0191419.

Siegel, R. L., K. D. Miller and A. Jemal. 2019. Cancer statistics. *CA Cancer J Clin* 69:7–34.

Skov, K. A., H. Adomat and N. P. Farrell. 1988. Effects of nickel-lapachol in hypoxic cells. In *Platinum and Other Metal Coordination Compounds in Cancer Chemotherapy: Proceedings of the Fifth International Symposium on Platinum and Other Metal Coordination Compounds in Cancer Chemotherapy*, 733–738. Abano, Padua, and Italy: Springer.

Skov, K. A., H. Adomat and N. P. Farrell. 1993. Radiosensitization by nickel lapachol. *Int J Radiat Biol* 64(6):707–713.

Srinivasa, C., S. Pradeep, S. M. Patil, R. Ramu, et al. 2022. Bio prospecting of Lapachol producing endophytic fungi. *Int J Health Allied Sci* 11(1):13. https://rescon.jssuni.edu.in/ijhas/vol11/iss1/13

Subramanian, S., M. M. C. Ferreira and M. A. Trsic. 1998. A structure-activity relationship study of lapachol and some derivatives of 1,4-naphthoquinones against carcinosarcoma walker 256. *Struct Chem* 9(1):47–57.

Tabrizi, L., F. Talaie and H. Chiniforoshan. 2017. Copper (II), cobalt (II) and nickel (II) complexes of lapachol: Synthesis, DNA interaction, and cytotoxicity. *J Biomol Struct Dyn* 35(15):3330–3341.

Takarabe, M., M. Kotera, Y. Nishimura, S. Goto and Y. Yamanishi. 2012. Drug target prediction using adverse event report systems: A pharmacogenomic approach. *Bioinformatics* 28: 1611–1618.

Thomson, R. H. 1971. Distribution and biogenesis. In *Naturally Occurring Quinones*. London: Academic Press, Elsevier.

Thota, S., D. A. Rodrigues, D. C. Crans and E. J. Barreiro. 2018. Ru(II) compounds: Next-generation anticancer metallotherapeutics? *J Med Chem* 61:5805–5821.

Tseng, C. H., C. M. Cheng, C. C. Tzeng, S. I. Peng, C. L. Yang and Y. L. Chen. 2013. Synthesis and anti-inflammatory evaluations of B-lapachone derivatives. *Bioorg Med Chem* 21:523–531.

Ursu, O., A. Rayan, A. Goldblum and T. I. Oprea. 2011. Understanding drug-likeness. *Wiley Interdis Rev Comp Mol Sci* 1(5):760–781.

Valand, J. H., D. Twine, M. Kyomukamaa, R. Atino, et al. 2022. Role of bioinformatics in cancer diagnosis. *Res Sq.* https://doi.org/10.21203/rs.3.rs-1299906/v2.

Vargas, M. D., A C. Pinto, C. A. Camara, et al. 2007. Natural naphthoquinones and semi-synthetic, partially hydrogenated derivatives of lapachol with cytotoxic and antitumor activity. *BR2005002766A*.

World Health Organization (WHO). 2022. *Cancer Fact Sheet*. www.who.int/news-room/fact-sheets/detail/cancer (accessed October 2022).

Yadav, P., A. Bandyopadhyay, A. Chakraborty and K. Sarkar. 2018. Enhancement of anticancer activity and drug delivery of chitosan-curcumin nanoparticle via molecular docking and simulation analysis. *Carbohydr Polym* 182:188–198.

Yarbro, J. W. 1992. The scientific basis of cancer chemotherapy. In M. C. Perry (ed) *The Chemotherapy Source Book*, 2–14. Baltimore, MD: Lippincott, Williams and Wilkins.

Yoshito, K. and S. Nobuhiro. 2002. Possible mechanisms for induction of oxidative stress and suppression of systemic nitric oxide production caused by exposure to environmental chemicals. *Environ Health Prev Med* 7(4):141–150.

Zhang, C., Y. Qu, Y. Jia, et al. 2016. α-Lapachol analog, its synthetic method and application as anticancer drug. *CN105503692A*. https://patents.google.com/patent/CN105503692A/en.

Zhavoronkov, A., Y. A. Ivanenkov, A. Aliper, et al. 2019. Deep learning enables rapid identification of potent DDR1 kinase inhibitors. *Nat Biotechnol* 37:1038–1040.

Zhu, T., Y. Wang, W. Ding, J. Xu, et al. 2015. Anticancer activity and DNA-binding investigations of the Cu(II) and Ni(II) complexes with coumarin derivative. *Chem Biol Drug Des* 85:385–393.

12 Transcriptome Analysis Identifies Genes Involved in Vitamin B Biosynthesis in *Solanum virginianum* Whole Fruit

*Megha Gowri Thippeswamy**,
*Sumachirayu Chitradurga Kubera***,
*Rajeshwara Achur**, *Ravikumar H****,
*Thoyajakshi Ramasamudhra Siddaraju*****,
*and Nagaraju Shivaiah***,†
*Department of Biochemistry, Jnana Sahyadri Kuvempu University, Shivamogga; **Department of Studies and Research in Biotechnology, Tumkur University, Tumakuru; ***Department of Life Science, Bangalore University, Bangalore, Karnataka, India; ****Department of Studies and Research in Biotechnology, Tumkur University, Tumakuru
†Corresponding Author: nagarajubiochem@gmail.com

ABBREVIATIONS

BLAST	Basic local alignment tool
CDS	Coding sequences, ZR: Zymo research
PCR	Polymerase chain reaction
QV	quality threshold
NCBI NR	National Center for Biotechnology Information Non redundant
GO	Gene ontology
COG	Clusters of Othrologous Groups
KEGG	Kyoto Encyclopedia of Genes and Genome
Pfam	Protein families
PE	Paired ends
GTP	Guanosine-5'-triphosphate
FAD	Flavin adenine dinucleotide
NAD+	Nicotinamide adenine dinucleotide
mRNA	Messenger Ribonucleic acid
CO_2	Carbon dioxide

DOI: 10.1201/9781003354437-12

pABA	Para-aminobenzoic acid
DHF	Dihydrofolate
THF	Tetrahydrofuran
DHFR	Dihydrofolate reductase
PLP	Pyridoxal 5-phosphate
KAPA	7-Keto-8-aminopelargonic acid
DAPA	7,8-diaminopelargonic acid
THP	Tetrahydrofolate.

12.1 INTRODUCTION

The enormous traditional systems of medicine and the pharmacological potential of plants have inspired scholars to go beyond the discovery of new drugs and uncover the underlying molecular processes. *Solanum virginianum L* (Syn.: *Solanum xanthocarpum*), known as wild eggplant or nightshade plant, is a prickly herb that can be found throughout Asia (Rane et al. 2014). In India, it mainly occurs in dry locations across all four geographical regions (the Himalayan Mountain Complex, the North Indian Plain, the Peninsular Plateau, and the Islands), but it is mostly found in tropical and subtropical areas (Subhash Patil and Amit Patil 2022). The various parts of the plant, particularly the roots, are widely used by traditional medicinal practitioners, including Ayurveda, to treat female infertility, leucoderma, scorpion bites, asthma, and chest pain. Seed oil is used in the treatment of arthritis, and dried fruit ash is used as an analgesic to treat toothaches (Tr et al. 2017). The seeds are aphrodisiac, anthelmintic, antipyretic, laxative, anti-inflammatory, and anti-asthmatic. Antihelmintic and indigestion-relieving seeds are eaten. Its fruit juice treats rheumatism and sore throats. The fruit paste is spread externally to reduce swelling and pimples. Charaka and Sushruta used Kantkari to cure bronchial asthma, tympanitis, misperistalsis, piles, dysuria, and as rejuvenating agent (Rane et al. 2014). Recent developments in next-generation sequencing (NGS) technology and bioinformatics have made a high-throughput molecular data collection available, allowing researchers to completely understand the genomic and transcriptome profiles of any species (Mohanty et al. 2020), researching and statistically characterizing worldwide changes in gene types and expression levels by transcriptome profiling (RNA-seq) (Wang, Gerstein, and Snyder 2009). In humans, these group of water-soluble vitamins known as the vitamin B complex are involved in blood cell synthesis and cellular metabolism (Hanna et al. 2022). Therefore, studying the biosynthetic pathway of the vitamin B complex in plants is essential for humans and animals, since the humans and other animals depend on plants for vitamin B (Roje 2007). The precise number or name of each vitamin, such as B_1 for thiamin, B_2 for riboflavin, and B_3 for niacin, is used to identify individual vitamin B supplements. In addition, some are typically identified by their name such as pantothenic acid, biotin, and folate (Hanna et al. 2022). The significance of the vitamin B complex occurs at all stages of the human life span. Eight different vitamin B complex requirements are examined throughout the human life cycle, from conception and pregnancy through adolescence and old age, with a focus on their interactions and underlying mechanisms of action. For the health of both mother and child, thiamin, riboflavin, niacin, pyridoxine, and folic acid are essential (Ali et al. 2022). Megaloblastic anaemia (MA) is a collection of metabolic, neurological, cardiovascular, pulmonary, gastrointestinal, and musculoskeletal diseases caused by the lack of any of these vitamin B complex components. The deficiency also leads to pellagra, a photosensitivity dermatitis, hemorrhage-associated intestinal mucosa, congestion, neurological disorders, skin disorders, eye diseases, various neuropsychiatric symptoms, and other clinical symptoms (Smith et al. 2021; Thakur et al. 2017; Ikenouchi-Sugita and Sugita 2015; Zucker 1958; Piraccini et al. 2019; Li et al. 2022a; Sijilmassi 2019). Therefore, the biosynthetic pathway of vitamin B and its functional annotations provide a mechanism for both systematic and predictive vitamin metabolism pathways, allowing evaluations of each species' capacity for vitamin biosynthesis.

A comprehensive transcriptome annotation, analysis, and comparison of *S. virginianum* whole fruit has been attempted here. The de novo transcriptome sequencing of the vitamin B biosynthetic pathway was carried out on an Illumina platform, and the data was analysed using a number of different bioinformatics programmes. Moreover, the findings from this study will pave the way for the recognition and comprehension of genes essential for vitamin B production.

12.2 MATERIALS AND METHODS

12.2.1 Plant Sample Collection

The plant sample was collected in the Chitradurga district, Karnataka, India. Fruits were picked from the plants and placed on dry ice until brought to the laboratory. RNA-seq sample processing requires pure, high-quality RNA. Since RNA is more unstable than DNA, tissue storage at −80°C is suggested for long-term storage.

12.2.2 Total RNA Isolation and Library Preparation

Total RNA was extracted from the fruit samples according to the manufacturer's instructions using ZR plant RNA Miniprep (ZYMO Research, California). Nanodrop was used to assess the quality of RNA isolated, and Agilent Tape station employing high sensitivity RNA Screentape (model 4200, Agilent Technologies, USA) was used to assess the amount of the obtained RNA. The RNA-Seq paired sequencing library was produced from the QC passed RNA sample using Illumina TruSeq Stranded mRNA sample Prep kit. The PCR enriched library was evaluated using 4200 Tape Station system (Agilent Technologies, USA) utilizing high-sensitivity D1000 Screen tape as per the manufacturer recommendations.

12.2.3 Transcriptome Sequencing, De Novo Assembly

Low-quality reads (reads with more than a 10% quality threshold [QV] 20 phred score) and ambiguous reads (reads with unidentified nucleotides "N" larger than 5%) were removed from the sequencing raw data for the fruit sample (Bolger, Lohse, and Usadel 2014). A de novo sample was developed using paired-end readings. For this study, transcripts were built from high-quality fruit sample readings using the Trinity de novo assembler (version 2.8.4) and a kmer value of 25 (Haas et al. 2013). CD-HIT-EST-4.6 was then used to cluster the assembled transcripts and remove any isoforms that had resulted from the assembly process (Fu et al. 2012). Sequence extensions are thus no longer possible. Unigenes are a type of sequence that could be used as a starting point for further research. Coding sequences were predicted using TransDecoder-v5.3.0 and the aforementioned unigenes (https://github.com/TransDecoder). TransDecoder finds potential coding areas within the sequences of unigenes (Tang, Lomsadze, and Borodovsky 2015).

12.2.4 Functional Annotation of CDS

The CDS was functionally annotated with the use of the DIAMOND programme, a BLAST-compatible local aligner for mapping translated DNA query sequences to a protein reference database. Using the BLASTX algorithm, DIAMOND compares the CDS sequence to the NCBI NR in order to detect CDS homologs (non-redundant protein database). (Buchfink, Xie, and Huson 2015).

12.2.5 Gene Ontology of CDS

Each CDS's function was determined by using BLAST2GO to search for similar sequences in the NR (NCBI non-redundant protein), Swiss-Prot, GO, COG (Clusters of Orthologous Groups), and KEGG databases (www.blast2go.com/) (Conesa et al. 2005).

12.2.6 Pathway Enrichment Analysis of CDS

Determining the metabolic and signal transduction processes involved in enriched uranium among CDSs, as well as the biological activities related to these pathways, can be done with the help of the Kyoto Encyclopedia of Genes and Genomes (KEGG) (Chen et al. 2017). All the fruit CDS were mapped to the KEGG reference canonical pathways to determine if they were involved in any of the biological processes (nightshade family).

12.3 RESULTS

12.3.1 Transcriptome Sequencing, De Novo Assembly

TransDecoder finds potential coding areas within the sequences of unigenes. High-quality paired-end data to the tune of 5.31 GB was produced, including 5,314,463,360 bases and 18,184,076 PE reads. There were 160,162 transcripts obtained from high-quality reads. During assembly, unigenes were eliminated using CD-HIT-EST-4.6, yielding 140,200 unigenes. Transcoder-v5.3.0 was used to predict nucleotide sequences from unigenes. This yields a total of 60,487 coding sequences (CDS), as shown in Table 12.1. A similar study reported de novo assembly and characterization

TABLE 12.1
High-Quality Read Statistics and Transcript Summary

High-Quality Read Statistics	
No. of PE reads	18,184,076
No. of bases	5,314,463,360
Transcript summary	
No. of transcripts	160,162
Total transcript length (bp)	173,343,596
N50 (bp)	1,905
Maximum transcript length (bp)	15,780
Minimum transcript length (bp)	201
Mean transcript length (bp)	1,082

of the fruit transcriptome in *Litchi chinensis Sonn*, as well as the genes that are differently regulated in reaction to shading, which were investigated by Li *et al.* (Li et al. 2013). They collected 57,050 unigenes from 53,437,444 paired-end reads totalling 4,007,808,300 bp.

12.3.2 Gene Ontology of CDS

Analysis of Gene Ontology (GO) Terms Annotations from NR and Pfam were used to successfully assign 54,259 CDSs to the GO word annotation, which enabled for their grouping into the broad categories of biological processes, cellular components, and molecular function. As can be seen in Table 12.2, the vast majority of CDSs were classified as belonging to molecular functions, followed by biological processes and cellular components. Figure 12.1 displays the results of a GO study performed using the B2G framework. The GO term "molecular function" was determined to have the most CDSs associated with it. A similar study was conducted in which Ong, Voo, and Kumar assembled, characterized, and annotated the pineapple fruit transcriptome using massively parallel sequencing (Ong, Voo, and Kumar 2012). They used Blast2GO to label the UTs against the non-redundant (nr) Genbank library. The nr-marked UTs were mapped against the GO database to derive GO terms. All 15,507 mapped UTs were assigned a total of 65,637 GO words, or 4 on average per UT. The most frequent GO term was molecular function, followed by biological process and cellular component.

12.3.3 Functional Annotation of CDS

Use of DIAMOND's BlastX mode against the NCBI "Nr" database allowed for functional annotation of the predicted CDS. Functional annotation is the inference and

TABLE 12.2
Unigenes Summary and CDS Statistics

Unigenes Summary	
No. of unigenes	140,200
Total unigene length (bp)	136,839,529
N50 (bp)	1,743
Maximum unigene length (bp)	15,780
Minimum unigene length (bp)	201
Mean unigene length (bp)	976
CDS Statistics	
No. of CDS	60,487
Total CDS length (bp)	55,354,977
N50 (bp)	1,176
Maximum CDS length (bp)	15,273
Minimum CDS length (bp)	255
Mean CDS length (bp)	915

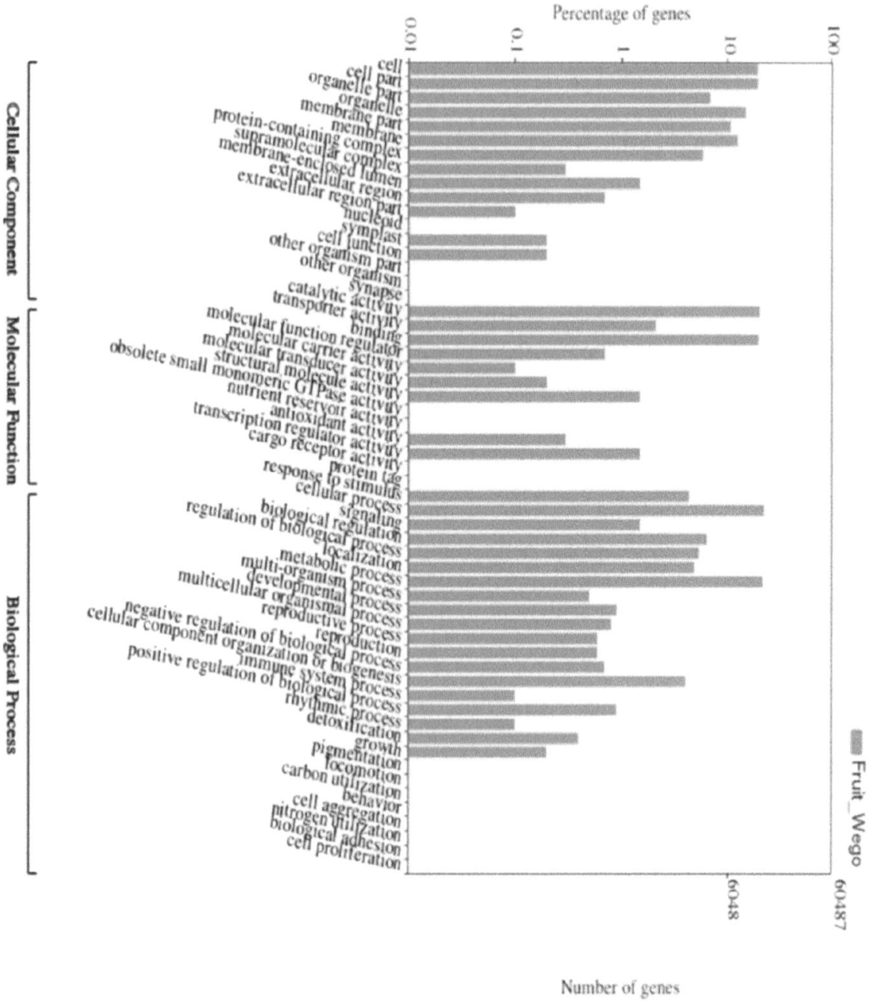

FIGURE 12.1 Histogram of the GO classifications. The ontology categories "Biological Processes," "Cellular Component," and "Molecular Function" were used to annotate the *Solanum virginianum* transcriptome.

assignment of information regarding the biological functionality of a sequence utilizing in silico approaches. The majority of the CDSs were discovered to be identical with *Solanum tuberosum*, which is in the same genus as *S. virginianum*. Fang *et al.* studied the characterization of full-length transcriptome and mechanisms of sucrose accumulation in *Annona squamosa* fruit, similar to our study (Fang et al. 2020). Comparing the FLNC transcript sequences with available genome sequenced plant species from the Nr database revealed that *A. squamosa* and *Nelumbo nucifera* shared the maximum number of transcripts.

12.3.4 Pathway Enrichment Analysis of CDS

We evaluated CDS with KEGG pathway data. Metabolic processes, genetic information processing, environmental information processing, cellular activities, and organismal systems were the five primary groups into which 7,283 CDS were placed. The majority of CDSs were found to be associated with signal transduction, as shown in Tables 12.3 and 12.4 (A, B, C, D). A total of 239 CDSs were found to be in the vitamin B biosynthesis, as shown in Figures 12.2, 12.3, 12.4, 12.5, 12.6, and 12.7. Li *et al.* identified

TABLE 12.3
GO Category Distribution of CDS for *Solanum virginianum* Whole Fruit

Sample Name	Total No. of Annotated CDSs	Biological Process	Cellular Component	Molecular Function
***Solanum virginianum* fruit**	54,259	17,918	16,071	20,270

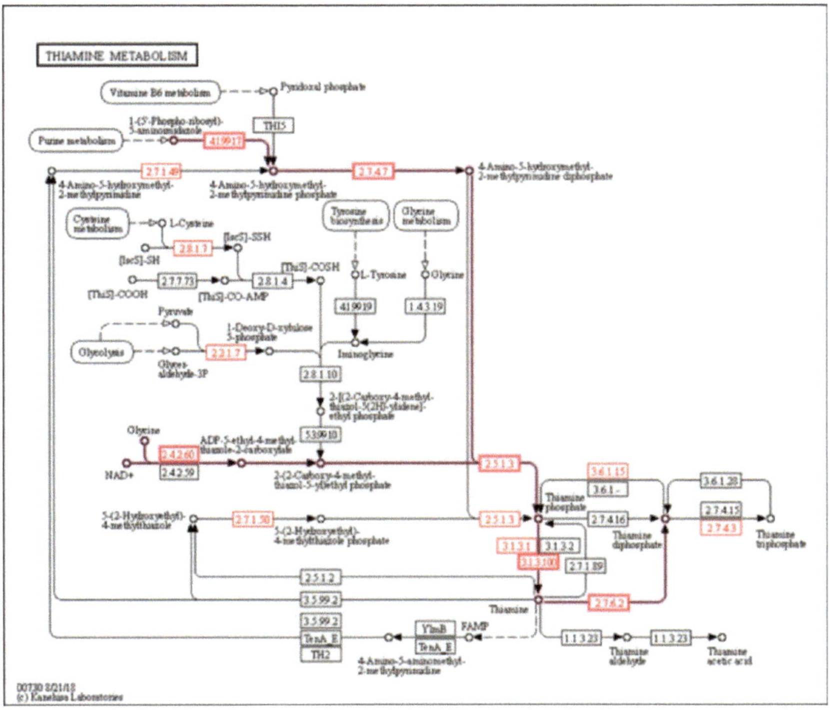

FIGURE 12.2 Thiamine metabolism pathway. Red indicates the thiamine biosynthetic pathway and 1-(5'-phosphor-ribosyl)-5-aminioimidazole, 4-amino-5-hydroxymethyl-2-methylpyrimidine phosphate, thiamine-phosphate pyro phosphorylase, cysteine-dependent adenosine diphosphate thiazole synthase, thiamine phosphate phosphatase, and thiamine pyro phosphokinase enzymes involved in the thiamine biosynthetic pathway.

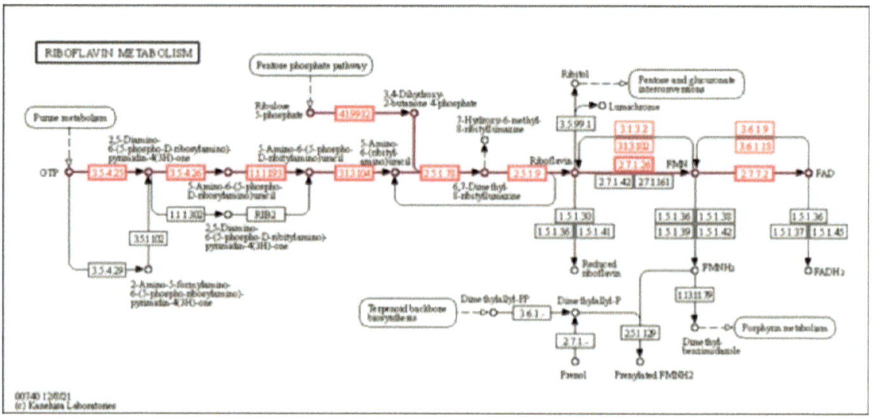

FIGURE 12.3 Riboflavin metabolism pathway. The colour red denotes the riboflavin biosynthesis route, which includes 3,4-dihydroxy 2-butanone 4-phosphate synthase, GTP cyclohydrolase II, diaminohydroxyphosphoribosylaminopyrimidine deaminase, 5-amino-6-(5-phosphoribosylamino)uracil reductase, 5-amino-6-(5-phospho-D-ribitylamino)uracil phosphatase, 6,7-dimethyl-8-ribityllumazine synthase, riboflavin synthase, and FAD synthetase enzymes involved in the riboflavin biosynthetic pathway.

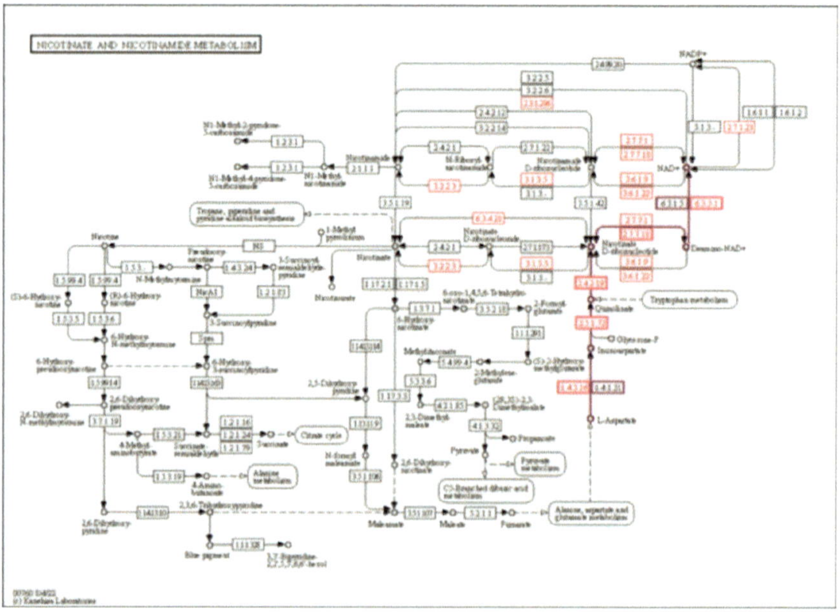

FIGURE 12.4 Nicotinate and nicotinamide metabolism pathway. Red denotes the nicotinate and nicotinamide biosynthesis route and L-aspartate oxidase, quinolinate synthase, nicotinate-nucleotide pyrophosphorylase (carboxylating), nicotinate-nucleotide adenylyltransferase, and NAD+ synthase (glutamine-hydrolysing) enzymes involved in the nicotinate and nicotinamide metabolic pathway.

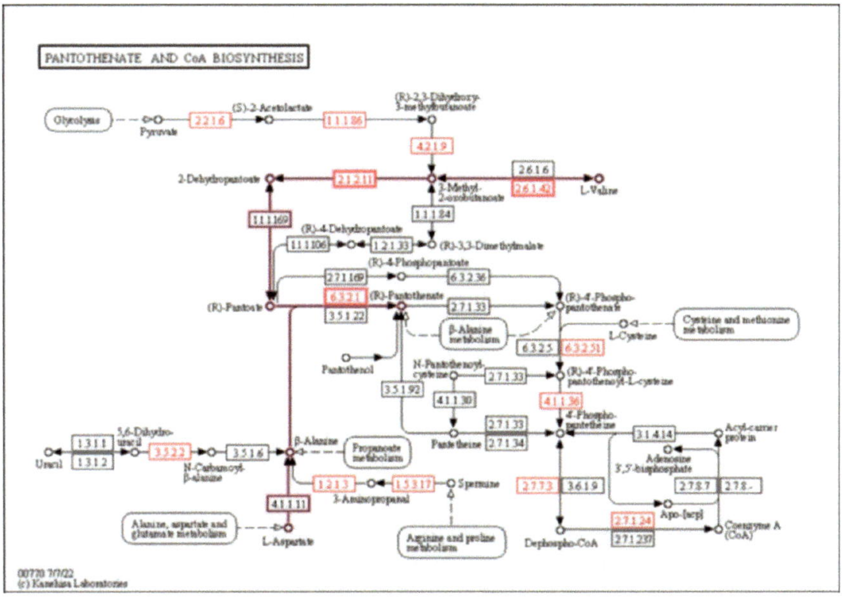

FIGURE 12.5 Pantothenate and CoA biosynthesis pathway. Red indicates the pantothenate biosynthetic pathway and 3-methyl-2-oxobutanoate hydroxymethyltransferase, pantoate–beta-alanine ligase, branched-chain amino acid aminotransferase, polyamine oxidase, and alcohol dehydrogenase (NAD+) enzymes involved in the pantothenate biosynthetic pathway.

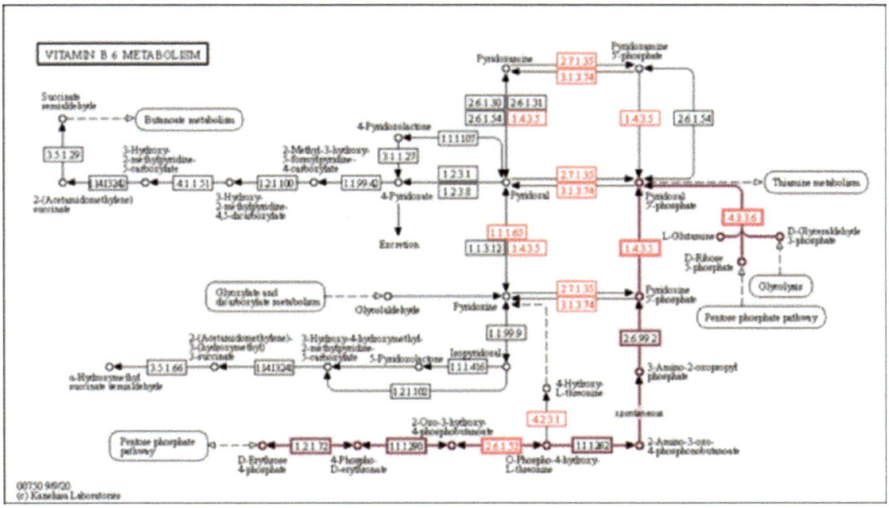

FIGURE 12.6 Vitamin B_6 metabolism pathway. Red indicates the pyridoxine biosynthetic pathway and pyridoxamine 5'-phosphate oxidase, phosphoserine aminotransferase, and pyridoxal 5'-phosphate synthase pdxT subunit enzymes involved in the pyridoxine biosynthetic pathway.

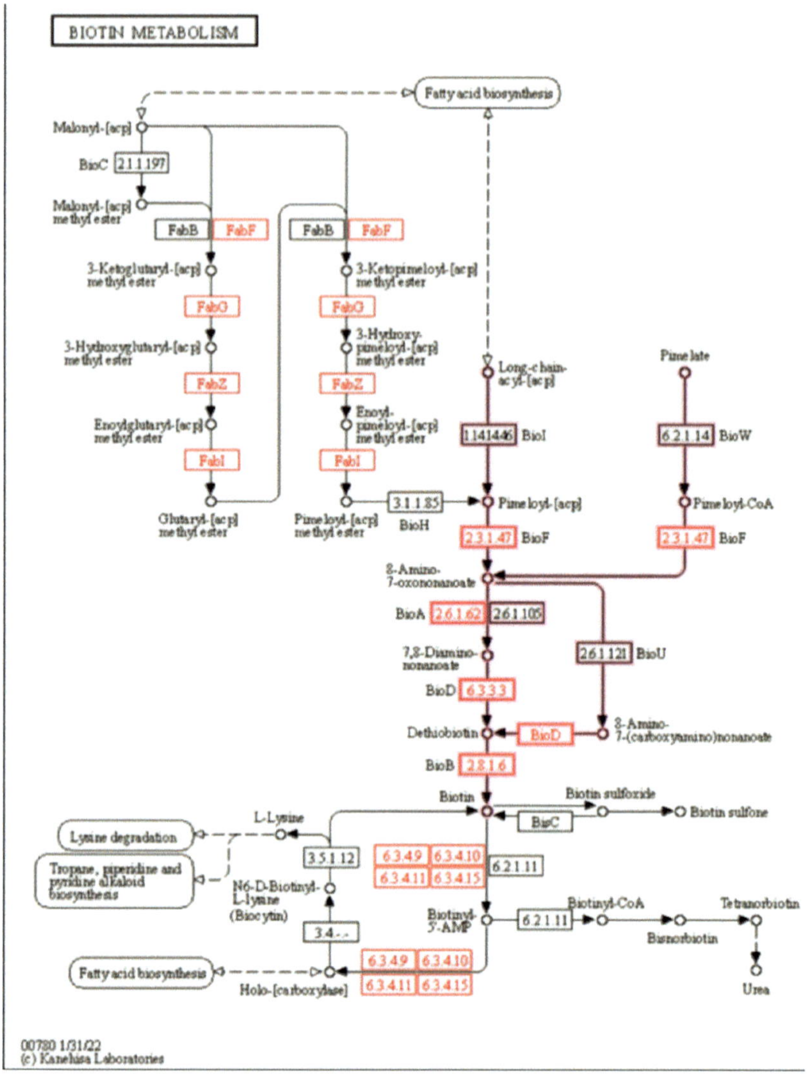

FIGURE 12.7 Biotin metabolism pathway. The biotin biosynthesis route and the 8-amino-7-oxononanoate synthase, bifunctional dethiobiotin synthetase, adenosylmethionine–8-amino-7-oxononanoate aminotransferase, and biotin synthase enzymes involved in the biotin biosynthetic pathway.

transcription factors that regulate anthocyanin biosynthesis in various parts of red-fleshed apple "May" fruit through transcriptome analysis (Li et al. 2022b). KEGG's analysis of DEGs revealed additional details about the biological functions of the identified DEGs, which are primarily related to phenylpropanoid biosynthesis, flavonoid biosynthesis, and phenylalanine metabolism, all of which result in anthocyanin biosynthesis.

12.3.5 Analysis of Biosynthetic Pathway Genes

The present study annotated the vitamin B complex biosynthesis pathway transcripts in the whole fruit transcriptome of *S. virginianum*. Identification of potential genes and important enzymes is a critical step in revealing the biosynthesis pathways of functional vitamin B complex in *S. virginianum*. For the genes involved in the thiamine biosynthesis pathway, there are between 1 and more than 8 CDSs that match the genes, depending on which enzyme is involved: adenosine diphosphate thiazole synthase, 1-(5'-phosphor-ribosyl)-5-aminioimidazole, 4-amino-5-hydroxymethyl-2-methylpyrimidine phosphate, cysteine-dependent adenosine diphosphate thiazole synthase, thiamine phosphate phosphatase, and thiamine pyro phosphokinase, as shown in Figure 12.2. Thirty-three CDSs were involved in the riboflavin metabolism pathway, 22 of which encode nine genes involved in the riboflavin biosynthesis pathway, including the 3,4-dihydroxy 2-butanone 4-phosphate synthase, GTP cyclohydrolase II, diaminohydroxyphosphoribosylaminopyrimidine deaminase, 5-amino-6-(5-phosphoribosylamino) uracil reductase, 5-amino-6-(5-phospho-D-ribitylamino)uracil phosphatase, 6,7-dimethyl-8-ribityllumazine synthase, riboflavin synthase, and FAD synthetase, as shown in Figure 12.3. The nicotinate and nicotinamide metabolism (vitamin B_3) pathway involved 37 CDSs, 8 of which encode five genes including L-aspartate oxidase, quinolinate synthase, nicotinate-nucleotide pyrophosphorylase (carboxylating), nicotinate-nucleotide adenylyltransferase, and NAD^+ synthase (glutamine-hydrolyzing), as shown in Figure 12.4. According to Figure 12.5, 13 of the 32 CDSs engaged in pantothenate and CoA biosynthesis (vitamin B_5) metabolism encode five genes involved in the pantothenate biosynthesis pathway, including 3-methyl-2-oxobutanoate hydroxymethyltransferase, pantoate–beta-alanine ligase, branched-chain amino acid aminotransferase, polyamine oxidase, and aldehyde dehydrogenase (NAD^+), as shown in Figure 12.5. There were 16 CDSs found to be involved in pyridoxine metabolism; 6 of these encode for three genes in the pyridoxine biosynthesis pathway (Figure 12.6). These three genes are phosphoserine aminotransferase, pyridoxamine 5'-phosphate oxidase, and pyridoxal 5'-phosphate synthase pdxT subunit. Figure 12.7 shows that 32 CDSs, of which 10 encode four genes for the biotin biosynthesis pathway, were necessary for biotin metabolism: bifunctional dethiobiotin synthetase, 8-amino-7-oxononanoate synthase, and 8-amino-7-oxononanoate aminotransferase. Five of the 60 CDSs implicated in folate metabolism, including GTP cyclohydrolase IA, alkaline phosphatase D, 7,8-dihydroneopterin aldolase, folylpolyglutamate synthase, and dihydrofolate synthase, are involved in folate biosynthesis. There are transcripts that have been traced to the biosynthetic route of thiamine, riboflavin, nicotinate, nicotinamide, pantothenate, pyridoxine, biotin, and folate, making up the plant's crucial vitamin B complex (Figure 12.8). A similar study was conducted in which Mansouri and Mohammadi identified the key genes involved in terpenoid and rosmarinic acid biosynthesis in lemon balm (*Melissa officinalis*) (Mansouri and Mohammadi 2021). They found the terpenoids biosynthesis was associated with 149 unigenes, including 75 unigenes involved in the methyl-erythritol phosphate and mevalonate pathway, terpenoid

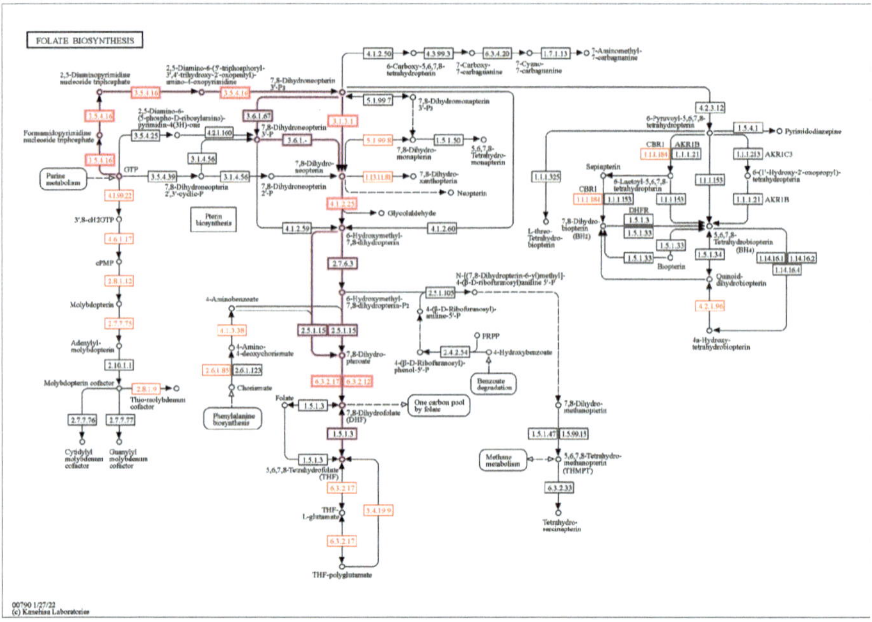

FIGURE 12.8 Folate biosynthesis pathway. The folate biosynthesis pathway is shown in red, along with the enzymes GTP cyclohydrolase IA, alkaline phosphatase D, 7,8-dihydroneopterin aldolase, folylpolyglutamate synthase, and dihydrofolate synthase.

backbone biosynthesis genes, and 74 unigenes associated with the terpene synthase. Additionally, they identified the 144 and 30 unigenes associated with the biosynthesis of phenylpropanoid and the rosmarinic acid pathway, respectively.

12.3.5.1 Discussion

S. virginianum whole fruit was sequenced and de novo assembly was done in the current work. A total of 60,487 CDSs were produced after a de novo assembly, with a N50 of 1,176 bp. A total of 54,259 CDSs were classified into categories as biological processes, molecular activities, and cellular components as part of the functional annotation of the transcriptome. There's a chance that some of the unlabelled CDSs still serve specialized roles for certain species.

Functional annotation employs *in silico* methods to infer a sequence's biological function. Functional annotation is usually applied to messenger RNAs (mRNAs), as the translated proteins execute biological activities (and so contribute to cell function). Classification of RNA and prediction of amino acid sequences are the foundations of functional annotation. (Raghavan et al. 2022). A total of 53,317 CDSs were functionally annotated in total. The majority of CDS were identified as being like those of *S. tuberosum*.

The cellular localization, molecular role, and involvement in biological process of a gene are all defined by the GO. GO uses ontology and annotation. Ontology hierarchizes concepts and their relationships. Gene annotation relates to ontology concepts. "GO annotation employs evidence codes to document gene-GO term links (Thomas 2017). By using the B2G framework to aim at GO, it was found that molecular function had the most CDSs associated with it.

Databases of pathways in the KEGG may be broken down into three distinct levels: category pathways, subclass pathways, and subsidiary pathways. Enrichment analysis tools primarily employ KEGG, as it helps to understand biological processes which are altered to identify the most affected pathway, further helping to prioritize the target for research and/or intervention (Du et al. 2016). CDS was KEGG-annotated. As part of the functional annotation of the transcriptome, 54,259 CDSs were divided into categories such biological processes, molecular activities, and cellular components. It's conceivable that some of the unlabelled CDS that are still present have unique functions for certain species. Signal transduction was seen in the majority of CDSs.

The high vitamin B content of *S. virginianum* makes transcriptome analysis a vital tool for discovering the genes involved in the production of vitamin B. This biosynthetic route for thiamine in plants is similar to the one seen in prokaryotes. Thiamine is produced separately from its constituent pyrimidine and thiazole moiety (Feng et al. 2019). In the biosynthesis of thiamin, the pyrimidine and thiazole ring moieties are synthesized independently and then combined to produce thiamin monophosphate (ThMP), which is then converted to the active form thiamin diphosphate (ThDP) (Guan et al. 2014).

Plants and eubacteria use the same chemical route to produce riboflavin, while fungi use a slightly different one. One molecule of riboflavin requires two molecules of ribulose 5-phosphate, one molecule of GTP, and one molecule of vitamin B_2. By hydrolyzing the imidazole ring of GTP, a 2,5-diaminopyrimidine is released, which is subsequently converted into 5-amino-6-ribitylamino-2,4(1H,3H)-pyrimidinedione by a sequence of side chain reduction, deamination, and dephosphorylation reactions. Combining ribulose 5-phosphate-derived 3,4-dihydroxy-2-butanone 4-phosphate with ribulose 5-phosphate-derived 5-amino-6-ribitylamino-2,4(1H,3H)-pyrimidinedione yields the cyclic amine 6,7-dimethyl-8-ribityllumazine. Dismutation of the lumazine derivative results in the formation of riboflavin and 5-amino-6-ribitylamino-2,4(1H,3H)-pyrimidinedione. (Fischer and Bacher 2006).

Niacinamide adenine dinucleotide (NAD), often known as vitamin B_3, nicotinamide, and nicotinic acid, is an essential redox cofactor involved in a wide variety of vital metabolic processes. Similarly to higher species, intestinal bacteria can produce vitamin B_3 from tryptophan, though they do so by a slightly different process (Hossain, Amarasena, and Mayengbam 2022).

Enzyme cofactors, such as the 4'-phosphopantetheine moiety of coenzyme A and acyl carrier protein, are required for the key metabolic and energy-producing pathways in all living things. The universal precursor for their production is pantothenate (vitamin B_5), which is synthesized primarily in microbes and plants from primitive steps. The biosynthetic pathway in microbes has been well established, while in plants the biosynthetic pathway has not been completely studied. Plants are a major source of dietary pantothenate and studying the vitamin B complex biosynthetic pathway has more significance. The enzyme ketopantoate hydroxymethyltransferase produces ketopantoate from ketoisovalerate in the first committed step. Ketopantoate reductase then converts ketopantoate to pantoate. From L-aspartate, alanine may be synthesized by the enzyme L-aspartate-decarboxylase. Pantothenate is a byproduct of pantoate and β-alanine's condensation process, which is mediated by pantothenate synthetase (Ottenhof et al. 2004).

Vitamin B_6 can be biosynthesized by plants from primitive steps. While vitamin B_6 is present in all parts of the plant, it is most concentrated in the metabolically active leaves. Two enzymes, a synthase (PDX1) and a glutaminase (PDX2), are all that are required for the de *novo* process to take place in the cytosol (Vanderschuren et al. 2013). *Escherichia coli* is expected to create the coenzyme pyridoxal 5'-phosphate (PLP) by condensing 4-(phosphohydroxy)-L-threonine and L-deoxy-D-xylulose. Certain enzymes, PdxA and PdxJ, are credited with catalyzing a condensation that yields either pyridoxine (vitamin B_6) or pyr (phosphonomethyl pyrophosphate) (Laber et al. 1999).

The enzymes that manipulate carbon dioxide (CO_2) in all three kingdoms of life need the cofactor biotin, often known as vitamin H or B_8 (Alban 2011). Studies of the biotin biosynthesis route in plants have centred on biotin synthase. It is the mitochondria that house the enzyme that catalyzes the last step of the route. Similarities exist between the pimeloyl-CoA–based metabolic pathway in bacteria and its counterpart in plants. All bacteria use a four-step enzymatic process including 7-keto-8-aminopelargonic acid (KAPA) synthase, 7,8-diaminopelargonic acid (DAPA) aminotransferase, dethiobiotin synthase, and biotin synthase to produce the cofactor from pimeloyl-CoA (Pinon et al. 2005).

Folates may be produced in plants, bacteria, and fungus, but mammals must get them from their food. Tetrahydrofolate (THF) and its derivatives are referred to collectively as "folates." The para-aminobenzoate (pABA), glutamate tail, and pterin ring make up the structure of the THF molecule. Dihydrofolate (DHF) and tetrahydrofolate (THF) are two naturally occurring folates that may be differentiated by the pterin ring's oxidation state. DHF must be reduced by dihydrofolate reductase before it can be used biologically, while THF is already in its active state (DHFR). The molecule of folic acid has a pterin ring that has been totally oxidatedf. After folic acid has been reduced twice, it may then be used by the system. One-carbon units in different oxidation states may be found in THF molecules. The N5 and or N10 locations of THF molecules are connected to one-carbon units with various oxidation states. The THF molecules' one-carbon unit types determine their metabolic functions. The number of glutamate residues in naturally occurring folates in plants is another way to identify individual folate molecules. (Gorelova et al. 2017).

12.4 CONCLUSION

NGS and bioinformatics enable high-throughput molecular data collection, enabling researchers to fully understand any species' genomic and transcriptome profiles. We can use the information from a transcriptome to determine which regions of the genome are used to code for active genes. After sequencing several transcriptomes under various growth or conditions, we could determine which genes are more essential in which biological processes. The vitamin B complex is essential for catabolic metabolism and anabolic metabolism and are cofactors for axonal transport, synthesis of neurotransmitters, and many cellular metabolic pathways. Based on the presence and absence of genome annotations, we predicted the transcripts involved in the vitamin B complex biosynthesis. We have performed a transcriptome analysis of *S. virginianum* fruit and discussed the features of the identified genes. Its fruits have been subjected to de novo sequencing and transcriptome analysis. Our findings reveal the transcriptome profile of a powerful medicinal plant used to treat female infertility and give additional benefits as an anti-inflammatory, analgesic, and antimicrobial. The current study will help identify the essential biosynthetic pathway of the vitamin B complex in traditional medicinal plants. The information will give insight into the biosynthetic processes that give the vitamin B complex its enrichment targets. More data on *S. virginianum* may be gained from the transcriptome profile, which reveals the genes involved in the vitamin B complex pathway.

12.5 COMPETING INTERESTS

The authors have no conflicts to disclose.

TABLE 12.4A
KEGG Pathway Classification Summary

Metabolism Pathways	CDS Count
Carbohydrate	679
Energy	413
Lipid	352
Nucleotide	129
Amino acid	440
Metabolism of other amino acids	186
Glycan biosynthesis and metabolism	170
Cofactor and vitamins	334
Terpenoids and polyketides	147
Biosynthesis of other secondary metabolites	198
Xenobiotics biodegradation and metabolism	85

TABLE 12.4B

Genetic Information Processing Pathways	CDS Count
Transcription	360
Translation	747
Folding, sorting, and degradation	572
Replication and repair	191

TABLE 12.4C

Environmental Information Processing Pathways	CDS Count
Membrane transport	31
Signal transduction	813
Pathways	**CDS Count**
Signalling molecules and interaction	1

TABLE 12.4D

Cellular Processes Pathways	CDS Count
Transport and catabolism	542
Cell growth and death	365
Cellular community-eukaryotes	109
Cell motility	59
Organismal systems pathways	**CDS Count**
Environmental adaptation	360

REFERENCES

Alban, Claude. 2011. 'Biotin (Vitamin B8) Synthesis in Plants'. In *Advances in Botanical Research*, 59:39–66. Elsevier. https://doi.org/10.1016/B978-0-12-385853-5.00005-2.

Ali, Mennatallah A., Hala A. Hafez, Maher A. Kamel, Heba I. Ghamry, Mustafa Shukry, and Mohamed A. Farag. 2022. 'Dietary Vitamin B Complex: Orchestration in Human Nutrition throughout Life with Sex Differences'. *Nutrients* 14 (19): 3940. https://doi.org/10.3390/nu14193940.

Bolger, Anthony M., Marc Lohse, and Bjoern Usadel. 2014. 'Trimmomatic: A Flexible Trimmer for Illumina Sequence Data'. *Bioinformatics* 30 (15): 2114–2120. https://doi.org/10.1093/bioinformatics/btu170.

Buchfink, Benjamin, Chao Xie, and Daniel H. Huson. 2015. 'Fast and Sensitive Protein Alignment Using DIAMOND'. *Nature Methods* 12 (1): 59–60. https://doi.org/10.1038/nmeth.3176.

Chen, Lei, Yu-Hang Zhang, ShaoPeng Wang, YunHua Zhang, Tao Huang, and Yu-Dong Cai. 2017. 'Prediction and Analysis of Essential Genes Using the Enrichments of Gene Ontology and KEGG Pathways'. Edited by Bin Liu. *PLoS ONE* 12 (9): e0184129. https://doi.org/10.1371/journal.pone.0184129.

Conesa, A., S. Gotz, J. M. Garcia-Gomez, J. Terol, M. Talon, and M. Robles. 2005. 'Blast2GO: A Universal Tool for Annotation, Visualization and Analysis in Functional Genomics Research'. *Bioinformatics* 21 (18): 3674–3676. https://doi.org/10.1093/bioinformatics/bti610.

Du, Junli, Manlin Li, Zhifa Yuan, Mancai Guo, Jiuzhou Song, Xiaozhen Xie, and Yulin Chen. 2016. 'A Decision Analysis Model for KEGG Pathway Analysis'. *BMC Bioinformatics* 17 (1): 407. https://doi.org/10.1186/s12859-016-1285-1.

Fang, Ren, Weixiong Huang, Jinyan Yao, Xing Long, Ji Zhang, Shuangyun Zhou, Biao Deng, Wenzhong Tang, and Zhenyu An. 2020. 'Characterization of Full-Length Transcriptome and Mechanisms of Sugar Accumulation in Annona Squamosa Fruit'. *Biocell* 44 (4): 737–750. https://doi.org/10.32604/biocell.2020.012933.

Feng, Xingxing, Suxin Yang, Kuanqiang Tang, Yaohua Zhang, Jiantian Leng, Jingjing Ma, Quan Wang, and Xianzhong Feng. 2019. 'GmPGL1, a Thiamine Thiazole Synthase, Is Required for the Biosynthesis of Thiamine in Soybean'. *Frontiers in Plant Science* 10 (November): 1546. https://doi.org/10.3389/fpls.2019.01546.

Fischer, Markus, and Adelbert Bacher. 2006. 'Biosynthesis of Vitamin B2 in Plants'. *Physiologia Plantarum* 126 (3): 304–318. https://doi.org/10.1111/j.1399-3054.2006.00607.x.

Fu, Limin, Beifang Niu, Zhengwei Zhu, Sitao Wu, and Weizhong Li. 2012. 'CD-HIT: Accelerated for Clustering the Next-Generation Sequencing Data'. *Bioinformatics* 28 (23): 3150–3152. https://doi.org/10.1093/bioinformatics/bts565.

Gorelova, Vera, Lars Ambach, Fabrice Rébeillé, Christophe Stove, and Dominique Van Der Straeten. 2017. 'Folates in Plants: Research Advances and Progress in Crop Biofortification'. *Frontiers in Chemistry* 5 (March). https://doi.org/10.3389/fchem.2017.00021.

Guan, Jiahn-Chou, Ghulam Hasnain, Timothy J. Garrett, Christine D. Chase, Jesse Gregory, Andrew D. Hanson, and Donald R. McCarty. 2014. 'Divisions of Labor in the Thiamin Biosynthetic Pathway among Organs of Maize'. *Frontiers in Plant Science* 5 (August): 370. https://doi.org/10.3389/fpls.2014.00370.

Haas, Brian J., Alexie Papanicolaou, Moran Yassour, Manfred Grabherr, Philip D. Blood, Joshua Bowden, Matthew Brian Couger, et al. 2013. 'De *Novo* Transcript Sequence Reconstruction from RNA-Seq Using the Trinity Platform for Reference Generation and Analysis'. *Nature Protocols* 8 (8): 1494–1512. https://doi.org/10.1038/nprot.2013.084.

Hanna, Mary, Ecler Jaqua, Van Nguyen, and Jeremy Clay. 2022. 'B Vitamins: Functions and Uses in Medicine'. *The Permanente Journal* 26 (2): 89–97. https://doi.org/10.7812/TPP/21.204.

Hossain, Khandkar Shaharina, Sathya Amarasena, and Shyamchand Mayengbam. 2022. 'B Vitamins and Their Roles in Gut Health'. *Microorganisms* 10 (6): 1168. https://doi.org/10.3390/microorganisms10061168.

Ikenouchi-Sugita, Atsuko, and Kazunari Sugita. 2015. 'Niacin Deficiency and Cutaneous Immunity'. *Japanese Journal of Clinical Immunology* 38 (1): 37–44. https://doi.org/10.2177/jsci.38.37.

Laber, Bernd, Wolfgang Maurer, Sandra Scharf, Karin Stepusin, Frank S. Schmidt. 1999. 'Vitamin B6 Biosynthesis: Formation of Pyridoxine 5′-Phosphate from 4-(Phosphohydroxy)-L-Threonine and 1-Deoxy-D-Xylulose-5-Phosphate by PdxA and PdxJ Protein'. *FEBS Letters* 449 (1): 45–48. https://doi.org/10.1016/S0014-5793(99)00393-2.

Li, Caiqin, Yan Wang, Xuming Huang, Jiang Li, Huicong Wang, and Jianguo Li. 2013. 'De *Novo* Assembly and Characterization of Fruit Transcriptome in Litchi Chinensis Sonn and Analysis of Differentially Regulated Genes in Fruit in Response to Shading'. *BMC Genomics* 14 (1): 552. https://doi.org/10.1186/1471-2164-14-552.

Li, Chen, Ying Guo, Zuomiao Xiao, Shi Luo, Xianchun Chen, Zhiqing Liu, and Dejun Xiao. 2022a. 'Megaloblastic Anemia Masked by an Unrecognized Hemoglobinopathy'. *Clinical Laboratory* 68 (09/2022). https://doi.org/10.7754/Clin.Lab.2021.211231.

Li, Hua, Shiyao Duan, Weilei Sun, Sifan Wang, Jie Zhang, Tingting Song, Ji Tian, and Yuncong Yao. 2022b. 'Identification, through Transcriptome Analysis, of Transcription Factors That Regulate Anthocyanin Biosynthesis in Different Parts of Red-Fleshed Apple "May" Fruit'. *Horticultural Plant Journal* 8 (1): 11–21. https://doi.org/10.1016/j.hpj.2021.07.001.

Mansouri, Mehdi, and Fatemeh Mohammadi. 2021. 'Transcriptome Analysis to Identify Key Genes Involved in Terpenoid and Rosmarinic Acid Biosynthesis in Lemon Balm (Melissa Officinalis)'. *Gene* 773 (March): 145417. https://doi.org/10.1016/j.gene.2021.145417.

Mohanty, Padmaja, Garima Ayachit, Preeti Sharma, Inayatullah Shaikh, Jatindra Nath Mohanty, Archana U. Mankad, Himanshu Pandya, and Jayashankar Das. 2020. 'De *Novo* Sequencing and Transcriptome Analysis of Indian Bael (Aegle Marmelos L.)'. *Gene Reports* 19 (June): 100671. https://doi.org/10.1016/j.genrep.2020.100671.

Ong, Wen Dee, Lok-Yung Christopher Voo, and Vijay Subbiah Kumar. 2012. 'De *Novo* Assembly, Characterization and Functional Annotation of Pineapple Fruit Transcriptome through Massively Parallel Sequencing'. Edited by Baohong Zhang. *PLoS ONE* 7 (10): e46937. https://doi.org/10.1371/journal.pone.0046937.

Ottenhof, Harald H., Jennifer L. Ashurst, Heather M. Whitney, S. Adrian Saldanha, Florian Schmitzberger, Hyun Soon Gweon, Tom L. Blundell, Chris Abell, and Alison G. Smith. 2004. 'Organisation of the Pantothenate (Vitamin B 5) Biosynthesis Pathway in Higher Plants'. *The Plant Journal* 37 (1): 61–72. https://doi.org/10.1046/j.1365-313X.2003.01940.x.

Pinon, Violaine, Stéphane Ravanel, Roland Douce, and Claude Alban. 2005. 'Biotin Synthesis in Plants. The First Committed Step of the Pathway Is Catalyzed by a Cytosolic 7-Keto-8-Aminopelargonic Acid Synthase'. *Plant Physiology* 139 (4): 1666–1676. https://doi.org/10.1104/pp.105.070144.

Piraccini, Bianca M., Enzo Berardesca, Gabriella Fabbrocini, Giuseppe Micali, and Antonella Tosti. 2019. 'Biotin: Overview of the Treatment of Diseases of Cutaneous Appendages and of Hyperseborrhea'. *Giornale Italiano Di Dermatologia e Venereologia* 154 (5). https://doi.org/10.23736/S0392-0488.19.06434-4.

Raghavan, Venket, Louis Kraft, Fantin Mesny, and Linda Rigerte. 2022. 'A Simple Guide to de *Novo* Transcriptome Assembly and Annotation'. *Briefings in Bioinformatics* 23 (2): bbab563. https://doi.org/10.1093/bib/bbab563.

Rane, Madhavi H., Neha K. Sahu, Sainin S. Ajgoankar, Nikhil C. Teli, and Deepa R. Verma. 2014. 'A Holistic Approach on Review of Solanum Virginianum. L'. *Journal of Pharmacy and Pharmaceutical Sciences* 3: 1–4.

Roje, Sanja. 2007. 'Vitamin B Biosynthesis in Plants'. *Phytochemistry* 68 (14): 1904–1921. https://doi.org/10.1016/j.phytochem.2007.03.038.

Sijilmassi, Ouafa. 2019. 'Folic Acid Deficiency and Vision: A Review'. *Graefe's Archive for Clinical and Experimental Ophthalmology* 257 (8): 1573–1580. https://doi.org/10.1007/s00417-019-04304-3.

Smith, Taryn J., Casey R. Johnson, Roshine Koshy, Sonja Y. Hess, Umar A. Qureshi, Mimi Lhamu Mynak, and Philip R. Fischer. 2021. 'Thiamine Deficiency Disorders: A Clinical Perspective'. *Annals of the New York Academy of Sciences* 1498 (1): 9–28. https://doi.org/10.1111/nyas.14536.

Subhash Patil, Dhanashree, and Swaroopa Amit Patil. 2022. 'Regeneration of Medicinal Plant Solanum Virginianum L. Via Somatic Embryogenesis from Seed Explant'. *Archives of Internal Medicine Research* 5 (4). https://doi.org/10.26502/aimr.0138.

Tang, Shiyuyun, Alexandre Lomsadze, and Mark Borodovsky. 2015. 'Identification of Protein Coding Regions in RNA Transcripts'. *Nucleic Acids Research* 43 (12): e78–e78. https://doi.org/10.1093/nar/gkv227.

Thakur, Kiran, Sudhir Kumar Tomar, Ashish Kumar Singh, Surajit Mandal, and Sumit Arora. 2017. 'Riboflavin and Health: A Review of Recent Human Research'. *Critical Reviews in Food Science and Nutrition* 57 (17): 3650–3660. https://doi.org/10.1080/10408398.2016.1145104.

Thomas, Paul D. 2017. 'The Gene Ontology and the Meaning of Biological Function'. In Christophe Dessimoz and Nives Škunca (Eds.), *The Gene Ontology Handbook*, 1446:15–24. Springer. https://doi.org/10.1007/978-1-4939-3743-1_2.

Tr, Prashith Kekuda, Raghavendra HL, Rajesh MR, Avinash HC, Ankith GN, and Karthik KN. 2017. 'Antimicrobial, Insecticidal, and Antiradical Activity of Solanum Virginianum L. (Solanaceae)'. *Asian Journal of Pharmaceutical and Clinical Research* 10 (11): 163. https://doi.org/10.22159/ajpcr. 2017.v10i11.20180.

Vanderschuren, Hervé, Svetlana Boycheva, Kuan-Te Li, Nicolas Szydlowski, Wilhelm Gruissem, and Teresa B. Fitzpatrick. 2013. 'Strategies for Vitamin B6 Biofortification of Plants: A Dual Role as a Micronutrient and a Stress Protectant'. *Frontiers in Plant Science* 4. https://doi.org/10.3389/fpls.2013.00143.

Wang, Zhong, Mark Gerstein, and Michael Snyder. 2009. 'RNA-Seq: A Revolutionary Tool for Transcriptomics'. *Nature Reviews Genetics* 10 (1): 57–63. https://doi.org/10.1038/nrg2484.

Zucker, Theodore F. 1958. 'Pantothenic Acid Deficiency and Its Effect on the Integrity and Functions of the Intestines'. *The American Journal of Clinical Nutrition* 6 (1): 65–74. https://doi.org/10.1093/ajcn/6.1.6.

13 Identification of Compounds Present in the Ethanolic Extract of *Cecropia pachyatachya* Trécul Leaves by CG-MS and *In Silico* Studies with the Enzymes 5-LOX and α-1-Antitrypsin

Penina S. Mourão, Rafael de O. Gomes*, Clara A. C. B. Costa**, Orlando F. da S. Moura**, Johnnatan D. de Freitas**, Francisco das C. A. Lima*, Wellington dos S. Alves*, and Valdiléia T. Uchôa**,†*

*State University of Piaui; **Federal Institute of Alagoas

†Corresponding Author: valdileiatexeira@ccn.uespi.br

ABBREVIATIONS

PreADMET	Predictions of Absorption, Distribution, Metabolism, Excretion and Toxicity
5-LOX	5-lipoxygenase enzyme
GC-MS	Gas chromatography coupled to a mass spectrum
COPD	Chronic Obstructive Pulmonary Disease
CPF	Ethanolic extract of the leaves of *C. pachystachya*
PDB	Protein Data Bank
ADT	Autodock Tools version 1.5.6
R_{T-}	Retention time
PPB	Plasma Protein Binding
BBB	Blood-Brain Barrier
HIA	Human Intestinal Absorption
PgP	P-glycoprotein

DOI: 10.1201/9781003354437-13

TA100 and TA1535	Ames test cell lines 100 and 1535
-S9	no metabolic activation
+S9	with metabolic activation
OECD 423	Test guideline for testing for Acute Oral Tosxidity using the Acute Toxic Class Method
DNA	deoxyribonucleic acid
CYP450	cytochrome P450
ΔG_{bind}	Interaction energy
Ki	Inhibition constant.

13.1 INTRODUCTION

The use of plants has been widely employed for the treatment of several diseases as an alternative and more accessible option (Rogério & Ribeiro, 2021). They are considered medicinal plants because they are capable of developing therapeutic action and have phytochemical compounds with biological activities, also known as secondary metabolites (Andrade et al., 2021b; Pedroso et al., 2021). They are used in the form of teas, licks, and others, but it is of utmost importance to conduct studies that prove such biological activities in order to standardize the use of these without affecting human health (Andrade et al., 2021b; Pedroso et al., 2021).

Among the varieties of medicinal plants, we have *Cecropia pachystachya* Trécul (Cecropeaceae), popularly known as "embaúba" and found in Central and South America and is abundant throughout Brazil (Andrade et al., 2021a; Pacheco et al., 2014). It is widely used in folk medicine for the treatment of colds, asthma, cough, hypertension, diabetes, and inflammation (Pacheco et al., 2014) and as a bronchodilator, antiseptic, expectorant, antispasmodic, and cardiotonic (Bigliani et al., 2010). The following secondary metabolites have already been reported to be present for *C. pachyastachya*: chlorogenic acid, isoorientin, orientin, catechin, epicatechin, isoquercitrin, isovitexin, sitosterol (Uchôa et al., 2010), and α-amyrin; ursolic, pomolic, oleanolic, and tormentic acids (Lima et al., 2016; Pacheco et al., 2014; Uchôa et al., 2010); and ethyl hexadecanoate, L-(+)-ascorbic acid-2,6-dihexadecanoate, (9E,12E)-octadec-9,12-dienoate, (Z)-octadec-9-enoate, ethyl octadecanoate, sitostenone, beccaridiol, lupeol, and syringaldehyde (Mourão et al., 2022).

Of its various parts, the leaves have been widely used in studies to prove the biological activities and determination of bioactive compounds present in this plant. These have been reported to have hypoglycemic, diuretic, anti-inflammatory, and antioxidant properties (Ferreira et al., 2021). The leaves present bronchodilator activity and cardiovascular effects, have cardiotonic and sedative actions, antioxidant properties and anti-inflammatory and apoptotic activity (Duque et al., 2016; Machado et al., 2021; Schinella et al., 2008; Velázquez et al., 2003).

In silico approaches are being widely used in the discovery of new drugs because they are a way to save both time and money with tests that are time-consuming but necessary for the classification of molecules as drugs/phytopharmaceuticals. It is emphasized that with *in silico* testing one can screen substances for *in vitro*, *in vivo*, and clinical testing, not that one should exclude such procedures. ADMET predictions are performed to verify administration, distribution, metabolization, excretion, and toxicity properties of substances (PreADMET, 2022). Molecular docking, on the other hand, seeks the best form of interaction between these substances and disease target enzymes, in a key-and-lock model in the analysis of values of interaction energies and hydrogen-bridge and hydrophobic interactions (Santos, 2021).

The enzymes 5-lipoxygenase (5-LOX) and α-1-antitrypsin are related to chronic obstructive pulmonary disease (COPD), which is characterized by chronic inflammation of the airways and destruction of the lung alveoli (Mourão et al., 2021). Among the factors that cause COPD we can mention active and/or passive smoking and the genetic deficiency of α-1-antitrypsin (Mourão et al., 2021). It is a progressive disease and has no cure, but its treatment is based on the use of corticoids such as Clenil A and N-acetylcysteine, and it is generally diagnosed in adults over 40 years of age (Carvalho et al., 2020; Dourado et al., 2006). 5-LOX acts in the development of inflammation as a catalyst of arachidonic acid oxygenation reaction, that is, in the biosynthesis of leukotrienes that in excess trigger inflammation (Radmark & Samuelsson, 2008). Of the leukotrienes that are best known and most active in inflammatory cells, we have polymorphonuclear leukocytes, neutrophils, monocytes, basophils, mast cells, eosinophils, and macrophages in different organs such as the lung, spleen, heart, and brain (Etienne et al., 2021).

On the other hand, α-1-antitrypsin is a circulating medium-sized glycoprotein encoded by the *SERPINA1* gene, and deficiency of this enzyme is caused by mutations in this gene. Such a fact leads to the development of studies for the discovery of precision prototype drugs for COPD, since it has an identifiable genetic basis, with specific epidemiological and clinical features (Sidhaye et al., 2018). In view of this, the aim of this work is to perform an identification study of bioactive compounds in the ethanolic extract of *C. pachystachya* leaves, verify their PreADMET properties, and analyze the interaction of these bioactive compounds with 5-LOX and α-1-antitrypsin enzymes. *C. pachystachya* was selected because it is a plant already used in folk medicine for the treatment of respiratory diseases. The solvent, in this case ethanol, was selected because it has good extraction properties and is polar, biodegradable, and non-toxic (Silva et al., 2019).

13.2 METHODOLOGY

13.2.1 Botanical Material

The leaves of *C. pachystachya* were collected in the city of Monsenhor Gil–Piauí (5°33'56.7"S 42°36'19.3"W) in the months of October and November 2020. The botanical identification was performed by the botanist Ivanilza Moreira de Andrade, and an exsiccate is deposited in the Herbarium Delta do Parnaíba of the Federal University of Parnaíba Delta (UFDPar) under voucher number 6727. The project for this work was registered on the SisGen platform (National System for Managing Genetic Heritage and Associated Traditional Knowledge) under number A46333F.

13.2.2 Extract Production

The leaves (495.14 g), were washed in running water, then dried at room temperature, crushed, weighed on an analytical balance (460.93 g), and stored in a glass container. Subsequently, the extract was made with 99% ethanol, by the maceration method, in a 1:3 ratio, under mechanical agitation for three times, at room temperature of 26°C ±1. The solvent was evaporated in a Fisatom R-801 rotary evaporator under reduced pressure with the aid of PRSIMATEC BBV-132 vacuum pumps at a temperature ≤40°C in the Natural Products Synthesis Laboratory of the Federal Institute of Piauí–Teresina Central Campus. The ethanolic extract obtained from the 21.75 g leaves (named ethanolic extract [CPF]), with yield of approximately 4.56%, was subjected to phytochemical prospection and gas chromatography coupled with mass spectrometry (GC-MS).

13.2.3 Preliminary Phytochemical Prospection

The phytochemical prospection followed the methodology of Matos (2009) to verify the presence of secondary metabolite classes such as tannins, steroids and triterpenes, flavonoids, saponins, and alkaloids through qualitative analysis of coloration and precipitation during reactions with ethyl extract (CPF). The tests were performed in two different ratios of extract to solvent: 1:1 and 2:1.

13.2.4 Gas Chromatography Coupled with Mass Spectrometry of the CPF Extract

This analysis was performed in a Shimadzu equipment (GC/MS-GCMS-QP2010CN Ultra), following the methodology reported by Bezerra et al. (2021) and Mourão et al. (2022). The carrier gas used was helium gas (1.69 mL/min, 100 KPa), ionization temperature 200°C and interface temperature 250°C. The mass spectrometer operated at 70 eV in full scan mode with temperature propagation 50°C/5 min, then 250°C (5°C/min for 35 min). CPF was prepared in 1 mg/mL solution (1 μL injected) and quantification calculation done by area normalization.

13.2.5 ADMET Prediction Analysis

The theoretical ADMET (absorption, distribution, metabolization, excretion and toxicity) properties of the molecules were performed in the free online software Pre-ADMET (PreADMET, 2022), in which we can obtain the pharmacokinetic and pharmacodynamic properties in order to reduce the financial expenses with experimental tests. The structural formulas of the phytochemical compounds identified in the ethanol extract (CPF) were drawn in the software itself and subjected to ADMET testing as represented in Figure 13.1 and Table 13.1 (Mourão et al., 2022).

13.2.6 Molecular Docking

The procedure followed the methodology described by Mourão et al. (2022), using software such as Autodock 4.2 (Goodsell, 2005), Autodock Tools (ADT) version

1.5.6 (Sanner, 1999), and Chimera (Pettersen et al., 2004), with each docking occurring with a total of 100 simulations in a 60 × 60 × 60 box. The enzymes were obtained from the Protein Data Bank (PDB) (Protein Data Bank, 2022), with codes 3V92 (5-lipoxygenase, 5-LOX) and 1KCT (α-1-antitrypsin) and the ligands obtained from the PubChem database, listed in Table 13.1 and structure shown in Figure 13.1. The active site of each enzyme corresponds to the vicinity of residue Phe177 for 5-LOX and residues Met358 and Ser359 for the enzyme α-1-antitrypsin.

TABLE 13.1
Descriptions of Bioactive Compounds from the Ethanolic Extract of *C. pachystachya* Leaves

Code	Molecule	PubChem CID	Molecular Description
32	Ethyl hexadecanoate	12366	$C_{18}H_{36}O_2$ (284.5 g/mol)
37	Phytol	5280435	$C_{20}H_{40}O$ (296.5 g/mol)
42	Linoleic acid	5280450	$C_{18}H_{32}O_2$ (280.4 g/mol)
43	2,2-Sichloroacetate tridec-2-inyl	531238	$C_{15}H_{24}Cl_2O_2$ (307.3 g/mol)
45	Ethyl octadecanoate	8122	$C_{20}H_{40}O_2$ (312.5 g/mol)

Code: identification number of the compounds in this work.

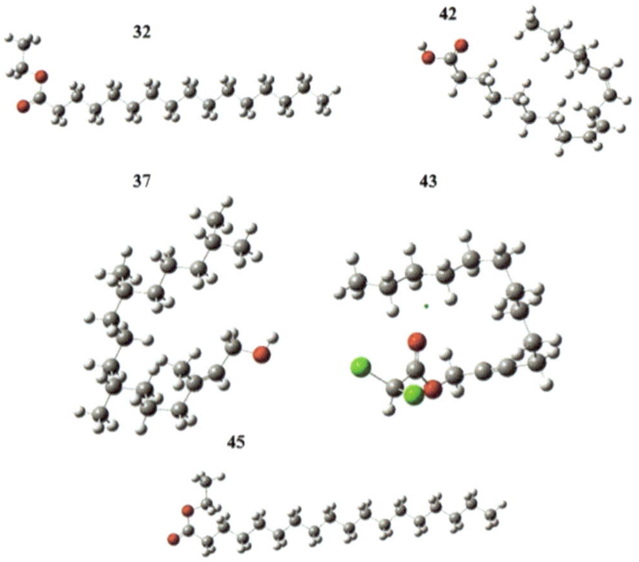

FIGURE 13.1 Bioactive compounds identified in the CPF ethanolic extract: 3D structure. 32. ethyl hexadecanoate, 37. phytol, 42. linoleic acid, 43. tridec-2-inyl 2,2-dichloroacetate, 45. ethyl octadecanoate; In gray: carbons, white: hydrogens, red: oxygen, and green: chlorine.

13.3 RESULTS AND DISCUSSION

13.3.1 Preliminary Phytochemical Prospection

The preliminary phytochemical prospection analysis was performed in order to identify the classes of secondary metabolites present in the ethanolic extract (CPF) in a qualitative way. With the interpretation of the results, the presence of saponins and alkaloids (2:1 ratio) and triterpenes, saponins, and alkaloids (1:1 ratio) was noted.

The phytochemical screening is a qualitative process of the recognition of substances present in a significant amount, it being more difficult to recognize metabolites in smaller quantities (Coelho et al., 2021). In the literature there are reports of the presence of tannins, alkaloids, and flavonoids for the aqueous extract of *C. pachystachya* leaves and of tannins, saponins, and steroids for the ethanolic extract of the same (Costa & Hoscheid, 2018).

Comparing the results, tannins were not identified in the extract studied. Saponins have an action on cell membrane permeability and when administered orally can exert hypocholesterolemic activity (Coelho et al., 2021). The triterpenes can have analgesic, antipyretic, hepatoprotective, and anti-inflammatory actions (Coelho et al., 2021). The alkaloids are widely used in the treatment and relief of pain, also presenting antitussive and antiviral activities (Coelho et al., 2021).

13.3.2 GC-MS Analysis of the Ethanolic Extract

The result of the analysis of the ethanolic extract (CPF) showed a chromatogram with 62 signals, and 54 compounds could be identified, as noted in Table 13.2. Of these 62 substances, we have 17 mixed functions, 22 esters, 5 hydrocarbons, 3 alcohols, 2 carboxylic acids, 1 diterpene, 1 ketone, and 11 unidentified compounds. The compounds ethyl hexadecanoate (32), phytol (37), linoleic acid (42), tridec-2-inyl 2,2-dichloroacetate (43), and ethyl octadecanoate (45) showed the most significant percent area values and received a highlight in this work. The lowest percent area values were obtained for the molecules 5-(hydroxymethyl)furan-2-carbaldehyde (04), 2-methyl-4-[(E)-oct-2-en-2-yl]-2H-furan-5-ane (27), shiobuane (51), isoamyl laurate (52), and 2,3-dihydroxypropyl (9Z, 12Z)octadeca-9,12-dienoate (56).

Among the compounds identified, the five with the highest percentage area value were highlighted in this work. Some of the compounds found in CPF have already been reported for the ethanolic extract of the roots of this same plant, such as ethyl hexadecanoate and ethyl octadecanoate (Mourão et al., 2022). Ethyl hexadecanoate (32) has already been reported in the liquid oily chloroform extract of seeds of *Juglans regia* (Pillai & Young, 2022), petroleum ether and methanol extract of the leaves of *Helicteres guazumifolia* Kunth (D'Armas et al., 2021), and essential oil of the aerial parts of *Salvia verbenaca* L. (from Italy) (Khouchlaa et al., 2022). Abarca-Vargas and Petricevich (2018) published a review article on the genus *Bougainvillea* and in their work reported ethyl hexadecanoate in *B. x buttiana* (which may develop antioxidant activity) and *B. spectabilis* (to which antioxidant and anti-inflammatory activities are attributed).

The phytol (**37** anti-close up except for anti-inflammatory) is a compound of the dipertene family, having a long and branched chain, characterized by being an acyclic alcohol (Mendonça, 2020). Used as an addition in food, it is non-mutagenic and

TABLE 13.2
Compounds Identified in the GC-MS Analysis of the Ethanolic Extract (CPF)

Peak N°	R_T (min)	Compound	Molecular Formula	Molecular Mass (u)	Relative Percentage of Area (%)
01	3.366	Ethyl 2-fluoroacetate	$C_4H_7O_2F$	106.10	1.46
02	3.861	Methyl 2-oxopraponoate	$C_4H_6O_3$	102.09	0.34
03	6.667	2,3-Dihydroxypropanal	$C_6H_{12}O_6$	180.16	0.22
04	18.197	5-(Hydroxymethyl)furan-2-carbaldehyde	$C_6H_6O_3$	126.11	0.18
05	22.460	Benzene-1,2,3-triol	$C_6H_6O_3$	126.11	1.64
06	23.094	Ethyl decanoate	$C_{12}H_{24}O_2$	200.32	0.45
07	24.243	2-Hydroxy-4-methylbenzaldehyde	$C_8H_8O_2$	136.15	0.23
08	25.069	Acetic acid [4-(1-hydroxy-1-methylethyl)]	$C_{31}H_{32}O_6$	500.6	0.25
09	26.455	Methyl dodecanoate	$C_{13}H_{26}O_2$	214.34	0.42
10	26.696	4,4,7a-Trimethyl-6,7-dihidro-5H-1-benzofuran-2-one	$C_{11}H_{16}O_2$	180.24	0.44
11	28.186	Ethyl dodecanoate	$C_{14}H_{28}O_2$	228.37	0.22
12	28.309	Heneicosane	$C_{21}H_{44}$	296.6	0.32
13	28.474	2-(Hydroxymethyl)-5-(2-hydroxypropan-2-yl)cyclohex-2-en-2-one	$C_{10}H_{16}O_3$	184.23	0.41
14	28.635	(2S,3S,4S,5S,6S)-2-Ethoxy-6-(hydroxymethyl)oxane-3,4,5-triol	$C_8H_{16}O_6$	208.21	0.56
15	30.657	(Unidentified)	$C_{21}H_{44}$	296.6	0.28
16	31.611	(Unidentified)	$C_{14}H_{22}O_3$	238.32	0.26
17	31.987	Tetradecanoic acid	$C_{14}H_{28}O_2$	228.37	0.35
18	32.251	[(*E*)-2-(2,2,6-Trimethyl-7-oxabicyclo[4.1.0]heptans-1-il)prop-1-enyl] acetate	$C_{14}H_{22}O_3$	238.32	0.75
19	32.734	(Unidentified)	-	-	0.59
20	32.885	Octadecane	$C_{18}H_{38}$	254.5	0.28
21	33.746	Phytol acetate	$C_{22}H_{42}O_2$	338.6	1.39
22	33.873	6,10,14-Trimethylpentadecan-2-one	$C_{18}H_{36}O$	268.5	0.72
23	34.275	(Unidentified)	$C_{22}H_{42}O_2$	338.6	0.33
24	34.407	Bis(2-methylpropyl) benzene-1,2-dicarboxylate	$C_{16}H_{22}O_4$	278.34	0.26
25	34.652	(*E*)-3,7,11,15-Tetramethylhexadec-2-en-1-ol	$C_{20}H_{40}O$	296.5	0.51
26	35.009	Eicosane	$C_{20}H_{42}$	282.5	0.22
27	35.159	2-Methyl-4-[(*E*)-oct-2-en-2-yl]-2H-furan-5-ane	$C_{13}H_{20}O_2$	208.3	0.16
28	35.554	Methyl hexadecanoate	$C_{17}H_{34}O_2$	270.5	0.75
29	36.283	L-(+)-Ascorbic acid-2,6-dihexadecanoate	$C_{38}H_{68}O_8$	652.9	6.65

30	36.520	(Unidentified)	$C_{18}H_{34}O_2$	282.5	0.16
31	36.807	(E)-Ethylhexadec-9-enoate	$C_{18}H_{34}O_2$	282.5	0.66
32	36.934	Ethyl hexadecanoate	$C_{18}H_{36}O_2$	284.5	10.56
33	37.032	(Unidentified)	$C_{20}H_{42}$	282.5	0.22
34	38.203	Heptadecanoic acid	$C_{17}H_{34}O_2$	270.5	0.20
35	38.894	Methyl (9Z, 12Z)-octadeca-9,12-dienoate	$C_{19}H_{34}O_2$	294.5	1.65
36	39.012	(E)-Octadec-9-methyl acetate	$C_{19}H_{36}O_2$	296.5	1.22
37	39.258	Phytol	$C_{20}H_{40}O$	296.5	18.72
38	39.490	Methyl octadecanoate	$C_{19}H_{38}O_2$	298.5	0.44
39	39.605	(Unidentified)	$C_{18}H_{32}O_2$	280.4	2.15
40	39.724	(Unidentified)	$C_{15}H_{24}O_2Cl_2$	310.5	3.67
41	40.002	(Unidentified)	$C_{22}H_{42}O_2$	338.6	0.36
42	40.154	Linoleic acid	$C_{18}H_{32}O_2$	280.4	11.12
43	40.278	2,2-Dichloroacetate tridec-2-inyl	$C_{15}H_{24}O_2Cl_2$	310.5	9.10
44	40.375	Ethyl (Z)-octadec-9-enoate	$C_{20}H_{38}O_2$	310.5	0.33
45	40.736	Ethyl octadecanoate	$C_{20}H_{40}O_2$	312.5	9.36
46	41.912	(E)-Pentatriacont-17-ene	$C_{35}H_{70}$	490.9	0.32
47	42.031	Tributyl 2-acetyloxypropane-1,2,3-tricarboxylate	$C_{20}H_{34}O_8$	402.5	0.19
48	43.595	5-Methyl-5-(4,8,12-trimethyltridecyl)oxolan-2-one	$C_{21}H_{40}O_2$	324.5	0.48
49	44.220	Ethyl (9Z, 12Z, 15Z)-octadeca-9,12,15-trienoate	$C_{20}H_{34}O_2$	306.5	1.01
50	44.317	Bis(2-ethylhexyl) hexanedioate	$C_{22}H_{42}O_4$	370.6	0.31
51	44.910	Shiobuano	$C_{15}H_{24}O$	220.35	0.13
52	45.090	isoamyl laurate	$C_{17}H_{34}O_2$	270.5	0.16
53	45.333	Gamma-sitosterol	$C_{29}H_{52}O_2$	432.7	0.56
54	46.185	1,3-Dihydroxypropan-2-yl hexadecanoate	$C_{19}H_{38}O_4$	330.5	0.33
55	47.013	Bis(2-ethylhexyl) benzene-1,2-dicarboxylate	$C_{24}H_{38}O_4$	390.6	0.88
56	50.155	2,3-Dihydroxypropyl (9Z, 12Z)octadeca-9,12-dienoate	$C_{21}H_{38}O_4$	354.5	0.11
57	50.252	2,3-Dihydroxypropyl (Z)-octadec-9-enoate	$C_{21}H_{40}O_4$	356.5	0.20
58	51.859	Bbis(2-ethylhexyl) benzene-1,3-dicarboxylate	$C_{24}H_{38}O_4$	390.6	1.12
59	54.644	Scalene	$C_{30}H_{50}$	410.7	1.79
60	55.640	Unidentified	$C_{27}H_{44}O_2$	400.6	0.32
61	56.490	Unidentified	$C_{27}H_{44}O_2$	400.6	0.31
62	70.761	Vitamin E	$C_{29}H_{50}O_2$	430.7	1.26

of great abundance in nature (Mendonça, 2020). It has already been identified in the essential oil of the leaves and flowers (Italy) of *S. verbenaca* (Khouchlaa et al., 2022), *Cleome serrata*, *Lantana radula*, aquatic alga *Hydrilla verticillata* (Mendonça, 2020), *C. difformis*, *C. odoratus*, and *C. alternifolius* (Al-mayyahi & Sosa, 2022). The pharmacological activities associated with phytol are antimicrobial, antiviral, cytotoxic in MCF-7 breast tumor and HeLa cervical cancer cell lines, antitumor, antiteratogenic, anti-inflammatory, antidiabetic and antioxidant (Mendonça, 2020).

Linoleic acid (42) has already been found in the oil and essential oil extract of the seeds of *S. verbenaca* (Tunisia) (Khouchlaa et al., 2022), crude methanolic extract of the stem barks of *Fagraea fragans*, and liquid oily chloroform extract of seeds of *J. regia* and is used in the treatment of reducing acute inflammatory pain, chronic blood glucose levels, elevating serum insulin and normalizing glycated hemoglobin levels (Pillai & Young, 2022). The fatty acids and esters have exhibited pharmacological activities, such as antioxidant and antifungal activities (Pillai & Young, 2022).

Tridec-2-inyl 2,2-dichloroacetate (43) is poorly reported in the literature, but has been described for *C. difformis* and *C. odoratus* species (Al-mayyahi & Sosa, 2022), *Hypha enethebaica* L. (Adekoyeni et al., 2019), and *Eclipta prostrata* (Zubair et al., 2017). Dichloroacetic acids are commonly used in peel treatments and tattoo removal and show activity against brain cancer cells (Roy et al., 2019). Ethyl octadecanoate (45) is described as a major component of the essential oil from *Z. spina-christi* leaves (Asgarpanah & Haghighat, 2012). It is also identified in the essential oil of the aerial parts of *Koelreuteria paniculata* Laxm (Andonova et al., 2020) and the ethanolic extract of *Elephantopus scaber* Linn. (Hiradeve & Rangari, 2014).

13.3.3 ADMET Prediction Analysis of Compounds Identified in the Ethanolic Extract

The molecule-plasma protein interaction is very important from pharmacokinetic, toxicological, and pharmacological point of view, as plasma protein binding (PPB) relates to drug distribution, half-life, and clearance (Ciura et al., 2021). PPB determines the fraction of drug available in free form to be distributed to various tissues, and human plasma contains 70% human serum albumin protein, acid alpha-l-glycoprotein, and lipoprotein as the major components (Megantara et al., 2018). All compounds showed PPB values above 90%, and with this it can be shown that these molecules have considerably strong interactions which influences their action and their efficacy. These and other predictions are shown in Table 13.3.

The blood-brain barrier (BBB) is a complex and highly selective structure located in blood vessels that supplies the brain and acts as a boundary protecting the central nervous system from toxins, pathogens, and other harmful molecules that can impair brain homeostasis. Upon crossing the BBB, metabolites with appropriate physicochemical properties can cause various damages in the brain (Carecho et al., 2020; Rashid et al., 2022). The bioactive compounds 32, 37, 42, 43, and 45 showed BBB potential value above >2.0, indicating that these have the possibility to freely cross the BBB (Bastos et al., 2020; Ma et al., 2005).

It is also important to assess skin permeability, an indispensable parameter when talking about transdermal administration of drugs and used in the pharmaceutical

TABLE 13.3
ADMET Predictions of Bioactive Compounds Identified in the Ethanolic Extract (CPF)

ADMET	32	37	42	43	45
Plasma protein binding (PPB) (%)	100	100	100	100	100
Penetration at the blood-brain barrier (BBB)	14.69	19.08	7.31	13.34	16.33
Skin permeability (logKp, cm/hour)	−0.57	−0.52	−0.54	−0.65	−0.53
Human intestinal absorption (HIA, %)	100	100	98.37	100	100
Permeability in cells CaCo-2 (nm/sec)	56.86	37.63	28.08	49.38	57.11
P-glycoprotein inhibition P	Inhibition	Inhibition	Inhibition	Inhibition	Inhibition
Solubility in water (mg/L)	5.83	1.45	645.76	4.75	1.55
Solubility in pure water (mg/L)	0.51	0.074	2.65	0.65	0.094
Ames test	Non-mutation	Non-mutation	Mutation	Non-mutation	Non-mutation
Ames TA100 (+S9)	Negative	Negative	Negative	Negative	Negative
Ames TA100 (-S9)	Negative	Negative	Negative	Negative	Negative
Ames TA1535 (+S9)	Negative	Negative	Negative	Negative	Negative
Ames TA1535 (-S9)	Negative	Negative	Negative	Negative	Negative
Carcinogenicity in mice	Positive	Positive	Positive	Positive	Positive
Carcinogenicity in rats	Negative	Negative	Positive	Negative	Negative
CYP2C19* inhibition	Inhibition	Inhibition	Inhibition	Inhibition	Inhibition
CYP2C9* inhibition	Inhibition	Inhibition	Inhibition	Inhibition	Inhibition
CYP2D6* inhibition	No	No	No	No	No
CYP2D6** inhibition	No	No	No	No	No
CYP3A4* inhibition	Inhibition	Inhibition	Inhibition	Inhibition	Inhibition
CYP3A4** inhibition	Weak	Substrate	No	Weak	Weak
Rule of Lipinski	Suitable	Suitable	Suitable	Suitable	Suitable

32. ethyl hexadecanoate, 37. phytol, 42. linoleic acid, 43. tridec-2-inyl 2,2-dichloroacetate, 45. ethyl octadecanoate; *Inhibitor; **Substrate.

industry to assess the danger of products when they come into contact with the skin (Mohan & Kirti, 2012; Nunes et al., 2020). It is related to the drug/skin interaction resulting in an increase or decrease in the penetration rate of the drug and can also interfere with the absorption of another therapeutic agent applied concomitantly (Mohan & Kirti, 2012; Nunes et al., 2020). The skin permeability rate predicted for the molecules were −0.57 (32), −0.52 (37), −0.54 (42), −0.65 (43), and −0.53 (45). Analyzing these values with the literature—Bastos et al. (2020) (<0.1 high permeability and >0.1 low permeability)—it is considered that these bioactive compounds are able to exert a high permeability in the skin, since they presented values below 0.1.

Human intestinal absorption (HIA) is related to the sum of bioavailability and absorption is assessed from the ratio of cumulative excretion or excretion in urine, bile, and feces (Megantara et al., 2018). This is important in the design, optimization, and selection of drug candidates due to its relationship to the absorption of orally administered drugs (Megantara et al., 2018). Analyzing the percentages predicted for this parameter, we see that all compounds showed a high percentage of intestinal absorption (value greater than 70%) (Bastos et al., 2020).

Caco-2 cells are derived from human colon adenocarcinoma and are involved in the drug transport cycle through epithelial cells of the small intestine, and in *vitro* models are reliable to predict oral absorption of drugs (pharmaceuticals, phytochemicals) (Megantara et al., 2018). The preADMET performs computational simulations (*in silico*) that also express the permeability coefficient in Caco-2. Among the analyzed compounds, all showed intermediate permeability—values between 4 and 70 nm/sec (Bastos et al., 2020; Yamashita et al., 2000).

Another parameter of drug absorption, distribution, and excretion that we may study is the inhibition of P-glycoprotein (PgP), which can be found in the cells of the small intestine, BBB, hepatocytes, and near the tubule of the kidney (Nunes et al., 2020). To perform the identification of molecules that interact with PgP requires very complex *in vitro* and *in vivo* studies, but using *in silico* predictions of PgP substrates can facilitate the identification and elimination of candidate phytopharmaceutical molecules (Khan et al., 2018). All substances can cause inhibition of P-glycoprotein, and thus may cause intracellular bioaccumulation of their substrates (Azeredo et al., 2009). The water solubility of each bioactive compound was evaluated, providing the values of 5.83, 1.45, 645.76, 4.75, and 1.55 mg/L for 32, 37, 42, 43, and 45, respectively. The predicted solubility in pure water for each molecule was 0.51 (32), 0.074 (37), 2.65 (42), 0.65 (43), and 0.094 mg/L (45).

Moving on to the toxicological analysis of the compounds, the mutagenicity test is the Ames test that uses *Salmonella typhimurium* strains in an *in vitro* model based on the exposure of mammalian cells to the compound under study and the observation of the nucleotide sequence in genes, number, and structure of chromosomes (Santana et al., 2020). The *in silico* predictions for the Ames test suggest the possibility of mutations carried out by substance 42 that was identified in the ethanolic extract (CPF). As for the Ames tests in specific lineages TA100 and TA1535 (-S9 and +S9), molecules 32, 37, 43, and 45 may not cause mutations, and substance 42 may cause mutation in TA1535 (-S9). Mendonça et al. (2016), in his work with the aqueous extract of *C. pachystachya*, reported that this does not show mutagenic action in tests with TA100 and TA1535, whether the metabolic activation (S9) is present or not. The crude extract and triterpene-enriched fractions from *C. pachystachya* leaves can develop a cytotoxic effect on the human prostate cancer PC3 cell line (Rosa et al., 2020).

The carcinogenicity in mice described by the ADMET software prescribes that all molecules can develop carcinogenic activity, and the carcinogenicity in rats can be caused by molecule 42. In the literature, there are reports that *C. pachystachya* extracts have a genotoxic effect (Pereira et al., 2020). Conjugated linoleic acid has been shown to be beneficial for health by decreasing oxidative stress values, micronucleus frequencies, and megakaryocytic emperipolesis and with effects on the proportion of polychromatic erythrocytes in bone marrow in a model of oxidative stress caused by oral administration of acreloin (Aydın et al., 2018). With this, this work highlighted the ability of this acid to exhibit antioxidant activity and prevent genetic damage (Aydın et al., 2018).

Cytochrome P450 plays a key role in the phase I metabolic cycle, and these are the strongest oxidizing agents known in living things (Choi et al., 2009). The isoenzymes of the CYP450 family are particularly prone to passible competitive inhibition due to their broad substrate specificity (Choi et al., 2009). Such inhibition can result in undesirable consequences: (1) increased toxicity caused by decreased rate of drug metabolism, (2) decreased formation of reactive prodrug metabolites, and (3) dual-drug interactions, which lead to decreased clearance of one of the drugs when two or more drugs are administered simultaneously (Choi et al., 2009). From *in silico* tests with CYP450 isoenzymes, all inhibit CYP2C19* and CYP3A4*; all molecules cause inhibition to CYP2C9*; none of them cause inhibition to CYP2D6 (* and **); compounds 32, 43, and 45 act weakly with CYP3A4**; and molecule 37 acts as a substrate in CYP3A4**. Nunes et al. (2020) describes that inhibition of the enzymes CYP2C19 and CYP2C9 tend to increase plasma concentrations and may cause adverse effects, CYP2D6 is responsible for the metabolism of many drugs and toxic chemicals, and the cytochrome CYP3A4 is an enzyme responsible for the oxidation of small organic molecules (xenobiotics).

The last parameter analyzed was the similarity of the compounds to drugs, which used the Lipinski rule (also known as the rule of five) and its guiding principles for such classification of oral drug availability. The rule of fives is based on the following principles: (1) molecular weight below 500 w.m.a.; (2) estimated octanol/water partition coefficient (log P) less than 5; (3) the number of hydrogen donors less than 5; and (4) the number of acceptors less than 10 (Fisli et al., 2021; Pollastri, 2010). All compounds follow the four criteria of the rule of five, which allows us to classify the molecules as drug-like, i.e., they have molecular weight less than 500 w.m.a., log P value less than 5, hydrogen donors value less than 5, and hydrogen receptors value less than 10.

13.3.4 Molecular Docking Analysis of Complexes Formed with the Compounds Identified in the Ethanolic Extract

The results of the *in silico* study performed with the enzyme 5-LOX are shown in Table 13.4. Among the complexes performed with this enzyme, 5-LOX/linoleic acid showed the best value of interaction energy, with −5.77 Kcal/mol and inhibition constant 59.03 μM, showing no hydrogen bridge bonds, but hydrophobic interactions with amino acid residues Phe177, Tyr181, Gln363, His367, Leu368, His372, Ile406, Ala410, Leu414, Leu420, Phe421, Ala424, Asn425, Trp599, Ala603, Leu607, and Ile673, as demonstrated in Figure 13.2A. In contrast, the 5-LOX/ethyl octadecanoate complex showed the highest energy value (−2.80 Kcal/mol) and the lowest inhibition constant value (8.88 μM), showing hydrogen bridge interaction with the amino acid Gln611 and hydrophobic interactions with the amino acid residues Phe169, Ser171, Gly174, Val175, Asn180, Lys183, Ala606, Gln609, Gln611, and Ile673.

The enzyme 5-LOX participates in the first step of the metabolic pathway of the leukotriene biosynthesis reaction as a catalyst. This reaction consists of the conversion of arachidonic acid into leukotrienes, which are metabolites involved in the inflammatory process (Delgado et al., 2021; Etienne et al., 2021). Gadnayak and

TABLE 13.4
Docking with the Enzyme 5-LOX (PDB: 3V92) and the Compounds Identified in the Ethanolic Extract (CPF)

Complex (Protein-Ligand)	ΔG_{bind}* (Kcal/mol)	Ki*	Number of Runs*	Number of Conformations*	Aminoacids that Interact by Hydrogen Bridges*	Aminoacids that Make Hydrophobic Interactions*
32 **5-LOX/ethyl hexadecanoate**	−3.74	1820 μM	100	33	Asn180	Phe169, Asp170, Ser171, Gly174, Val175, Asn180, Phe402, Ala606, Leu607, Gln609, Gln611, Ala672 e Ile673
37 **5-LOX/phytol**	−3.3	3790 μM	100	38	Lys161	Cys159, His160, Lys161, Glu172, Lys173, Asp176, Val178, Lys409, Glu412, Gln413, Cys418, Glu419 e Leu420
42 **5-LOX/linoleic acid**	−5.77	59.03 μM	100	32	-	Phe177, Tyr181, Gln363, His367, Leu368, His372, Ile406, Ala410, Leu414, Leu420, Phe421, Ala424, Asn425, Trp599, Ala603, Leu607 e Ile673
43 **5-LOX/tridec-2-inyl 2,2-dichloroacetate**	−4.6	426.03 μM	100	43	Gln611	Phe169, Asp170, Ser171, Val175, Asn180, Trp605, Ala606, Gln609, Gln611, Ala672 e Ile673
45 **5-LOX/ethyl octadecanoate**	−2.80	8.88 μM	100	37	Gln611	Phe169, Ser171, Gly174, Val175, Asn180, Lys183, Ala606, Gln609, Gln611 e Ile673

*Values shown are for the lowest and best value of ΔG_{bind} in each docking, ΔG_{bind}: Interaction energy, Ki: Inhibition constant.

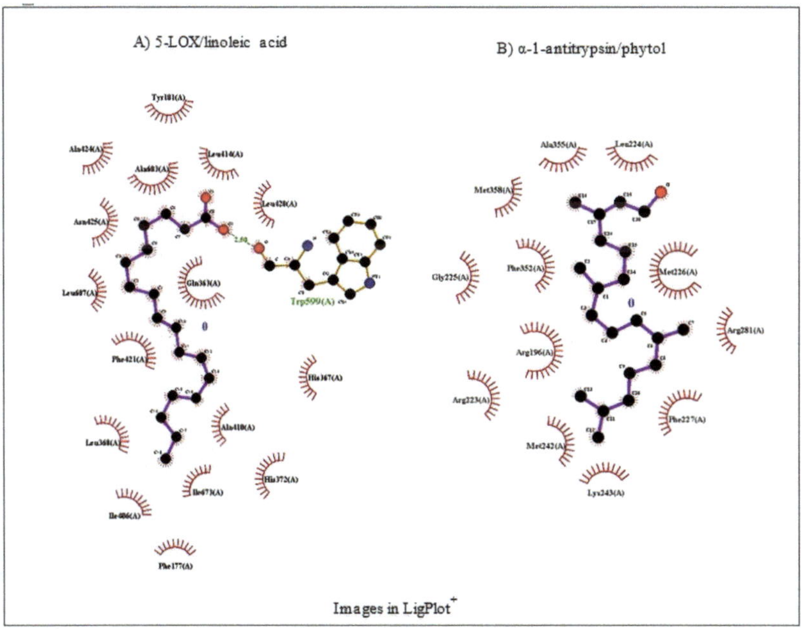

FIGURE 13.2 Complexes that performed best in molecular docking calculations with A) 5-LOX enzyme and B) α-1-antitrypsin. Imagens in LigPlot+ (www.ebi.ac.uk/thornton-srv/software/LIGPLOT/) (Wallace et al., 1996).

colleagues (2022) conducted a multicomposite study to select more potential 5-LOX inhibitors from the essential oil components of *Curcuma* species oil and to elucidate their mechanisms of action using computational biology approaches. The molecules α-turmerone, β-turmerone, α-terpineol, and dihydrocarveol showed the best binding affinity with 5-LOX (PDB: 308Y). By analyzing the energy of the catechin complex, identified in the ethyl extract of *C. pachystachya*, with 5-LOX, it showed a satisfactory result, and by showing interactions with amino acids close to the Phe177 residue, the molecule was effectively inserted in the active site of the enzyme. Drugs and phytochemicals isolated from plants that inhibit 5-LOX have gained prominence in the treatment of chronic respiratory diseases, as they will inhibit the generation of inflammatory mediators from the arachidonic acid pathway (Gadnayak et al., 2022).

Regarding the complexes performed with α-1-antitrypsin, presented in Table 13.5, the α-1-antitrypsin/phytol complex showed the best value of interaction energy (−4.84 Kcal/mol, constant 281.28 μM), without hydrogen bridging and hydrophobic interactions with amino acid residues (Table 13.5) as shown in Figure 13.2B. And the complex with ethyl octadecanoate also showed the highest value, −3.54 Kcal/mol, and the lowest inhibition constant value, 2.54 μM. Such a complex reported hydrophobic interactions with residues Arg223 and Met226 and hydrophobic interactions with some amino acid residues described in Table 13.5. The complexes with ethyl hexadecanoate and ethyl octadecanoate with both enzymes have already been

TABLE 13.5
Docking with the Enzyme α-1-Antitrypsin (PDB:1KCT) and the Compounds Identified in the Ethanolic Extract (CPF)

	Complex (Protein-Ligand)	ΔG_{bind}* (Kcal/mol)	Ki*	Number of Runs*	Number of Conformations*	Amino Acids that Interact by Hydrogen bridges*	Amino Acids that Make Hydrophobic Interactions*
32	**α-1-antitripsina/ ethyl hexadecanoate**	−4.00	1160 μM	100	27	Arg223, Agr223 e Met226	Arg196, Arg223, Leu224, Gly225, Met226, Arg281, Met351, Phe352, Glu354, Ala355 e Met358
37	**α-1-antitripsina/ phytol**	−4.84	281.28 μM	100	39	-	Arg196, Arg223, Leu224, Gly225, Met226, Phe227, Arg281, Met242, Lys243, Phe352 e Ala355
42	**α-1-antitripsina/ linoleic acid**	−4.28	723.17 μM	100	29	Arg223 e Met226	Arg223, Leu224, Gly225, Met226, Phe352, Ala355 e Met358
43	**α-1-antitripsina/ tridec-2-inyl 2,2-dichloroacetate**	−3.87	1460 μM	100	43	Arg223	Arg223, Leu224, Met226, Phe227, Arg281, Met351, Phe352, Glu354, Ala355 e Met358
45	**α-1-antitripsina/ ethyl octadecanoate**	−3.54	2.54 μM	100	39	Arg223 e Met226	Arg196, Arg223, Leu224, Gly225, Met226, Ser283, Phe352, Met358, Ser359 e Ile360

*Values shown are for the lowest and best value of ΔG_{bind} in each docking, ΔG_{bind}: Interaction energy, Ki: Inhibition constant.

studied in previous work by Mourão et al. (2022) and showed similar results to those found in this work.

The enzyme α-1-antitrypsin is an important protease inhibitor of the human body and belongs to the family of serpins; its deficiency is one of the pathological factors of COPD that generates an imbalance between neutrophil elastase and antielastase activity, thus triggering the progressive and irreversible destruction of lung tissue (Luna et al., 2020; Song et al., 1995). The presence of interaction with residues near the amino acids Met358 and Ser359 are indicative that the bioactive compounds used as ligands were in the reactive site of the enzyme. Therefore, it is possible that the extract of *C. pachystachya* leaves may be able to develop antioxidant and anti-inflammatory biological activities, as well as being a candidate for alternative treatment for chronic respiratory diseases, associating such pharmacological properties to the various compounds identified in this extract. The importance of conducting experimental tests in a model of COPD treatment with this extract, and consequently with its bioactive compounds, is emphasized in order to reaffirm the good results obtained in this work.

13.3.5 Future Perspectives

The results presented in this work suggest that *C. pachystachya* can be used in the treatment of chronic respiratory diseases, but in order to make this statement true, we have for future perspectives the realization of more studies using *in vivo* test models of COPD and treatment with ethanolic extract of *C. pachystachya* leaves, as well as *in vivo* tests with compounds isolated from this plant.

13.4 CONCLUSION

C. pachystachya is a plant known throughout Brazil, which presents a very broad and diverse chemical composition of compounds, which gives them the ability to perform various biological activities. In this work, 62 compounds were identified by GC-MS, with 5 having the highest percentage of area: ethyl hexadecanoate, phytol, linoleic acid, tridec-2-inyl 2,2-dichloroacetate, and ethyl octadecanoate.

ADMET predictions were determined for each compound, and they show pharmacokinetic properties with favorable results and can be classified as a drug according to Lipinski's criteria. Molecular docking calculations were also performed for each of the bioactive substances, and the compounds linoleic acid and phytol showed better interactions with the enzymes 5-LOX and α-1-antitrypsin, respectively. With this, we have results of great scientific importance in terms of the composition and pharmacological properties of the embaúba, and further studies (*in vivo* and *in vitro*) are necessary to better understand the mechanism of action in relation to the treatment of chronic respiratory diseases.

13.5 ACKNOWLEDGMENTS

Thanks to FAPEPI-Brazil (Fundação de Amparo à Pesquisa do Piauí—Brazil) and to the Natural Products Laboratories of Instituto Federal de Alagoas (IFAL), Universidade Federal do Piauí (UFPI), Instituto Federal do Piauí (IFPI—Campus Teresina Central) and the Computational Quantum Chemistry and Drug Planning Research Group (GPQQCPF).

13.6 DISCLOSURE STATEMENT

The authors declare that there is no conflict of interest.

13.7 FINANCING

This work was supported by Fundação de Amparo à Pesquisa do Piauí—Brazil.

ORCID

Penina S. Mourão https://orcid.org/0000-0001-7504-7258
Rafael de O. Gomes https://orcid.org/0000-0003-4774-9839
Clara A. C. B. Costa https://orcid.org/0000-0002-6474-221X
Orlando F. da S. Moura https://orcid.org/0000-0002-1055-8564
Johnnatan D. de Freitas http://orcid.org/0000-0002-6977-3322
Francisco das C. A. Lima https://orcid.org/0000-0002-0447-4911
Wellington dos. S. Alves https://orcid.org/0000-0003-1114-773X
Valdiléia T. Uchôa https://orcid.org/0000-0001-8080-6335

REFERENCES

Abarca-Vargas, R., and V. L. Petricevich. 2018. *Bougainvillea* genus: A review on phytochemistry, pharmacology, and toxicology. *Evidence-Based Complementary and Alternative Medicine*, 9070927, 1–17. https://doi.org/10.1155/2018/9070927

Adekoyeni, O. O., A. F. Adegoke, and F. F. Ajayi. 2019. GC-MN analysis and identification of pharmacological components of doum palm nuts. *Nigerian Journal of Scientific Research*, 18(5), 571–578.

Al-mayyahi, T. F., and A. A. Sosa. 2022. Chemical study of some species for *Cyperus* L. (Cyperaceae) in Diwaniyah river using Gas Chromatography—Mass spectrometry. *International Journal of Academic Management Science Research*, 6(3), 17–33.

Andonova, T., I. Dimitrova-Dyulgerova, I. Slavov, et al. 2020. A comparative study of *Koelreuteria paniculata* laxm. Aerial parts essential oil composition. *Journal of Essential Oil Bearing Plants*, 23(6), 1363–1370. http://doi.org/10.1080/0972060X.2020.1853610

Andrade, B. R. D., A. C. Silva, J. B. Souza, et al. 2021a. Avaliação do potencial antimicrobiano do extrato Etanólico de Folhas da *Cecropia pachysrachya* t. (Embaúba). *Research, Societ and Development*, 10(10), 1–7. http://doi.org/10.33448/rsd-v10i10.18679

Andrade, N. D., B. M. Almeida, R. M. S. Sousa, and M. S. Araújo. 2021b. Uso das plantas medicinais para fns terapêuticos por estudantes do Ensino médio. *Research, Societ and Development*, 10(4), 1–11. http://doi.org/10.33448/rsd-v10i4.14484

Asgarpanah, J., and E. Haghighat. 2012. Phytochemistry and pharmacologic properties of *Ziziphus spina christi* (L.) Willd. *African Journal of Pharmacy and Pharmacology*, 6(31), 2332–2339. http://doi.org/10.5897/AJPP12.509

Aydın, B., Z. A. Şekeroğlu, and V. Şekeroğlu. 2018. Acrolein-induced oxidative stress and genotoxicity in rats: Protective effects of whey protein and conjugated linoleic acid. *Drug and Chemical Toxicology*, 41(2), 225–231. https://doi.org/10.1080/01480545.2017.1354872

Azeredo, F. J., F. T. Uchôa, and T. D. Costa. 2009. P-glycoprotein role on drug pharmacokinetics and interactions. *Revista Brasileira de Farmacognosia*, 19, 321–326.

Bastos, K. Z. C., A. H. da S. Cortêz, T. H. C. Cortêz, et al. 2020. *In silico* analysis of the pharmacokinetic and toxicological profile of research drugs for the treatment of COVID-19. *Research, Society and Development*, 9, e529119450. https://doi.org/10.33448/rsd-v9i11.9450

Bezerra, M. de S. S., H. G. de Sousa, M. J. dos P. Santos, et al. 2021. Identification of bioactive compounds present in ethanol and hexanic extracts of *Moringa oleifera* Lam. *Revista Virtual de Química*, 13, 1303–1318. https://doi.org/10.21577/1984-6835.20210078

Bigliani, M. C., E. Grondona, P. M. Zunino, and A. A. Ponce. 2010. Effects of *Cecropia pachystachya* and *Larrea divaricata* aqueous extracts in mice. *Human and Experimental Toxicology*, 29(7), 601–606. http://doi.org/10.1177/0960327109358613

Carecho, R., D. Carregosa, and C. N. Santos. 2020. Low molecular weight (poly) phenol metabolites across the blood-brain barrier: The underexplored journey. *Brain Plasticity*, 6, 193–214. http://doi.org/10.3233/BPL-200099

Carvalho, G. F. S., L. K. Marques, H. G. Sousa, et al. 2020. Phytochemical study, molecular docking, genotoxicity and therapeutic efficacy of the aqueous extract of the stem bark of *Ximenia americana* L. in the treatment of experimental COPD in rats. *Journal of Ethnopharmacology*, 247, 112259. https://doi.org/10.1016/j.jep.2019.112259

Choi, I., S. Y. Kim, H. Kim, et al. 2009. Classification models for CYP450 3A4 inhibitors and non-inhibitors. *European Journal of Medicinal Chemistry*, 44, 2354–2360. http://doi.org/10.1016/j.ejmech.2008.08.013

Ciura, K., J. Fedorowicz, H. Kapica, et al. 2021. Interaction between antifungal isoxazolo[3,4-b] pyridin 3(1H)-one derivatives and human serum proteins analyzed with biomimetic chromatography and QSAR approach. *Processes*, 9(512). https://doi.org/10.3390/pr9030512

Coelho, A. C. B., B. F. Borges, E. C. C. Pinheiro, et al. 2021. Analysis of secondary metabolites of *mangifera indica* linneaus as na alternative treatment possibility for the post-covid-19 syndrome. *Brazilian Journal of Development*, 7(10), 95673–95692. http://doi.org/10.34117/bjdv7n10-65

Costa, J. C. and J. Hoscheid. 2018. Phytochemical profile and evaluation of antimicrobial activity of aqueous and ethanolic extracts from leaves of *Cecropia pachystachya*. *Revista Fitos*, 12, 175–185. https://doi.org/10.5935/2446-4775.20180016

D'Armas, H., V. Vásquez, S. Moreno, and G. Ordaz. 2021. Identification of some constituents of *Helicteres guazumifolia* Kunth (Malvaceae) leaves from Sucre state, Venezuela. *Journal of Pharmacognosy and Phytochemistry*, 10(2), 96–103. https://doi.org/10.22271/phyto

Delgado, Y. B., J. R. Vargas, I. M. González, and H. M. Quevedo. 2021. Evaluación *in silico* del efecto de compuestos fenólicos de *Pleurotus ostreatus* sobre la enzima 5-lipoxigenasa (5-LOX). *Rev Cubana Invest Bioméd*, 40, e678.

Dourado, V. Z., S. E. Tanni, S. A. Vale, et al. 2006. Systemic manifestations in chronic obstructive pulmonary disease. *Journal of Brazilian Pulmonology*, 32, 161–171. https://doi.org/10.1590/S1806-37132006000200012

Duque, A. P. do N., N. de C. C. Pinto, R. de F. Mendes, et al. 2016. *In vivo* wound healing activity of gels containing *Cecropia pachystachya* leaves. *Journal of Pharmacy and Pharmacology*, 68, 128–138. https://doi.org/10.1111/jphp.12496

Etienne, R., F. P. D. Viegas, and C. Viegas Jr. 2021. Pathophysiological aspects of inflammation and drug design: An updated overview. *Revista Virtual de Química*, 13, 167–191. https://doi.org/10.21577/1984-6835.20200138

Ferreira, S., R. G. Tavares, A. F. Raimundo, et al. 2021. *Cecropia pachystachya* protection against preproIAPP cytotoxicity is independent of Ca^{2+} homeostasis: lessons learned using a novel yeast model of preproIAPP-induced Ca^{2+} intracellular dysregulation. *Biomedical and Biopharmaceutical Research*, 18(2), 1–17. http://doi.org/10.19277/bbr.18.272

Fisli, H., A. Hennig, M. L. Chelaghmia, and M. Abdaoui. 2021. The relationship between solvatochromic properties and *in silico* ADME parameters of new chloroethylnitrosourea derivatives with potential anticancer activity and their b-Cyclodextrin complexes. *Spectrochimica Acta Part A: Molecular and Biomolecular Spectroscopy*, 253, 119579.

Gadnayak, A., B. Dehury, and A. Nayak. 2022. Mechanistic insights into 5-lipoxygenase inhibition by active principles derived from essential oils of *Curcuma* species: Molecular docking, ADMET analysis and molecular dynamic simulation study. *PLoS ONE*, 17(7), e0271956. https://doi.org/10.1371/journal.pone.0271956

Goodsell, D. S. 2005. Computational docking of biomolecular complexes with Auto-Dock, in: E. A. Golemis and P. D. Adams (Eds.), *Protein-Protein Interact. A Mol. Cloning Man*, Second Edition, Cold Spring Harbor Laboratory Press, New York.

Hiradeve, S. M. and V. D. Rangari. 2014. *Elephantopus scaber* Linn.: A review on its ethnomedical, phytochemical and pharmacological profile. *Journal of Applied Biomedicine*, 12, 49–61.

Khan, M. F., N. Nahar, R. B. Rashid, et al. 2018. Computational investigations of physicochemical, pharmacokinetic, toxicological properties and molecular docking of betulinic acid, a constituent of *Corypha taliera* (Roxb.) with Phospholipase A2 (PLA2). *BMC Complementary and Alternative Medicine*, 18(48). http://doi.org/10.1186/s12906-018-2116-x

Khouchlaa, A., A. Et-Touys, F. Lakhdar, et al. 2022. Ethnomedicinal use, phytochemistry, pharmacology, and toxicology of *Salvia verbenaca* L.: A review. *Biointerface Research in Applied Chemistry*, 12(2), 1437–1469. https://doi.org/10.33263/BRIAC122.14371469

Lima, E. C. S., M. B. S. Feijó, E. R. Santos, et al. 2016. Characterization of nutrients in the leaves and fruits of embaúba (*Cecropia Pachystachya*) trécul. *Journal of Regulatory Science*, 4, 29–37.

Luna, M. M., A. R. Granados, R. I. L. Pacheco, et al. 2020. Enfermedad pulmonar obstructiva crónica (EPOC). *Revista de la Facultad de Medicina UNAM*, 63, 28–35. https://doi.org/10.22201/fm.24484865e.2019.63.3.06

Ma, X. L., C. Chen, and J. Yang. 2005. Predictive model of blood-brain barrier penetration of organic compounds. *Acta Pharmacologica Sinica*, 26, 500–512. https://doi.org/10.1111/j.1745-7254.2005.00068.x.

Machado, C. D., L. M. Klider, C. A. S. Tirloni, et al. 2021. Ethnopharmacological investigations of the leaves of *Cecropia pachystachya* Trécul (Urticaceae): A native Brazilian tree species. *Journal of Ethnopharmacology*, 270, 113740. https://doi.org/10.1016/j.jep.2020.113740

Matos, F. J. A. 2009. *Introduction to Experimental Phytochemistry*. Edições UFC, Fortaleza.

Megantara, S., J. Levita, M. I. Iwo, and S. Ibrahim. 2018. Absorption, distribution and toxicity prediction of andrographolide and its derivatives as anti-HIV drugs. *Research Journal of Chemistry and Environment*, 22.

Mendonça, E. D., J. da Silva, M. S. dos Santos, et al. 2016. Genotoxic, mutagenic and antigenotoxic effects of *Cecropia pachystachya* Trécul aqueous extract using *in vivo* and *in vitro* assays. *Journal of Ethnopharmacology*, 193, 214–220. https://doi.org/10.1016/j.jep.2016.07.046

Mendonça, G. A. 2020. *O potencial terapêutico do fitol: uma revisão bibliográfica. 35 f. Monografia (Curso de Graduação em Farmácia)—Centro de Educação e Saúde/Universidade Federal de Campinas Grande—UFCG*, Cuité, PB, 2020.

Mohan, A. and N. Kirti. 2012. *In silico* molecular docking and ADME-toxicity studies on Berberine derivatives against NS3 protein of Zika vírus. *International Journal of Therapeutic Applications*, 8, 28–32.

Mourão, P. S., R. O. Gomes, C. A. C. B. Costa, et al. 2022. *Cecropia pachystachya* Trécul: identification, isolation of secondary metabolites, in silico study of toxicological evaluation and interaction with the enzymes 5-LOX and α-1-antitrypsin. *Journal of Toxicology and Environmental Health, Part A*, 85. https://doi.org/10.1080/15287394.2022.2095546

Mourão, P. S., V. T. Uchôa, W. dos S. Alves, et al. 2021. Medicinal plants used in the treatment of chronic respiratory diseases: period from 2010 to 2020. *Research, Society and Development*, 10, e29710817179. https://doi.org/10.33448/rsd-v10i8.17179

Nunes, A. M. V., F. das C. P. Andrade, L. A. Figueiras, et al. 2020. PreADMET analysis and clinical aspects of dogs treated with the Organotellurium compound RF07: A possible control for canine visceral leishmaniasis? *Environmental Toxicology and Pharmacology*, 80, 103470. https://doi.org/10.1016/j.etap.2020.103470

Pacheco, N. R., N. De C. C. Pinto, J. M. Da Silva, et al. 2014. *Cecropia pachystachya*: A species with expressive *in vivo* topical anti-inflammatory and *in vitro* antioxidant effects. *BioMed Research International*, Article ID 301294. https://doi.org/10.1155/2014/301294

Pedroso, R. S., G. Andrade, and R. H. Pires. 2021. Plantas medicinais: uma abordagem sobre o uso seguro e racional. *Physis: Revista de Saúde Coletica*, 31(2), 1–19. http://doi.org/10.1590/S0103-73312021310218

Pereira, E. D. de M., J. da Silva, P. da S. Carvalho, et al. 2020. *In vivo* and *in vitro* toxicological evaluations of aqueous extract from *Cecropia pachystachya* leaves. *Journal of Toxicology and Environmental Health, Part A*, 83, 659–671. https://doi.org/10.1080/15287394.2020.1811817

Pettersen, E. F., T. D. Goddard, C. C. Huang, et al. 2004. UCSF Chimera--a visualization system for exploratory research and analysis. *Computational Chemistry*, 1605–1612.

Pillai, M. K., and D. J. Young. 2022. Phytochemical characterization of extracts from *Fagraea Fragrans* and *Juglans Regia* by GC-MS analysis. *Fine Chemical Engineering*, 3, 107–120. https://doi.org/10.37256/fce.3120221334

Pollastri, M. P. 2010. Overview on the rule of five. *Current Protocols in Phamacology*, 49. http://doi.org/10.1002/0471141755.ph0912s49

PreADMET/Tox—Prediction of Absorption, Distribution, Metabolization, Excretion and Toxicity. 2022. Disponível em: https://preadmet.qsarhub.com/ Acesso em: 14 de março 2022.

Protein Data Bank (PDB). 2022. Disponível em: www.rcsb.org/ Acesso em: 22 de março 2022.

Rådmark, O. and B. Samuelsson. 2008. 5-Lipoxygenase: mechanisms of regulation. *Journal of Lipid Research*, 50, S40–S45. https://doi.org/10.1194/jlr.R800062-JLR200

Rashid, M., H. Rashid, S. Andleeb, and A. Ali. 2022. Evaluation of blood-brain-barrier permeability, neurotoxicity, and potential cognitive impairment by *Pseudomonas aeruginosa*'s virulence factor pyocyanin. *Oxidative Medicine and Cellular Longevity*, 3060579. https://doi.org/10.1155/2022/3060579

Rogério, L. V. F. and J. C. Ribeiro. 2021. Uso de plantas medicinais e medicamentos fitoterápicos em insônia: uma revisão bibliográfica. *Brazilian Journal of Health and Pharmacy*, 3(2), 35–44. https://doi.org/10.29327/226760.3.2-4

Rosa, H. H., P. Carvalho, C. F. Ortmann, et al. 2020. Cytotoxic effects of a triterpene-enriched fraction of *Cecropia pachystachya* on the human hormone-refractory prostate cancer PC3 cell line. *Biomedicine & Pharmacotherapy*, 130, 110551. https://doi.org/10.1016/j.biopha.2020.110551

Roy, S. J., P. S. Baruah, L. Lahkar, et al. 2019. Phytochemical analysis and antioxidant activities of *Homalomena aromatica* Schott. *Journal of Pharmacognosy and Phytochemistry*, 8(1), 1379–1385.

Sanner, M. F. 1999. Python: A programming language for software integration and development. *Journal of Molecular Graphics and Modelling*, 17, 57–61.

Santana, L. E. G. S., I. K. I. Miranda, and J. A. Sousa. 2020. *In silico* analysis of the pharmacokinetics, pharmacodynamics and toxicity of two compounds isolated from *Moringa oleífera. Research, Society and Development*, 9(11), e81991110469. http://doi.org/10.33448/rsd-v9i11.10469

Santos, L. H. 2021. Molecular docking: In search of the perfect and affordable fit. *BIOINFO—Rev Bras Bioinform.* https://doi.org/10.51780/978-6-599-275326-09

Schinella, G., S. Aquila, M. Dade, et al. 2008. Anti-inflammatory and apoptoic activities of pomolic acid isolated from *Cecropia pachystachya. Planta Medica*, 74, 215–220. https://doi.org/10.1055/s-2008-1034301

Sidhaye, V. K., K. Nishida, and F. J. Martinez. 2018. Precision medicine in COPD: Where are we and where do we need to go? *European Respiratory Review*, 27, 180022. https://doi.org/10.1183/16000617.0022-2018

Silva, L. R. C., M. B. M. Ribeiro, A. D. Oliveira, et al. 2019. Destilação solar do solvente etanol proveniente da extração de óleo de coco. *Brazilian Journal of Development, Curitiba*, 5(12), 28964–28982, ISSN 2525–8761. https://doi.org/10.34117/bjdv5n12-066

Song, H. K., K. N. Lee, K.-S. Kwon, et al. 1995. Crystal structure of an uncleaved al-antitrypsin reveals the conformation of its inhibitory reactive loop. *FEBS Letters*, 377, 150–154. https://doi.org/10.1016/0014-5793(95)01331-8

Uchôa, V. T., R. C. de Paula, L. G. Krettli, et al. 2010. Antimalarial activity of compounds and mixed fractions of *Cecropia pachystachya*. *Drug Development Research*, 71, 82–91. https://doi.org/10.1002/ddr.20351

Velázquez, E., H. A. Tournier, P. M. Buschiazzo, et al. 2003. Antioxidant activity of Paraguayan plant extracts. *Fitoterapia*, 74, 91–97. https://doi.org/10.1016/s0367-326x(02)00293-9

Wallace, A. C., R. A. Laskowski, and J. M. Thornton. 1996. LIGPLOT: A program to generate schematic diagrams of protein-ligand interactions. *Protein Engineering*, 8, 127–134. [PubMed id: 7630882]

Yamashita, S., T. Furubayashi, M. Kataoka, et al. 2000. Optimized conditions for prediction of intestinal drug permeability using Caco-2 cells. *European Journal of Pharmaceutical Sciences*, 10, 195–204.

Zubair, M. F., S. O. Ajibade, A. Z. Lawal, et al. 2017. GC-MS analysis, antioxidant and antimicrobial properties of *Eclipta prostrata* leaves. *International Journal of Chemical and Biochemical Sciences*, 11, 25–43.

14 Computational Biology Approach in Viticulture

Yogita Ranade,† and Pranav Deepek Pathak**
*MIT School of Bioengineering Science and Research,
MIT Art, Design and Technology University, Pune, India
†Corresponding Author: Yogita.ranade@mituniversity.edu.in

14.1 INTRODUCTION

Vitis vinifera is one of the most important plants in modern agriculture. The grapevine (*V. vinifera*) is a member of the Vitaceae family, which includes numerous species. Iran and the Black Sea were the first places where grapes were domesticated (Terral et al., 2010). Grapes are consumed as fresh fruit or used to produce wine across the world. There are several ways to propagate grapevine, including grafting, softwood cutting, and *in vitro* shoot apex culture. Annual grapevine growth is described by Eichorn-Lorenz (E-L) stages, which are characterized by crucial developmental phases (Coombe, 1992). Sugars, organic acids, antioxidants, minerals, pectic chemicals, and various aromatic compounds make up a significant group of chemical constituents in grapes. An invasion of many diseases and pests affects grape cultivation. Changes in the climate make it easier for several pathogens to infect grapes, which might result in the crop being completely destroyed. Abiotic stress such as drought, salinity, desertification, high temperature, and excessive rainfall affect the growth, quality, and production of grapes (George and Haynes, 2014). Fungicides are a key component in the management of diseases. However, many pathogens have shown resistance to the majority of them. As an alternative, various biological control agents that manage the diseases and are relatively less harmful to the environment are used. In the previous few decades, pesticide use has contributed to the increased production of both food and non-food commodities. There are indications that certain pesticides may be hazardous to both individuals and the environment.

Information technology and life science techniques are vital in agriculture and related industries. The use of various bioinformatics software has revolutionized data interpretation and interference, enriching scientific study (Pereira et al., 2020). Computational biology has the potential to be crucial in the elucidation of experimental data and the identification of several genes and pathways in plants that have yet to be fully understood. The omics cascade, which is used to characterize the profile of grapevines, includes the fields of genomics, transcriptomics, proteomics, and metabolomics. (Figure 14.1). Numerous research projects on grape genetics have been influenced by the grape genome. Many biological functions of grapes are focused on the genetics of grapes.

Transcriptome analysis, proteomics, gene expression and transcriptional profiling, and metagenomics approaches have particular value for grape improvement.

DOI: 10.1201/9781003354437-14

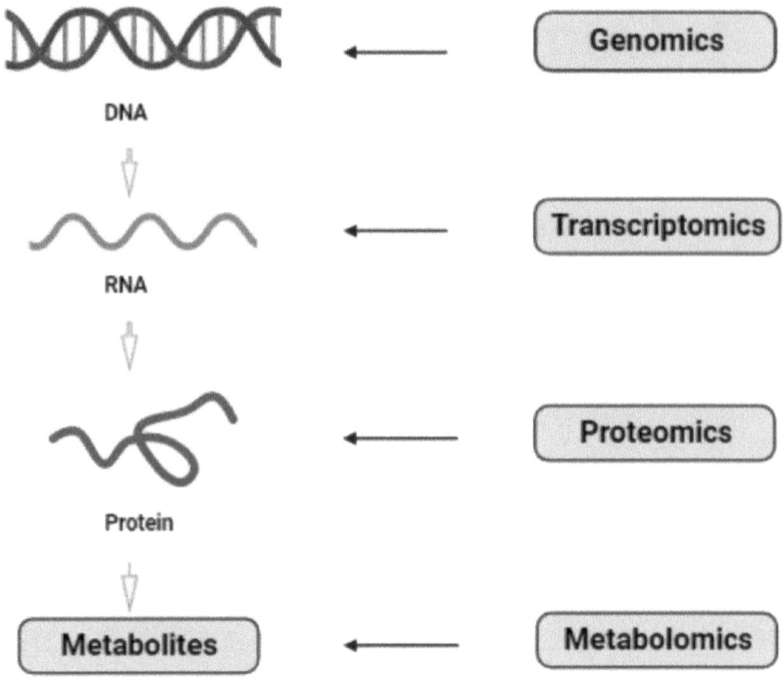

FIGURE 14.1 Illustration of omics cascade

14.2 GRAPEVINE

14.2.1 Physiology

The onset of seasonal growth and grape production is marked by bud burst, which is well recognized to be significantly influenced by temperature. In order to improve canopy management and crop forecasting, bud burst is essential since the timing and coordination of this event have a significant impact on flowering, fruit set, and ripening. The growth of the shoot starts during bud burst, when the leaves begin to alternate on the two sides of the shoot (Morgani et al., 2022). Typically, inflorescences start to form opposite a leaf at the third to sixth node from the shoot base. Self-pollination after cap fall results in the formation of seeds and fruits. Different stages of berry development mark grapevine development. Initially, the berry is pea size. The berry is hard and grows by cell division, and its size increases rapidly. This is followed by a lag phase during which the embryo grows quickly, and the size of the berry increases slowly. The berry growth resumes at veraison, and the fruit softens (Rogiers et al., 2017). Finally, at harvest, the berries are ready to be picked.

14.2.2 Chemical Composition

Sugars, organic acids, antioxidants, minerals, pectic chemicals, and various aromatic compounds make up a significant group of chemical constituents in grapes

(Batista-Silva et al., 2018; González-Barreiro et al., 2015). The concentration of sugar in grapes determines how delicious they are. Ripe grapes of various types exhibit variation in the ratio of glucose to fructose. Acidity is a key parameter for assessing the quality of grapes and is represented in terms of titratable acidity.

14.2.3 Disease and Pests

Grapevine is susceptible to different pests and diseases (Fand et al., 2020; Ranade et al., 2021; Salini and Yadav, 2011). The primary method of disease management is through the use of chemical and biological insecticides and pesticides. Overuse of chemical pesticides can lead to the development of resistance in pathogens. Downy mildew, powdery mildew, and anthracnose are the three grape diseases that are the most common. Mealybugs, thrips, wood borer, and mites are important insects affecting grapevines.

14.3 DEVELOPMENT OF COMPUTATIONAL BIOLOGY APPROACH IN VITICULTURE

Computational biology is a field that studies and models the structures and functioning of living organisms using computers and computer technology (Knüpfer et al., 2013). It involves applying computational techniques, such as algorithms, on an extremely large scale for describing and simulating biological systems and interpreting experimental data. Computational biology and bioinformatics are frequently used interchangeably. Examples of traditional bioinformatics data analysis include DNA sequencing, protein amino acid sequencing, protein three-dimensional structure, and nucleic acids complexes. Studies in grapevine using different omics approach is listed in Table 14.1.

14.3.1 Genomics

Genomics is a branch of "omics" science that deals with the study of complete genetic information of an organism. The application of genomics to agriculture and breeding programs could improve efforts to produce superior fruits, vegetables, and flowers with appealing phenotypes. Knowledge of the grape genome is necessary for the improvement of a cultivar of grapevine. Sanger sequencing has historically been used to decipher DNA sequencing results (Sanger et al., 1977). The French-Italian Public Consortium for Grapevine Genome Characterization completed the first *V. vinifera* genome sequencing in 2007. (Jaillon et al., 2007). Whole-genome resequencing has distinctly classified the variations between single-nucleotide variation (SNV) and insertion/deletion (InDel) (Tanaka et al., 2020). The sequencing of the whole genome and genotyping array is frequently used for the study of the grapevine genome (Myles et al., 2010). Utilizing Denovo MAGIC3, the whole genome sequence of a table grape derived from an interspecific hybrid revealed potential differences in structural and gene sequences when compared to other *Vitis* genera that could aid in the development of novel interspecific hybrid varieties in the future (Shirasawa et al., 2022). Grapes with a small market could be improved by utilizing multi-locus genome-wide association study (GWAS) analysis and whole-genome

TABLE 14.1
Omics Studies in Grapevine

Omics Approach	Study in Grapes	Reference
Transcriptomics	Berry development and ripening	(Campayo et al., 2021; Zhong et al., 2020; Ma and Yang, 2019)
	Growth of leaves, stem, and flowers	(Pucker et al., 2020; Vannozzi et al., 2021; Livigni et al., 2019; Royo et al., 2016)
	Adaptation to abiotic stress	(Campayo et al., 2021; Prinsi et al., 2020; Upadhyay et al., 2018; George and Haynes, 2014)
	Grapevine pathogen interaction	(Brasili et al., 2021; Zhang et al., 2019; Li et al., 2015)
	Agricultural practices	(Zenoni et al., 2020; Pastore et al., 2017)
Proteomics	Proteome dynamic during berry ripening	(Kambiranda et al., 2014)
	Proteome of skin, flesh and seed	(Tian et al., 2015)
	Vacuolar proteome profile	(Kuang et al., 2019)
	Proteomic expression during post-harvest withering of grapes	(Di Carli et al., 2011)
	Wine proteomic	(Albuquerque et al., 2023)
	Pathogen-related (PR) proteins	(Liu et al., 2021; Tian and Harrison, 2021)
	Effect of stress on the metabolite profile	(Reshef et al., 2018; Herrera et al., 2017; Pinasseau et al., 2017; Hochberg et al., 2015)
Metabolomics	Grape polyphenols	(Grant et al., 2021; Ruocco et al., 2017)
	Flavanols and flavanols profile	(Degu et al., 2015)
	Flavonoid profile	(VanderWeide et al., 2018)
	Emission of grape volatile metabolites	(Vrhovsek et al., 2014)
	Biomarkers in plant-pathogen interaction	(Adrian et al., 2017; Negrel et al., 2018; Negri et al., 2017)

sequencing. (Park et al., 2022). Phenotypic variations in grapes are directly related to their genomic variations. Sequencing of the DNA by the Illumina protocol depicted differences in wine grapes at the genetic level with variations related to geography and the environment (Magris et al., 2021). In comparison to other cultivars, recent genomic characterization of Japanese "Koshu" grapes demonstrated considerable heterogeneity on chromosome 7 (Tanaka et al., 2020). Utilizing numerous genomic studies connected to genome and marker-associated selection would aid in the improvement of wine cultivars. The interaction of numerous genes related to hormones, receptors, and transcription factors were used to explain the genetic regulation of the grape berry shape (Zhang et al., 2019). Grapevine is associated with a large microbial community. Different culturally dependent and culture-independent methods for isolation have been used to characterize the microbial populations of grapevine plant parts, including the leaves and berries. Technology advancements in high-throughput sequencing have fundamentally altered how transcriptomes' functional complexity can be investigated by enabling the sequencing of total cDNA (Zenoni et al., 2020). A culture-dependent method makes use of different culture media to isolate the microbes (Ranade et al., 2023). Culture-independent methods utilize several computational technologies, such as high-throughput DNA sequencing techniques (HTS).

14.3.2 Transcriptomics

When examining important physiological and metabolic functions of plants, the integration of different methods has recently become of the highest importance. In the context of crop and fruit enhancement, our knowledge of grapevine physiology has expanded through the research pointing to the transcriptome's expression or the abundance of grape metabolites that are already well-known. (Cramer et al., 2020). The E-L phenological scale is widely used by viticulturists to describe different growth stages of the vine. Different growth stages characterize grape berry development. However, different cultivars may have differences in the development of berries depending upon the type of cultivars and abiotic factors. Poni et al. (2019) explained the precise progression of berry growth and ripening in pinot noir and cabernet sauvignon varieties. They developed a transcriptomic model of berry development by performing RNA-seq analysis. The model clearly revealed that this strategy might effectively coordinate the growth stage of berries from the same cultivar sampled in several vintages and of various phonologies. Minio et al. (2019) studied the grape berry's development while comparing cabernet sauvignon's annotated gene space to other grape varieties. Their transcriptomic model built with Iso-Seq data showed that there were more than 1500 cultivar-specific genes. As the degradation process of chlorophyll and other macromolecules increases, there is an increase in the genes related to this process. Grape berry ripening is an important stage and is accompanied by several biochemical changes which result in changes in the cell wall's flexibility and enhance the organoleptic characteristic of berry and transcriptional increase in the gene expression (Brasili et al., 2021). These changes in the gene expression were related to gene ontology, chemical signaling, and metabolism during the late stages of ripening, particularly the gene involved in ethylene signaling pathway (Cramer et al., 2020; Cramer et al., 2014). According to the study, ethylene is more crucial than originally believed, particularly during the latter stages of ripening when taste is developed. The transcriptomic study has also revealed that the type of rootstock influences berry maturation. Zombardo et al. (2020) investigated the effect of different rootstocks on berry skin phenotype and gene expression. RNA- and miRNA-seq analyses showed that in the berries of the vines grafted on 1103 Paulsen rootstock, the transcriptional level increased at the end of berry maturation as compared to the transcriptome at veraison.

The majority of research on transcriptome analysis in grapes focuses on abiotic variables affecting grapevine. Environmental factors and climate change significantly affect vine growth phenology, berry development, composition, and yield. Water stress can affect the quality of berries and wines. The differential response of two table grapes, Italia and Autumn Royal varieties, under water deficiency, revealed that both the varieties had genes related to plant stress response (Catacchio et al., 2019). Italia differentially expressed more than 1500 genes than Autumn Royal varieties under stress conditions. The specific adaptation of each cultivar to the environment is what determines the observed responses to drought stress, which is strictly genotype-dependent. Removing the basal leaves allows more sunshine to reach the grape cluster, which reduces fruit rot and boosts quality. A transcriptomic analysis study indicated that after the basal leaves are removed, the exposure to sunshine upregulates the genes related to stress response to prevent grape injury (He et al., 2020). These types of results help the viticulturist to plan better cultivation strategies to get the desired yield. According to research by Lee et al. (2019), "Kyoho" grapevines are sensitive to high temperatures during the vegetative growing period and face a variety of physiological problems, which leads to decreased production and poor fruit quality. To better understand the process of grapevine temperature tolerance, it is important to identify the genes that are differently expressed in response to high temperatures (Pastore et al., 2017). Genes that are selectively expressed by high temperatures can be utilized as molecular markers to identify grape types that are heat tolerant and to understand better how fruit plants defend themselves against high temperatures. Recently, Wang et al. (2022) carried out a comprehensive transcriptome analysis of Crimson Seedless grapes infected with grapevine berry inner necrosis virus (GINV). The study revealed that the GINV infection was a complicated process involving 1700 differently expressed genes (DEGs), with 846 upregulated and 854 downregulated genes. Zhang et al. (2019) studied the transcriptome profile of grapevine infected with *Lasiodiplodia theobromae*. It was possible to comprehend the plant response to pathogens in terms of their molecular interaction by identifying differentially expressed genes.

14.3.3 Proteomics

Proteomic analysis methods are developing continuously, and high-throughput analysis has been made possible by improvements in mass spectrometry equipment, sample preparation methods, and bioinformatics tools. In grapevine, proteomic responses have been investigated in grape berries, shoots, cell culture, and roots using techniques such as iTRAQ and TMT and label-free quantitation methods (George and Haynes, 2014). Proteomics analysis using mass spectrometry (MS), liquid chromatography coupled to electrospray ionization (LC-ESI-MS), matrix-assisted laser desorption ionization (MALDI)/time of flight (TOF), and high resolution (HR)-MS have all made progress in the identification of proteins with high sensitivity, accuracy, resolution, and speed of analysis (Hines et al., 2015). The world's highest level of grape production is used to make wine. Environmental factors such as soil, weather, and abiotic stress significantly impact wine's proteome. Silvaner wine's proteome was profiled to identify proteins involved in metabolism, signaling, defence, and structure that would aid in characterizing the wine proteome for potential future applications (Albuquerque et al., 2023). Different strains of *Brettanomyces bruxellensis* collected from wineries in Croatian winegrowing regions were analyzed using proteomic analysis, and it was discovered that they contained proteins that could be used as biomarkers, as well as those that were involved in nitrogen metabolism, protein synthesis, ubiquitin conjugation pathway, and carbohydrate metabolism (Križanović et al., 2019). Such proteomic fingerprinting would help identify a particular microbial strain and understand its capacities to cause wine spoilage. Tian and Harrison (2021), detected pathogenesis-related (PR) protein in white wine using nano-high performance liquid chromatography (HPLC)/tandem mass spectrometry. Protein research revealed the need for a different strategy to eliminate these PR proteins. Recently, Liu et al. (2021), studied the incompatible and compatible interactions at an early stage of *Plasmopara viticola* infection in grapevine using iTRAQ technique. This would make it easier to comprehend the molecular chain of events resulting in *P. viticola* resistance in grapes as well as develop control methods. Grapevine response to abiotic stress like draught (Azri et al., 2022), salt (Prinsi et al., 2020), temperature (Liu et al., 2021), and herbicides (Castro et al., 2005) has been investigated using the proteomic analysis technique. The ripening process makes significant changes in the grape berry proteome. Kambiranda et al. (2014) analyzed the berry proteome of the muscadine grape during ripening using the iTRAQ-Based Quantitative Proteomics approach. Their study discovered antimicrobial proteins which may offer protection as the fruit ripens. Plant cell cultures offer an alluring substitute for whole plants for several physiological and biochemical studies (Kuang et al., 2019; Sharathchandra et al., 2011). The dynamics of berry development and ripening were studied using the proteomic technique, which revealed proteins from berries that were expressed differently and exhibited the same patterns as ripening berries on vines. Additionally, the cultures discovered proteins with a lower abundance that had not previously been found in berries. Chitosan is a polysaccharide that is of importance in agriculture. Proteomic and metabolic analysis revealed that enhancement of phenylpropanoid and mevalonate pathways by chitosan spray treatment at the cluster level would allow researchers to understand better how the vine responds to diseases. (Bavaresco et al., 2017).

14.3.4 Metabolomics

Metabolomics is a commonly used experimental tool to study the metabolic complement of the cell. Vineyards and grapevines are the sources of valuable bioactive compounds. The complexity of the matrix is a well-known obstacle in the study of wine. Analyses are complicated because there are hundreds of different chemical families of various substances (Josep et al., 2021). Assorted grape metabolites with similar physical and chemical properties are studied using various analytical techniques. To differentiate wines based on their origins in different regions and vine varieties, various wine metabolites can be utilized as a fingerprint. Mass spectroscopy and NMR are two important tools for analyzing wine metabolomics (Son et al., 2009). Le Mao et al. (2021) recently used 1H-NMR metabolomics and multivariate analysis to investigate wine metabolites and their impact on wine production and quality. Variation in wine metabolites from different regions and varieties has been studied previously using ultra-high-pressure liquid chromatography (UHPLC)/quadrupole time of flight mass spectrometry (QTOF MS) and SPME-GC-MS/MS for metabolomics analysis (Tzachristas et al., 2021; Awale et al., 2021; Raúl et al., 2019; Bokulich et al., 2016). Their investigations showed that depending on the rootstock, cultivar, and region, there are differences in the wine's microbial terroir, wine aroma, and metabolic component. Metabolomics investigations were carried out to compare the primary metabolites of leaves and fruits, with and without stress (Garrido et al., 2021; Maoz et al., 2019). Other studies have focused on the plasticity of berries (Anesi et al., 2015), the identification of biomarkers (Ciubotaru et al., 2021), and the susceptibility of vines to pathogens (Brasili et al., 2021).

14.4 FUTURE SCOPE AND LIMITATIONS

The improvement of crops and fruits through knowledge of grapevine physiology has been increased by thorough research pointing to the transcriptome's expression or the abundance of the already-known grape metabolites. Most molecular and omics research is focused on wine grapes, but table grape berries eaten as fresh fruit differ from wine grapes in many ways. A significant amount of research must also be done on table grapes. Only some studies have examined the early inflorescence and berry setting, while studies using the computational approach emphasize the late berry development. During early stages, the berries are more metabolically active, necessitating the need for a transcriptomic or metabolomics study. All omics studies must now have access to raw data supported by a large collection of metadata. It is crucial to share data at many levels in order to increase reproducibility and transparency.

14.5 CONCLUSION

The practice of growing grapes has a long history. Earlier, the lack of understanding of the mechanisms involved in plant development and breeding was a disadvantage. However, the cultivation of grapevines has greatly improved because of inventions and applications of new molecular techniques. The introduction of new omics techniques brought about a new revolution in grape farming. The study of grapes using genomes, proteomics, transcriptomics, and metabolomics provided a new avenue for grapevine development. It was possible to study the gene and gene expression of grapes with respect to location, cultivar, rootstock, biotic and abiotic stress, and associated microbiome. These investigations helped us learn more about the grape genome and develop crucial strategies for vine improvement. With the use of an omics approach, the future of grape development seems promising. An integrative study that goes beyond single omics methods is required in the modern age of molecular systems biology.

REFERENCES

Adrian, M., Lucio, M., Roullier-Gall, C., Heloir, M.C., Trouvelot, S., Daire, X., Kanawati, B., Lemaitre-Guillier, C., Poinssot, B., Gougeon, R., Schmitt-Kopplin, P. 2017. Metabolic Fingerprint of PS3-Induced Resistance of Grapevine Leaves against Plasmopara Viticola Revealed Differences in Elicitor-Triggered Defenses. *Frontiers in Plant Science*. 8: 101.

Albuquerque, W., Ghezellou, P., Seidel, L., Burkert, J., Will, F., Schweiggert, R., Spengler, B., Zorn, H., Gand, M. 2023. Mass Spectrometry-Based Proteomic Profiling of a Silvaner White Wine. *Biomolecules*. 13: 650.

Anesi, A., Stocchero, M., Dal Santo, S., Commisso, M., Zenoni, S., Ceoldo, S., Tornielli, G.B., Siebert, T.E., Herderich, M., Pezzotti, M., Guzzo, F. 2015. Towards a Scientific Interpretation of the Terroir Concept: Plasticity of the Grape Berry Metabolome. *BMC Plant Biology*. 15: 191.

Awale, M., Liu, C., Kwasniewski, M.T. 2021. Workflow to Investigate Subtle Differences in Wine Volatile Metabolome Induced by Different Root Systems and Irrigation Regimes. *Molecules*. 26.

Azri, W., Jardak, R., Cosette, P., Guillou, C., Riahi, J., Mliki, A. 2022. Physiological and Proteomic Analyses of Tunisian Local Grapevine (*Vitis Vinifera*) Cultivar Razegui in Response to Drought Stress. *Functional Plant Biology*. 49: 25–39.

Batista-Silva, W., Nascimento, V.L., Medeiros, D.B., Nunes-Nesi, A., Ribeiro, D.M., Zsögön, A., Araújo, W.L. 2018. Modifications in Organic Acid Profiles During Fruit Development and Ripening: Correlation or Causation? *Frontiers in Plant Science*. 9: 1689.

Bavaresco, L., Zamboni, M., Squeri, C., Xu, S., Abramowicz, A., Lucini, L.J.B.W.C. 2017. Chitosan and Grape Secondary Metabolites: A Proteomics and Metabolomics Approach. *BIO Web of Conferences*. 9: 01004.

Bokulich, N.A., Collins, T.S., Masarweh, C., Allen, G., Heymann, H., Ebeler, S.E., Mills, D.A. 2016. Associations among Wine Grape Microbiome, Metabolome, and Fermentation Behavior Suggest Microbial Contribution to Regional Wine Characteristics. *mBio*. 7:

Brasili, E., Donati, L., Sciubba, F., Ferretti, L., Miccheli, A., Pasqua, G. 2021. Comparative Transcriptomics and Metabolomics in Vitis Vinifera 'Malvasia' and Vitis Rupestris 'Du Lot' Cultured Cells Provide Insights in Possible Innate Resistance Against Pathogens. *Plant Biosystems—An International Journal Dealing with all Aspects of Plant Biology*. 155: 557–566.

Campayo, A., Savoi, S., Romieu, C., Lopez-Jimenez, A.J., Serrano de la Hoz, K., Salinas, M.R., Torregrosa, L., Alonso, G.L. 2021. The Application of Ozonated Water Rearranges the Vitis Vinifera L. Leaf and Berry Transcriptomes Eliciting Defence and Antioxidant Responses. *Scientific Reports*. 11: 8114.

Castro, A.J., Carapito, C., Zorn, N., Magne, C., Leize, E., Van Dorsselaer, A., Clement, C. 2005. Proteomic Analysis of Grapevine (Vitis Vinifera L.) Tissues Subjected to Herbicide Stress. *Journal of Experimental Botany*. 56: 2783–2795.

Catacchio, C.R., Alagna, F., Perniola, R., Bergamini, C., Rotunno, S., Calabrese, F.M., Crupi, P., Antonacci, D., Ventura, M., Cardone, M.F. 2019. Transcriptomic and Genomic Structural Variation Analyses on Grape Cultivars Reveal New Insights into the Genotype-Dependent Responses to Water Stress. *Scientific Reports*. 9: 2809.

Ciubotaru, R.M., Franceschi, P., Zulini, L., Stefanini, M., Skrab, D., Rossarolla, M.D., Robatscher, P., Oberhuber, M., Vrhovsek, U., Chitarrini, G. 2021. Mono-Locus and Pyramided Resistant Grapevine Cultivars Reveal Early Putative Biomarkers Upon Artificial Inoculation with Plasmopara Viticola. *Frontiers Plant Science*. 12: 693887.

Coombe, B.G. 1992. Research on Development and Ripening of the Grape Berry. *American Journal of Enology and Viticulture*. 43: 101–110.

Cramer, G.R., Cochetel, N., Ghan, R., Destrac-Irvine, A., Delrot, S. 2020. A Sense of Place: Transcriptomics Identifies Environmental Signatures in Cabernet Sauvignon Berry Skins in the Late Stages of Ripening. *BMC Plant Biology*. 20: 41.

Cramer, G.R., Ghan, R., Schlauch, K.A., Tillett, R.L., Heymann, H., Ferrarini, A., Delledonne, M., Zenoni, S., Fasoli, M., Pezzotti, M. 2014. Transcriptomic Analysis of the Late Stages of Grapevine (Vitis Vinifera cv. Cabernet Sauvignon) Berry Ripening Reveals Significant Induction of Ethylene Signaling and Flavor Pathways in the Skin. *BMC Plant Biology*. 14: 370.

Degu, A., Morcia, C., Tumino, G., Hochberg, U., Toubiana, D., Mattivi, F., Schneider, A., Bosca, P., Cattivelli, L., Terzi, V., Fait, A. 2015. Metabolite Profiling Elucidates Communalities and Differences in the Polyphenol Biosynthetic Pathways of Red and White Muscat Genotypes. *Plant Physiology and Biochemistry.* 86: 24–33.

Di Carli, M., Zamboni, A., Pè, M.E., Pezzotti, M., Lilley, K.S., Benvenuto, E., Desiderio, A. 2011. Two-Dimensional Differential in Gel Electrophoresis (2D-DIGE) Analysis of Grape Berry Proteome during Postharvest Withering. *Journal of Proteome Research.* 10: 429–446.

Fand, B.B., Amala, U., Yadav, D.S., Rathi, G., Mhaske, S.H., Upadhyay, A., Ahammed Shabeer, T.P., Kumbhar, D.R. 2020. Bacterial Volatiles from Mealybug Honeydew Exhibit Kairomonal Activity Toward Solitary Endoparasitoid Anagyrus Dactylopii. *Journal of Pest Science.* 93: 195–206.

Garrido, A., Engel, J., Mumm, R., Conde, A., Cunha, A., De Vos, R.C.H. 2021. Metabolomics of Photosynthetically Active Tissues in White Grapes: Effects of Light Microclimate and Stress Mitigation Strategies. *Metabolites.* 11.

George, I.S., Haynes, P.A. 2014. Current Perspectives in Proteomic Analysis of Abiotic Stress in Grapevines. *Frontiers in Plant Science.* 5: 686.

González-Barreiro, C., Rial-Otero, R., Cancho-Grande, B., Simal-Gándara, J. 2015. Wine Aroma Compounds in Grapes: A Critical Review. *Critical Reviews in Food Science and Nutrition.* 55: 202–218.

Grant, E., Johnson, L., Prodromidis, A., Giannoudis, P.V. 2021. The Impact of Peer Support on Patient Outcomes in Adults with Physical Health Conditions: A Scoping Review. *Cureus.* 13: e17442.

He, L., Xu, X.Q., Wang, Y., Chen, W.K., Sun, R.Z., Cheng, G., Liu, B., Chen, W., Duan, C.Q., Wang, J., Pan, Q.H. 2020. Modulation of Volatile Compound Metabolome and Transcriptome in Grape Berries Exposed to Sunlight Under Dry-Hot Climate. *BMC Plant Biology.* 20: 59.

Herrera, J.C., Hochberg, U., Degu, A., Sabbatini, P., Lazarovitch, N., Castellarin, S.D., Fait, A., Alberti, G., Peterlunger, E. 2017. Grape Metabolic Response to Postveraison Water Deficit Is Affected by Interseason Weather Variability. *Journal of Agricultural and Food Chemistry.* 65: 5868–5878.

Hines, K.M., Ford, G.C., Klaus, K.A., Irving, B.A., Ford, B.L., Johnson, K.L., Lanza, I.R., Nair, K.S. 2015. Application of High-Resolution Mass Spectrometry to Measure Low Abundance Isotope Enrichment in Individual Muscle Proteins. *Analytical and Bioanalytical Chemistry.* 407: 4045–4052.

Hochberg, U., Batushansky, A., Degu, A., Rachmilevitch, S., Fait, A. 2015. Metabolic and Physiological Responses of Shiraz and Cabernet Sauvignon (Vitis Vinifera L.) to Near Optimal Temperatures of 25 and 35 degrees C. *International Journal of Molecular Sciences.* 16: 24276–24294.

Jaillon, O., Aury, J.M., Noel, B., Policriti, A., Clepet, C., Casagrande, A., Choisne, N., Aubourg, S., Vitulo, N., Jubin, C., Vezzi, A., Legeai, F., Hugueney, P., Dasilva, C., Horner, D., Mica, E., Jublot, D., Poulain, J., Bruyère, C., Billault, A., Segurens, B., Gouyvenoux, M., Ugarte, E., Cattonaro, F., Anthouard, V., Vico, V., Del Fabbro, C., Alaux, M., Di Gaspero, G., Dumas, V., Felice, N., Paillard, S., Juman, I., Moroldo, M., Scalabrin, S., Canaguier, A., Le Clainche, I., Malacrida, G., Durand, E., Pesole, G., Laucou, V., Chatelet, P., Merdinoglu, D., Delledonne, M., Pezzotti, M., Lecharny, A., Scarpelli, C., Artiguenave, F., Pè, M.E., Valle, G., Morgante, M., Caboche, M., Adam-Blondon, A.F., Weissenbach, J., Quétier, F., Wincker, P. 2007. The Grapevine Genome Sequence Suggests Ancestral Hexaploidization in Major Angiosperm Phyla. *Nature.* 449: 463–467.

Josep, F., Grégoire, L., Tristan, R. 2021. MS- and NMR-Metabolomic Tools for the Discrimination of Wines: Applications for Authenticity. In P. Pétriacq, A. Bouchereau (Eds.), *Advances in Botanical Research* (vol. 98, pp. 297–357). Academic Press.

Kambiranda, D., Katam, R., Basha, S.M., Siebert, S. 2014. iTRAQ-Based Quantitative Proteomics of Developing and Ripening Muscadine Grape Berry. *Journal of Proteome Research.* 13: 555–569.

Knüpfer, C., Beckstein, C., Dittrich, P., Le Novère, N. 2013. Structure, Function, and Behaviour of Computational Models in Systems Biology. *BMC Systems Biology.* 7: 43.

Križanović, S., Gracin, L., Cindrić, M., Tomašević, M., Kelšin, K., Lukić, K., Kovačević Ganić, K. 2019. Comparison of Proteomic, Metabolic, and Growth Profiles of Brettanomyces Bruxellensis Isolates from Croatian Wines. *American Journal of Enology and Viticulture.* 70: 77–87.

Kuang, L., Chen, S., Guo, Y., Ma, H. 2019. Quantitative Proteome Analysis Reveals Changes in the Protein Landscape During Grape Berry Development with a Focus on Vacuolar Transport Proteins. *Frontiers in Plant Science.* 10: 641.

Lee, J., Kim, S., Ahn, S.H.Y. 2019. Differential Expression of Genes in Response to Temperature Conditions Selected by Transcriptome Analysis of Grapevine Leaves. *Horticultural Science and Technology*: 437–447.

Le Mao, I., Martin-Pernier, J., Bautista, C., Lacampagne, S., Richard, T., Da Costa, G. 2021. (1)H-NMR Metabolomics as a Tool for Winemaking Monitoring. *Molecules.* 26.

Li, X., Wu, J., Yin, L., Zhang, Y., Qu, J., Lu, J. 2015. Comparative Transcriptome Analysis Reveals Defense-Related Genes and Pathways Against Downy Mildew in Vitis Amurensis Grapevine. *Plant Physiology and Biochemistry.* 95: 1–14.

Liu, G.T., Wang, B.B., Lecourieux, D., Li, M.J., Liu, M.B., Liu, R.Q., Shang, B.X., Yin, X., Wang, L.J., Lecourieux, F., Xu, Y. 2021. Proteomic Analysis of Early-Stage Incompatible and Compatible Interactions Between Grapevine and P. Viticola. *Horticuture Research.* 8: 100.

Livigni, S., Lucini, L., Sega, D., Navacchi, O., Pandolfini, T., Zamboni, A., Varanini, Z. 2019. The Different Tolerance to Magnesium Deficiency of Two Grapevine Rootstocks Relies on the Ability to Cope with Oxidative Stress. *BMC Plant Biology.* 19: 148.

Ma, Q., Yang, J. 2019. Transcriptome Profiling and Identification of the Functional Genes Involved in Berry Development and Ripening in Vitis Vinifera. *Gene.* 680: 84–96.

Magris, G., Jurman, I., Fornasiero, A., Paparelli, E., Schwope, R., Marroni, F., Di Gaspero, G., Morgante, M. 2021. The Genomes of 204 Vitis Vinifera Accessions Reveal the Origin of European Wine Grapes. *Nature Communications.* 12: 7240.

Maoz, I., De Rosso, M., Kaplunov, T., Vedova, A.D., Sela, N., Flamini, R., Lewinsohn, E., Lichter, A. 2019. Metabolomic and Transcriptomic Changes Underlying Cold and Anaerobic Stresses after Storage of Table Grapes. *Scientific Reports.* 9: 2917.

Minio, A., Massonnet, M., Figueroa-Balderas, R., Vondras, A.M., Blanco-Ulate, B., Cantu, D. 2019. Iso-Seq Allows Genome-Independent Transcriptome Profiling of Grape Berry Development. *G3 (Bethesda).* 9: 755–767.

Morgani, M.B., Peña, J.E.P., Fanzone, M., Prieto, J.A. 2022. Pruning After Budburst Delays Phenology and Affects Yield Components, Crop Coefficient and Total Evapotranspiration in Vitis Vinífera L. Cv. 'Malbec' in Mendoza, Argentina. *Scientia Horticulturae.* 296: 110886.

Myles, S., Chia, J.-M., Hurwitz, B., Simon, C., Zhong, G.Y., Buckler, E., Ware, D. 2010. Rapid Genomic Characterization of the Genus Vitis. *PLoS ONE.* 5: e8219.

Negrel, L., Halter, D., Wiedemann-Merdinoglu, S., Rustenholz, C., Merdinoglu, D., Hugueney, P., Baltenweck, R. 2018. Identification of Lipid Markers of Plasmopara Viticola Infection in Grapevine Using a Non-targeted Metabolomic Approach. *Frontiers in Plant Science.* 9: 360.

Negri, S., Lovato, A., Boscaini, F., Salvetti, E., Torriani, S., Commisso, M., Danzi, R., Ugliano, M., Polverari, A., Tornielli, G.B., Guzzo, F. 2017. The Induction of Noble Rot (Botrytis cinerea) Infection during Postharvest Withering Changes the Metabolome of Grapevine Berries (Vitis vinifera L., cv. Garganega). *Frontiers in Plant Science*. 8: 1002.

Park, M., Darwish, A.G., Elhag, R.I., Tsolova, V., Soliman, K.F.A., El-Sharkawy, I. 2022. A Multi-Locus Genome-Wide Association Study Reveals the Genetics Underlying Muscadine Antioxidant in Berry Skin. *Frontiers in Plant Science*. 13: 969301.

Pastore, C., Dal Santo, S., Zenoni, S., Movahed, N., Allegro, G., Valentini, G., Filippetti, I., Tornielli, G.B. 2017. Whole Plant Temperature Manipulation Affects Flavonoid Metabolism and the Transcriptome of Grapevine Berries. *Frontier in Plant Science*. 8: 929.

Pereira, R., Oliveira, J., Sousa, M. 2020. Bioinformatics and Computational Tools for Next-Generation Sequencing Analysis in Clinical Genetics. *Journal of Clinical Medicine*. 9: 132.

Pinasseau, L., Vallverdú-Queralt, A., Verbaere, A., Roques, M., Meudec, E., Le Cunff, L., Peros, J.-P., Ageorges, A., Sommerer, N., Boulet, J.-C., Terrier, N., Cheynier, V. 2017. Cultivar Diversity of Grape Skin Polyphenol Composition and Changes in Response to Drought Investigated by LC-MS Based Metabolomics. *Frontiers in Plant Science*. 8: 1826.

Poni, S., Fasoli, M., Richter, C.L., Zenoni, S., Sandri, M., Zuccolotto, P., Dal Santo, S., Pezzotti, M., Dokoozlian, N., Tornielli, G.B. 2019. Towards the Definition of a Detailed Transcriptomic Map of Berry Development. *BIO Web of Conferences*. 13: 01001.

Prinsi, B., Failla, O., Scienza, A., Espen, L. 2020. Root Proteomic Analysis of Two Grapevine Rootstock Genotypes Showing Different Susceptibility to Salt Stress. *International Journal of Molecular Sciences*. 21: 1076.

Pucker, B., Pandey, A., Weisshaar, B., Stracke, R. 2020. The R2R3-MYB Gene Family in Banana (Musa Acuminata): Genome-Wide Identification, Classification and Expression Patterns. *PLoS ONE*. 15: e0239275.

Ranade, Y., Pathak, P., Chandrashekar, M., Saha, S. 2023. Diversity Analysis of Culturable Epiphytic Microbial Consortia of Table Grape Berry Surface. *Food Biotechnology*. 37: 54–73.

Ranade, Y., Sawant, I., Saha, S., Chandrashekar, M., Pathak, P. 2021. Epiphytic Microbial Diversity of Vitis vinifera Fructosphere: Present Status and Potential Applications. *Current Microbiology*. 78: 1086–1098.

Raúl, G-D, Ana, S., Ángeles, F-R. 2019. Metabolomics: An Emerging Tool for Wine Characterization and the Investigation of Health Benefits. In A.M. Grumezescu, A.M. Holban (Eds.), *Engineering Tools in the Beverage Industry* (pp. 315–350). Woodhead Publishing.

Reshef, N., Agam, N., Fait, A. 2018. Grape Berry Acclimation to Excessive Solar Irradiance Leads to Repartitioning between Major Flavonoid Groups. *Journal of Agricultural and Food Chemistry*. 66: 3624–3636.

Rogiers, S.Y., Coetzee, Z.A., Walker, R.R., Deloire, A., Tyerman, S.D. 2017. Potassium in the Grape (Vitis Vinifera L.) Berry: Transport and Function. *Frontiers in Plant Science*. 8: 1629.

Royo, C., Carbonell-Bejerano, P., Torres-Perez, R., Nebish, A., Martinez, O., Rey, M., Aroutiounian, R., Ibanez, J., Martinez-Zapater, J.M. 2016. Developmental, Transcriptome, and Genetic Alterations Associated with Parthenocarpy in the Grapevine Seedless Somatic Variant Corinto Bianco. *Journal of Experimental Botany*. 67: 259–273.

Ruocco, S., Stefanini, M., Stanstrup, J., Perenzoni, D., Mattivi, F., Vrhovsek, U. 2017. The Metabolomic Profile of Red Non-V. Vinifera Genotypes. *Food Research International.* 98: 10–19.

Salini, S., Yadav, D.S.J.P.M.I.H.E. 2011. Occurrence of Stromatium Barbatum (Fabr.) (Coleoptera: Cerambycidae) on Grapevine in Maharashtra, India. *Pest Management in Horticultural Ecosystems.* 17: 48–50.

Sanger, F., Nicklen, S., Coulson, A.R. 1977. DNA Sequencing with Chain-Terminating Inhibitors. *Proceedings of the National Academy of Sciences of the United States of America.* 74: 5463–5467.

Sharathchandra, R.G., Stander, C., Jacobson, D., Ndimba, B., Vivier, M.A. 2011. Proteomic Analysis of Grape Berry Cell Cultures Reveals that Developmentally Regulated Ripening Related Processes Can Be Studied Using Cultured Cells. *PLoS ONE.* 6: e14708.

Shirasawa, K., Hirakawa, H., Azuma, A., Taniguchi, F., Yamamoto, T., Sato, A., Ghelfi, A., Isobe, S.N. 2022. De Novo Whole-Genome Assembly in an Interspecific Hybrid Table Grape, 'Shine Muscat'. *DNA Research.* 29: 1–9.

Son, H.-S., Hwang, G.-S., Kim, K.M., Ahn, H.-J., Park, W.-M., Berg, F., Hong, Y.-S., Lee, C.-H. 2009. Metabolomic Studies on Geographical Grapes and Their Wines Using H-1 NMR Analysis Coupled with Multivariate Statistics. *Journal of Agricultural and Food Chemistry.* 57: 1481–1490.

Tanaka, K., Hamaguchi, Y., Suzuki, S., Enoki, S. 2020. Genomic Characterization of the Japanese Indigenous Wine Grape Vitis sp. cv. Koshu. *Frontiers in Plant Science.* 11: 532211.

Terral, J.F., Tabard, E., Bouby, L., Ivorra, S., Pastor, T., Figueiral, I., Picq, S., Chevance, J.B., Jung, C., Fabre, L., Tardy, C., Compan, M., Bacilieri, R., Lacombe, T., This, P. 2010. Evolution and History of Grapevine (Vitis Vinifera) Under Domestication: New Morphometric Perspectives to Understand Seed Domestication Syndrome and Reveal Origins of Ancient European Cultivars. *Annals of Botany.* 105: 443–455.

Tian B, Harrison R. 2021. Pathogenesis-Related Proteins in Wine and White Wine Protein Stabilization. In F. Cosme, F.M. Nunes, L. Filipe-Ribeiro (Eds.), *Winemaking – Stabilization, Aging Chemistry and Biochemistry.* IntechOpen.

Tian, B., Harrison, R., Morton, J., Deb-Choudhury, S. 2015. Proteomic Analysis of Sauvignon Blanc Grape Skin, Pulp and Seed and Relative Quantification of Pathogenesis-Related Proteins. *PLoS ONE.* 10: e0130132.

Tzachristas, A., Dasenaki, M.E., Aalizadeh, R., Thomaidis, N.S., Proestos, C. 2021. Development of a Wine Metabolomics Approach for the Authenticity Assessment of Selected Greek Red Wines. *Molecules.* 26.

Upadhyay, A., Gaonkar, T., Upadhyay, A.K., Jogaiah, S., Shinde, M.P., Kadoo, N.Y., Gupta, V.S. 2018. Global Transcriptome Analysis of Grapevine (Vitis Vinifera L.) Leaves Under Salt Stress Reveals Differential Response at Early and Late Stages of Stress in Table Grape cv. Thompson Seedless. *Plant Physiology and Biochemistry.* 129: 168–179.

VanderWeide, J., Medina-Meza, I.G., Frioni, T., Sivilotti, P., Falchi, R., Sabbatini, P. 2018. Enhancement of Fruit Technological Maturity and Alteration of the Flavonoid Metabolomic Profile in Merlot (Vitis vinifera L.) by Early Mechanical Leaf Removal. *Journal of Agricultural and Food Chemistry.* 66: 9839–9849.

Vannozzi, A., Palumbo, F., Magon, G., Lucchin, M., Barcaccia, G. 2021. The Grapevine (Vitis Vinifera L.) Floral Transcriptome in Pinot Noir Variety: Identification of Tissue-Related Gene Networks and Whorl-Specific Markers in Pre- and Post-Anthesis Phases. *Horticulture Research.* 8: 200.

Vrhovsek, U., Lotti, C., Masuero, D., Carlin, S., Weingart, G., Mattivi, F. 2014. Quantitative Metabolic Profiling of Grape, Apple and Raspberry Volatile Compounds (VOCs) Using a GC/MS/MS Method. *Journal of Chromatography B: Analytical Technologies in the Biomedical and Life Sciences.* 966: 132–139.

Wang, X., Liu, Y., Guo, L., Shen, J., Hu, H., Zhou, R. 2022. Transcriptome Analysis of Crimson Seedless Grapevine (Vitis Vinifera L.) Infected by Grapevine Berry Inner Necrosis Virus. *Current Research in Virological Science.* 3: 100024.

Zenoni, S., Amato, A., D'Incà, E., Guzzo, F., Tornielli, G.B. 2020. Rapid Dehydration of Grape Berries Dampens the Post-Ripening Transcriptomic Program and the Metabolite Profile Evolution. *Horticulture Research.* 7: 141.

Zhang, W., Yan, J., Li, X., Xing, Q., Chethana, K.W.T., Zhao, W. 2019. Transcriptional Response of Grapevine to Infection with the Fungal Pathogen Lasiodiplodia Theobromae. *Scientific Reports.* 9: 5387.

Zhong, H., Zhang, F., Pan, M., Wu, X., Zhang, W., Han, S., Xie, H., Zhou, X., Wang, M., Ai, C.M., He, T. 2020. Comparative Phenotypic and Transcriptomic Analysis of Victoria and Flame Seedless Grape Cultivars During Berry Ripening. *FEBS Open Bio.* 10: 2616–2630.

Zombardo, A., Crosatti, C., Bagnaresi, P., Bassolino, L., Reshef, N., Puccioni, S., Faccioli, P., Tafuri, A., Delledonne, M., Fait, A., Storchi, P., Cattivelli, L., Mica, E. 2020. Transcriptomic and Biochemical Investigations Support the Role of Rootstock-Scion Interaction in Grapevine Berry Quality. *BMC Genomics.* 21: 468.

15 Screenings of the Inhibitory Ability of Vietnamese Medicinal Plant-Based Substances and Protein-Related Structures

Computation-Pharmacological Experiment Correlations

Nguyen Thi Ai Nhung, Nguyen Thi Xuan Dieu**, and Nguyen Thanh Triet***,†*
*Department of Chemistry, University of Sciences, Hue University, Vietnam; **Faculty of Pharmacy, University of Medicine and Pharmacy at Ho Chi Minh City, Ho Chi Minh City, Vietnam; ***Faculty of Traditional Medicine, University of Medicine and Pharmacy at Ho Chi Minh City, Ho Chi Minh City, Vietnam; All authors contributed equally to this chapter
†Corresponding Author: nguyenthanhtriet1702@ump.edu.vn

15.1 INTRODUCTION

15.1.1 The Biodiversity of Vietnamese Medicinal Plants

Vietnam is a tropical monsoon country in Southeast Asia with favorable climatic conditions for the development of an extremely diverse and rich biological system, estimated to possess about 20,000 to 30,000 species of vascular plants. Previous survey data showed that this place is home to about 11,458 species of fauna and 21,017 species of flora. However, of the plant species found, only 6,000 species are used for human purposes, such as medicine, food, materials and other purposes. Moreover, Vietnam is said to be home to 10% of the world's wild plant and animal species. Vietnam, similarly to other countries in Asia, also possesses an invaluable treasure of traditional and folk medicine knowledge, with about 80% of the population using it in the primary health care system (Ha et al. 2007). The fact is that the biodiversity of plant resources along with

DOI: 10.1201/9781003354437-15

the experience of using them passed down through generations have contributed to sustainable livelihoods, food security and local people's health care, especially those who live in remote and isolated areas and are directly dependent on resource exploitation. Many investigations into the indigenous knowledge of ethnic minority communities living in Vietnam have recorded thousands of medicinal plants and hundreds of traditional remedies used by the Dao, Nung, Tay and H'mong people in the locality. Traditional practices play an important role in protecting nature and preserving precious and unique medicinal plants of the country (Ministry of Natural Resources and Environment 2008).

Traditional Vietnamese medicine (TVM) uses medicines made from animals, plants and mineral products. However, most of the medicinal materials used in herbal remedies are derived from plants, even those with animal ingredients as the main ingredient also need plant ingredients to regulate the taste and increase the overall effect as well as reduce the side effects of the drug. According to the records, depending on the plant and the remedy, various parts of the plant can be used (roots, rhizomes, bark, stems, leaves, flowers, fruits, resin and seeds). In many cases, the same plant can produce many different medicines from the parts used, such as Lien diep (lotus leaf), Lien tu (lotus stamens) and Lien thach (lotus fruit) (Van and Tap 2008).

With the favor of nature along with a long history of traditional medicine, Vietnam has used many species of plants as medicine. Previous surveys showed that there are about 1,863 herbal plants used in VTM. Of these, several plants are common, many are valuable and some special plants are rare or at high risk of extinction. The Vietnamese government has promulgated and applied a national policy on medicinal herbs, encouraging the use of traditional medicine in combination with modern medicine in the treatment of diseases. That gave impetus to the development of research on medicinal plants resulting in a large number of monographs on medicinal plants being published (Kurian 2012).

Vietnam is a multi-racial country, home to 54 different ethnic groups living together. Each of these ethnic groups has their own experience and traditional knowledge in using locally available plant and animal species for health promotion, disease prevention and treatment. Many remedies and methods of using traditional medicine of some ethnic minorities (for example, the Dao people, the H'mong people in the northwest mountainous provinces, the Ca Tu and Van Kieu people in Nam Dong, Thua Thien province) has been studied, while many traditional remedies of other ethnic groups are part of their cultural life and are still kept secret (Van and Tap 2008).

In this chapter, we include several plants with antibacterial and antiviral effects from our previous published papers, such as *Melaleuca cajuputi* L., *Piper betle* L., *Ageratum conyzoides* L., *Cleistocalyx operculatus* L. and *Allium sativum* L. In addition, we also cite some results of our previous studies on antibacterial and anti-α-glucosidase effects from *Distichochlamys citrea* M.F. Newman species as a good example for combining experimental studies *in vitro* and docking simulation. These medicinal plants were selected because they are easy to find, widely distributed, have a high biomass and are endemic in Vietnam, which have been used in folk medicine for infections and diabetes.

15.1.2 Medicinal Plants Used in Vietnamese Traditional Medicine for Antibacterial, Antiviral and Antidiabetic Activities

Natural products, isolated from living organisms have been considered to be a valuable source for the manufacture of medicines and drugs thanks to their bioactivities and physiocompatibility (Byler et al. 2016; Bindseil et al. 2001; Teixeira et al. 2014). Their extensive availability in the natural reservoir means that they could be either exploited directly by folk medicine or investigated for continuing development (Teixeira et al. 2014). The former is justified by the fact that natural compounds have been under rigorous natural selection in order to gain the evolved value making up their existence. Furthermore, they have also been proven to be more favorable to humans than their synthetic counterparts (Byler et al. 2016). In contrast to this, natural substances, especially newly identified compounds, can serve as lead structures for preparation of their derivatives, which perform elevated efficacy or even have a novel property. This may confirm the important for developing new antiviral agents (Teixeira et al. 2014; Newman and Cragg 2012; Quy et al. 2021).

It is well known that essential oils are hydrophobic liquids containing volatile fragrant aroma compounds which have also been studied and reviewed for a long time. For instance, essential oils from *Melaleuca cajuputi*, *Piper betle* L., *Ageratum conyzoides* L., *Cleistocalyx operculatus* L. and garlic essential oil (Figure 15.1) in Vietnam have been carried studied for antioxidant, antimicrobial, anticancer, antidiarrheal, antihypertensive, antidiabetic, anti-inflammatory and immunomodulatory properties (Chauhan et al. 2016; Thuy, My, et al. 2020). *Melaleuca cajuputi* can be used as fuelwood and as piles and pillars in construction. *M. cajuputi* L. flowers attract honey bees, and its wood is used for pulp and paper, fiber and particle board Moreover, its wood also produces qualified charcoal and possible sawn timber (Doran and Turnbull 1997). Especially, the essential oil of *M. cajuputi* is widely used for medicinal application (Barbosa et al. 2013). Traditionally, cajeput ntial oil is further used in herbal medicinal products to relieve symptoms of coughs, colds, as a laxative and as a general muscle relaxant and sedative (Oyen and Nguyen Xuan 1999). The *P. betle* essential oil is used for treatment of various ailments since ancient times and has been proven to possess anticancer, antiallergic, antibacterial, antifungal and antioxidant activities (Paridhi et al. 2018). The *A. conyzoides* essential oil is used as antimalarial, antidiabetic and anthelmintic agents (V et al. 2010), while the *C. operculatus* essential oil is well documented to show antioxidant, antihyperglycemic, hypolipidemic and cardiotonic effects (Stéphane, Koffi, and Bernard 2013) and exhibits a strong antimicrobial activity and cytotoxicity to several cancer cell lines (Dosoky, Pokharel, and Setzer 2015).

Recently, pharmacological researches indicated that essential oil of garlic is an exceptional source of organosulfur compounds, possessing strong antioxidant, antibacterial, antifungal, anticancer and antimicrobial properties. It is also proven to be beneficial for hypoglycemia, hypotension, antithrombotic, immunomodulatory and prebiotic therapy. In addition, allicin is a typical reactive sulfur species found in the essential oil. The compounds in the garlic essential oil inhibited the angiotensin-converting enzyme 2 (ACE2) protein, causing the virus to lose the host receptor and attack the protease of the COVID-19 virus, preventing protein maturation of the virus and the spread of infection in the *in silico* studies (Thuy, My, et al. 2020).

Influenza is a common and serious public health problem. In some cases, the disease can not only progress to become severe leading to death but also a significant economic burden. According to estimates by the World Health Organization (WHO), every year this acute respiratory infection causes more than 3 million severe cases and 650,000 deaths worldwide. In Vietnam, due to its location in the tropical

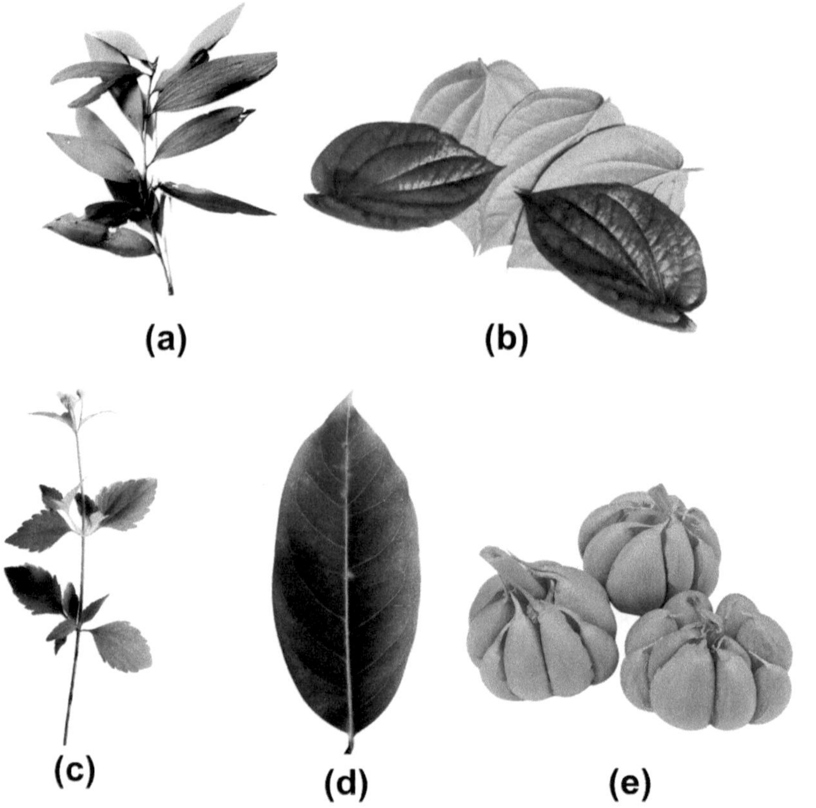

FIGURE 15.1 Picture of (a) *Melaleuca cajuputi* L., (b) *Piper betle* L., (c) *Ageratum conyzoides* L., (d), *Cleistocalyx operculatus* L. and (e) *Allium sativum* L.

monsoon climate, infectious diseases are very common and were the cause of more than 16,000 deaths in 2018 according to the latest report of the WHO (Organization 2021). Note that a new flu subtype could eventually cause a pandemic. Currently, vaccines are still an effective weapon in the fight against influenza, but they are facing many challenges. Furthermore, SARS-CoV-2 is a new strain of a large family of human pathogens known by the name coronavirus, the well-known agents causing common colds in humans. The latest caused a severe pandemic worldwide, which is due to the infection by SARS-CoV-2. Therefore, demands for the discovery of sufficient medicines or effective medication-assisted agents for treatment of the infection are of great and urgent concern to researchers around the world. SARS-CoV-2 infection is based upon a virus-host interaction of two proteins. ACE2 in humans is an integral membrane glycoprotein, known for the highest expression in tissues such as the kidney, endothelium, lungs and heart. However, it was speculated that the protein is the host receptor of the SARS-CoV-2 and SARS-CoV. Therefore, if the ACE2 protein can be temporarily inhibited, infection caused by SARS-CoV-2 to humans would be deferred. The structure of the ACE2 protein (DOI: 10.2210/pdbACE2/pdb) can be referenced from UniProtKB. The SARS-CoV-2 main protease functions as a proteolytic enzyme, cutting polyproteins into functional pieces (Wang et al. 2020), which was defined and archived at the Worldwide Protein Data Bank with the PDB entry-ID is 6LU7 (DOI: 10.2210/pdb6LU7/pdb). More importantly, SARS-CoV-2 utilizes a spike glycoprotein to gain entry into its targeted cells (Krammer et al. 2018; Gong et al. 2018).

Diabetes mellitus (DM) is a non-communicable metabolic disease involving impaired glucose consumption and metabolism in the body, with the main feature being abnormally high blood glucose levels (Association 2017). In 2021, according to estimates by the International Diabetes Federation (IDF), the global prevalence of diabetes in the 20–79 age group was 10.5% (536.6 million) and by 2045, it is expected to reach 12.2% (783.2 million). Taxonomically, diabetes can be classified into the two most common groups: type 1 diabetes is characterized by destruction of pancreatic β-cells that reduce insulin secretion, while type 2 diabetes is specifically characterized by a combination of decreased insulin secretion and peripheral insulin resistance. Diabetes can be caused by genetic abnormalities (especially type 1 diabetes) and can also be caused by other medical disorders or clinical conditions, or gestational diabetes (American Diabetes Association Professional Practice 2022). The enzyme α-glucosidase is an essential enzyme of digestion involved in the hydrolysis of polysaccharides into glucose for absorption (Tomasik and Horton 2012). α-Glucosidase belongs to the group of enzymes that catalyze the hydrolysis of α-(1–4)-glucoside links to liberate α-glucose from complex polymers. The release of glucose molecules from the N-glycans (Glc3Man9GlcNAc2) of the endoplasmic reticulus glycoprotein is carried out by two different α-glucosidases, glucosidase 1 (Gls1) and glucosidase 2 (Gls2) produced by *Saccharomyces cerevisiae* (Hossain et al. 2016). The structure of α-glucosidase MAL12 extracted from *S. cerevisiae* was published for UniProt under entry ID P53341. Several herbs have been shown to be effective in improving diabetes symptoms with the advantage of decreased cost and fewer side effects than synthetic drugs (Alam et al. 2018). Based on previous studies, bioactive compounds of plants origin, e.g., phenolic compounds, phytosterols, alkaloids, etc., have shown antiallergic, anticancer, antibacterial, anti-inflammatory, antidiabetic and antioxidant activities (Blahova et al. 2021). Various compounds belonging to these classes have been shown to improve insulin sensitivity in many studies. In Vietnam, some previous studies on essential oils which were extracted from leaves and rhizomes of a number of indigenous medicinal herbs containing the main active ingredients such as 1,8-cineole, α-citral, β-citral, geraniol, geranyl acetate, terpinen-4-ol, linalool and α-terpineol detected by GC-MS showed this activity (Viet et al. 2017; Huong et al. 2017). Natural compounds are known to have great potential in the treatment of infections related to diseases and diabetes (Van Chen et al. 2022).

In silico studies are currently seeing a gain in popularity since they can reduce the cost and time of laboratory experiments significantly. The approaches are based on computational simulation and computing analysis as prescreening research, predicting the controlled compounds with undesirable properties and the most promising candidates. Regarding ligands-proteins interaction, molecular docking simulation is an effective method to investigate the potency of ligands as inhibitors towards theis targeted proteins by calculating ligands-proteins' binding energies and static stability of the inhibitory systems. The docking method was used to consider the interaction between the compounds and proteins in which the active compounds were docked into the protein systems; that means, we had to calculate how the compounds interact with the protein and inhibit the protein, as well as make the proteins become weaker than the state without the compounds' inhibitory effects. The steady state of proteins and ligands/compounds are always assessed through docking score energy (DS) and root-mean-square deviation (RMSD) values as presented in the manuscript. Note that the more negative the DS value, the more stable the interaction and cohesion of the compound into the proteins; that means the effects of the active compounds exhibit strong protein inhibition. The docking analysis exhibited the strong inhibitory effects of the DS values. Moreover, the DS energy and RMSD between ligands and proteins were shown through hydrogen bonds, cation-π, π-π bonds, ionic interactions, interactions distance between amino acids and the active sites in the molecules into proteins. From this it follows that the stability of the protein has been checked when it is bounded with compounds after docking.

It must be recognized that diverse chemical frameworks from natural compounds can serve as a great library for screening potential compounds for drug discovery. In addition, medicinal herbs and compounds of natural origin have long been applied as medicines to treat acute respiratory infections, especially in children thanks to their few side effects, cost savings and safety. Among the active ingredients commonly found in medicinal herbs, alkaloids and flavonoids have received great attention because of their high structural diversity, wide distribution in the plant kingdom and rich biological activities, especially antiviral properties. Compared with experiments performed in the laboratory, the molecular data–based approach provides the possibility of identifying compounds with strong inhibitory activity and designing novel active compounds on frameworks discovered quickly and with great efficiency. In turn, classical assays help validate the outcomes predicted through those computational methods (Lucas et al. 2019; Harborne and Williams 1975; Qiu et al. 2014; Huang and Zou 2010; Bui et al. 2022).

In this chapter, molecular docking simulation was carried out to investigate static inhibitability, hydrogen-bonding interactions and shape complementarity of the natural compounds and protein interactions of some natural compounds towards influenza A/X-31(H3N2) virus hemagglutinin 2VIU (Protein Data Bank) and SARS-CoV-2 main protease 6LU7 (Protein Data Bank) and protein P53341 of α-glucosidase from *S. cerevisiae*. UniProtKB-P53341 (MAL12_YEAST) (Uniprot) which is referenced from Worldwide Protein Data Bank.

15.2 METHODOLOGY OF MOLECULAR DOCKING SIMULATION

Molecular docking analysis was obtained using MOE 2015.10 to consider the interaction between the ligand and protein (Tarasova, Poroikov, and Veselovsky 2018; Thai et al. 2015; Ngo et al. 2016). Intermolecular-complex configurations, DS energy, RMSD, types of interactions and respective distances between the potential compounds and proteins were included. The figure is yielded by the free-energy sum of all individual intermolecular interactions, whose affinity stems from hydrophilic

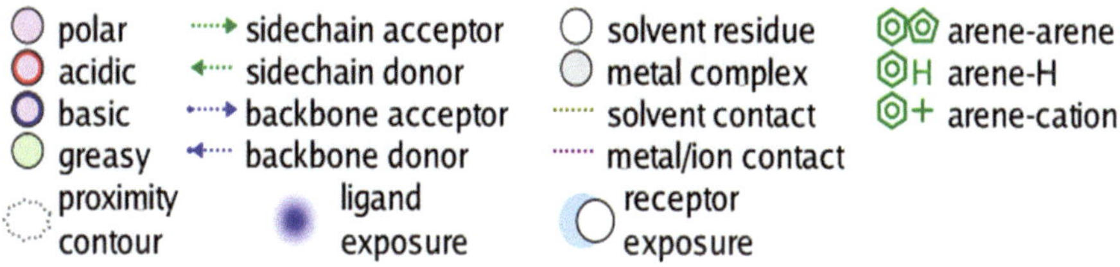

FIGURE 15.2 Types of interactions projected by MOE2015.10 for molecular docking analysis.

bonding, i.e., various hydrogen bonds types, and hydrophobic binding, i.e., van der Waals interactions. Figure 15.2 shows the types of interactions calculated by MOE2015.10 for molecular docking analysis.

In a typical procedure, molecular docking simulation follow four steps:

a. *Pre-docking preparation*
    - Proteins selected in Protein Data Bank: the crystal structures of influenza (H3N2) virus hemagglutinin 2VIU, SARS-CoV-2 main protease 6LU7, and protein P53341 of α-glucosidase from *Saccharomyces cerevisiae*. UniProtKB-P53341 (MAL12_YEAST) (Uniprot), were referenced from Worldwide Protein Data Bank.
    - Positional determination of bonding between ligands and proteins: The ligand position in the 4.5 Å radius and the existence of important amino acids were selected as the active regions of the protein. Before re-establishing the active sites of the enzyme, water was removed and then the structure of the amino acids was examined.
    - The state of lowest energy: The mismatched values of bond lengths, bond angles, bending angles and unusual non-bonding interactions will be then corrected through the optimization of the 3D molecular structure of the compounds.
    - Plotting chemical structures the compounds: The protein 3D-protonation structures were prepared by Quickprep tool following configuration: Tether—Receptor with the strength of 5000; Refine of 0.0001 $kcal{\cdot}mol^{-1}{\cdot}Å^{-1}$; The active zones were determined based on the ligand position within a radius of 4.5 Å as well as the presence of important amino acids. The program automatically iterated five times to find the various configurations needed and then the minimized energies were observed again to determine steric energies.

b. *Docking investigation*

    After preparing the input data, the intermolecular interactions were simulated, using the MOE 2015.10 system with the configuration including retained positions to probe the intermolecular interactions = 10; max solution per iteration = 1000; max solution per fragment = 200. Simulated protein-ligand inhibitory structures were saved in *.sdf format.

c. *Re-docking*

Re-docking of ligands-protein cocrystal structures: the re-docking of protein-ligand complex cocrystal structures aims to assess the suitability of docking parameters. The process was carried out with three structures of compounds as follows:

(i) Separation of investigated compounds from homogenized complexes in target proteins.
(ii) Separation of investigated compounds from homogeneous complexes and re-preparation.
(iii) Preparation of the new compounds via structure drawing, structural optimization parameters on minima energies.

Root-mean-square deviation (RMSD) values reflects the deviation of investigated compounds structures after docking compared to available structures in the crystal structure and comparing the interactions of studied compounds in the crystal structure after docking. The docking parameters are considered reliable when the RMSD value is < 2 Å and the interactions between studied compounds and the initial enzymes/proteins are nearly similar.

d. *Docking results analysis*

Docking score (DS) energy indicates the Gibbs free energy of the respective ligand-protein inhibitory systems, which is considered as the primary indicator of the duo-system inhibitability. Intermolecular interactions formed between the ligands and in-pose amino acids of the proteins include hydrophilic binding, electron-transferring, cation-arene, arene-arene, and ionic and hydrophobic interaction, and van der Waals interactions.

15.3 METHODOLOGY OF *IN VITRO* PHARMACOLOGICAL STUDIES OF VIETNAMESE MEDICINAL PLANTS

In vitro biological assays are used to screen the antibacterial and hypoglycemic effects of some medicinal plants in Vietnam. Initial studies are aimed at screening and demonstrating the effects according to modern medicine of plants commonly used in VTM to treat infections and diabetes according to the experience of local people.

15.3.1 Inhibitory Activity *In Vitro* Against Bacteria of Vietnamese Medicinal Plants

Extracts and secondary metabolites isolated from some selected Vietnamese herbal plants were screened for antibacterial effects on a number of disease-matched bacterial strains targeted through docking. Effective extracts or purified substances will be evaluated for activity by minimum inhibitory concentration (MIC) value. This concentration was determined by the broth microdilution method. The process can be summarized as follows: 100 L of suspension containing 1×10^6 CFU/mL of bacteria is inoculated into the wells of a 96-well plate containing 100 L of solution of the extract or pure substances at various concentrations, ranging from small to high ones. The tested samples were incubated, using 96-well plates at 37 °C for 24 h, before absorbance at 630 nm was measured by a microplate reader. The MIC concentrations of antimicrobial agents were defined as the minimum concentrations that totally inhibited bacterial growth. The common antibiotics, such as gentamicin or penicillin, were used as a positive control (Dat et al. 2022).

15.3.2 *In Vitro* α-Glucosidase Inhibitory Assay of the Extracts from Vietnamese Medicinal Plants

The α-glucosidase inhibitory activity of the plant extracts and pure compounds was performed according to the method described based on the measurement of the absorbance of the colored product formed (Van Chen et al. 2022). The anti-glucosidase activity was experimentally performed on a 96-well plate; a reaction mixture consisting of 60 µl of sample solution, 50 µL solution containing 0.1 M phosphate buffer adjusted at pH 6.8 and the enzyme α-glucosidase (0.2 U/mL) was incubated at 37 °C for 10 min. After incubation, a reaction substrate of 50 µL solution of 5 mM p-nitrophenyl-α-D-glucopyranoside (p-NPG) in buffer was added. The mixture was further incubated under the same conditions for another 20 minutes. The absorbance of result obtained was measured at 405 nm as the maximum absorption wavelength of the product with a Biotek microplate reader (USA). Acarbose was used as a positive control for the assay. The inhibitory effect of α-glucosidase was exhibited as the percentage inhibition obtained from the following formula:

$$\text{Inhibition of } \alpha-\text{glucosidase activity} (\%) = 1 - \frac{(A_c - A_{oc}) - (A_t - A_{ot})}{(A_c - A_{oc})} \times 100$$

in which

- A_c is the absorbance of the control (with enzyme but no sample);
- A_{oc} is the absorbance of the sample containing the reactants but without both the enzyme and the tested extract;
- A_t is the absorbance of the test sample containing all the components of the reaction;
- A_{ot} is the absorbance of the non-enzymatic sample;
- The α-glucosidase inhibitory activity of the tested samples was evaluated based on IC_{50} values (µg mL^{-1}).

15.3.3 Statistical Analysis

All experimental samples were performed in triplicate. The obtained results are expressed as mean ± SD. Calculations, analysis and plotting of data presentation were performed using the Microsoft Excel software. All statistical analyses were performed according to the analysis of variance (ANOVA) method.

15.4 RESULTS AND DISCUSSION OF MOLECULAR DOCKING ANALYSIS INHIBITABILITY

15.4.1 Docking Simulation of Natural Compounds in Garlic Essential Oil and Cajeput Essential Oil into PBD-6LU7 Protein of SARS-CoV-2

This was the first successful demonstration of the model describing the docking molecules of compounds in the garlic essential oil into the complex structure of protein 6LU7 (Thuy, My, et al. 2020). It has been found that sulfur-content compounds had strong interactions with amino acid in the target protein 6LU7. Note that the interactions mainly took place with the molecule groups that containing sulfur in the compounds

The DS and RMSD between ligands and proteins were shown through van der Waals interactions, hydrogen bonds, cation-π, π-π bonds, ionic interactions, interaction distance between amino acids and the active sites in the molecules of the garlic essential oil (Thuy, My, et al. 2020).

It was also found that the compounds allyl disulfide and allyl trisulfide exhibited the strongest anti-coronavirus activity into 6LU7 protein. The five compounds of allyl disulfide, allyl trisulfide, allyl methyl trisulfide, diallyl tetrasulfide and trisulfide, 2-propenyl propyl obtained the strongest anti-coronavirus activity out of 17 compounds (Thuy, My, et al. 2020) presented the visual presentation and in-pose interaction map of representative compounds of garlic essential oil and 6LU7 inhibitory structures. The DS was negative, in the range from −15.3 kcal.mol^{-1} for allyl disulfide to −11.6 kcal.mol^{-1} for trisulfide,2-propenyl propyl. Interactions with amino acids include Pro 565, Gln 102, Glu 208, Asn 210, Gly 205, Gln 98, Trp 566, Lys 94, Val 209, Gln 101, Asp 206, Asn 103, Ser 563, Ala 396 and Lys 562. The docking simulation results are excellent evidence of sulfur compounds in garlic essential oil for SARS-CoV-2 resistance.

The literature review indicated the major constituents of the cajeput essential oil are 1,8-cineol and α-terpineol (Doran and Turnbull 1997), which have antibacterial, antifungal and antiparasitic activities. In fact, *Melaleuca* oil has been used in Vietnam for respiratory and infectious diseases; it has also been shown to have antifungal, anti-inflammatory and antioxidant activities (Zhang et al. 2019). According to some folk remedies, people use cajeput essential oil to help improve resistance, inhibit some bacteria and viruses and freshen the air in the room, which is especially suitable for newborn babies and women who are unable to use menthol related to respiratory depression in the infants (My et al. 2020; Jedlicková, Mottl, and Serý 1992). The PDB6LU7 protein of the SAR-CoV-2 docked with terpineol, guaiol and linalool of the cajeput essential oil brought the strongest inhibitory effects (My et al. 2020).

Previous studies have confirmed the strong inhibitory effect of terpineol on PDB6LU7 protein with docking simulation results with DS of −10.9 kcal.mol-1 and RMSD for 1.16 Å and site-site binding interaction between—OH and the amino acid His 163 is 2.38 Å. Terpineol is a monoterpene alcohol easily found in a number of essential oils such as petitgrain oil, cajeput oil and pine oil (My et al. 2020). It has a pleasant aroma and is commonly used in perfumery ingredients, cosmetics and fragrances (Khaleel, Tabanca, and Buchbauer 2018). In addition, in the field of medicine, α-terpineol also attracts great attention from scientists because of its effectiveness in inhibiting pathogenic viruses to help protect health, treat insect bites or wounds, relieve itching and discomfort, reduce swelling quickly and cure respiratory infections.

The inhibitory effects of guaiol on the PDB-6LU7 protein are not much different compared to the terpineol in which the docking results show a DS of −10.9 kcal.mol^{-1} and RMSD of 0.84 Å. Note that guaiol is a sesquiterpenoid alcohol, and its molecule has the –OH group and it has strong interactions with amino acids Asn 103 and His 163 of the 6LU7 protein. Other studies indicated that guaiol is also present in the oil of guaiacum and cypress pine (Eppenberger, Galassi, and Rühli 2017). This can be affirmed in the docking simulation map, which gave clear evidence for this activity of guaiol.

After that linalool was docked with the 6LU7 protein and showed quite good interactions with amino acid Asn 210 of the LU7 protein with the docking results of DS of −11.1 kcal.mol^{-1}, RMSD value of 1.18 Å and site-site bonding interaction between –OH and amino acid Gly 143 (2.89 Å) and Cys 145 (2.82 Å). It can be seen that linalool is a monoterpenoid having a very flexible –OH group at the C3 position, which is the active center of the compound with protein interaction. Moreover, linalool is also a major ingredient in some essential oils and is used to produce perfumes, pharmaceuticals and cosmetics (Peana et al. 2002).

15.4.2 Docking Simulation on Inhibitability of Some Alkaloids Against Influenza Virus Hemagglutinin

The investigation of the binding affinity of some alkaloid derivatives, including berberine, lycorine, hemanthamine, aloperin and dendrobine (Figure 15.3) towards influenza A/X-31(H3N2) virus hemagglutinin 2VIU was investigated (Bui et al. 2022, Protein Data Bank).

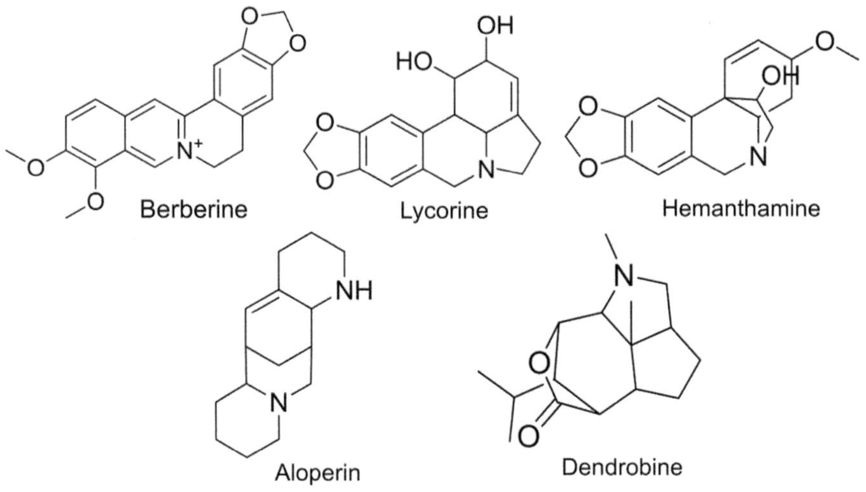

FIGURE 15.3 Structural formula of alkaloidal derivatives: berberine, lycorine, hemanthamine, aloperin and dendrobine.

Research data on the 2VIU inhibitory effects of some structures (Bui et al. 2022) suggested that interpretations of the static stability of the ligand-protein inhibitory structure have good support for the general prediction of inhibitory effect in this order: hemanthamine –2VIU (DS –12.9 kcal.mol^{-1}; RMSD 1.02 Å) > lycorine-2VIU (DS –12.2 kcal.mol^{-1}; RMSD 1.05 Å) > berberine-2VIU (DS –10.5 kcal.mol^{-1}; RMSD 1.01 Å) > dendrobine-2VIU (DS –10.3 kcal.mol^{-1}; RMSD 1.24) > aloperin-2VIU (DS –9.4 kcal.mol^{-1}; RMSD 1.78 Å). Compound-binding studies have found H-donor and acceptor interactions, noting that inhibition of berberine-2VIU finds a particular hydrophilic (π-cation) binding to an energetic free Gibbs bond is –10.9 kcal.mol^{-1} and between an aromatic cyclohexene of the ligand and a nitrogen atom of Lys A326. This value is significant and is detected for the first time among our previous similar studies. This means that although the berberine-2VIU complex is generally not highly structurally stable and structurally rigid, berberine is still capable of transmitting sufficient strain force to the tertiary structure of the protein through binding, thereby inducing denaturation and inhibition of shape-based activity. It was shown that berberine could be a very promising inhibitor of influenza virus hemagglutinin (2VIU) for further studies to develop this lead compound.

15.4.3 α-Glucosidase Inhibitability of Some Natural Compounds of the EtOAc Extract of *Distichochlamys citrea* Rhizomes Using Molecular Docking Analysis

Some major chemical constituents in the EtOAc extract of *Distichochlamys citrea* rhizomes were determined by gas chromatography–mass spectrometry (Van Chen et al. 2022), presented in Table 15.1. Analytical results detected the major compounds, including 5-hydroxy methyl furfural (20.89%), **3-deoxy-D-mannoic lactone** (16.39 %), 2,3-dihydro-3,5-dihydroxy-6-methyl-4H-pyran-4-one (7.12%), monoacetin (6.77%), maltol (4.95%), γ-decalactone (3.76%), propyl valerate (2.08%), 4-chloroanisole (1.50%), 1-(3-thiomorpholinyl)ethanone (1.49%), *p*-meth-1-en-3,8-diol (1.49%) and vanillic acid (1.21%). Other compounds were also detected in small quantities, such as methyl-6-oxoheptanoate (0.38%) and 1,3,3-trimethyl-2-oxabicyclo[2.2.2]octan-6-yl isobutyrate (0.72%). These compounds have been investigated *in silico* using molecular docking simulations (Van Chen et al. 2022).

The ligand-protein inhibition was performed by *in silico* screening, and the structures of compounds detected in the EtOAc extract of *D. citrea* rhizomes and the α-glucosidase crystal structure (UniProtKB—P53341) were selected to conduct molecular docking simulations. The results presented the selected data of molecular docking simulation. Accordingly, the most effective (DS < –10 kcal.mol^{-1}) ligand-protein inhibitory structures might be in the following order: 1-(3-thiomorpholinyl)ethanone -P53341 with DS is –13.6 kcal.mol^{-1} and RMSD is 1.31 Å > **3-deoxy-D-mannoic lactone** -P53341 with DS –12.8 kcal.mol^{-1} and RMSD 0.94 Å > monoacetin-P53341 gives DS –12.6 kcal.mol^{-1} and RMSD 0.59 Å > 2,3-dihydro-3,5-dihydroxy-6-methyl-4H-pyran-4-one-P53341 has DS –11.3 kcal.mol^{-1} and RMSD 0.88 Å) > vanillic acid-P53341 with DS –10.4 kcal.mol^{-1} and RMSD 1.41 Å) > *p*-meth-1-en-3,8-diol-P53341 gives DS –10.1 kcal.mol^{-1} and RMSD 1.45 Å. This initially specifies 1-(3-thiomorpholinyl)ethanone (i.e., structure of 1-(3-thiomorpholinyl)ethanone) and monoacetin

TABLE 15.1
Major Volatile Bioactive Compounds Detected in EtOAc Fraction of *Distichochlamys citrea* Rhizomes by GC-MS

No.	Substance Investigated	Formula
1	Maltol	$C_6H_6O_3$
2	Methyl 6-oxoheptanoate	$C_8H_{14}O_3$
3	1-(3-Thiomorpholinyl)ethanone	$C_6H_{11}NOS$
4	2,3-Dihydro-3,5-dihydroxy-6-methyl-4H-pyran-4-one	$C_6H_8O_4$
5	γ-Decalactone	$C_{10}H_{18}O_2$
6	5-Hydroxy methyl furfural	$C_6H_6O_3$
7	Monoacetin	$C_5H_{10}O_4$
8	Propyl valerate	$C_8H_{16}O_2$
9	4-Chloroanisole	C_7H_7ClO
10	*p*-Meth-1-en-3,8-dio*l*	$C_{10}H_{18}O_2$
11	Vanillic acid	$C_8H_8O_4$
12	**3-Deoxy-D-mannoic lactone**	$C_6H_{10}O_5$
13	1,3,3-Trimethyl-2-oxabicyclo[2.2.2]octan-6-yl isobutyrate	$C_{14}H_{24}O_3$

(i.e., structure of monoacetin) as the most promising inhibitors against *α*-glucosiase, yet the synergic effects of other components are still unknown. In the other works on the inhibitory effectiveness of semi-synthesised derivatives from *Dolichandrone spathacea* iridoids and *Dipterocarpus alatus* dipterocarpol towards diabetes-related proteins, docking data exhibited DS values at −13 to −15 kcal.mol^{-1}. Therefore, these compounds, especially 1-(3-thiomorpholinyl)ethanone and monoacetin, are very promising for isolation and performing *in vitro* bioassays.

The projections of the interaction map and in-pose morphology also provide certain leads to further development of the ligands. The high-continuous contours in the former indicated the complementarity of the ligands to the in-pose features of their targeted protein sites. This means they are already leading frameworks regarding topographical fitting. It can be confirmed that significant further modification on the investigated compounds were not justifiably favorable in terms of spatial capacity (Van Chen et al. 2022).

15.5 RESULTS AND DISCUSSION OF *IN VITRO* STUDIES

15.5.1 The Inhibitory Activity of *n*-Hexane Extract from *Distichochlamys citrea* M.F. Newman Rhizome Against *Streptococcus pyogenes*

The *n*-hexane extract of the rhizome of *D. citrea* has been demonstrated against *Streptococcus pyogenes in vitro.* A common antibiotic, penicillin G, was chosen as a positive control for activity evaluation and model checking.

The results showed that *n*-hexane extract has antibacterial potential against *S. pyogenes.* At a concentration of 200 mg.mL^{-1}, the inhibitory diameter is ca. 14 ± 2.0

mm. The MIC value of the *n*-hexane fraction was determined as 156.25 μg.mL^{-1}. Compared with the simulation results of docking the anti-*S. pyogenes* effect of substances in *n*-hexane extract, this extract has potential in searching for substances effective against against *S. pyogenes* (Thuy, Hieu, et al. 2020).

15.5.2 The α-Glucosidase Inhibitory Activity of the Sub-Fraction from *Distichochlamys citrea* M.F. Newman Rhizome

In the tested extracts, the EtOAc extract exhibited significant inhibition of α-glucosidase, with an inhibition of over 57% at a concentration of 187.5 g mL^{-1}. In addition, other fractionated extracts, such as *n*-hexane, $CHCl_3$, *n*-BuOH and water demonstrated weaker α-glucosidase inhibition when tested at four different concentrations of 750, 375, 750 and 1125 g mL^{-1}, respectively. Inhibitory activity against α-glucosidase of all tested extracts showed concentration dependence. The anti–α-glucosidase activity was exhibited in the following order: EtOAc fraction (IC_{50} = 115.75 μg mL^{-1}), followed by $CHCl_3$ fraction (IC_{50} = 371.37 μg mL^{-1}), *n*-BuOH fraction (IC_{50} = 545, 98 μg mL^{-1}), *n*-hexane (IC_{50}= 621.37 μg mL^{-1}) and the lowest water fraction (IC_{50} = 965.70 μg mL^{-1}). In addition, the IC_{50} value of the acarbose positive control against α-glucosidase was also calculated: 58.51 μg mL^{-1}. This proves that the model used in the study is appropriate. The EtOAc extract showed the most promising anti-α-glucosidase activity, so its components were identified through GC-MS analysis, and the activity was also evaluated through docking simulation. The results showed that the active ingredients identified in this extract are also capable of inhibiting the activity of α-glucosidase quite well (as described in Section 15.4.3). Therefore, there is an active match between the docking simulation and the *in vitro* assay (Van Chen et al. 2022).

15.6 BIOASSAY-GUIDED ISOLATION LED TO THE DISCOVERY OF NEW PLANT AGENTS FOR INFECTIOUS AND DIABETIC DISEASES

Bioactivity-guided fractionation and isolation is a useful tool for the discovery of active constituents from natural products. This technique has been extensively used in natural product research to identify and isolate active compounds from complex mixtures such as plant extracts or microbial cultures and has led to the discovery of many well-known drugs such as penicillin, berberine, artemisinin, taxol and so on (Heinrich et al. 2012). The bioactivity-guided separation and isolation approach typically includes a systematic process of extraction, followed by fractionation and biological evaluation of natural products such as extracts, fractions and subfractions to identify the compound(s) responsible for a particular biological activity. The observed bioactivity of evaluated natural products (extracts, fractions, subfractions, etc.) plays an important role in navigating the subsequent separation steps (Colegate and Molyneux 2007).

In drug discovery, bioactivity-guided isolation is a powerful approach because it directs researchers to focus their time and efforts on the most promising compounds in natural products. In general, the composition of natural products is often complex with hundreds or thousands of different compounds, and it can be challenging to determine which compounds are responsible for a particular bioactivity. Bioactivity-guided isolation allows researchers to systematically evaluate the bioactivity of each fraction from a natural product and then further purify and test the active fractions until a single active compound is identified. This approach is particularly sped up when combined with modern analytical techniques such as high-performance liquid chromatography (HPLC) and high-resolution mass spectrometry (HR-MS). These combined techniques (bioactivity-based molecular networking) sometimes even allow researchers to quickly predict and identify the structures of the active components in the complex matrix of the extracts before the isolation step (Nothias et al. 2018). With the continued development of analytical techniques and the growing interest in natural products as a potential source of new drugs, bioactivity-guided isolation is likely to remain a helpful tool in drug discovery for the near future.

However, bioactivity-guided isolation still has several limitations. One of the main drawbacks is the evaluation of the bioactivity of interest. In some cases, the activity may be difficult to measure or may require specialized assays that are not widely available. Furthermore, bioactivity may come from a complex interaction between multiple components in the natural product, making it challenging to isolate a single active compound (Nothias et al. 2018).

15.6.1 Isolation Techniques Used in the Discovery of New Promising Plant-Derived Substances for Infectious and Diabetic Diseases

First, total extraction is performed aiming at obtaining the highest yield of phytochemicals. Plant material is ground or crushed and extracted with a suitable solvent (in general, methanol or ethanol is mostly used for total extraction). Depending on circumstances, conventional methods such as cold maceration, hot extraction, percolation, reflux extraction, decoction, infusion or ultrasonic extraction or microwave-assisted extraction can be chosen. Recently, according to the concept of "green chemistry", several modern extraction approaches can also be applied, e.g., pressurized liquid extraction, supercritical fluid extraction, pulsed electric field extraction, solvent-free microwave extraction or enzyme-assisted extraction (Zhang, Lin, and Ye 2018). The extract is then removed (usually by evaporation at low pressure using a rotary evaporator) to gain a crude extract. The resulting extract is often a complex mixture of compounds. In the next step, normally liquid-liquid extraction is carried out to separate the total extract quickly and inexpensively into simpler fractions. This is a separation technique based on the distribution of compounds between two different immiscible solvents, usually an aqueous phase and organic phase. The crude extract is suspended in distilled water and then partitioned sequentially with different solvents from non-polar to polar solvent gradient such as petroleum ether/n-hexan, dichloromethane/chloroform/diethyl ether and ethyl acetate followed by *n*-butanol/isopropanol. Each of the combined organic layers as well as aqueous layer are evaporated to afford the respective fractions. After that, obtained fractions are tested on bioassays to direct the isolation. The most promising fractions are selected for further separation. Many different separation techniques can be applied such as adsorption column chromatography (e.g., silica gel column chromatography), partition chromatography (e.g., counter-current chromatography, reversed-phase chromatography), gel filtration chromatography (e.g., Sephadex column chromatography), ion-exchange chromatography, etc. These techniques can be flexibly applied to efficiently separate the fractions into much simpler subfractions thanks to the combination of many complicated separation mechanisms. The obtained subfractions are tested for their potential effects. The active subfractions are fractionated to isolate the active compounds. If necessary, subfractions or enriched substances will be purified by recrystallization, preparative TLC, semi-preparative HPLC or other suitable chromatographic techniques. The purity of all isolated compounds is normally determined by LC-PDA and LC-MS. The chemical structures of the isolated compounds will be determined by NMR spectroscopy (1H, 13C, DEPT, COSY, HMBC, HSQC, etc.) and mass spectrometry. In some cases, the structure determination of compounds is not limited to the identification of the constitution but also addresses conformation and configuration. Absolute configuration can be assigned by several techniques and approaches, including X-ray diffraction (XRD), electronic and vibrational circular dichroism (ECD and VCD) and Raman optical activity (ROA). Finally, all isolated and identified compounds will be evaluated for their biological properties.

15.6.1.1 Extraction Methods

The selection of a suitable extraction method for bioactivity-guided isolation is based on many factors, such as the available apparatus, the nature of plant materials, the target compounds and so on (Heinrich et al. 2012). Researchers should carefully consider the advantages and disadvantages of each method and choose the most appropriate method for their specific research needs (Bucar, Wube, and Schmid 2013).

First, the features of plant materials should be considered. The target compounds that need to be extracted are also critical in choosing the suitable extraction methods. Medicinal plants contain a wide diversity of compounds, including phenolics, alkaloids, terpenes, steroids and so on. Each group of compounds has a unique chemical structure and physicochemical properties that affect the choice of extraction methods. For instance, polar compounds, such as saponin, glycosides and alkaloids are better extracted with polar solvents such as hot water, methanol and ethanol, while less polar compounds, such as terpenes and aglycones, are best extracted with less polar solvents such as *n*-hexane and petroleum ether. In addition, the extraction efficiency and selectivity of the method should also be considered. The good extraction method should have a high yield (high percentage of the target compound extracted from the medicinal plant), while still extracting the target compounds selectively without or less co-extracting unwanted compounds. For example, some extraction methods, such as Soxhlet extraction and maceration, have high extraction efficiency but low selectivity, which can result in contamination of the extract with unwanted compounds. In contrast, methods such as solid-phase extraction and supercritical fluid extraction have high selectivity but lower extraction efficiency. Furthermore, consideration of the cost and availability of the method is also critical; sometimes it is the decisive factor in choosing extraction methods. Some extraction methods, such as solvent-free microwave extraction, pressurized liquid extraction, supercritical fluid extraction and pulsed electric field extraction, require specialized equipment and skilled personnel, which can increase the cost and limit the availability. In contrast, methods such as cold maceration, hot extraction, percolation, reflux extraction and ultrasound-assisted extraction are cost-effective and easy to handle but may have lower extraction efficiency and selectivity. Therefore, selection of a suitable extraction method in natural product research requires careful consideration of various factors. Researchers should choose the most appropriate method to ensure the quality and quantity of the extract and to achieve the desired outcomes in their research.

15.6.1.2 Fractionation and Separation Methods

15.6.1.2.1 Liquid-Liquid Extraction

Liquid-liquid extraction is a countercurrent separation process frequently used in natural products research. The separation principle behind liquid-liquid extraction is based on the different solubility or distribution of the solute in the two immiscible liquids (e.g., aqueous and organic solvent). The extract dissolved or suspended in a solvent (normally water) is first placed in a separating funnel and a second solvent (usually an organic solvent) is added. The mixture is then shaken and allowed to separate into two layers. Sometimes, instead of using a separating funnel, an agitator is used to stir the mixture. In that way, the compounds transfer from one layer to the other based on the solubility in each solvent. The separated layers can be easily collected, and the solute can be further purified or analyzed. Generally, in natural product research, a set of solvents with polarity gradient is used. Due to the complexity of natural product mixtures, their isolation and purification can be challenging, and liquid-liquid extraction is usually performed as a first separation step thanks to its cost-effective, simple and fast properties.

15.6.1.2.2 Chromatography (Heinrich et al. 2012)

Chromatography has become an indispensable technique in natural product research, allowing the separation and isolation of components from complex mixtures of compounds.

15.6.1.2.2.1 Column Chromatography Column chromatography is a classical and powerful technique used to separate and isolate natural products based on their physicochemical properties, such as polarity, size and charge. The mixture of compounds is loaded onto the top of the column and then eluted through a stationary phase packed into the column using a mobile phase. The stationary phase is typically a solid material such as silica gel or alumina, while the mobile phase is normally a liquid (a solvent or a mixture of solvents) or sometimes a gas that flows through the stationary phase. When the mobile phase passes through the column, the components of the mixture interact with the stationary phase and the mobile phase in different ways, resulting in different rates of migration through the column.

The selection of stationary phase depends on the physical and chemical properties of the mixture to be separated and the aim of separation. Silica gel is the most commonly used stationary phase in column chromatography, but other materials such as

Sephadex, RP18, cellulose and ion-exchange resins can also be used. The selection of mobile phase depends on the nature (mostly the polarity) of the sample being separated and the desired selectivity and resolution.

One of the key advantages of column chromatography is its wide array of applications. The technique can be used to separate and isolate a diverse array of groups of compounds, including alkaloids, flavonoids, terpenoids, saponins, coumarins and so on. However, the technique is not without limitations, such as low separation efficiency, time-consuming process and the need for large amounts of stationary phase material as well as solvents used. In addition, sometimes column chromatography requires careful attention when choosing the mobile phase, which can be challenging and even impossible in several cases such as separation and isolation of isomers.

There are many ways to classify column chromatography, e.g., based on the mechanism of separation or the type of stationary phase or the type of chromatography (GC, HPLC, TLC). Some of the common mechanisms used in natural product research include adsorption column chromatography, partition chromatography, gel filtration chromatography and ion-exchange chromatography. Each type has its own unique features and applications.

15.6.1.2.2.2 Adsorption Chromatography (Sometimes Referred to as Normal Phase Chromatography) In adsorption chromatography, the stationary phase is a polar material, such as silica gel or alumina, and the mobile phase is a nonpolar to polar solvent gradient, such as hexane, chloroform or ethyl acetate or a mixture of organic solvents. The separation is based on the polarity of the molecules in the mixture, which affects their ability to engage in polar interactions with the adsorbent (Zhang, Lin, and Ye 2018). The more polar components interact more strongly with the stationary phase; therefore, they are eluted later than less polar compounds. Adsorption chromatography is sometimes referred to as normal phase chromatography. The term "normal phase" indicates the stationary phase is more polar than the mobile phase.

The most commonly used stationary phase in adsorption chromatography is silica gel (Zhang, Lin, and Ye 2018). Silica gel is a porous, amorphous form of silica that contains hydroxyl groups on its surface. Silica gel with a high surface area can interact with a wide array of compounds through hydrogen bonding, Van der Waals forces and electrostatic interactions. The mobile phase is important for separation efficiency and selectivity of the column chromatography. In normal phase chromatography, a less polar solvent system is typically used for the initial elution, followed by a more polar solvent system to elute the more polar components.

15.6.1.2.2.3 Partition Chromatography (Sometimes Referred to as Reverse Phase Chromatography) Contrasted to normal phase chromatography, in reversed phase chromatography, the stationary phase is a modified silica substrate with long hydrophobic long chains such as C8 or C18-bonded silica gel (the stationary phase is actually a liquid film coated on those packing materials), while the mobile phase is mainly water, methanol or acetonitrile from a polar to nonpolar solvent gradient. The elution order of solutes is also different with polar components of the mixture eluted first, and less polar or non-polar components retained longer. The separation mechanism in reversed phase chromatography is based on the differential hydrophobicities of the compounds in the mixture, with more hydrophobic compounds interacting more strongly with the stationary phase and eluting later. Reverse phase chromatography is also known as hydrophobic interaction chromatography (HIC). The term "reverse phase" refers to chromatographic techniques in which a nonpolar stationary phase is used together with a polar mobile phase (Ahmad Dar, Sangwan, and Kumar 2020).

15.6.1.2.2.4 Size Exclusion Chromatography (Gel Filtration Chromatography) The separation in size exclusion chromatography is based on the size of the components in the mixture or their molecular weight (Ahmad Dar, Sangwan, and Kumar 2020; Zhang, Lin, and Ye 2018). The stationary phase is a porous material, typically a gel or a resin, with defined pore sizes. The size or molecular weight of the compound determines the degree to which it is excluded from the pores in the stationary phase and the rate at which it moves through the column. Large molecules, such as triterpenes and saponins, will be excluded from the pores and elute from the column first, while smaller molecules, such as flavonoids or coumarins, will elute later.

15.6.1.2.2.5 Ion Exchange Chromatography The separation in ion exchange chromatography is based on differences in charge, size and shape of the molecules (Ahmad Dar, Sangwan, and Kumar 2020). This technique is suitable for separation and isolation of charged compounds, such as alkaloids, peptides and polysaccharides. The stationary phase is typically made up of resin beads or membranes that contain either positive or negative charged functional groups, such as carboxyl, sulfonic or amino groups, while the mobile phase is a buffer solution with a pH and ionic strength chosen to promote the desired interactions. These functional groups interact with oppositely charged components in the sample. Compounds are separated based on their net charge (Zhang, Lin, and Ye 2018), with compounds that have a greater affinity for the stationary phase eluting later. For example, positively charged analytes will bind more strongly to a negatively charged stationary phase than negatively charged analytes, while smaller analytes will elute later than larger analytes due to their greater interaction with the stationary phase.

Depending on the properties of the sample to be separated, each particular separation and desired selectivity and resolution, each of these methods can be flexibly combined by applying different types of stationary phase materials or by changing the mobile phase systems, allowing for a wide range of applications in natural product research.

15.6.1.2.2.6 Preparative Thin Layer Chromatography (Prep-TLC) TLC is also a technique used routinely in natural product research. In this technique, a sample is spotted onto a thin layer of stationary phase, typically silica gel or alumina. The plate is then put in a chamber containing a mobile phase (a solvent or a mixture of solvents), which moves up the plate by capillary action, carrying the components of the mixture with it. The separated compounds can then be detected using a variety of techniques, such as UV or reagents.

Preparative TLC is a scaled-up version of analytical TLC. In preparative TLC, a larger amount of the sample is loaded onto the plate, typically from a few milligrams to several grams. The fractions are collected based on the R_f values of the compounds, which can be determined by cutting the plate into sections or by using a detection system such as UV or fluorescence. The collected fractions are then analyzed by other techniques, such as NMR, IR or mass spectrometry, to identify the purified compounds. In comparison with preparative HPLC, preparative TLC is more cost-effective. The success of preparative TLC depends on the optimization of the stationary phase and the mobile phase, the loading and spotting of the sample and the collection and analysis of the fractions.

15.7 FUTURE PROSPECTS AND LIMITATIONS

Traditional medicine has been playing a very important role in disease prevention and treatment in developing countries, especially in Southeast Asia, including Vietnam. Many medicinal plants and remedies are used by the Vietnamese people for the primary health care system, but most are based on experience or lack scientific evidence. Therefore, evidence-based medicine is currently being valued in order to promote the use value of medicinal herbs and modernize dosage forms from traditional usage methods to bring about therapeutic efficacy and safety as well as contributing to the commercialization and globalization of medicinal plant-based products. The bioactivity screenings are often the first step in further studies such as bioactivity-guided isolation of potential targeted metabolites, *in vivo* animal experiments and clinical trials. The combination of docking simulation and *in vitro* biological activity testing methods demonstrate the effects of medicinal plants in Vietnam in the light of modern science. *In vitro* screening methods and *in silico* simulations have the advantage of being fast and can be performed in a short time with a large sample size, so they can save time and suggest the effects be experimentally tested at further stages. However, *in vitro* evaluation does not always yield the desired results when conducting further *in vivo* studies such as animals or clinical trials due to substances entering the body influenced by many host factors such as absorption, distribution, metabolism and excretion (pharmacokinetics) and interactions with the gut microbiota. Therefore, in order for these initial studies to be put into application, more follow-up studies need to be carried out in animals as well as in humans. In addition, further studies for chemical and pharmaceutical forms and quality control of products should be conducted. Since then, the use value of medicinal herbs has been enhanced or opened a new therapeutic direction, contributing to preserving and promoting the treasure of indigenous knowledge and characteristics of VTM.

15.8 CONCLUSIONS

The results are the initial basis for the deployment of more powerful research tools, such as molecular dynamics simulations, to elucidate the possible inhibitory effects of natural compounds on with the enzymatic function of 2VIU (against influenza virus hemagglutinin), SARS-CoV-2 and α-glucosidase and further investigation for drug development relating to infection and diabetic diseases.

In addition, currently *in vitro* assays are also quite developed and diverse. *In vitro* screenings of bioactivities of medicinal plants have the advantage of being fast and convenient and can perform screening of multiple samples at the same time. However, further studies in animals and humans as well as the investigation of the products according to the oriented therapeutic effects need to be carried out in the future.

REFERENCES

Ahmad Dar, A., P. L. Sangwan, and A. Kumar. 2020. "Chromatography: An Important Tool for Drug Discovery." *J Sep Sci* 43 (1):105–119. https://doi.org/10.1002/jssc.201900656.

Alam, F., M. A. Islam, M. A. Kamal, and S. H. Gan. 2018. "Updates on Managing Type 2 Diabetes Mellitus with Natural Products: Towards Antidiabetic Drug Development." *Curr Med Chem* 25 (39):5395–5431. https://doi.org/10.2174/0929867323666160813222436.

American Diabetes Association Professional Practice, Committee. 2022. "2. Classification and Diagnosis of Diabetes: Standards of Medical Care in Diabetes-2022." *Diabetes Care* 45 (Suppl 1):S17–S38. https://doi.org/10.2337/dc22-s002.

Association, American Diabetes. 2017. "2. Classification and Diagnosis of Diabetes: Standards of Medical Care in Diabetes—2018." *Diabetes Care* 41 (Supplement_1):S13–S27. https://doi.org/10.2337/dc18-S002.

Barbosa, Luiz Cláudio Almeida, Cléber José da Silva, Róbson Ricardo Teixeira, Renata Maria Strozi Alves Meira, and Antônio Lelis Pinheiro. 2013. "Chemistry and Biological Activities of Essential Oils from Melaleuca L. Species." *Agriculturae Conspectus Scientificus* 78 (1):11–23.

Bindseil, K. U., J. Jakupovic, D. Wolf, J. Lavayre, J. Leboul, and D. van der Pyl. 2001. "Pure Compound Libraries; A New Perspective for Natural Product Based Drug Discovery." *Drug Discov Today* 6 (16):840–847. https://doi.org/10.1016/s1359-6446(01)01856-6.

Blahova, J., M. Martiniakova, M. Babikova, V. Kovacova, V. Mondockova, and R. Omelka. 2021. "Pharmaceutical Drugs and Natural Therapeutic Products for the Treatment of Type 2 Diabetes Mellitus." *Pharmaceuticals (Basel)* 14 (8). https://doi.org/10.3390/ph14080806.

Bucar, Franz, Abraham Wube, and Martin Schmid. 2013. "Natural Product Isolation—How to Get from Biological Material to Pure Compounds." *Natural Product Reports* 30 (4):525–545. https://doi.org/10.1039/C3NP20106F.

Bui, Thanh Q., Nguyen Thi Thanh Hai, Tran Van Chen, Phan Tu Quy, Ly Nguyen Hai Du, To Dao Cuong, Nguyen Thanh Triet, Nguyen Thi Thu Thuy, and Nguyen Thi Ai Nhung. 2022. "Theoretical Study on Inhibitability of Some Natural Alkaloids Against Influenza Virus Hemagglutinin and SARS-CoV-2 Main Protease." *Vietnam J Chem* 60 (4):502–517. https://doi.org/https://doi.org/10.1002/vjch.202100175.

Byler, K. G., J. T. Collins, I. V. Ogungbe, and W. N. Setzer. 2016. "Alphavirus Protease Inhibitors from Natural Sources: A Homology Modeling and Molecular Docking Investigation." *Comput Biol Chem* 64:163–184. https://doi.org/10.1016/j.compbiolchem.2016.06.005.

Chauhan, Ekta Singh, Jaya Aishwarya, Akriti Singh, and Anamika Tiwari. 2016. "A Review: Nutraceuticals Properties of Piper." *Am J Phytomedicine Clin Ther* 4 (2):28–41.

Colegate, Steven M., and Russell J. Molyneux. 2007. *Bioactive Natural Products: Detection, Isolation, and Structural Determination*, Second Edition. CRC Press.

Dat, Ton That Huu, Le Canh Viet Cuong, Dao Viet Ha, Phung Thi Thuy Oanh, Nguyen Phuc Khanh Nhi, Hoang Le Tuan Anh, Phan Tu Quy, Thanh Q. Bui, Nguyen Thanh Triet, and Nguyen Thi Ai Nhung. 2022. "The Study on Biological Activity and Molecular Docking of Secondary Metabolites from Bacillus sp. Isolated from the Mangrove Plant Rhizophora Apiculata Blume." *Reg Stud Mar Sci* 55:102583. https://doi.org/10.1016/j.rsma.2022.102583.

Doran, John C., and John W. Turnbull. 1997. *Australian Trees and Shrubs: Species for Land Rehabilitation and Farm Planting*, Australian Centre for International Agricultural Research (ACIAR).

Dosoky, Noura Sayed, Suraj K. Pokharel, and William N. Setzer. 2015. "Leaf Essential Oil Composition, Antimicrobial and Cytotoxic Activities of *Cleistocalyx operculatus* from Hetauda, Nepal." *Am J Essent Oil Nat Prod* 3:34–37.

Eppenberger, P., F. Galassi, and F. Rühli. 2017. "A Brief Pictorial and Historical Introduction to Guaiacum—From a Putative Cure for Syphilis to an Actual Screening Method for Colorectal Cancer." *Br J Clin Pharmacol* 83 (9):2118–2119. https://doi.org/10.1111/bcp.13284.

Gong, Y. N., R. L. Kuo, G. W. Chen, and S. R. Shih. 2018. "Centennial Review of Influenza in Taiwan." *Biomed J* 41 (4):234–241. https://doi.org/10.1016/j.bj.2018.08.002.

Ha, Nguyen Manh, Vu Van Dung, Nguyen Van Song, Hoang Van Thang, Nguyen Huu Dung, Pham Ngoc Tuan, Than Thi Hoa, and Doan Canh. 2007. *Report on the Review of Vietnam's Wildlife Trade Policy*. CRES/FPD/UNEP/CITES/IUED, Hanoi, Vietnam.

Harborne, J. B., and C. A. Williams. 1975. "Flavone and Flavonol Glycosides." In *The Flavonoids*, 376–441. Springer.

Heinrich, Michael, Joanne Barnes, Jose Prieto-Garcia, Simon Gibbons, and Elizabeth Williamson. 2012. *Fundamentals of Pharmacognosy and Phytotherapy*, Churchill Livingstone (Elsivier).

Hossain, T. J., Y. Harada, H. Hirayama, H. Tomotake, A. Seko, and T. Suzuki. 2016. "Structural Analysis of Free N-Glycans in α-Glucosidase Mutants of Saccharomyces Cerevisiae: Lack of the Evidence for the Occurrence of Catabolic α-Glucosidase Acting on the N-Glycans." *PLoS ONE* 11 (3):e0151891. https://doi.org/10.1371/journal.pone.0151891.

Huang, S. Y., and X. Zou. 2010. "Advances and Challenges in Protein-Ligand Docking." *Int J Mol Sci* 11 (8):3016–3034. https://doi.org/10.3390/ijms11083016.

Huong, Le Thi, Dao T. M. Chau, Nguyen V. Hung, Do N. Dai, and Isiaka A. Ogunwande. 2017. "Volatile Constituents of Distichochlamys Citrea MF Newman and Distichochlamys Orlowii K. Larsen MF Newman (Zingiberaceae) from Vietnam." *J Med Plants Res* 11 (9):188–193. https://doi.org/10.5897/JMPR2016.6337.

Jedlicková, Z., O. Mottl, and V. Serý. 1992. "Antibacterial Properties of the Vietnamese Cajeput Oil and Ocimum Oil in Combination with Antibacterial Agents." *J Hyg Epidemiol Microbiol Immunol* 36 (3):303–309.

Khaleel, Christina, Nurhayat Tabanca, and Gerhard Buchbauer. 2018. "α-Terpineol, a Natural Monoterpene: A Review of Its Biological Properties." *De Gruyter* 16 (1):349–361. https://doi.org/10.1515/chem-2018-0040.

Krammer, Florian, Gavin J. D. Smith, Ron A. M. Fouchier, Malik Peiris, Katherine Kedzierska, Peter C. Doherty, Peter Palese, Megan L. Shaw, John Treanor, Robert G. Webster, and Adolfo García-Sastre. 2018. "Influenza." *Nat Rev Dis Primers* 4 (1):3. https://doi.org/10.1038/s41572-018-0002-y.

Kurian, J. C. 2012. "Ethno-Medicinal Plants of India, Thailand and Vietnam." *J Biodivers* 3 (1):61–75. https://doi.org/10.1080/09766901.2012.11884737.

Lucas, S., M. J. Leach, S. Kumar, and A. C. Phillips. 2019. "Complementary and Alternative Medicine Practitioner's Management of Acute Respiratory Tract Infections in Children—A Qualitative Descriptive Study." *J Multidiscip Healthc* 12:947–962. https://doi.org/10.2147/jmdh.S230845.

Ministry of natural resources and environment. 2008. *4th Country Report Vietnam's Implementation of the Biodiversity Convention.* Report to the Biodiversity Convention Secretariat, Ha Noi.

My, T. T. A., H. T. P. Loan, N. T. T. Hai, L. T. Hieu, T. T. Hoa, B. T. P. Thuy, D. T. Quang, N. T. Triet, T. T. V. Anh, N. T. X. Dieu, N. T. Trung, N. V. Hue, P. V. Tat, V. T. Tung, and N. T. A. Nhung. 2020. "Evaluation of the Inhibitory Activities of COVID-19 of Melaleuca Cajuputi Oil Using Docking Simulation." *ChemistrySelect* 5 (21):6312–6320. https://doi.org/10.1002/slct.202000822.

Newman, David J., and Gordon M. Cragg. 2012. "Natural Products as Sources of New Drugs Over the 30 Years from 1981 to 2010." *Journal of Natural Products* 75 (3):311–335. https://doi.org/10.1021/np200906s.

Ngo, T. D., T. D. Tran, M. T. Le, and K. M. Thai. 2016. "Computational Predictive Models for P-Glycoprotein Inhibition of In-House Chalcone Derivatives and Drug-Bank Compounds." *Mol Divers* 20 (4):945–961. https://doi.org/10.1007/s11030-016-9688-5.

Nothias, L. F., M. Nothias-Esposito, R. da Silva, M. Wang, I. Protsyuk, Z. Zhang, A. Sarvepalli, P. Leyssen, D. Touboul, J. Costa, J. Paolini, T. Alexandrov, M. Litaudon, and P. C. Dorrestein. 2018. "Bioactivity-Based Molecular Networking for the Discovery of Drug Leads in Natural Product Bioassay-Guided Fractionation." *J Nat Prod* 81 (4):758–767. https://doi.org/10.1021/acs.jnatprod.7b00737.

Organization, World Health. 2021. "Influenza (Seasonal)." www.who.int/vietnam/health-topics/influenza-seasonal.

Oyen, L. P. A., and Dung Nguyen Xuan. 1999. *Plant Resources of South-East Asia No. 19: Essential-Oil Plants.* Backhuys Publishers.

Paridhi, Bhargava, Uppoor S. Ashita, Pralhad Swati, and Naik G. Dilip. 2018. "An Invitro Study of Determination of Anti-Bacterial, Antioxidant, Anti-Inflammatory Potential of Piper Betel Essential Oil: Piper Betel Essential Oil." *Natl J Integr Res Med* 6 (2):37–44.

Peana, A. T., P. S. D'Aquila, F. Panin, G. Serra, P. Pippia, and M. D. Moretti. 2002. "Anti-Inflammatory Activity of Linalool and Linalyl Acetate Constituents of Essential Oils." *Phytomedicine* 9 (8):721–726. https://doi.org/10.1078/094471102321621322.

Protein Data Bank. www.rcsb.org/structure/2VIU.

Qiu, S., H. Sun, A. H. Zhang, H. Y. Xu, G. L. Yan, Y. Han, and X. J. Wang. 2014. "Natural Alkaloids: Basic Aspects, Biological Roles, and Future Perspectives." *Chin J Nat Med* 12 (6):401–406. https://doi.org/10.1016/s1875-5364(14)60063-7.

Quy, Phan Tu, Tran Thi Ai My, Thanh Q. Bui, Huynh Thi Phuong Loan, Tran Thi Van Anh, Nguyen Thanh Triet, Duong Tuan Quang, and Nguyen Thi Ai Nhung. 2021. "Molecular Docking Prediction of Carvone and Trans-Geraniol Inhibitability Towards SARS-CoV-2." *Vietnam J Chem* 59 (4):457–466. https://doi.org/10.1002/vjch.202000175.

Stéphane, Doh Koffi, N'guessan Koffi, and Aké Claude Bernard. 2013. "Effect of Aqueous Extract of *Ageratum conyzoides* Leaves on the Glycaemia of Rabbits." *Pharm Innov J* 2:1–8.

Tarasova, O., V. Poroikov, and A. Veselovsky. 2018. "Molecular Docking Studies of HIV-1 Resistance to Reverse Transcriptase Inhibitors: Mini-Review." *Molecules* 23 (5). https://doi.org/10.3390/molecules23051233.

Teixeira, Róbson Ricardo, Wagner Luiz Pereira, Ana Flávia Costa da Silveira Oliveira, Adalberto Manoel Da Silva, André Silva De Oliveira, Milene Lopes Da Silva, Cynthia Cânedo Da Silva, and Sérgio Oliveira De Paula. 2014. "Natural Products as Source of Potential Dengue Antivirals." *Molecules* 19 (6):8151–8176.

Thai, K. M., D. P. Le, N. V. Tran, T. T. Nguyen, T. D. Tran, and M. T. Le. 2015. "Computational Assay of Zanamivir Binding Affinity with Original and Mutant Influenza Neuraminidase 9 Using Molecular Docking." *J Theor Biol* 385:31–39. https://doi.org/10.1016/j.jtbi.2015.08.019.

Thuy, Bui Thi Phuong, Le Trung Hieu, Tran Thi Ai My, Nguyen Thi Thanh Hai, Huynh Thi Phuong Loan, Nguyen Thi Thu Thuy, Nguyen Thanh Triet, Tran Thi Van Anh, Nguyen Thi Xuan Dieu, Phan Tu Quy, Nguyen Van Trung, Duong Tuan Quang, Lam K. Huynh, and Nguyen Thi Ai Nhung. 2020. "Screening for *Streptococcus Pyogenes* Antibacterial and Candida Albicans Antifungal Bioactivities of Organic Compounds in Natural Essential Oils of *Piper Betle* L., *Cleistocalyx Operculatus* L. and *Ageratum Conyzoides* L." *Chem Papers*:1507–1519.

Thuy, Bui Thi Phuong, Tran Thi Ai My, Nguyen Thi Thanh Hai, Le Trung Hieu, Tran Thai Hoa, Huynh Thi Phuong Loan, Nguyen Thanh Triet, Tran Thi Van Anh, Phan Tu Quy, Pham Van Tat, Nguyen Van Hue, Duong Tuan Quang, Nguyen Tien Trung, Vo Thanh Tung, Lam K. Huynh, and Nguyen Thi Ai Nhung. 2020. "Investigation into SARS-CoV-2 Resistance of Compounds in Garlic Essential Oil." *ACS Omega* 5 (14):8312–8320. https://doi.org/10.1021/acsomega.0c00772.

Tomasik, P., and D. Horton. 2012. "Enzymatic Conversions of Starch." *Adv Carbohydr Chem Biochem* 68:59–436. https://doi.org/10.1016/b978-0-12-396523-3.00001-4.

V, Ukwe Chinwe, Ekwunife Obinna I, Epueke Ebele A, and Ubaka Chukwuemeka M. 2010. "Antimalarial Activity of Ageratum Conyzoides in Combination with Chloroquine and Artesunate." *Asian Pac J Trop Med* 3 (12):943–947. https://doi.org/10.1016/S1995-7645(11)60005-9.

Van, Nguyen Dao Ngoc, and Nguyen Tap. 2008. *An Overview of the Use of Plants and Animals in Traditional Medicine Systems in Viet Nam.* Traffic Southeast Asia.

Van Chen, Tran, To Dao Cuong, Phan Tu Quy, Thanh Q. Bui, Le Van Tuan, Nguyen Van Hue, Nguyen Thanh Triet, Duc Viet Ho, Nguyen Chi Bao, and Nguyen Thi Ai Nhung. 2022. "Antioxidant Activity and α-Glucosidase Inhibitability of Distichochlamys Citrea M.F. Newman Rhizome Fractionated Extracts: In Vitro and in Silico Screenings." *Chem Papers* 76 (9):5655–5675. https://doi.org/10.1007/s11696-022-02273-2.

Viet, Ty Pham, Truong Van, Nhan Dang, Quoc Hung Vo, and Duc Viet Ho. 2017. "Chemical Composition of the Essential Oils of *Distichochlamys Citrea* Leaves Collected from Central Vietnam." *Vietnam J Chem* 55 (4E23):358–362.

Wang, Manli, Ruiyuan Cao, Leike Zhang, Xinglou Yang, Jia Liu, Mingyue Xu, Zhengli Shi, Zhihong Hu, Wu Zhong, and Gengfu Xiao. 2020. "Remdesivir and Chloroquine Effectively Inhibit the Recently Emerged Novel Coronavirus (2019-nCoV) in Vitro." *Cell Res* 30 (3):269–271.

Zhang, J., H. Wu, D. Jiang, Y. Yang, W. Tang, and K. Xu. 2019. "The Antifungal Activity of Essential Oil from Melaleuca Leucadendra (L.) L. Grown in China and Its Synergistic Effects with Conventional Antibiotics Against Candida." *Nat Prod Res* 33 (17):2545–2548. https://doi.org/10.1080/14786419.2018.1448979.

Zhang, Qing-Wen, Li-Gen Lin, and Wen-Cai Ye. 2018. "Techniques for Extraction and Isolation of Natural Products: A Comprehensive Review." *Chin Med* 13 (1):20. https://doi.org/10.1186/s13020-018-0177-x.

Index

U

V

W